Recent Results in Cancer Research 68

Fortschritte der Krebsforschung
Progrès dans les recherches sur le cancer

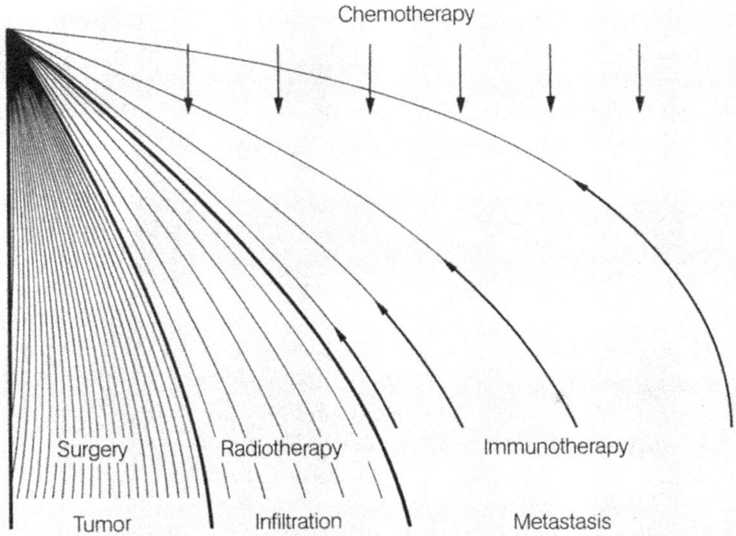
Chemotherapy
Surgery
Radiotherapy
Immunotherapy
Tumor
Infiltration
Metastasis

Adjuvant Therapies and Markers of Post-Surgical Minimal Residual Disease II

Adjuvant Therapies of the Various Primary Tumors

Edited by
G. Bonadonna G. Mathé S. E. Salmon

With 181 Figures and 218 Tables

Springer-Verlag
Berlin Heidelberg New York 1979

1978 Annual Plenary Meeting of the European Organization for Research on Treatment of Cancer, Paris, June 1978

Professor Gianni Bonadonna
Istituto Nazionale dei Tumori,
Via Venezian 1
I-20133 Milano

Professor Georges Mathé
Institut de Cancérologie et d'Immunogénétique
Hôpital Paul-Brousse, 14–16, Avenue Paul-Vaillant-Couturier
F-94800 Villejuif

Professor Sydney E. Salmon
University of Arizona Cancer Center
1501 North Campbell Ave.
Tucson, Arizona 85724/USA

Sponsored by the Swiss League against Cancer

ISBN-13: 978-3-642-81334-4 e-ISBN-13: 978-3-642-81332-0
DOI: 10.1007/ 978-3-642-81332-0

Library of Congress Cataloging in Publication Data. European Organization for Research on Treatment of Cancer. Adjuvant therapies and markers of post-surgical minimal residual disease I & II. (Recent results in cancer research; 67–68 "1978 annual plenary meeting of the European Organization for Research on Treatment of Cancer, Paris, June 1978." "Sponsored by the Swiss League against Cancer." Bibliography: p. Includes index. 1. Cancer-Congresses. 2. Cancer-Surgery-Congresses. 3. Tumor proteins-Congresses. 4. Therapeutics-Congresses. I. Bonadonna, G., 1934 – II. Mathé, Georges, 1922 – III. Salmon, Sydney E. – IV. Schweizerische Nationalliga für Krebsbekämpfung und Krebsforschung. – V. Title. VI. Series. RC261.R35 no. 67-68 [RC270.8] 616.9'94'008s 79-9998 [616.9'94'06]

Softcover reprint of the hardcover 1st edition 1979

Typesetting: Carl Ritter & Co./Wiesbaden

2125/3140–543210

Contents

D. Ovary, Uterus and Testis Cancer

List of Participants see Volume 67, pp. XII–XVIII

Contents of Volume 67

Adjuvant Therapies and Markers of Post-Surgical Mininal Residual Disease I

II. Adjuvant Therapies of Post-Surgical Minimal Residual Disease

A. Rational and Experimental Basis of Post-Surgical Residual Therapies

B. Wilms' Tumor and Sarcomas

Wilms' Tumor: Assessment and Treatment of Residual Disease

J. Lemerle, M. F. Tournade, and C. Patte

Wilms' tumor is a very good model for the study of residual disease in pediatric oncology. It is one of the commonest solid tumors of childhood, it has been extensively studied during the past 10 years, and its treatment has become significantly more successful during this period. Surgery alone can cure a small proportion of these patients, probably 20%–25%. Surgery is still a keystone of the treatment in all the cases and is still the only treatment that is necessary in a small number of well-defined cases where the risk of recurrences can be considered to be very small. The addition of preoperative or postoperative radiotherapy to the tumor or the tumor bed has been followed by a rise in the cure rates, which came close to 50% in the early 1950s. Then chemotherapy was introduced into the treatment schedules, first with actinomycin D alone, then with various combinations of actinomycin D and vincristine. This resulted in another very significant increase in the cure rate, which is close to 80% in all recently published series of cases. These clear-cut data obviously indicate the following:

1. Surgery alone is not a radical treatment in the majority of cases: there is usually some residual disease when the surgeon has completed the operation;
2. Radiotherapy to the area of the primary tumor has improved the results only slightly; the residual disease is not only there.
3. The main problem is the metastatic spread, which is present, although undetected, at the time of surgery.

In considering the treatment of Wilms' tumor, we must keep in mind that we are dealing with young children, the majority being 2–5 years old, so that we must make as little use as possible of the aggressive means of treatment at our disposal, and only when necessary. Therefore, the first question is how residual disease can be assessed in Wilms' tumor, or how recurrences can be predicted and the patients at risk identified.

Biologic markers, at this time, are not helpful. There is no available equivalent to catecholamines of α-fetoprotein that could help in detecting residual or recurrent disease at a subclinical level in Wilms' tumor. In 1970, however, Allerton and co-workers [1] published several papers mentioning the presence in the serum of patients with Wilms' tumor of an abnormal mucopolysaccharide, suggesting that it could be helpful in the diagnosis and follow-up of these patients. We repeated their studies in a large number of children bearing various tumors. We found that the test described was very inconsistently positive in Wilms' patients, and occasionally positive in controls. Therefore, it is of no practical value and is not used.

The tumor-associated antigens found by different authors [4], which seemed to be more specific, are more interesting. But none of these antigens can be considered as a biologic marker for very small amounts of residual tumor. Finally, the best way of predicting recurrences came out of statistical retrospective and prospective studies of large series of cases in which clinical, surgical, and pathologic data were carefully collected and systematically correlated with survival. We have published the results of such a retrospective study, made on 248 cases treated in our institution from 1952 to 1967 [9]. These results are consistent with those of other similar studies [3, 6] and also with the large amount of information being collected from the study conducted by the International Society of Pediatric Oncology (SIOP).

Two important prognostic indicators are available at the time of diagnosis, before surgery is performed, i.e., age and size of tumor. Patients under 2 years of age have higher 2-year relapse-free survival and 5-year survival rates ($P < 0.05$) [9]. All the most important studies confirm this finding but do not explain it. It is worth noting that this is true for patients treated in very different manners, with or without maintenance chemotherapy. The size of the tumor is also an important prognostic factor, which is easier to understand. This has been established in different studies. Breslow, analyzing the results of the National Wilms' Tumor Study (NWTS) No 1, conducted in the United States from 1969 to 1973 [3], found that the weight of the tumor-bearing kidney was significantly correlated with outcome. The smallest tumors, with specimen weight < 250 g, led to fewer abdominal relapses and deaths. Tumors over 250 g, i.e., the vast majority, had an equivalent outcome whatever their actual weight, which varied from 250 g to 100+ g. The SIOP study has obtained a similar result, the only difference being that the size of the tumor is estimated by measuring its horizontal and vertical diameters on diagnostic IVP, giving the "area" of the total mass. This simple method has proved to give results comparable to those derived from the weight of the tumor. This is important from a practical point of view for the SIOP studies, in which the majority of patients now receive preoperative treatments; this makes it impossible to take into account the weight of the pathologic specimen, which has usually shrunk considerably.

The size of the tumor, as estimated from pretreatment IVP, has been proposed for definition of the clinical T in the official TNM classification of Wilms' tumor. The surgical and pathologic stage takes into account all available information on the tumor extent as collected after surgery. The staging system designed for the NWTS is convenient although necessarily imperfect and is widely used. Stage I tumors are limited to the kidney, well encapsulated and totally resected. In stage II the tumors extend locally beyond the kidney, but can be totally resected. Stage III defines cases where residual nonhematogenous tumor confined to the abdomen is identified. Stage IV embraces patients with distant metastases identified at diagnosis, and stage V those with bilateral renal involvement.

In our retrospective study [9], stage was very well correlated with relapse-free survival and survival, except for bilateral tumors, which are associated with a survival rate between those of stages II and III. This study was made in patients who had received no or little chemotherapy and no "maintenance" treatments. In our more recent series, in which subjects were treated with efficient long-term maintenance chemotherapy, it appears that the difference between stages I and II has disappeared, and that only stages III and IV have significantly worse results. If we consider the lymph node involvement at histologic examination separately, we can make two observations. The first is that in a large proportion of the cases there is no available information, because radical lymph node dissection is not routinely performed in Wilms' tumor and probably should not be recommended. The second observation is that the lymph node involvement, when ascertained, is of high prognostic value but is closely linked to other pathologic findings defining the stage. This is another reason not to make aggressive lymph node dissections, since pathologic examination of the renal capsule, for instance, may give similar information regarding prognosis.

Histologic grading of Wilms' tumor has been extensively studied. Analyzing our institution's material [9], we have found that a favorable clinical course is related to the number of different varieties of epithelial differentiation found in the tumor, whatever the abundance of each of them. Several authors have made comparable findings [7]. BECKWITH and PALMER, reviewing the pathologic material collected in the NWTS No. 1 [2] have described a small group (11.5% of all cases) with especially bad prognosis. This group, defined by anaplasia and/or sarcomatous pattern, had a 57% death rate, while only 6.9% of the other patients have died. In many cases where a preoperative treatment is given, especially radiotherapy, it appears that pathologic grading of the tumor is difficult.

Prognostic indicators should be used in a practical way to adjust treatment to each individual patient so as to give him the exact amount of therapy he needs to be cured, without useless damage to normal tissues, which is difficult in a given case if these factors are considered separately. Therefore, attempts are made to combine these factors so as to define a reasonably small number of groups significantly different in terms of risk of recurrence. In our above-mentioned retrospective study [9], survival in such groups ranged from 100% to 17%. In the SIOP material, "good" cases are patients under 2 years of age with small tumors in stage I or II and patients over 2 years with large tumors in later stages are "bad" cases. But with this classification, the majority of patients fall into a "middle" group, which should be further analyzed.

The results of the treatment of residual disease in Wilms' tumor have improved very significantly during the past 10 years. Cure rates in our patients have risen from 50% to 80% (all cases combined). This change in survival has been obtained in two steps, which can be clearly separated. First the treatment of metastases has become more aggressive, better standardized, and more efficient. All metastatic cases received large amounts of chemotherapy, and up to 70% of the lung metastases in our series were cured. This first step brought the cure rates from 50% to approximately 65%. But these aggressive treatments were associated with significant morbidity and resulted in severe sequelae in those patients who could be cured. Pulmonary, skeletal, and intestinal late effects of treatment were predominant, not to mention second malignancies possibly associated with previous treatment.

During this period, the SIOP has undertaken a first clinical trial [8], which showed the merits of preoperative radiotherapy to shrink the tumor and make surgery safer, thus avoiding surgical rupture of the tumor. Another trial in the same patients failed to show any improvement in survival and relapse-free survival in patients treated with multiple courses of actinomycin D over those treated with a single course. Meanwhile, NWTS No. 1 was complete [5] and showed that maintenance treatment with two drugs, vincristine and actinomycin D, significantly increased freedom from relapse in Wilms' patients, with results with either vincristine or actinomycin D given as a single agent. The second step in bringing the survival rate of our patients to 80% was the result of the application of the conclusions drawn from SIOP No. 1 and NWTS No. 1 trials to our patients. The important point is that, in our latest series of cases, recurrence-free survival has reached 75%. This means that, today, the 80% cure rate we obtain is due to so-called prevention of metastases, which is in fact treatment of occult residual disease rather than treatment of overt metastases. In terms of treatment-associated morbidity and sequelae, the advantage is obvious and can be measured.

Coming back to prognostic indicators, we can see that not all patients have benefited from the changes in treatment. Stage III patients, for instance, still have a comparatively high metastatic rate, while stages I and II patients seem to be almost completely free of recurrences. This is an indication that we may have reached the point where treatment can be more accurately individualized. Cautiously decreasing the amount of therapy given to good cases can now be considered, as well as increasing the burden of treatment given to the now better known bad cases. This kind of adjustment is likely to be the aim of future trials of SIOP and NWTS, which are now being actively prepared.

References

1. Allerton, S. E., Beierle, J. W., Powars, D. R.: Abnormal extra-cellular components in Wilms' tumor. Cancer Res. *30*, 679–682 (1970)
2. Beckwith, J. B., Palmer, N. F.: Histopathology and prognosis of Wilms' tumor. Results from the first National Wilms' Tumor Study. Cancer *41*, 1937–1948 (1978)
3. Breslow, N. E., Palmer, N. F., Hill, L. R. et al.: Wilms' tumor: Prognostic factors for patients without metastases at diagnosis. Results of the National Wilms' Tumor Study. Cancer *41*, 1577–1589 (1978)
4. Burtin, P., Gendron, M. C.: A tumor-associated antigen in human nephroblastomas. Proc. Natl. Acad. Sci. USA *70*, 2051–2054 (1973)
5. Dangio, G. J., Evans, A. E., Breslow, N. et al.: The treatment of Wilms' tumor. Results of the National Wilms' Tumor Study. Cancer *38*, 633–646 (1976)
6. Jereb, B., Sandstedt, B.: Structure and size versus prognosis in nephroblastoma. Cancer *31*, 1473–1481 (1973)
7. Lawler, W., Marsden, H. B., Palmer, M. K.: Wilms' tumor: Histologic variation and prognosis. Cancer *36*, 1122–1126 (1975)
8. Lemerle, J., Voute, P. A., Tournade, M. F. et al.: Preoperative versus postoperative radiotherapy, single versus multiple courses of actinomycin D, in the treatment of Wilms' tumor. Cancer *38*, 647–654 (1976)
9. Lemerle, J., Tournade, M. F., Gerard-Marchant, R. et al.: Wilms' tumor, natural history and prognostic factors. Cancer *37*, 2557–2566 (1976)

Adjuvant Therapy in the Management of Osteosarcoma: Need for Critical Reassessment

K. Breur and E. van der Schueren

"I suppose it was only one more indication of a human being's capacity for self-deception, our baseless optimism that is so much more appalling than our despair."
Graham Greene, 1938

Introduction

Until about 8 years ago, the prognosis for patients with osteosarcomas used to be extremely bad [3, 9, 14] in spite of the fact that the control of the primary tumor is usually achieved. As about 90% of these tumors arise in the long bones of the limbs, ablative surgery can usually be performed as a radical procedure and local recurrences are fairly rare. In some centers, mainly in France, radiotherapy is used as an alternative. As osteosarcomas are rather radioresistant tumors, very high radiation doses are necessary. Even though such treatment regimens sometimes lead to complications in the normal tissues, some local recurrences still do occur. However, both the sequelae and the tumor regrowth can usually be managed without great difficulty with ablative surgery. Although this policy is much more complicated and requires intensive follow-up of the patient, the possibility to preserve the limb in a fraction of the patients merits serious consideration.

After treatment of the primary tumor, 75%–80% of the patients developed distant metastases, usually to the lungs [6, 13, 14]. As the interval between primary treatment and appearance of the metastases is very short (0–24 months) with a limited median survival (6 months) after appearance of metastases, the need for a mutilating radical approach as the primary treatment has sometimes been questioned. In an attempt to select a group of patients with a better long-term prognosis before amputation, Cade proposed to irradiate the primary tumor and, after a delay of 6 months, to operate only those patients without distant metastases. In this way, a useless mutilation could be prevented for the group of patients that already had a disseminated tumor process at the start. It has been found that the different approaches for the treatment of the primary tumor did not influence the final survival rate. As the fate of these patients depends on the appearance of distant metastases, it is clear that prognosis can only be improved by suppressing the development of metastases, especially those in the lungs.

It must be assumed that all metastases appearing after radical treatment of the primary tumor were present in a subclinical phase at the time of the initial treatment. The concept of the relation between number of tumor cells and possibility of tumor control has stimulated the development of the elective or adjuvant treatment. Already within 6 months, 40% of the patients in follow-up have demonstrable lung metastases and 60% within 1 year. Of all patients developing lung metastases, only 20% do so after 1 year. Appearance of secondaries after 2 years is relatively rare [3, 13].

It is clear that the metastases that do appear within the first 6 months of follow-up, although smaller than the volume of ± 1 cc needed to become visible on the chest X-ray, already contained a great number of tumor cells at the time of diagnosis, while those appearing after an interval of 1 year or longer must have been very small at the time the primary tumor was treated. Extrapolation of the exponential growth curves of lung metastases toward the date of the first treatment of the primary also indicated that most of the patients already had lung deposits containing 10^7–10^9 cells, which means that these were just subvisual on the X-rays. In about a quarter of the cases, the number of cells estimated to be present at the time of diagnosis was 10^5 or lower.

Experience has taught that metastases that are clinically detectable can hardly be controlled with radiotherapy as the necessary radiation dose cannot be tolerated by the normal long tissue. Assuming a D_{10} (dose necessary to reduce the number of proliferating tumor cells with a factor of 10) of 400 rad, the generally accepted tolerance dose of 2000 rad in 2 weeks would cope with tumor deposits up to about 10^5 cells.

Based on this principle, the cooperative group on radiotherapy of the EORTC started a prospective randomized clinical trial in 1970 to evaluate the possibility of lung irradiation in patients with osteosarcoma of the limbs without clinically detectable lung metastases. At about the same time, the efficacy of some cytostatic drugs was demonstrated in metastatic disease. Efforts were immediately started to use these drugs as an adjuvant therapy after treatment of the primary. In the following, we will discuss the results of the EORTC trial, the published data on adjuvant chemotherapy, and the protocol for a recently started clinical trial of the EORTC and the SIOP (International Society of Pediatric Oncology).

EORTC Trial (O_2) on the Value of Elective Lung Irradiation in Patients with Osteosarcoma of the Limbs

The results of this trial have been published recently [1] and will only be briefly reviewed here. The general concept was to randomize the patients after radical treatment of an osteosarcoma in a limb into one group with no additional treatment and one with lung irradiation. The radiotherapy on the lungs consisted of a dose of 1750 rad in ten sessions over 12 days, without correction for the lesser absorption in the lungs, resulting in a actual dose of about 2000 rad. The treatment was given through one anterior and one posterior field encompassing the total thoracic cavity. The choice of the treatment modalities for the primary tumor was left to the treating center. Three different policies were followed: direct ablative surgery (13 patients), radiotherapy to a dose of about 6000 rad followed by ablative surgery in those patients who did not develop metastases after a delay of 6 months (16 patients, 9 of whom underwent surgery), and "high dose" radiotherapy to 8000–9000 rad (57 patients, secondary surgery in 23). This last method was used mainly in France, while the Cade method was usually practiced in the Netherlands.

Between 1970 and January 1975, 86 patients were included from six French and two Dutch centers: Institut Gustave Roussy, Villejuif (37), Centre Léon Bérard, Lyon (12), Centre Claudius Regaud, Toulouse (9), Centre François Baclesse, Caen (2), Hospices Civils, Strasbourg (3), Rotterdams Radiotherapeutisch Instituut (10), and Antoni van Leeuwenhoek Ziekenhuis, Amsterdam (13). Based on a follow-up of at least 2 years, and in the vast majority of patients 3 years, a final evaluation of the results can now be done. The radiotherapy group of the EORTC has refrained from earlier publication of seemingly interesting results so as not to provoke undue optimism.

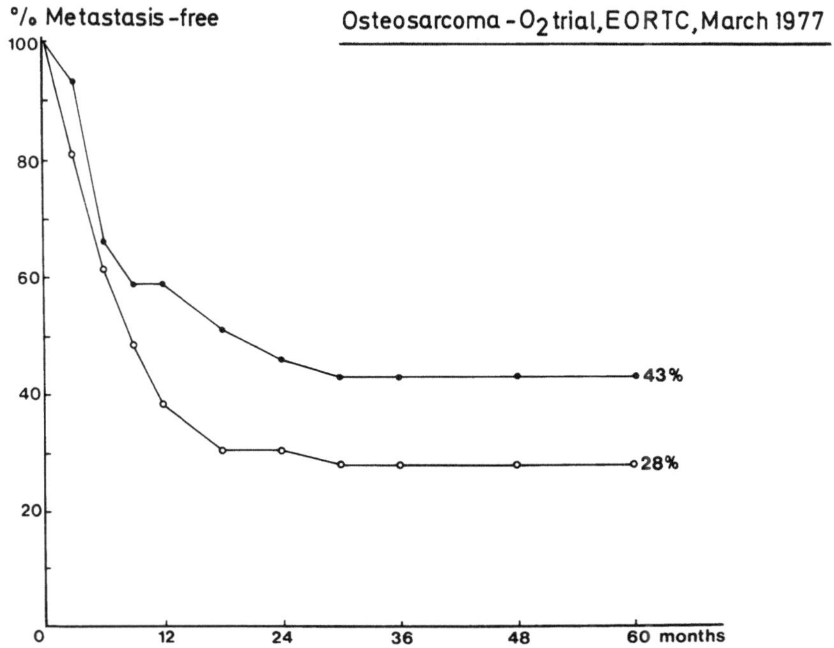

Fig. 1. Actuarial curves for metastases-free periods (%) for group O_2A without adjuvant lung irradiation and group O_2B with adjuvant lung treatment. (Europ. J. Cancer)

In Fig. 1 the percentage of metastases-free patients is shown as a function of the time of follow-up. In the first 6 months after treatment, there is only very little difference in the appearance rate of metastases between the irradiated group and the control group. Between the 6th and 30th months, the lines clearly diverge, suggesting that the lung metastases that still do appear are delayed by the irradiation. No new metastases developed in either treatment group after the 30th month of follow-up, with a tendency toward earlier appearance of metastases in the nonirradiated patients. The level at which patients finally remain metastases-free, which is the main criterion for adjuvant treatment, is 43% for the irradiated patients and 28% for the nonirradiated patients. The value of this difference was calculated according to the method of MANTEL and was $P_1 = 0.059$, indicating that it is significant at the 6% level.

The results of adjuvant lung irradiation are even better in the younger age group. There were 65 patients under 17 years of age. While the number of the disease-free patients in the control group was the same as in the total nonirradiated group, the irradiated patients did better (48% remained metastases-free). This difference is statistically significant ($P_1 = 0.02$). Taking 72% as the percentage of patients who do develop metastases when non lung irradiation is given, one can calculate in how many cases of metastases the development is suppressed by lung irradiation. In the total group, this would be 15/72 (about 20%) and in the children 20/72 (28%). This means that between 20% and 30% of the patients with disseminated disease carry metastases containing a number of cells small enough to be eradicaced by a radiation dose of 2000 rad.

These results correlate very well with the numbers that had been calculated beforehand on the basis of the available radiobiologic data of radiosensitivity and cell number. It thus seems that only the cell-killing ability of ionizing radiation has to be taken into account to explain the

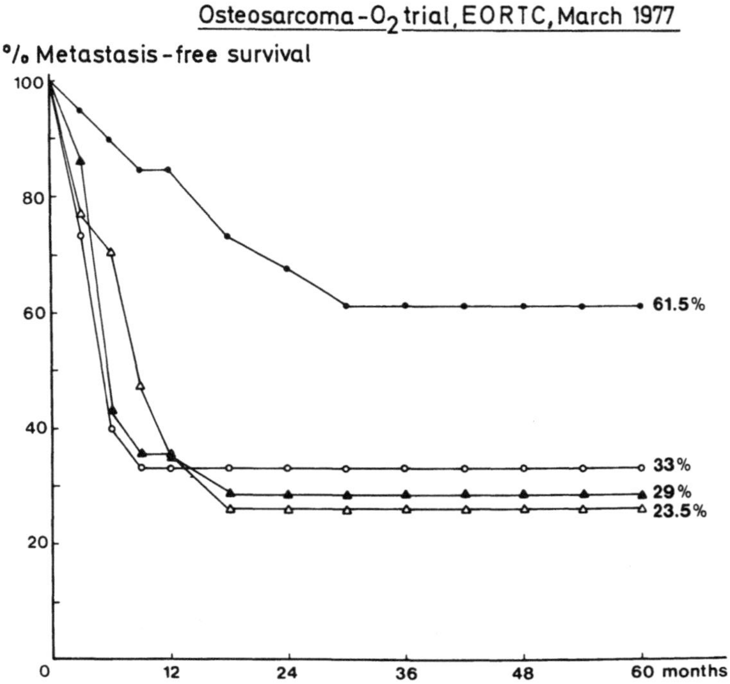

Fig. 2. Patients under 17 years of age (16 years or younger). Metastases-free survival curves (%) for patients treated in the Institut Gustave-Roussy (Paris) and the combined group of patients treated in other centers (except Paris); comparison of groups with or without lung irradiation (L.I.). (Europ. J. Cancer)

effectiveness of the lung irradiation and that no role has to be assumed for helpful immune reactions. The hypothesis put forward again by STJERNSWÄRD during this symposium that elective radiation would adversely affect treatment results by immune depression is also not supported by this study. The lack of any rise in the percentage of extrapulmonary metastases in the lung irradiated group makes STJERNSWÄRD's supposition highly improbable in this model.

The effectiveness of the radiation can also be measured by the delay it produces in the appearance time of the metastases. It was already suggested that only very little delay is produced in the metastases that do appear soon after treatment but that the metastases that would have appeared later are delayed to a larger extent. This might indicate that the smaller tumor deposits are much more radiosensitive than the larger metastases, which are just subvisual and contain 10^8–10^9 cells. Using the delay in appearance and an estimate of the growth rate, the range of D_{10} can be estimated to be as wide as 200–1200 rad.

While the difference between the treated and untreated groups was fairly large, remarkable differences were found when the results of some of the centers were evaluated separately. This was most easily done for the Institut Gustave Roussy (Villejuif), which entered 38 patients. Here, nearly no beneficial effect could be demonstrated by lung irradiation as 73% of the control group and 67% of the treated group developed metastases. This, however, also means that in the group of patients from all centers except Paris a very high number of irradiated patients did remain disease-free (50%). For the patient group under 17 years of age (Fig. 2),

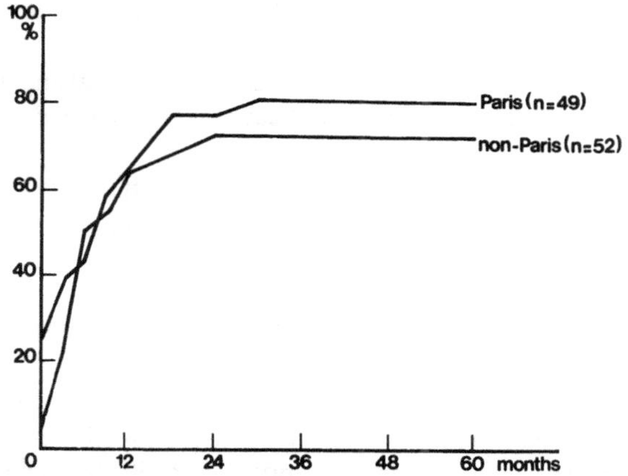

Fig. 3. Appearance rate of lung metastases in patients registered in the trial as having no metastases. Follow-up begins at the time of randomization so that the numbers of 24% (Paris) and 4% (other centers) at time zero are the fraction of patients developing metastases in between the time of referral and the moment of randomization

this difference is even more striking as lung irradiation raises the percentage of disease-free patients from 23% to 33% in Paris and from 29% to 61% in the other centers. This last difference is significant at the 1% level. No apparent differences could be found between the patient groups in Paris or in the other centers with regard to tumor and host characteristics. Also, no evidence was obtained indicating an influence of the type of primary treatment on the results of adjuvant therapy.

It thus seems likely that the center from Villejuif had received a selection of patients with more advanced disease for which the elective irradiation proved to be less effective. This impression is supported by the study of the appearance rate of metastases in the total group of patients referred to this center (Fig. 3). In Villejuif, 12 of 49 initially registered patients did develop metastases before they reached the time of randomization. In the other centers, only 3 of 52 patients had to be dropped from the trial before randomization due to the appearance of metastases. The cumulative curve of appearance of metastases also seems to be slightly shifted to an earlier period for the group of patients treated in Paris. While it is very difficult to draw any significant conclusions from these data, they stress again the great influence of the selection by which patients are referred to a particular center. The same trial done in Paris only or in the other centers would have led to either disappointing or overoptimistic conclusions.

It is still too early to estimate the influence of the adjuvant treatment on survival as some patients with metastases are still alive due to aggressive treatment with cytostatics and thoracotomy with metastatectomy. This last procedure was carried out in eight patients (five untreated and three irradiated patients) and seems to have been successful in four cases (two in each group) although longer follow-up is still necessary in some of these cases. The main conclusions from this trial seem to be that:

1. A dose of 2000 rad on both lungs applied in 2 weeks significantly decreases the percentage of patients in whom metastases later become apparent. This holds true especially for patients under the age of 17 years;
2. Results of adjuvant therapy can be influenced by the selection of patients offered to a particular center. This should warn us that exceptionally good results obtained in a

particular center, e.g., with adjuvant chemotherapy, may not be within reach for another center;
3. The relatively high metastases-free survival and actual survival rate in the control group of our trial (30%—40%) indicate that the use of data from historical series as controls can be highly misleading;
4. The evaluation of the final results with regard to permanent control should be postponed until at least 2 years after the end of the adjuvant therapy.

Role of Chemotherapy in Adjuvant Treatment of Osteosarcoma

The observation in the late 1960s that metastases of osteosarcoma did respond to some cytostatic drugs led immediately to the use of these agents in an adjuvant setting after radical treatment of the primary tumor. Three different schedules were used: high dose methotrexate with citrovorum rescue [10, 17], adriamycin as single agent [5, 9, 18] and a combination of several agents [24]. As early as 1974, euphoric reports were published claiming marked improvements in the fraction of patients remaining disease-free in comparison to historical series [11, 21, 25, 28]. The development of the high dose methotrexate regimens was stimulated mainly for the treatment of this disease.
The supposedly excellent results were so widely published that it was even considered unethical not to give the adjuvant chemotherapy with the result that within a very short time this form of treatment became established without a single prospective randomized study as support. The pressure was so high that the trial on lung irradiation that was being carried out by the EORTC had to be terminated. However, already at that time, serious objections were made against the validity of the results [2] Relatively small groups of selected patients were evaluated for very short follow-up times. Usually, the larger part of the patients were still receiving treatment when the first therapy results were already published. One has to question whether such premature reports are ethically justifiable.
The first in the scope of chemotherapy should require a different approach from the medical oncologist in evaluating his results. While in palliative treatment or in phase II studies tumor regressions or tumor growth delays may be interesting parameters, tumor cure should be the main criterion for adjuvant therapy. It seems that the burden of such a treatment on a group of patients without clinical evidence of tumor, some of whom do not even have any residual tumor, is only justified if the percentage of patients ultimately remaining disease-free is significantly increased. A reliable evaluation of such an effect can only be performed with a sufficiently long-follow-up period after the end of the adjuvant cytostatic therapy. The occurrence of so-called late metastases as have been reported should thus not have been surprising at all. In untreated patients, most metastases are detected within 24 months. However, if an efficient chemotherapy given during 12—18 months would result only in arrest of tumor growth, this would result in an extra delay in the appearance of metastases, at least equal to the length of time of the adjuvant therapy. If tumor regressions occur under chemotherapy, even longer delays would be found. It thus seems that follow-up periods of 3 years after the end of chemotherapy will be necessary to allow an exact estimate of the final number of patients remaining disease-free. This has indeed been proved to be the case as the percentage of metastases-free patients has been found to be more dependent on the length of the follow-up than on the treatment schedule uses. In only one large series with reasonable follow-up has the percentage of disease-free patients remained above 50%, i.e., the Conpadri I trial (55%) [23, 26], but the same group of investigators has been much less successful with

subsequent analogous treatment schemes. In both the Conpadri II and III trials, after initial glowing reports [22, 24], the percentage of disease-free patients has already decreased to about 40% [23]. Comparable and even worse results after longer follow-up have been recently published by the groups in New York [20], Boston [12], Stanford [7], Memphis [16], and Milano [8] and the CALGB group [4].

Parallel to these less optimistic results, some doubts began to arise about the validity of the historical control groups. The publication by the Mayo clinic of a disease-free survival of 40% in their most recent group of patients without adjuvant treatment [27] showed that the use of small patient groups with historical controls is a dangerous exercise. Analogous results were obtained in the EORTC trial in which about 30% of the untreated patients remained disease-free. All these numbers are a far cry from the 15%–20% that has usually been employed as a reference series in many studies. It should be pointed out, however, that Sutow did not find such an improvement in the natural prognosis of osteosarcoma in his material from the M.D. Anderson Hospital [22]. This again could be due to selection of patients referred to different centers.

In conclusion, it can be said that most published chemotherapy studies still show higher numbers of disease-free patients than were previously reported without adjuvant therapy. However, when compared to more recent control series, the difference is probably only small. Moreover, most chemotherapy series involve fairly small numbers of patients and these are probably selected on a more stringent basis than before due to increased interest of the treating doctors in this disease. Ultimately, the real value of this therapy can only be determined by new prospective randomized clinical trials.

Concept of the New EORTC/SIOP Trial (O_3)

The best that can be said is that the amount of hard data that is now available concerning the adjuvant therapy of osteosarcoma is in no way related to the tremendous effort that has been put into it. As Muggia [15] said at the 1977 osteosarcoma meeting in the NCI, the present studies have generated more questions than answers. These answers will only be provided by prospective randomized studies. In conceiving a new trial, a critical reassessment of the results obtained to date is necessary.

The effect of radiotherapy has received some support from our previous trial. However, while the difference in the younger age groups between irradiated and control groups was statistically significant, this was only marginally so when the older patients were also considered. This was, among other things, due to the fact that the trial was discountinued prematurely resulting in an insufficient number of patients included. It is also important to point out that two other studies on the value of lung irradiation were carried out by other groups with mixed results. In the Mayo clinic, no improvement in the disease-free percentage was found with lung irradiation [19]. A slightly lower dose was used and there were less patients in this study than in the EORTC trial.

In a nonrandomized study, Newton obtained results after lung irradiation comparable to our trial (personal communication). It can be said that fairly good evidence is available to show the efficacy of irradiation in suppressing lung metastases. In view of the relatively small numbers and the negative trial in the Mayo clinic, it would be good to repeat this treatment to broaden the experience with this type of therapy.

The data on chemotherapy were extensively discussed before and seem to lead to similar conclusions. With some of the regimens, interesting results were obtained but more patients

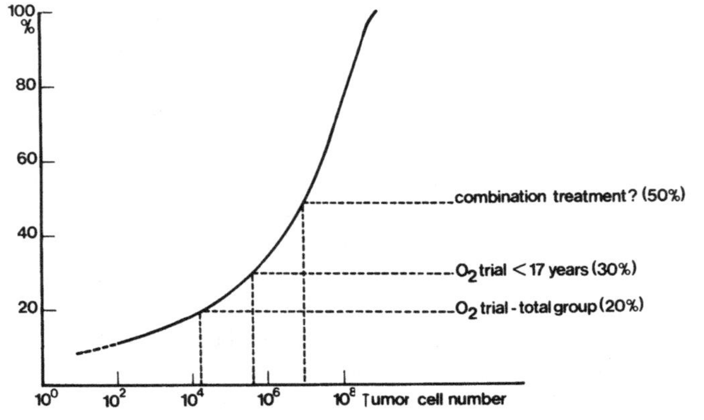

Fig. 4. Cumulative percentage of the number of cells present in the largest subvisual metastasis at the moment of treatment of the primary tumor. To calculate this curve, data are used from patients without metastases at diagnosis and those who develop metastases afterward. The moment of appearance of the metastases, the distribution of the growth rates, the relation between time of appearance and growth rate, and the size of the metastasis at diagnosis are used (calculated by HART, Amsterdam)

would be necessary, this time in a randomized setting to affirm the value of this type of treatment. The best way to confirm the value of these two modalities would have been to compare them to a group of patients receiving no adjuvant therapy. However, it still proved impossible in 1977 to get the approval of a majority of participating centers to start such a trial. It is hoped that the Mayo clinic, which is presently carrying out a study comparing chemotherapy with no adjuvant treatment, will provide some information. The direct comparison between chemotherapy and radiotherapy, however, should also provide interesting results. The final effect of the two treatment modalities seems to be similar in different studies, with disease-free fractions around 40%. Chemotherapy, being much more toxic and expensive, should in such a prospective study be significantly better to make it a valid alternative to radiotherapy.

A second important point of comparison between radiotherapy and chemotherapy will be the distribution of metastases. It had been expected that the suppression of lung metastases by irradiation would lead to a relative increase in skeletal metastases. Although the numbers from the O_2 trial were fairly small, no significant difference could be demonstrated. More data will be necessary to answer this question. As the effectiveness of both radiotherapy and chemotherapy was suggested by available data, an estimation was made of the possible gain that could be expected from a combination of these two treatment modalities. Using the appearance rate of lung metastases and the distribution of volume doubling times, it was possible to estimate the number of cells that are present in the largest subvisual metastases at the time of treatment of the primary tumor, which was also the start of possible adjuvant therapy (Fig. 4).

About 20% of the patients have less than 5×10^4 cells in the largest metastases, and in 30% of the patients this would be 5×10^5 cells of less. As these values approximately represent the percentage of patients who can be rendered disease-free by lung irradiation, this proves that such numbers of cells can be killed by a dose of 2000 rad. Taking into account that the metastases are usually multiple, this would bring the number of cells amenable to radiotherapy to about 10^6 cells, which would mean a D_{10} of about 300 rad.

Table 1. Osteosarcoma study (O-3) EORTC and SIOP: schedule of chemotherapy

	M/V[a]	A[b]	M/V	A	M/V	C[c]	A	C	M/V
CFA						↓		↓	
ADR		↓		↓			↓		
VCR	↓		↓		↓				↓
MTX CF	↓		↓		↓				↓
Week	1	3	5	7	9	11	13	15	17
Week						19	21	23	25
Week						27	29	31	33
Week						35	37	39	41

MTX = Methotrexate 6000 mg/m²/6-h infusion; CF = Citrovorum factor 15 mg/6 h/×12; VCR = Vincristine 1.5 mg/m²/IV (max. 2 mg); ADR = Adriamycin 70 mg/m²/IV; C = Cyclophosphamide 1200 mg/m²/IV.
[a] M/V = Methotrexate/Vincristine.
[b] A = Adriamycin.
[c] C = Cyclophosphamide.

If the number of cells killed could be increased by a factor of 10 or 20, for instance, by giving a course of chemotherapy before the radiotherapy, this would mean the sterilization of 5×10^6 to 10^7 cells, which would cure 50% of all patients with potentially developing metastases. This would reduce the number of recurring patients from 70% to 35% or 65% of the total group remaining free of lung metastases.

This theoretical reasoning would only be valid if radiotherapy would be equally effective on all tumor deposits. We have, however, already suggested on the basis of the diverging slopes of the metastases-free periods that larger metastases are probably less radiosensitive. This would mean that progress would be harder to come by than expected as the additional metastases that we are now trying to suppress could be definitely less sensitive to treatment. The theoretically enticing possibility of the combination treatment was retained as the third regimen for our trial, which will consist of:

a) Chemotherapy (Table 1) 42 weeks with a combination of methotrexate (MTX) (60 g/m² + citrovorum rescue), vincristine (1.5 mg/m²), adriamycin (70 mg/m²), and cytoxan (1200 mg/m²). The chemotherapy will consist of a heavy induction therapy with only MTX and adriamycin, followed after 9 weeks by a lighter maintenance therapy with cytoxan alternating with the MTX and adriamycin;
b) Lung irradiation, 2000 rad after correction for the air in the lungs, to be given in ten fractions in 12 days, with anterior and posterior fields covering the whole thoracic cavity;
c) Combined treatment: a short chemotherapy course of 9 weeks consisting of the induction therapy of trial group a), followed by the radiotherapy of group b).

In an ancillary study, the possibilities of metastatectomies will be evaluated as a function of the previously given adjuvant therapy. This trial is a common venture of the EORTC and the SIOP. Already more than 20 European centers have expressed their wish to participate, which should ensure a reasonable accrual rate that will be necessary for a three-arm trial in a disease where most groups have even been reluctant to start a two-arm study.

References

1. Breur, K., Cohen, P., Schweisguth, O., Hart, A. M. M.: Irradiation of the lungs as an adjuvant therapy of osteosarcoma of the limbs. E.O.R.T.C. randomized study. Eur. J. Cancer *14*, 461–471 (1978)
2. Burchenal, J. H.: A giant step forward – if ..... N. Engl. J. Med. *291*, 1029–1031 (1974)
3. Cohen, P.: Osteosarcoma of the long bones. Eur. J. Cancer. (in press) (1978)
4. Cortes, E. O., Holland, J. F., Glidewell, O.: Amputation and adriamycin in primary osteosarcoma: A 5-year report. Cancer Treat. Rep. *62*, 271–277 (1978)
5. Cortes, E. P., Holland, J. F., Wang, J. J., Sinks, L. F.: Doxorubicin in disseminated osteosarcoma. JAMA *221*, 1132–1138 (1972)
6. Dahlin, D., Coventry, M.: Osteogenic sarcoma: A study of 600 cases. J. Bone Joint Surg. A *49*, 101–110 (1967)
7. Etcubanas, E., Wilbur, J. R.: Adjuvant chemotherapy for osteogenic sarcoma. Cancer Treat. Rep. *62*, 283–298 (1978)
8. Fossati Bellani, F., Gasparini, M., Gennari, L., Fontanillas, L., Bonadonna, G.: Adjuvant treatment with adriamycin in primary operable osteosarcoma. Cancer Treat. Rep. *62*, 279–281 (1978)
9. Friedman, M. A., Carter, S. K.: The therapy of osteogenic sarcoma: Current status and thoughts for the future. J. Surg. Oncol. *1*, 482–510 (1972)
10. Jaffe, N.: Recent advances in the chemotherapy of metastatic osteogenic sarcoma. Cancer *30*, 1627–1631 (1972)
11. Jaffe, N., Frei, E. III, Traggis, D., Bishop, Y.: Adjuvant methotrexate and citrovorum-factor treatment of osteogenic sarcoma. N. Engl. J. Med. *291*, 994–997 (1974)
12. Jaffe, N., Frei, E. III, Watts, H., Traggis, D.: High-dose methotrexate in osteogenic sarcoma: A 5-year experience. Cancer Treat. Rep. *62*, 259–264 (1978)
13. Jeffree, G. M., Price, D. H. G., Sissons, H. A.: The metastatic patterns of osteosarcoma. Br. J. Cancer *32*, 87–107 (1975)
14. Marcove, R. C., Mike, V., Hajek, J. V., Levin, A. G., Butter, R. V. P.: Osteogenic sarcoma, under the age of twenty-one. J. Bone Joint Surg. A *52*, 411–423 (1970)
15. Muggia, F. M., Louie, A. C.: Five years of adjuvant treatment of osteosarcoma: more questions than answers. Cancer Treat. Rep. *62*, 301–305 (1978)
16. Pratt, C. B., Rivera, G., Shanks, E., Mahesh Kumar, A. P., Green, A. A., George, S.: Combination chemotherapy for osteosarcoma. Cancer Treat. Rep. *62*, 251–257 (1978)
17. Pratt, C. B., Roberts, D., Shanks, E., Loehr, E.: Clinical trials and pharmacokinetics of intermittent highdose methotrexate-leucovorin rescue for children with malignant tumors. Cancer Res. *34*, 3326–3331 (1974)
18. Pratt, C. B., Shanks, E. C.: Doxorubicin in treatment of malignant solid tumors in children. Am. J. Dis. Child. *127*, 534–536 (1974)
19. Rab, G. T., Ivins, J. C., Childs, D. S. (Jr.), Cupps, R. E., Pritchard, D. J.: Elective whole lunirradiation in the treatment of osteogenic sarcoma. Cancer *38*, 939–942 (1976)
20. Rosen, G., Marcove, R. C., Caparros, B., Cahill, L., Huvos, A. G.: Primary osteogenic sarcoma: the rationale for preoperative chemotherapy and delayed surgery. Cancer (in press) (1978)

21. Rosen, G., Suwansirikul, S., Kwon, C.: Highdose methotrexate with citrovorum factor rescue and adriamycin in childhood osteogenic sarcoma. Cancer *33,* 1151–1163 (1974)
22. Sutow, W. W.: Perspectives in the management of osteosarcoma and rhabdomyosarcoma in children. Management of primary bone and soft tissue tumors. pp. 25–34, Year book medical publishers, Chicago, 1977
23. Sutow, W. W., Gehan, E. A., Dyment, P. G., Vietti, T., Miale, T.: Multidrug adjuvant chemotherapy for osteosarcoma: Interim Report of the Southwest Oncology Group Studies. Cancer Treat. Rep. *62,* 265–269 (1978)
24. Sutow, W. W., Gehan, E. A., Vietti, T. J., Frias, A. E., Dyment, P. G.: Multidrug chemotherapy in primary treatment of osteosarcoma. J. Bone Joint Surg. A *58,* 629–633 (1976)
25. Sutow, W. W., Sullivan, M. P., Fernbach, D. J.: Adjuvant chemotherapy in primary treatment of osteogenic sarcoma. Proc. Am. Assoc. Cancer Res. *15,* 20 (Abs.) (1974)
26. Sutow, W. W., Sullivan, M. P., Fernbach, D. J., Gangir, A George, S. L.: Adjuvant chemotherapy in primary treatment of osteogenic sarcoma. Cancer *36,* 1598–1602 (1975)
27. Taylor, W. F., Ivins, J. C., Dahlin, J. V., Pritchard, D. J.: Osteogenic sarcoma experience at Mayo Clinic, 1963–1974. Immunotherapy of cancer: present status of trials in man. Terry, W. D., Windhorst, D. (eds.), pp. 257–269. New York: Raven Press 1978
28. Wilbur, J. R., Etcubanas, E., Long, T., Glatstein, E., Leavitt, T.: Drug therapy and irradiation in primary and metastatic osteogenic sarcoma. Proc. Am. Assoc. Cancer Res. *15,* 188 (Abs.) (1974)

Adjuvant Therapy of Operable Primary Osteosarcoma-Cancer and Leukemia Group B Experience

E. P. Cortes, J. F. Holland, and O. Glidewell

Introduction

The major therapeutic approach to primary osteogenic sarcoma has, for many years, been radical surgery. Despite differences in pretherapeutic work-up, surgical techniques, and demography, the overall survival rates in the review of FRIEDMAN and CARTER was 19.7% (253 of 1286 patients) [8]. The range was fairly small, 16%–23% in the series published. Radiologic evidence of pulmonary metastases occurs at a median of 8.5 months after potentially curative amputation [10]. The patient usually dies within 6 months from the onset of detectable pulmonary metastases [13].

In the 1960s, the role of chemotherapy in metastatic osteogenic sarcoma was minimal. Although gratifying objective responses were occasionally seen with mitomycin-C, L-phenylalanine mustard, cyclophosphamide, or actinomycin-D, these results were exceptional and usually brief [8]. In the 1970s, two active regimens were uncovered for metastatic osteosarcoma.

The first approach involved an old drug, methotrexate given in massive doses in combination with citrovorum factor rescue. The rationale for this approach is that citrovorum factor is a reduced folate that bypasses the biochemical block caused by methotrexate. Thus, citrovorum factor rescue allows the use of very large doses of methotrexate that produces high drug concentrations in tumor cells while the systemic toxicity is prevented. JAFFE reported a 40% response rate (four of ten patients) with this combination [9].

The second approach involves a relatively new antitumor antibiotic, adriamycin, originally developed in Italy by the Farmitalia Company. In 1972 we initially reported objective responses of adriamycin in 7 of 17 patients (41%) with pulmonary metastases from osteogenic sarcoma [1, 2]. Encouraged by this therapeutic result in metastatic disease, the Cancer and Leukemia Group B (CALGB) reported the preliminary results of a study initiated in 1971 using intermittent adriamycin treatment shortly after radical surgical amputation of primary osteosarcoma [3, 4, 6]. The present paper reports the 6-year follow-up of amputation and adriamycin in primary osteogenic sarcoma undertaken by the CALGB.

Methods and Materials

The criteria for entry in the study included:

a) Histologically proven osteosarcoma, characterized by osteoid or bone opposed to tumor cells. Patients were excluded if they had parosteal osteosarcoma, chondrosarcoma, fibrosarcoma, radiation-induced osteosarcoma, soft-tissue osteosarcoma, and osteosarcoma after Paget's disease, all of which have different clinical courses [7];
b) Surgically resectable primary tumor without roentgenologic evidence of metastases;
c) A minimum leukocyte count of 4000/mm^3 and platelet count of 100,000/mm^3;
d) BUN and creatinine levels 25 and 1.5 mg/100 ml, respectively.

Hematologic, biochemical, and electrocardiographic examinations, chest roentgenogram and tomography, and bone survey were conducted before, during, and after therapy to monitor for possible tumor recurrence and drug toxicity.

Drug Dosage and Schedule

Four to 14 days after amputation of the primary lesion, or as soon as wound healing was complete, adriamycin was given at a dose schedule of 30 mg/m^2/day for 3 successive days repeated every 4–6 weeks for six courses. The total cumulative dose of adriamycin was 540 mg/m^2 over a period of 5–7 months. Thereafter, patients remained untreated. The response to therapy was measured by the disease-free interval after the first course of adriamycin. Treatment failure was defined as unequivocal roentgenologic evidence of disease recurrence.

Having demonstrated earlier in our report the steep dose response of adriamycin in advanced osteogenic sarcoma [1, 2], no dose adjustment was to be made if the leukocyte count nadir was $> 1000/mm^3$ unless an accompanying severe complication such as septicemia occurred. Any reduction of adriamycin dose if this leukocyte nadir was not reached was considered a protocol dose deviation. A leukocyte count nadir of $< 1000/mm^3$ however, called for the reduction of succeeding doses of adriamycin to 25 mg/m^2/day for 3 days.

The participating medical oncologists had no control as to the type of surgical procedure performed for the primary lesion although the protocol recommended radical amputation, i.e., complete removal of the involved bone. Cross-bone amputation of the involved long bone was considered an inadequate procedure and is therefore a protocol surgery deviation. From November 1971 to December 1975, 102 patients from 21 institutions were entered in the study. Fourteen patients were disqualified; six had overt metastases, four never received adriamycin, and one each had parosteal osteosarcoma, osteosarcoma arising from Paget's disease, inadequate records, and sequential adriamycin and high dose methotrexate treatment. The remaining 88 patients form the basis of this report.

Results

The clinical characteristics of 88 patients are shown in Table 1. There were 52 males and 36 females with their ages ranging 4–66 (mean, 17; medium 16 years) and 7–60 years (mean, 15; medium 14 years), respectively.

The primary sites of osteosarcoma in 65 patients (73%) was localized around the knee joint. While the femoral and tibial lesions predominated in both sexes of either age group, the incidence of tibial lesion in males under 16 years of age was lesser than in patients over 16 years. This observation was not noted in females of either age group.

Forty-six of 88 patients (52.2%) treated with adjuvant adriamycin therapy had relapsed (40 pulmonary metastases, three local recurrences, and three bone metastases). Relapses were seen in 26 of 52 (50%) males and 20 of 36 (55.5%) females. The median disease-free interval in both sexes was 20 months. Forty-nine percent of the male and 38% of the female patients were expected to be free of disease at 5 years as determined by the life table method.

Pulmonary metastases occurred in 14 of 88 patients before the completion of six courses of adriamycin therapy. Of 37 patients who have been observed for more than 2 years, only one

Table 1. Clinical characteristics of 88 primary osteosarcoma treated by adriamycin according to sex and age group

Category	Male			Female	
Age in years					
Range	4–66			7–60	
Mean	17			15	
Median	16			14	
Tumor site	Age group				
	Total No.	No. < 16	No. > 16	No. < 16	No. > 16
Femur	47	17	13	11	6
Tibia	26	4	10	7	5
Humerus	6	2	1	1	2
Fibula	4	1	0	2	1
Rib	3	0	3	0	0
Mandible	0	0	0	1	0
Iliac spine	1	1	0	0	0
Total	88	25	27	22	14

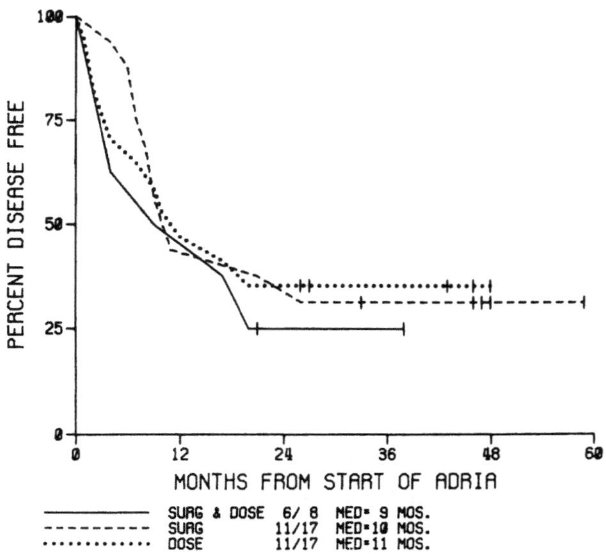

Fig. 1. Percent of patients with osteosarcoma remaining disease-free after subradical surgery, low dose adriamycin or subradical surgery and low adriamycin dose (vertical lines-individual patients free of disease from the last relapsing patient)

(2.7%) has developed pulmonary metastases, and this occurred at 42 months after the start of adriamycin.

For reasons unrelated to a nadir of leukocytes < 1000/mm³, 17 of the 88 patients had their adriamycin dose reduced. Eleven of these 17 (64.7%) have relapsed. Of 17 patients whose involved bones were not completely removed and eight who had both inappropriate dose reduction of adriamycin and a subradical surgical procedure, 11 (64.7%) and 6 (75%) have relapsed, respectively. Figure 1 shows the disease-free status of these patients as projected by the life-table method at 5 years: (a) adriamycin dose deviation, 34% (median disease-free = 11 months); (b) surgery deviation, 31% (median disease-free = 10 months); (c) adriamycin dose and surgery deviations, 25% (median disease-free = 9 months). In contrast, only 18 of the 46 patients (39%) who adhered to the protocol in terms of adriamycin dose or extent of amputation, have relapsed. Figure 2 shows the disease-free interval at 5 years of these 46 patients, which is projected to be 53% (median disease-free = not yet reached) as compared to 31% (median disease-free = 11 months) in 42 patients with various protocol deviations. The probability that the total groups with protocol adherence and protocol deviations would have this disparate relapse rate by chance alone is remote ($P < 0.003$).

Table 2 shows the site of recurrences according to protocol adherence. Pulmonary metastasis is the predominant site of recurrence regardless of surgical procedure performed. There are only three local recurrences (one of 21 femur, one of one iliac spine, and one of one mandibular lesion) out of 25 patients who had subradical surgery. In this same group of patients, 14 of 25 (56%) have pulmonary metastases. This is in contrast to 26 of 63 (41%) patients with radical surgery, regardless of adriamycin dose.

The shorter disease-free interval of patients deviating from the protocol compared to those who were properly treated held true irrespective of primary site, sex, and age group. Such factors as femur versus tibia-fibula, male versus female, and patient's age group of < 16 versus > 16 years old did not show significant difference in disease-free interval. Primary lesions

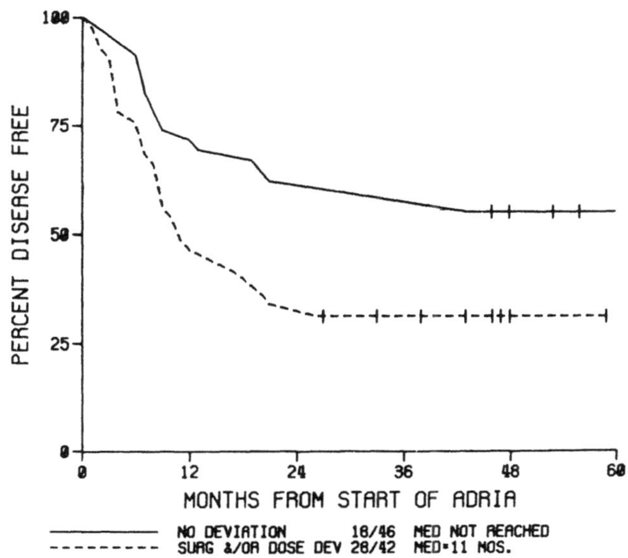

Fig. 2. Percent of patients with osteosarcoma remaining disease-free after radical surgery and full adriamycin dose versus subradical surgery and/or dose of adriamycin deviation

Table 2. Breakdown of recurrence site according to protocol adherence by primary site

	No deviation		Protocol deviation by								
			Surgery			Drug dose			Dose and surgery		
	No. cases	Relapse site Lung	No. cases	Relapse site		No. cases	Relapse site		No. cases	Relapse site	
				Lung	Local		Lung	Bone		Lung	Local
Femur	18	9	14	9		8	3	1	7	4	1
Tibia	17	5	2	1		7	4	2			
Humerus	4	2				2	1				
Fibula	4	1									
Rib	3	1									
Iliac spine			1		1						
Mandible									1		1
Total	46	18	17	10	1	17	8	3	8	4	2

ranging 5–10 cm in maximum diameter had a higher projected disease-free status than patients with primary lesions measuring < 5 or > 10 cm in diameter as shown in Fig. 3. Explanations for this apparent discrepancy are complex. The disease-free status as projected by the life table method at 5 years in all patients with measured primary lesion regardless of protocol adherence are: (a) less than 5 cm diameter 40%, (b) 5–10 cm diameter 62%, and (c) over 10 cm diameter 38%.

The characteristics of the primary tumors arising from the femur in 47 patients with or without protocol deviation are shown in Table 3. A greater number of cases and a higher

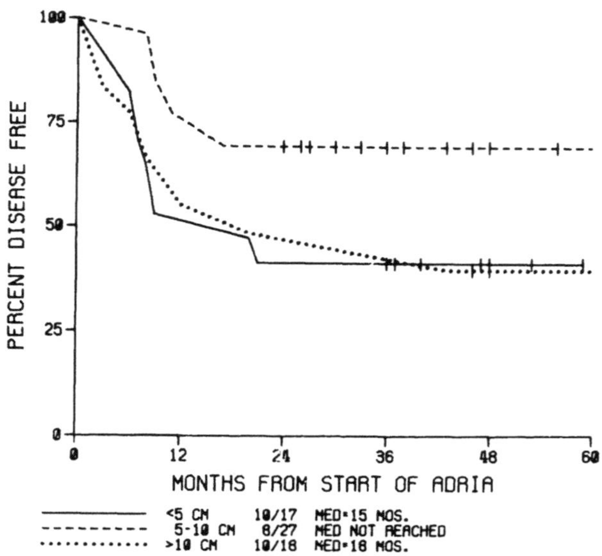

Fig. 3. Percent of patients with osteosarcoma remaining disease-free after surgery and adriamycin (all patients) according to primary tumor size

Table 3. Characteristics of 47 osteosarcomas arising from the femur according to protocol adherence

Category	Number of patients (%)	
	Protocol adherence	Protocol deviation
Total	18	29
Sex		
Males	12 (66)	18 (62)
Females	6 (33)	11 (38)
Age (years)		
16	9 (50)	19 (65.5)
16	9 (50)	10 (34.4)
Mean	20	14
Median	15	14
Tumor size (cm)		
5	2 (14)	5 (26)
5–10	7 (50)	9 (47)
10	5 (30)	5 (26)
Size not recorded	4	10

percentage of patients < 16 years old with tumor size < 5 cm in diameter were found in the protocol deviation group compared to the protocol adherence group. The remaining listed characteristics seemed to be comparable between the two groups including mean days from diagnosis to surgery, mean days from surgery to start of adriamycin therapy, ratio of males to females, and percentage of tumor lesions ranging 5–10 cm in diameter. At 5 years the

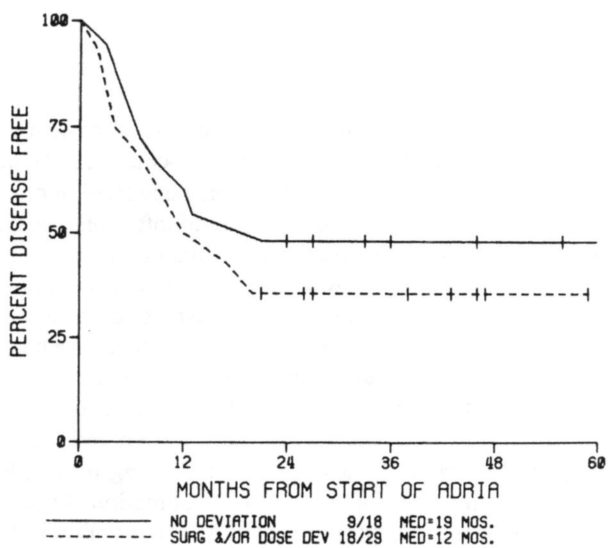

Fig. 4. Percent of patients remaining disease-free with osteosarcoma arising from femur with or without surgery and/or adriamycin dose deviation

Table 4. Alkaline phosphatase changes and relapse rate of primary osteosarcoma during adriamycin therapy

Alkaline phosphatase changes		No. cases	No. relapse	Rate
Before	After			
Normal	Normal	17	3	17.6
Elevated	Normal	11	7	63.6
Elevated	Elevated	21	16	76
Normal	Elevated	3	3	100
Total		52	29	

disease-free interval in the protocol deviation group was predicted to be 36%, whereas in the protocol adherence group it was 49%, as shown in Fig. 4.

Fifty-two patients had their serial serum alkaline phosphatase determinations before, during, and after adriamycin therapy. Table 4 shows the relapse incidence of osteosarcoma in relation to the changes of subsequent alkaline phosphatase levels. Only 3 of 17 patients have relapsed whose enzymes were not elevated initially and remained in the normal range during the course of continued observations. In contrast, those patients whose alkaline phosphatase levels were elevated before the start of adriamycin, and subsequently either became normal or persisted at high levels, as well as those patients with normal levels initially who had a rising titer following therapy relapsed in 26 of 35 (74%) cases. In three patients, elevation of the alkaline phosphatase alone preceded the onset or discovery of pulmonary metastases by 2–4 months. In another patient, roentgenologic evidence of pulmonary metastases occurred simultaneously with the rise of alkaline phosphatase.

Toxicity

The toxicity from adriamycin was tolerable. Transient capital alopecia occurred in 100% of the patients, leukopenia (< 3000/mm^3) occurred in 60%, nausea and vomiting in 50%, and stomatitis occurred in 45%. Pneumonia occurred in one patient. In another patient, delayed wound healing complicated by a wound infection was noted during adriamycin administration. Transient electrocardiographic changes in the form of premature atrial and ventricular beats occurred in 10%. Twenty of the 88 patients did not finish the six courses of adriamycin because of relapse (18 patients) or refusal (two patients). Of the 68 patients who finished the six courses of adriamycin, two developed congestive heart failure. One patient had a simultaneous onset of fatal pulmonary metastases and congestive heart failure 2 months after the completion of 540 mg/m^2 of adriamycin. At autopsy, a mural thrombus in the ventricle and interstitial fibrosis of the myocardium were noted. The other patient developed irreversible congestive heart failure 3 months after 540 mg/m^2 of adriamycin was completed. She died 1 month after the onset of myocardial dysfunction. At autopsy, metastatic lesions to the heart and lungs were demonstrated that had not been previously noted by roentgenologic studies. A girl who completed the six courses of adriamycin at 16 years of age delivered a normal child at age 21 years.

Discussion

Our data clearly indicate that adriamycin administration following radical amputation of primary osteogenic sarcoma delays of lessens the onset of metastases as compared to the historical control of multiple published series treated by amputation alone [8]. The favorable results are most striking in patients who were treated with full dose adriamycin following complete surgical removal of the involved bone.

Having demonstrated earlier the steep dose response of adriamycin in advanced osteosarcoma [1, 2], it is not surprising to note that inappropriate reduction of adriamycin even in an adjuvant setting had a projected disease-free status in substantially fewer patients than in patients appropriately treated with full doses of adriamycin.

The same relapse rate is true for patients with incomplete removal of the involved bone despite full adriamycin doses. The higher relapse rate in this group of patients is not clear to us. It has been reported, however, that simultaneous, secondary, smaller foci of osteosarcoma, anatomically separate from the primary lesion, known as "skip" metastases, do occur [7]. Although gross local recurrence was only seen in 3 of 25 patients with subradical surgery in our series, it is possible that the remaining unresected involved bone contained skip lesions or micrometastases not completely eradicated by adriamycin, which were responsible for the pulmonary metastases upon termination of therapy in 14 of 25 patients.

Other prognostic factors such as sex seem not to influence the disease-free interval of patients treated with adriamycin. This is in contrast to one series of amputation alone, which was reported to show a better prognosis in females than in males with primary osteogenic sarcoma [12]. Of special interest is the influence of tumor size in the disease-free interval. In the series reported by McKenna et al. [11], osteosarcoma patients with lesions < 5 cm in diameter had a 40% 5-year survival rate as compared to 17%, 4%, and 0% survivals in patients with lesions 5–10, 10–15, and > 15 cm, respectively. In our present report, it is uncertain why patients with a tumor of < 5 cm in diameter had a shorter disease-free interval than those with lesions ranging 5–10 cm. As might be expected, adriamycin-treated patients with lesions > 10 cm in diameter had the worst prognosis. The projected disease-free status for a tumor greater than 10 cm at 5 years is 38%, which is much higher than those patients treated by amputation alone.

The conclusion that full doses of adriamycin and complete removal of the involved bone in osteosarcoma are the most effective ways to assure successful adjuvant therapy is supported by a longer disease-free interval in patients with protocol adherence compared to those with protocol deviation in every prognostic category. This conclusion is reinforced by the effect of therapy in lesions of a single site, the femur, wherein the disease-free interval in the protocol adherence group is still significantly longer than in patients who deviated from the protocol.

The significance of serial serum alkaline phosphatase determinations in osteogenic sarcoma undergoing adjuvant therapy has never been emphasized before. In this series we have not analyzed preamputation values of alkaline phosphatase and cannot therefore use this for prognostication. Pre- and postadriamycin determinations of the enzymes, however, were done in 52 cases. In general, the initial and subsequent levels of alkaline phosphatase are of value in predicting the recurrence of osteosarcoma. Four patterns of alkaline phosphatase changes were observed during the course of the disease: (a) normal level initially remaining normal during therapy, (b) elevated initially with a drop to normal following therapy, (c) elevated initially with succeeding values intermittently low and high, and (d) normal initially with subsequent elevation. Normal levels of alkaline phosphatase throughout implies a better prognosis compared to the other patterns of enzyme changes. Most significantly, in some cases alkaline phosphatase elevation alone precedes the onset of overt metastases suggesting strongly that a thorough search for an active potentially resectable lesion is mandatory.

The toxicity from adriamycin has been well-tolerated. The high risk of serious cardiomyopathy in patients receiving a total cumulative dose of adriamycin over 550 mg/m^2 made us limit the cumulative dose to 540 mg/m^2 in this study [5]. Two of 68 patients receiving 540 mg/m^2 developed congestive heart failure. Both these patients were found to have pulmonary metastases, and cardiac involvement was noted in one, which may have contributed to the heart failure.

Whether the delayed recurrence observed for up to 6 years in this report will result in cure remains to be proved by time. The fact that only a single patient has relapsed after 2 years of observation lends credence to this proposition. The failure to adhere to the protocol by some doctors, and the appearance of metastases in approximately half the patients despite meticulous application of the treatment, clearly indicate that this is only one step along the way. Other programs building on this experience are under intensive investigation at present.

References

1. Cortes, E. P., Holland, J. F., Wang, J. J. et al.: Doxorubicin in disseminated osteosarcoma. JAMA *221*, 1132–1138 (1972)
2. Cortes, E. P., Holland, J. F., Wang, J. J. et al.: Chemotherapy of advanced osteosarcoma. Colston paper No. 24. In: Bone-certain aspects of neoplasia price, CHG, Rose, F. G. M. (eds.), pp. 265–280. London: Butterworth 1972
3. Cortes, E. P., Holland, J. F., Wang, J. J. et al.: Amputation and adriamycin in primary osteosarcoma. N. Engl. J. Med. *291*, 998–1000 (1974)
4. Cortes, E. P., Holland, J. F., Wang, J. J. et al.: Adriamycin (NSC-123127) in 87 patients with osteosarcoma. Cancer Chemother. Rep. (Part 3) *6*, 305–313 (1975)
5. Cortes, E. P., Lutman, G., Wanka, J. et al.: Adriamycin (NSC-123127) cardiotoxicity: a clinicopathologic correlation. Cancer Chemother. Rep. (Part 3), *6*, 215–225 (1975)
6. Cortes, E. P., Holland, J. F., Glidewell, O.: Amputation and adriamycin in primary osteosarcoma: a 5-year report. Cancer Treat. Rep. *62*, 271–277 (1978)
7. Enneking, R. W. F., Kagan, A.: "Skip" metastases in osteosarcoma. Cancer *36*, 2192–2205 (1975)
8. Friedman, M. A., Carter, S. K.: The therapy of osteogenic sarcoma: current status and thoughts for the future. J. Surg. Oncol. *4*, 482–510 (1972)
9. Jaffe, N.: Recent advances in the chemotherapy of metastatic osteogenic sarcoma. Cancer *30*, 1627–1631 (1972)
10. Marcove, R. C., Mike, V., Hajek, J. V. et al.: Osteogenic sarcoma in childhood. NY State J. Med. *71*, 855–859 (1971)
11. McKenna, R. J., Schwinn, C. P., Soong, K. Y. et al.: Sarcoma of the osteogenic series (osteosarcoma, fibrosarcoma, chondrosarcoma, parosteal osteogenic sarcoma, and sarcomata arising in abnormal bone): an analysis of 552 cases. J. Bone Joint Surg. *48*, 1–26 (1966)
12. Scranton, P. E., De Cicco, F. A., Totten, R. S. et al.: Prognostic factors in osteosarcoma. Cancer *36*, 2179–2191 (1975)
13. Sweetnam, R.: Amputation in osteosarcoma. J. Bone Joint Surg. *55 B*, 189–192 (1973)

Adriamycin in the Adjuvant Treatment of Operable Osteosarcoma

F. Fossati-Bellani, M. Gasparini, and G. Bonadonna

Since adriamycin (ADM) has been reported to be one of the most effective drugs in the treatment of clinically metastatic osteogenic sarcoma, this drug was selected in our institute for the combined treatment of childhood and adult osteosarcoma. The preliminary results were reported in 1978 [2]. The scope of this paper is to update the initial findings.

Patients, Methods, and Results

From March 1974 to May 1978, a total of 17 consecutive patients with the histologic features of classic osteogenic sarcoma were treated with ADM following amputation. Two other patients with the histologic diagnosis of parosteal osteosarcoma were also treated with this approach.

In the first series of 15 patients, including those with parosteal osteosarcoma, ADM was injected in a single IV dose of 75 mg/m^2. In the absence of relapse, treatments were repeated every 4 weeks for a total of eight cycles, without exceeding the total dose of 600 mg/m^2. The median follow-up period of this group is 23 months (range: 8—48$^+$ months). Because numerous treatment failures were documented, since March 1977 ADM has been administered according to the dose schedule utilized by Cortes et al. [1], i.e., 30 mg/m^2 for 3 consecutive days and treatments repeated every 4 weeks for a total of six cycles. So far, four patients have been treated in accordance with this dose schedule, and their median follow-up period is 11 months (range: 1$^+$—14$^+$ months).

As of 1 June 1978, a total of 10 of 19 (53%) patients have shown treatment failure. In most instances the first sign of metastatic disease was documented in the lungs. So far, relapse has been observed only in the first series of patients (10 of 15, or 67%), including one patient with parosteal osteosarcoma. The median time to relapse was 10 months (range: 1—32 months). In particular, two of ten patients relapsed while receiving chemotherapy. Five others of this group remain disease-free after 21$^+$ to 48$^+$ months. In the second series all four patients remain disease-free after 1$^+$—14$^+$ months. Figure 1 shows the actuarial analysis of disease-free survival for the total series of 19 patients. The present findings indicate that amputation followed by intermittent treatment with the maximum tolerated doses of ADM has not significantly improved the 2-year relapse rate over that obtained with surgery alone. Only a moderate increase in the disease-free status was achieved, and our results appear definitely inferior to those reported by other authors utilizing ADM as adjuvant therapy [3].

Treatment at first relapse could not be uniform in all patients for a number of clinical reasons. Resection of pulmonary metastases was performed in two children. Three patients were given methotrexate (50 mg/kg q 2 weeks) with citrovorum factor. In this group, disease progression was observed after 1, 2, and 7 months from the beginning of secondary treatment. No objective tumor response was observed in three patients treated with CCNU. All patients who relapsed were dead within 8 months from the diagnosis of primary treatment failure.

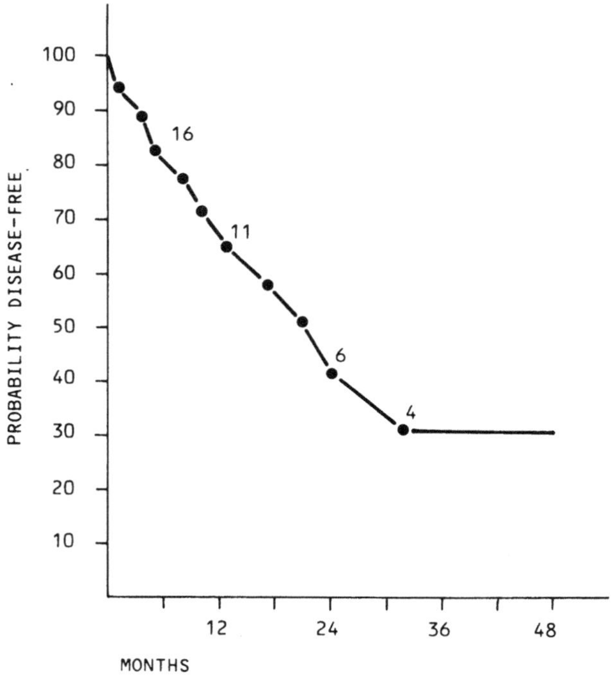

Fig. 1. Disease-free survival after adjuvant ADM

In general, treatment with ADM was well tolerated, and dose reductions for persisting myelosuppression were seldom required [2]. All patients developed complete alopecia, but no episodes of infection were observed. In the group treated with 75 mg/m^2, three patients developed electrocardiographic abnormalities and in one the ECG changes persisted for some time. One of four children treated with the dose of 90 mg/m^2 developed a severe cardiomyopathy after a cumulative dose of 450 mg/m^2. The patient is still alive and under treatment with digitalis, 6$^+$ months after the episode of congestive heart failure.

Conclusion

Our limited experience does not confirm that ADM alone is a particularly effective adjuvant treatment following amputation for clinically localized osteogenic sarcoma, since only a moderate increase in the disease-free status was observed. Treatment failure was apparently not related to age, sex, site, or extent of primary disease [2]. No relapse has yet been observed in the for patients treated with the dose regimen found successful by Cortes et al. [1]. However, both the limited number of patients and the short follow-up period prevent an adequate comparison either with our own first series treated with ADM or with that of Cortes. It is important to note that 90 mg/m^2 of ADM can increase the incidence of clinical manifestations of drug-induced cardiomyopathy. Adriamycin remains a potentially useful agent for the adjuvant treatment of osteogenic sarcoma. However, as in other neoplastic diseases, it should be properly combined with other agents to achieve a better improvement of disease-free survival.

References

1. Cortes, E. P., Holland, J. F., Glidewell, O.: Amputation and adriamycin in primary osteosarcoma: a 5-year report. Cancer Treat. Rep. *62,* 271–277 (1978)
2. Fossati-Bellani, F., Gasparini, M., Gennari, L., Fontanillas, L., Bonadonna, G.: Adjuvant treatment with adriamycin in primary operable osteosarcoma. Cancer Treat. Rep. *62,* 279–281 (1978)
3. Proceedings of the osteosarcoma study group meeting. Cancer Treat. Rep. *62,* 187–312 (1978)

Randomized Trial of Adjuvant Chemotherapy in Osteogenic Osteosarcoma: Comparison of Altering Sequential Administrations of High Doses of Adriamycin, Methotrexate, and Cyclophosphamide with a 6-Month Administration of High-Dose Adriamycin Followed by a Low-Dose Semicontinuous Chemotherapy

EORTC Osteosarcoma Working Party Group presented by C. Jasmin[1]

Introduction

In the past few years, a great impetus has been given to adjuvant chemotherapy of osteogenic osteosarcomas, particularly after the publication by JAFFE et al. [3] of promising preliminary results concerning the use of high-dose methotrexate with folinic acid rescue. CORTES et al. [2] reported the efficacy of adriamycin in adjuvant therapy and have shown that large doses of adriamycin (around 90 mg/m^2) are more efficient than small doses. Other groups have obtained significant results with various drug combinations [5, 6], most often including Alkeran or cyclophosphamide, adriamycin, high-dose methotrexate, and vincristine. Actually, most if not all of these trials have not been repeated; they often concern small groups of patients, and it is difficult to decide which protocol should be recommended. Our group has decided to make a randomized trial to compare (1) a relatively heavy and prolonged chemotherapeutic schedule, similar to the one proposed by ROSEN et al., including high-dose methotrexate, adriamycin, and cyclophosphamide with (2) high-dose adriamycin for 6 months, followed by a light ambulatory semicontinuous chemotherapy combined with the use of low-dose methotrexate.

Patients and Methods

The criteria of entry into this study included histologically proven osteogenic osteosarcomas. All anatomopathologic preparations were reviewed by A. MAZABRAUD, Fondation Curie, Paris. Parosteal osteosarcoma, nonosteogenic osteosarcomas, radiation-induced osteosarcoma, and osteosarcoma after Paget's disease were excluded. This study concerned only patients with bone tumors located in the limbs. Before entering the study, each patient had chest roentgenograms and tomography, a blood count, measurement of serum creatinine,

1 Participating Centers: A. MAZABRAUD (Fondation Curie, Paris); D. BERTEAUX, R. ROY-CAMILLE (La Pitié, Paris); C. CHENAL (Salpêtrière, Paris); R. BROSSEL (Tenon, Paris); GARETTA (Val-de-Grâce, Paris); G. MATHÉ (Institut de Cancérologie et d'Immunogénétique and Institut Gustave Roussy, Villejuif, France); G. MEYNARD (Bordeaux); D. DURAND, B. HOERNI (Fondation Bergonié, Bordeaux); M. WALLAERT (Centre Hospitalier, Lens); P. CAPPELAERE (Oscar-Lambret, Lille); VERHAEGHE (Faculté de Médecine, Lille); D. LIEGEY-BAGARRY, G. MEYER, G. ROUX (CRACM, Marseille); A. TRIFAUD (La Conception, Marseille); B. SERROU (Paul-Lamarque, Montpellier); P. FUMOLEAU, B. LE MEVEL (René-Gauducheau, Nantes); D. GUERIN (C. H. U., Rennes); D. HOFFSTETTER, R. METZ, J. STINES (Alexis-Vautrin, Vandoeuvre-les-Nancy).

urea, alkaline phosphatases, calcium, an electrocardiogram, and bone and liver scans. Patients were excluded if they had lung metastases detected at the time of randomization.

Treatment Protocols

This study was initiated in May 1976. Patients were randomized into two groups, just before treatment of the primary tumor. This treatment consisted of either (1) radical surgery for large tumors when the function of the limb was definitely compromised by large soft tissue invasion or by articular dysfunction or (2) radiotherapy treatment of small tumors and tumors on the superior limb, 8000 rad in 8 weeks on the tumoral zone and 6000 rad over a 10-cm zone above and below the limits of the tumour.

If hematologic effects had cleared, patients from group A received, successively, at intervals of 3 weeks:

1. 1.4 mg/m^2 vincristine (maximum 2 mg) IV followed, 6 h later, by 4.5 g/m^2 methotrexate given during a 6-h perfusion, followed, after 3 h, by the administration of 12.5 mg citrovorum factor every 3 h for 24 h IV, then 25 mg every 6 h for 48 h. For the first cycle, the dose of methotrexate was reduced to 3 g/m^2.
2. Adriamycin 75 mg/m^2 IV.
3. Cyclophosphamide 1.2 g/m^2. Methotrexate and cyclophosphamide were administered during 18 months. Adriamycin administration was discontinued after seven cycles.

In Group B. patients received adriamycin (45 mg/m^2/day) every 4 weeks for 2 consecutive days over a period of 24 weeks followed by a semicontinuous chemotherapy with methotrexate 30 mg/m^2 by IM injection every week associated with cyclophosphamide 150 mg/m^2 per os every day from day 1 to day 7 and Alkeran 2 mg/m^2 every day from day 15 to day 21. This cycle was repeated every 4 weeks for 12 months. In both groups, the treatment was delayed if there were less than 3000 leukocytes/mm^3 and less than 100,000 platelets/mm^3 in the peripheral blood. Twenty-seven patients entered this study, 15 in protocol A and 12 in protocol B. However, because of allergy to high-dose methotrexate, one patient initially randomized in group A was transferred to group B, after the first cycle of treatment.

Results

Table 1 summarizes the main characteristics of these patients. There were seven females and seven males in group A and six females and seven males in group B. Their ages ranged from 9 to 48 years with a mean and median age of 24 and 18 years, respectively. The primary tumor was located in the majority of patients either on the distal femur or in the proximal tibia. No significant difference was found between groups A and B. In group A, four patients were treated by radical surgery and ten patients by radiotherapy. In group B, only two patients were treated by surgery. The time interval between the first symptoms and diagnosis ranged from less than 1 to 7 months with a mean of 2.4 and 2.1 months for groups A and B, respectively. The time between diagnosis and the beginning of treatment ranged from a few days to 3 months, but the mean and the median was less than 1 month. The disease-free interval of both groups is shown in Fig. 1. Although the period of observation is relatively short, it appears that in group A less than 50% were disease-free at 1 year in contrast to 60% in

Table 1. Characteristics of patients

	Group A	Group B
Male/female	7/7	6/7
Mean age (years)	18	17
Age range	9–27	11–28
Mean delay between first symptoms and diagnosis (months)	2.4	2.1
Range	0–7	1–7
Localization of the primary tumor		
Distal femur	9	5
Proximal femur	1	0
Proximal tibia	3	4
Proximal fibula	0	3
Proximal humerus	1	1

group B. It is too early and the number of patients is too small to determine if a plateau in the curve has been reached. It should be noted that in group A lung metastasis occurred in three patients less than 3 months after randomization in contrast to one case of early metastasis in group B. The difference between the two curves is not statistically significant.

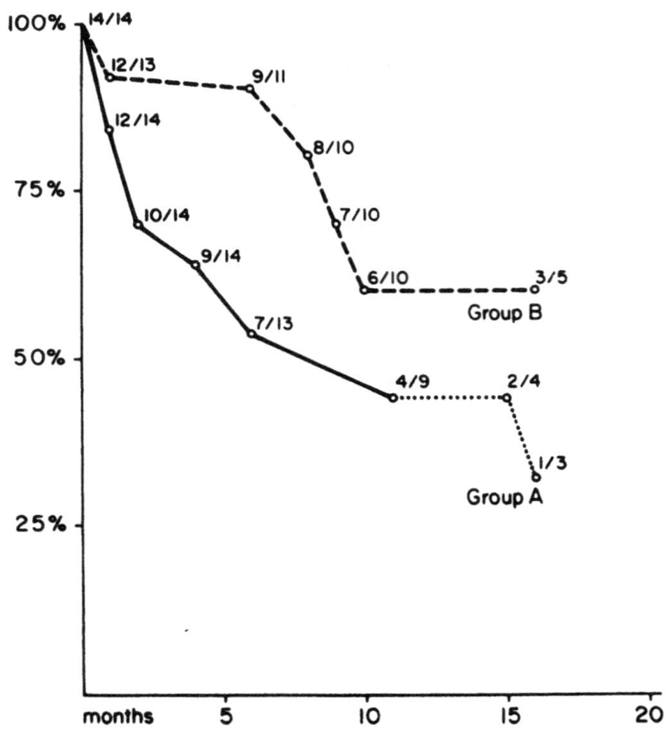

Fig. 1. Disease-free interval of patients with osteosarcoma treated by adjuvant chemotherapy (direct curve)

Toxicity

Protocol A was generally not as well tolerated by patients as protocol B because of a 2-day hospitalization for the high-dose methotrexate administration. One toxic death with severe aplasia and septicemia and severe mucosal toxicity was provoked by administration of high-dose methotrexate. Because of a severe cutaneous allergy to methotrexate, one patient from group A was changed to group B after the first injection of high-dose methotrexate. In group B, one patient refused to continue the injections of adriamycin and stopped treatment after the third cycle. Otherwise, protocol B was easier to administer than protocol A and better accepted by patients. No cardiotoxicity due to adriamycin was detected. The hematologic tolerance was good in both grous.

Discussion and Conclusions

Our results indicate that, although the number of patients is relatively small, chemotherapy with a succession of high-dose methotrexate, high-dose cyclophosphamide, and relatively high doses of adriamycin gives rather disappointing results. Our patients are mostly young adults and only a few children, but we cannot be sure that our protocol A of adjuvant therapy has done better than no treatment at all. Osteogenic osteosarcomas are so rare and have such a bad prognosis that a control group is not possible, but the difference between the results of group A and historical controls is not significant.

The results of protocol B are better and seem comparable to the results published by CORTES et al. We have not enough patients to determine whether the semicontinuous chemotherapy has had any additional beneficial effects. However, even for protocol B, the overall results are not fully satisfactory, considering that we have a maximum of 2 years follow-up and that the risk of late metastases persists. The tolerance and toxic cost of protocol A is also not negligible and was ascribed mainly to the use of high-dose methotrexate. The tolerance was better in protocol B.

In conclusion, our results underline the necessity of determining the validity of the results obtained with new protocols by different groups and also that adjuvants of osteogenic osteosarcoma remain a great problem. We hope that the combination of prophylactic lung irradiation, which has also given conflicting results [1, 4], with adjuvant chemotherapy during the first months of treatment (probably the most determinant period of the disease) may provide better results.

Summary

Twenty-seven patients with osteogenic osteosarcoma were treated with adjuvant chemotherapy. The first group was treated by intermittent high-dose methotrexate (4.5 g/m^2) for 18 months with citrovorum factor rescue, followed after 3 weeks by adriamycin 75 mg/m^2 and 3 weeks later by cyclophosphamide 1.2 g/m^2, etc. The second group of patients received adriamycin (90 mg/m^2) for 6 months every 4 weeks for 24 weeks, followed by semicontinuous chemotherapy with low-dose methotrexate, low-dose cyclophosphamide and Alkeran.
Actual results show that in the first group only 44% of patients were disease-free after 1 year in contrast to 60% in the second group. The difference is not statistically significant. Although

the number of patients is limited, the overall results, especially in the first group using high-dose methotrexate, are not very satisfactory. We are, therefore, now using the combination of chemotherapy and lung irradiation in the early phase of adjuvant therapy.

References

1. Breur, K., Cohen, P., Schweisguth, O., Hart, A. M. M.: Irradiation of the lung as an adjuvant therapy in the treatment of osteosarcoma of the limb. (in press) (1978)
2. Cortes, E. P., Holland, J. F., Wang, J. J., Clidewell, O.: Adriamycin (NSC-123127) in 87 patients with osteosarcoma. Cancer Treat. Rep. *6,* 305–313 (1975)
3. Jaffe, N., Frei, E., Traggis, D., Bishio, Y.: Adjuvant Methotrexate and citrovorum factor treatment of osteogenic sarcoma. N. Engl. J. Med. *291,* 994–997 (1974)
4. Rab, G. T., Ivin, J. C., Childs, O. S., Cupps, R. E., Pritchard, D. J.: Elective whole lung irradiation in the treatment of osteogenic sarcoma. Cancer *38,* 939 (1976)
5. Rosen, G., Murphy, M. L., Huvos, A. G., Guttierez, M., Marcove, R. C.: Chemotherapy in bloc, resection and prosthetic bone replacement in the treatment of osteogenic sarcoma. Cancer *37,* 1–11 (1976)
6. Sutow, W. W., Sullivan, M. P., Fernbach, D. J., Cangir, A., George, S. L.: Adjuvant chemotherapy in primary treatment of osteogenic sarcoma. Cancer *36,* 1598–1602 (1975)

Biochemistry of the Citrovorum Factor Rescue Effect in Normal Bone Marrow Cells After High-Dose Methotrexate Treatment: Implications for Therapy[1]

W. Wilmans, H. Sauer, and A. Schalhorn

High dose methotrexate therapy followed by citrovorum factor rescue (HDMTX/CF) therapy is based on the assumption that primary resistant tumors have an impaired active membrane transport system for folate compounds that is normally shared by methotrexate (MTX). At very high MTX serum concentrations, however, the drug can enter these cells by passive diffusion independent of the active transport system, resulting in cytocidal intracellular MTX concentrations [2, 3, 7]. Normal, rapidly proliferating tissues with an intact active transport system for folates can be protected from death by MTX by the application of relatively small doses of the antidote citrovorum factor (CF = leucovorin). This is the so-called rescue effect of CF. Since essentially no CF can enter the cells by passive diffusion at low serum concentrations, tumor cells lacking the active transport system do not benefit from the rescue effect.

For a better insight into this therapy, the MTX effect and CF rescue must be explained in more detail. The most important biochemical steps involved are shown in Fig. 1. Dihydrofolate reductase reduces dihydrofolic acid (FH_2) to tetrahydrofolic acid (FH_4). FH_4 is converted by serine hydroxymethyl transferase to 5-10-methylene-tetrahydrofolic acid, which is the main source for the pool of the activated one-carbon units. Thus, MTX, a potent inhibitor of the dihydrofolate reductase, reduces the pool of the activated one-carbon units and causes a

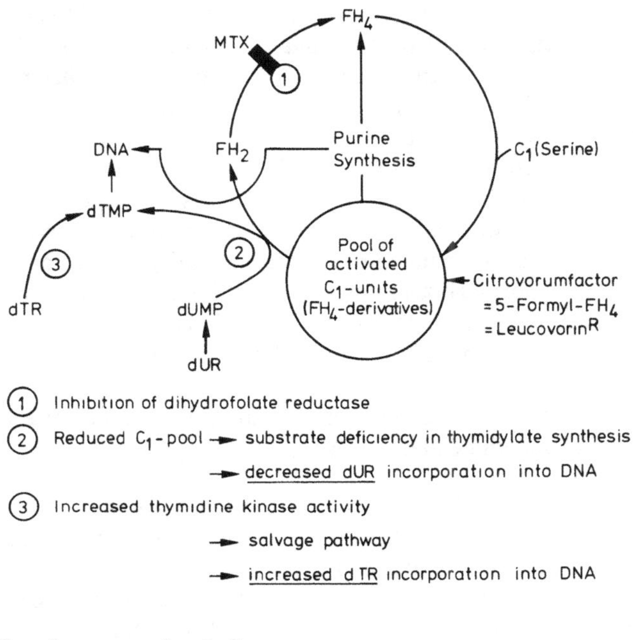

Fig. 1. Biochemical effects of methotrexate (MTX)

---

1 With the aid of the Deutsche Forschungsgemeinschaft.

substrate deficiency in the thymidylate synthetase reaction. The result is a decreased production of deoxythymidine monophosphate (dTMP). During the transfer from 5-10-methylene-FH_4 to deoxyuridine monophosphate (dUMP), the methylene group is reduced to methyl and the folate molecule is oxidized to FH_2. Activated folate is thus lost in this reaction and must be regenerated by dihydrofolate reductase [11]. On the other hand, during the enzymatic one-carbon transfer reactions in de novo purine synthesis, the FH_4 is not oxidized and can immetiately be reused for the activation of new one-carbon units. For this reason MTX affects the production of dTMP much more than the de novo purine synthesis.

If one offers exogenous tritium-labeled deoxyuridine (dRU) $^{(+)}$ to MTX-treated cells and measures its incorporation into the DNA, it is possible to monitor the effect of MTX in a biochemical way. The incorporation of dUR must be decreased, because after intracellular phosphorylation to deoxyuridine monophosphate (dUMP) the production of thymidine monophosphate (dTTP) is blocked. This lack of intracellular dTTP releases the normal feedback inhibition of the thymidine kinase reaction, which catalyzes the phosphorylation of thymidine (dTR) to dTMP. This activation of the thymidine kinase, the so-called salvage pathway, results in an increased production of dTMP and dTTP. By offering exogenous tritium-labeled dTR $^{(+)}$ to MTX-treated cells and measuring its increased incorporation into the DNA, one has another possibility for biochemically monitoring the MTX effect [21, 22]. Thus, both the decrease of the dUR incorporation and the increase of the dTR incorporation into the DNA serve as biochemical parameters of the MTX effect [18]. Normally, the incorporation rates of dUR and dTR are almost equal. The quotient dUR/dTR lies near 1.0 (normal range 0.7–1.3 [18]). Under MTX this value falls below the normal range and becomes less than 0.1 at high MTX concentrations. The quotient dUR/dTR has proved to be a direct indicator for the effectiveness of MTX.

The described biochemical effects of MTX can be corrected by the administration of its antidote citrovorum factor (CF) since this activated folate derivative directly enters the pool of the activated one-carbon units [17]. Thus, dTMP synthesis and de novo purine synthesis can resume although the dihydrofolate reductase is still inhibited by MTX. Biochemically, the rescue effect of CF is indicated by the normalization of the dUR/dTR quotient. It is established on an empiric basis that HDMTX/CF treatment of malignant tumors is successful [1, 2, 4, 6, 8, 12, 13–16, 20]. The rescue effect, however, has never been a subject of further biochemical investigation and questions as to the interval between MTX and CF administration, and the optimal CF dose necessary to protect the normal tissues from undesirable MTX side-effects still remain unanswered. In this presentation, the biochemical aspect of the CF rescue in normal bone marrow cells after HDMTX treatment is described for the first time in an attempt to answer the two most interesting questions:

1. At which time after the MTX infusion does the DNA synthesis in bone marrow cells regain normal activity?
2. At which MTX serum concentrations is CF really effective when given in the conventionally recommended doses?

The principles of the metabolic changes that are characteristic for the effects of MTX and CF were worked out with the model system of the permanent growing lymphoblast culture LS_2. The results are shown in Fig. 2.

In comparison to the control, 5-formyl-tetrahydrofolate (= citrovorum factor = CF) alone has no significant effect either on the cell growth or on the incorporation rates of ^{3}H-dTR and ^{3}H-dUR. Under normal conditions, the incorporation rates for these two nucleosides are nearly equal. The quotient dUR/dTR lies within the normal range of 0.7–1.3. As expected

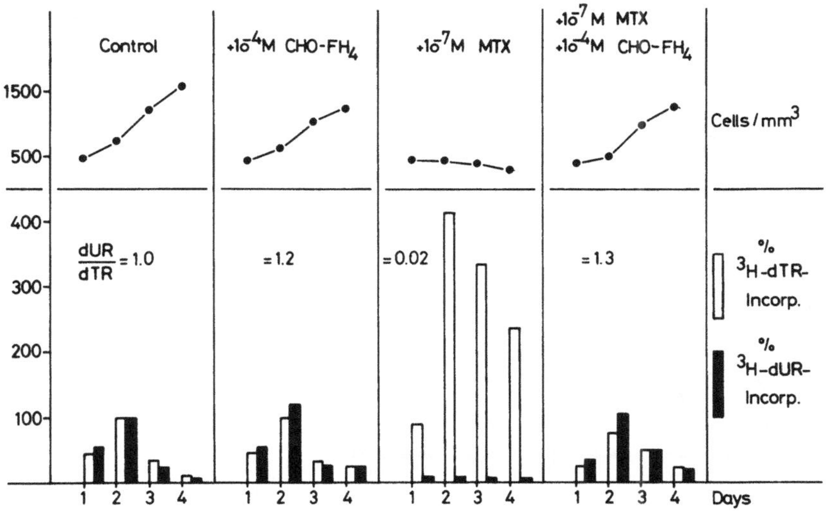

Fig. 2. DNA metabolism in cultured human lymphoblasts (LS_2). Effects of methotrexate (MTX) and citrovorum factor (leucovorin = $CHO\text{-}FH_4$)

from the biochemical mechanism, the dUR incorporation falls almost to zero after MTX whereas the dTR incorporation increases considerably. As a sign of a marked MTX effect, the dUR/dTR quotient falls below 0.1.

The DNA-metabolism of the cells is disturbed sufficiently that reproduction can no longer occur. After 4 h preincubation with 10^{-7} *M* MTX, the addition of CF normalizes the incorporation rates. The quotient dUR/dTR rises again to the normal value of 1.3. Culture growth is now normal again.

The same parameters as in the model culture were estimated in bone marrow cells of patients receiving MTX therapy. Figure 3 presents schematically the regimen of HDMTX/CF treatment. Two milligrams of vincristine are injected IV. Half an hour later the MTX infusion is started and the total dose is administered over a period of 6 h. Two hours later CF is given

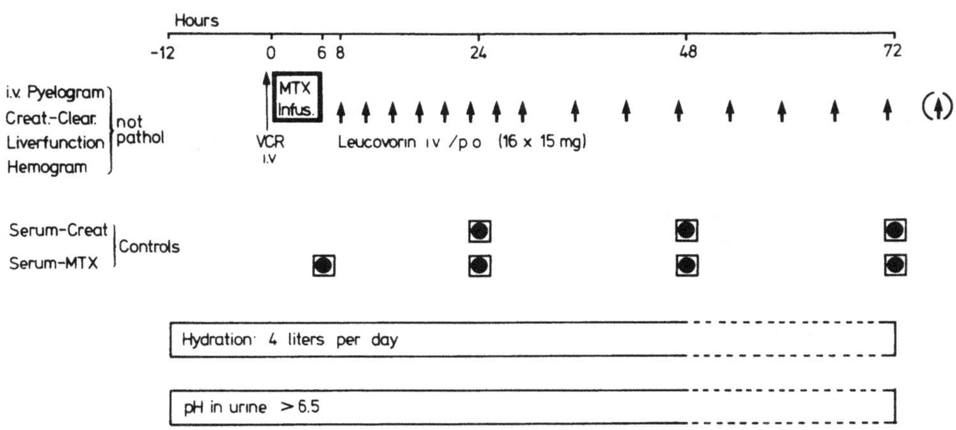

Fig. 3. High dose methotrexate/citrovorum factor (leucovorin) regimen (HDMTX/CF)

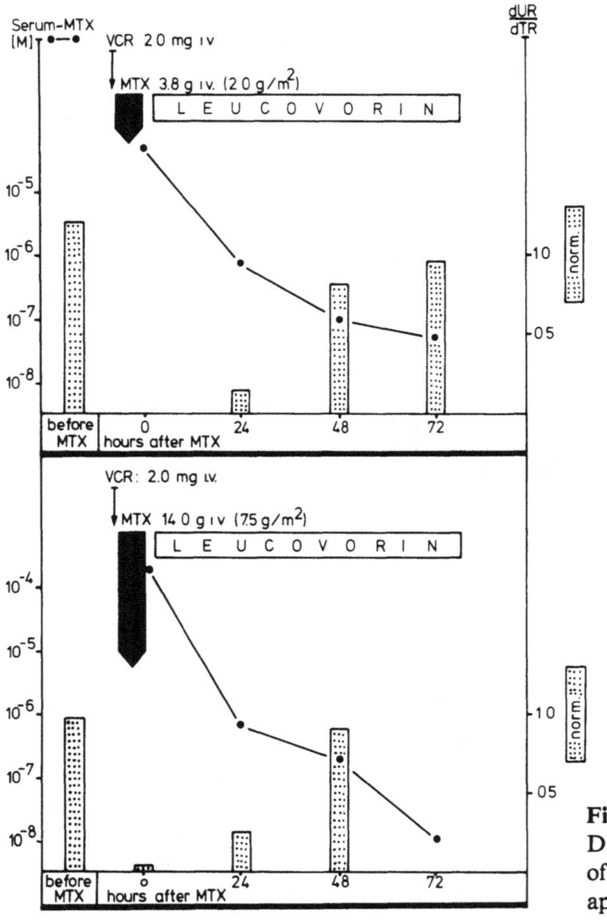

Fig. 4. MTX serum concentrations and DNA metabolism in bone marrow cells of a patient under HDMTX/CF therapy

IV in a dose of 15 mg every 3 h (eight times) and then every 6 h (eight times). This treatment is repeated every 2 weeks. During the first three courses, the MTX dose is increased from 3 g/m^2 to 6 g/m^2 and to 7.5 g/m^2. Then it is maintained at the latter dose for the following courses. The MTX serum concentration is determined enzymatically at the end of the MTX infusion and later on three times every 24 h. At these times bone marrow is aspirated for the examination of the DNA metabolism. Normal renal function is a most important precondition for HDMTX/CF therapy. Moreover, the urine must be alkalinized and a high fluid intake must be guaranteed. Figure 4 shows the results of the dUR/dTR quotient and the corresponding MTX serum levels in a patient with metastatic osteosarcoma who received 3.8 and 14.0 g of MTX as an adjuvant therapy for minimal residual disease after operation. Even 24 h after the end of the MTX infusion in both cases the DNA metabolism in the bone marrow cells shows a clear MTX effect although up to that time already seven doses of CF (15 mg each) have been injected. At 24 h the values of the dUR/dTR quotients are 0.14 and 0.25 and so considerably below the normal range.

Only after 48 h, when the MTX serum concentration decreased to the region of 10^{-7} *M*, did the dUR/dTR quotients (0.81 and 0.90, respectively) and DNA metabolism return to normal. A different course of another patient is demonstrated in Fig. 5.

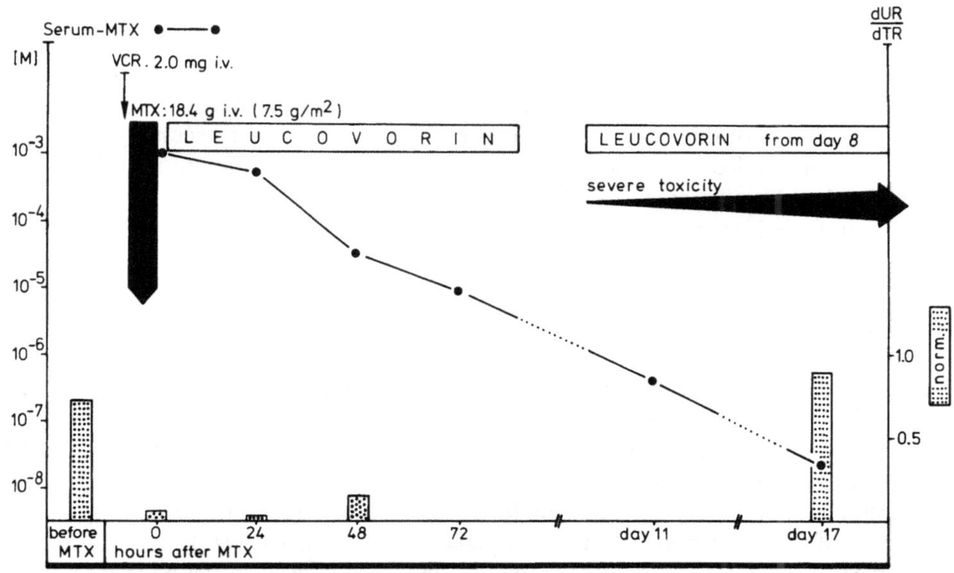

Fig. 5. Impaired MTX elimination and toxic reaction under HDMTX/CF therapy. No biochemical rescue for the bone marrow

As expected, again the dUR/dTR quotient after MTX administration falls to 0.06. Although CF is given regularly until the 48th h, there is no significant increase in the dUR/dTR quotient. For unknown reasons the MTX elimination from the patient's plasma is considerably retarted. On the 3rd day after the MTX infusion, the drug concentration in the serum is still 10^{-5}, M and even on the 11th day a pharmacologically effective level of 2×10^{-7} M is noted. At that time measurement of DNA metabolism was impossible because of a totally empty bone marrow. On the 17th day the bone marrow, had regenerated. Now under continued CF administration at a serum MTX concentration of 3×10^{-8} M, the dUR/dTR quotient was again within the normal range. In spite of reinitiation of CF treatment at the first signs of toxic side-effects (exanthema, leukopenia, thrombocytopenia), the patient developed very severe bone marrow depression, and despite intensive supportive care (antibiotics, platelet and granulocyte transfusions) he died due to sepsis and renal insufficiency. Other patients were treated with 35 courses of HDMTX/CF without any complications.

By the results demonstrated, it is shown that the usually administered doses of about 100 mg of CF per day are not sufficient for an effective rescue for the bone marrow cells as long as the MTX serum concentration is equal or higher than 10^{-6} M. At MTX serum concentrations of 10^{-7} M, CF is effective in these doses and leads to the normalization of the dUR/dTR quotient. According to these results, early CF application before the 24th or 36th h after the MTX infusion is not effective and seems to be of no benefit although this is required in most of the published schedules for HDMTX/CF therapy.

Should MTX elimination be retarded and MTX serum levels remain above 10^{-6} M for more than 48 h, the usually recommended CF doses are not sufficient to produce a significant rescue effect. In these patients, CF rescue with "normal" doses is ineffective since both MTX and CF enter the cell by the same active transport mechanism and inhibit one another

competitively [10]. Thus, high MTX concentrations nearly totally prevent the transport of low CF doses into the cell.
To save these patients from perhaps lethal damage of the bone marrow and/or the intestinal mucosa, the CF dose must be increased so much that the serum concentration of CF equals that of the MTX. For this purpose several grams of CF per day are necessary, as has been recently recommended by DJERASSY [5]. In critical cases the monitoring of the DNA metabolism in the bone marrow cells by means of the dUR/dTR quotient can determine if the CF dose used is high enough to prompt the desired rescue effect.

Summary

The decrease of the quotient of ^{3}H-deoxiuridine (dUR) and ^{3}H-thymidine (dTR) incorporation into the DNA of the cells is a good biochemical parameter for estimating the methotrexate (MTX) effect on rapidly proliferating cell systems like lymphoblast cultures and bone marrow. Using this indicator it could be shown that the usually administered doses of citrovorum factor (CF) are not sufficient for an effective rescue for the bone marrow cells as long as the MTX serum concentration is equal or higher than 10^{-6} *M*. In critical cases with retarded MTX elimination, the monitoring of DNA metabolism in the bone marrow cells by means of the dUR/dTR quotient can determine if the CF dose used is high enough to prompt the desired rescue effect.

Acknowledgement

The authors acknowledge the excellent technical help by Mrs. SARKAR, Miss HEIL and Miss STUPP-PUTOT.

References

1. Bender, R. A.: Anti-folate resistance in leukemia: treatment with "high-dose" methotrexate and citrovorum factor. Cancer Treat. Rev. *2,* 215–224 (1975)
2. Bleyer, W. A.: Methotrexate: clinical pharmacology, current status and therapeutic guidelines. Cancer Treat. Rev. *4,* 87–101 (1977)
3. Djerassi, I.: High-dose methotrexate (NSC-104) and citrovorum factor (NSC-3590) rescue: background and rationale. Cancer Chemother. Rep. *6,* 3–6 (1975)
4. Djerassi, I., Kim, J. S.: Methotrexate and citrovorum factor rescue in the management of childhood lymphosarcoma and reticulum cell sarcoma (non-Hodgkin's lymphomas). Cancer *38,* 1043–1051 (1976)
5. Djerassi, I., Kim, J. S., Nayak, N., Ohanissian, H., Adler, S., Hesieh, S.: New "rescue" with massive dose of citrovorum factor for potentially lethal methotrexate toxicity. Cancer Treat. Rep. *61,* 749–750 (1977)
6. Djerassi, I., Rominger, J., Kim, J. S., Ruchi, J., Suvansri, U., Hughes, D.: Phase I study of high doses of Methotrexate with citrovorum factor in patients with lung cancer. Cancer *30,* 22–30 (1972)
7. Frei, E.: Methotrexate revisited. Med. Ped. Oncol. *2,* 227–241 (1976)
8. Frei, E., Jaffe, N., Tattersall, M. H. N., Pitman, S., Parker, L.: New approaches to cancer chemotherapy with methotrexate. N. Eng. J. Med. *292,* 846–851 (1975)

9. Höffken, K., Seeber, S., Gallmeier, W. M., Bruntsch, U., Hossfeld, D. K., Schmidt, C. G.: Chemotherapie maligner Knochentumoren. Chirurg *48,* 274–279 (1977)
10. Huennekens, F. J., Rader, J. I., Neef, V., Otting, F., Jackson, R., Niethammer, D.: Folate antagonists: transport and target site in leukemic cells. In: Erythrocytes, thrombocytes, leukocytes. Gerlach, E., Moser, K., Deutsch, E., Wilmans, W. (eds.), pp. 496–503. Stuttgart: Thieme 1973
11. Jaenicke, L., Wilmans, W.: Der Stoffwechsel der Folsäure und der Einkohlenstoffeinheiten. Klin. Wochenschr. *41,* 1029–1038 (1963)
12. Jaffe, N.: The potential of combined modality approaches for the treatment of malignant bone tumors in children. Cancer Treat. Rev. *2,* 33–53 (1975)
13. Jaffe, J., Frei, E., Traggis, D., Watts, H.: Weekly highdose methotrexate-citrovorum factor in osteogenic sarcoma. Cancer *39,* 45–50 (1977)
14. Lustig, R. A., DeMare, P. A., Kramer, S.: Adjuvant Methotrexate in the radiotherapeutic management of advanced tumors of the head and neck. Cancer *37,* 2703–2708 (1976)
15. Pratt, C., Shanks, E., Hustu, O., Rivera, G., Smith, J., Kumar, M.: Adjuvant multiple drug chemotherapy for osteosarcoma of the extremity. Cancer *39,* 51–57 (1977)
16. Rosen, G., Murphy, M. L., Huvos, A. G., Gutierrez, M., Marcove, R. C.: Chemotherapy, en bloc resection, and prosthetic replacement in the treatment of osteogenic sarcoma. Cancer *37,* 1–11 (1976)
17. Sauer, H., Jaenicke, L.: Zur Aufhebung des zytostatischen Effekts von Amethopterin (Methotrexat®) durch Methyl-Tetrahydrofolsäure. Blut *28,* 321–326 (1974)
18. Sauer, H., Wilmans, W.: Cobalamin dependent methionine synthesis and methyl-folate-trap in human vitamin B_{12}deficiency. Br. J. Haematol. *36,* 189–198 (1977)
19. Townsend, C. M., Eilber, F. R., Morton, D. L.: Skeletal and soft tissue sarcomas: results of surgical adjuvant chemotherapy. Proc. Am. Soc. Clin. Onc. *17,* 265–270 (1976)
20. Vahrson, H., Gorges, P.: Enterale und parenterale Leucovorin-Medikation nach Methotrexat-Stoßbehandlung maligner Tumoren. Med. Klinik *71,* 1720–1723 (1976)
21. Wilmans, W.: Dihydrofolat-Reduktase und Thymidin-Kinase im Knochenmark unter Einwirkung von Folsäureantagonisten. Klin. Wochenschr. *45,* 987–994 (1967)
22. Wilmans, W., Kehr, D.: DNS-Synthese in Leukämiezellen unter der Einwirkung von Methotrexat, 5-Fluoro-Uracil und Cytosin-Arabinosid in vitro. Pharmacol. Clin. *2,* 161–167 (1970)

Adjuvant Interferon Treatment of Human Osteosarcoma

H. Strander, U. Adamson, T. Aparisi, L. Å. Broström, K. Cantell, S. Einhorn, K. Hall, S. Ingimarsson, U. Nilsonne, and G. Söderberg

Introduction

The 5-year survival rate for osteosarcoma patients is around 20% after primary surgery [7]. The short-term survival rate for patients given high dose adjuvant chemotherapy has been reported to be higher [5]. This communication deals with a clinical trial at the Karolinska Hospital where we are giving exogenous leukocyte interferon therapy to a consecutive series of osteosarcoma patients [1, 9, 11].

Case Series

The interferon group comprises all patients given interferon therapy to date; at present it numbers 33. Only patients without signs of metastases on admission are included in both groups.

The *contemporary control group* comprises the rest of all the osteosarcoma patients aged up to 30 years registered at the Cancer Registry at the National Board of Health and Welfare of Sweden during the period 1972–1975. They received no adjuvant therapy with the exception of six patients who received adjuvant high dose chemotherapy and were excluded from this study. All the patients in this group were treated elsewhere than at the Karolinska Hospital; the group numbers 30.

Pathologic Features

The pathology of most of the patients has been checked by an independent American group of investigators. The patients collected since May 1976 have not yet been checked by independent specialists but all had classic osteosarcomas according to the criteria established by the American group. Histologic typing was always performed by the method of Dahlin [4], according to which grade I and II tumors are well-differentiated and grades III and IV tend to be more anaplastic. The tumors were designated as either osteoblastic, chondroblastic, or fibroblastic osteosarcomas.

Endocrinologic Study

It has been suggested that hormonal mechanisms may be involved in the pathogenesis of osteosarcoma and also that such mechanisms have a bearing on the cause of the disease. The time incidence of the disease coincides with the puberty growth spurt, and the tumor is usually localized in the methaphyseal region of the long bones in the vicinity of the growth zones. The patients included in the present trial were analyzed for growth and dental development. Nineteen of the patients could be followed during childhood from birth to onset of the disease. No preponderance of tall individuals could be noted nor any significant difference from expected growth curves at the time of diagnosis. The latter finding could be confirmed from teeth eruption curves, which show a high correlation with somatic development. Some patients simultaneously displayed insulin resistance and an elevated level of somatomedins A and B in the plasma. This endocrinologic study is continuing.

Prognostic Factors

A study was undertaken to ascertain whether the two groups of patients were comparable with reference to prognostic factors. An analysis was made of age, sex, type of and frequency of symptoms, time period from first symptom to biopsy, time period from first symptom to treatment, localization of the tumors, largest diameter of tumor on radiogram, pathologic type, elapse period between the last negative and the first pulmonary X-ray, the type of operation performed, and the frequency and dose of irradiation. Except for the fact that local resections were made to a large extent on the interferon-treated group, there were no significant differences in the prognostic factors listed.

Interferon Preparations

Human leukocyte interferon was prepared as described previously [2, 3]. This type of interferon is produced by human leukocytes exposed to Sendai virus in tissue culture. The interferon released into the medium surrounding the cells is concentrated and purified. Two types of preparations have been used, one being more pure (P-IF) than the other (C-FI). The properties of these preparations have been described in detail previously [8].

In Vitro Studies

Nine established osteosarcoma cell lines were tested for their sensitivity to the cell multiplication inhibitory activity of the interferon employed for the clinical trial. The more specific details of this study have been presented earlier [12]. An inhibition of growth was recorded for all the cell lines, and the degree of inhibition was dose dependent. It is of interest that the serum levels of interferon achieved in the patients were shown to cause an inhibition of growth of all cell lines tested in tissue culture.

Administration of Interferon

The interferon was administered according to a standardized schedule [1]. Over a period of 1 month in hospital a daily dose of 3×10^6 standard interferon units was given by intramuscular injection. The preparation was then given on an ambulatory basis – 3×10^6 interferon standard units three times weekly for a further 17 months. All patients were started on the less purified interferon, C-IF, and if any side-effects were reported some of the patients were given the more purified interferon, P-IF.

Side-effects of Interferon

The six most commonly encountered side-effects recorded during the C-IF therapy were fever, local pain at the injection site, shivers, transient hair loss, itching erythema, and coryza. No major discomfort was reported. Due to the reported side-effects, however, most patients were given P-IF. Further details will be reported later. All the patients could be given interferon on an ambulatory basis, and it was not necessary in any case to abandon the treatment because of the side-effects.

Immunologic Findings

Prolonged treatment with exogenous interferon did not change the peripheral lymphocyte count in vivo or the mitogenic response of the patients' lymphocytes in vitro, nor did the interferon sensitivity of the lymphocytes alter during the therapy. The spontaneous cytotoxicity of the peripheral lymphocytes was shown to be enhanced after exposing them to human leukocyte interferon in vitro. Five patients were also studied for their spontaneous cytotoxicity in vivo. Four of these patients' lymphocytes exhibited spontaneous cytotoxicity before the injection of interferon. After the first injection there was an initial decrease of cytotoxicity followed by a larger increase to 1.5—5 times above the preinjection level and reaching a peak at 12 h. In three of these four patients the spontaneous cytotoxicity was still elevated after 24 h. The lymphocytes of the fifth patient had a very low spontaneous cytotoxicity before the injection and this did not markedly change thereafter. This study is continuing.

Infections

An impression of the incidence, duration, and severity of acute infections in osteosarcoma patients during interferon therapy was obtained from monthly questionnaires. For comparison, the incidence of infections among members of the patient's household was also noted. A preliminary account of the findings reported had been given elsewhere [10]. The incidence of infections was lower in the interferon-treated group. An analysis is now being made of recorded symptoms to see whether they are due to acute *viral* infections. The results of all these tests will be reported in due course.

Irradiation Therapy

Prior to operation, high dose irradiation of the primary site (> 4500 rad) was performed in 18% and low dose irradiation (1000—4500 rad) in 12% of the patients comprising the interferon group. None of the interferon group has been given preoperative irradiation therapy during the last 3 years and it is intended to discontinue this form of treatment. Of the control group 40% were given high dose and 3% low dose irradiation. Irradiation does not appear to be a significant prognostic factor in osteosarcoma [6].

Surgical Treatment

Surgical treatment for osteosarcoma has almost invariably consisted of amputation. We have preferred a local tumor resection when this is anatomically practicable, and in the interferon series this procedure was used on 44% of the patients. Owing to extensive involvement of the soft tissues by the tumor, amputation could not always be avoided and it was resorted to in 53%. Where the diaphyseal or adjoining metaphyseal region was involved, a block resection was performed, the defect being replaced by an autogenous bone graft. When the tumor was localized to the metaphyseal region or encroached on the epiphysis, the block resection also took in the joint surface compartment. For reconstruction, autogenous grafts and/or artificial implants were used.

Metastases and Survival Rate

A comparison of the interferon and the contemporary groups of patients was done with respect to the development of metastases and the survival rate. The interferon group consisted of 33 patients and the control group of 30. None of the patients in either groups were given chemotherapy until after development of metastases. According to life table analysis, 58% of the patients given interferon should still be free from metastases after 3 years, compared to 37% of the contemporary group. A similar analysis of survival, to some extent affected by chemotherapy given to some patients, showed that 68% of the interferon group should still be living after 3 years in contrast to 35% of the concurrent control group. These results are promising but the follow-up period is at present too short to warrant any definitive inferences. The study is being continued and the groups are constantly being added to.

Summary

This paper outlines results obtained to date in a clinical trial whose purpose is to examine the efficacy of exogenous leukocyte interferon therapy for osteosarcoma patients. This type of therapy has a low toxicity, and preliminary results indicate that most of the reported side-effects of the treatment disappear on further purification of interferon. The incidence of metastases is lower and the survival rate is better for the interferon group than for the contemporary control group. The study is being continued.

Acknowledgement

This study was supported by the Swedish Cancer Society, the Cancer Society of Stockholm, and Dagmer Hasselgren's Fund.

References

1. Adamson, U., Aparisi, T., Broström, L.-Å., Cantell, K., Einhorn, S., Hall, K., Ingimarsson, S., Nilsonne, U., Strander, H., Söderberg, G.: Interferon treatment of human osteosarcoma. Study week of the Pontificial Academy of Sciences, Vatican City, Oct. 17–21, 1977 (in press)

2. Cantell, K., Hirvonen, S., Mogensen, K. E., Pyhälä, L.: Human leukocyte interferon: Production, purification, stability and animal experiments. In: The production and use of interferon for the treatment and prevention of human virus infection (in vitro). Waymouth, M. C. (ed.), pp. 35–38. Culture Association Workshop. Rockville: Tissue Culture Association 1974
3. Cantell, K., Strander, H.: Human leukocyte interferon for clinical use. In: Blood leukocytes – function and use in therapy. Högman, C. F., Lindahl-Kiessling, K., Wigzell, H. (eds.), pp. 73–75. Uppsala: 1977
4. Dahlin, D. C.: Bone tumors – general aspects and data on 3987 cases, 2nd ed. Springfield (Ill.): C. C. Thomas 1973
5. Frei, III, E., Jaffe, N., Skipper, H. E., Gero, M. G.: Adjuvant chemotherapy of osteogenic sarcoma: progress and perspectives. In: Adjuvant therapy of cancer. Salmon, S. E., Jones, S. E. (eds.), pp. 49–64. Amsterdam: Elsevier North-Holland Biomedical 1977
6. Friedman, M. A., Carter, S. K.: The therapy of osteogenic sarcoma: current status and thoughts for the future. J. Surg. Oncol. *4,* 482–510 (1972)
7. Handelsman, H., Carter, S. K.: Current therapies in osteosarcoma. Cancer Treatm. Rev. *2,* 77–83 (1975)
8. Mogensen, K. E., Cantell, K.: Production and preparation of human leukocyte interferon. Pharmacol. Ther. [C.] *1,* 369–381 (1977)
9. Strander, H.: Interferons: Anti-neoplastic drugs? Blut *35,* 277–288 (1977)
10. Strander, H., Cantell, K., Carlström, G., Ingimarsson, S., Jakobsson, P. Å, Nilsonne, U.: Acute infections in interferon-treated patients with osteosarcoma: Preliminary report of a comparative study. J. Infect. Dis. *133,* A245–248 (1976)
11. Strander, H., Cantell, K., Ingimarsson, S., Jakobsson, P. Å., Nilsonne, U., Söderberg, G.: Interferon treatment of osteogenic sarcoma – a clinical trial. Fogarty Int. Center Proc. *28,* 377–381 (1977)
12. Strander, H., Einhorn, S.: Effect of human leukocyte interferon on the growth of human osteosarcoma cells in tissue culture. Int. J. Cancer *19,* 468–473 (1977)

Current Results With a Combined Treatment Approach to Localized Ewing's Sarcoma

M. Gasparini, F. Fossati-Bellani, and G. Bonadonna

Introduction

Like many malignant tumors of childhood and adolescence, Ewing's sarcoma should be considered a systemic disease, at least in the majority of patients. Multiple foci of neoplastic cells scattered throughout the body, mainly in the bones and lungs, are present at the time of initial diagnosis. In approximately 25% of patients metastases are clinically detectable, while in 75% they cannot be detected with the diagnostic tools currently available. In this latter group we generally detect one single bone lesion, which is considered to be the primary tumor. The concept of distant micrometastases has led clinical investigators to abandon mutilating surgical procedures and to adopt high-energy radiotherapy as the treatment of choice for the primary site [1]. Long-term results after radiation were similar to those obtained with radical surgery (cure rate: 10%–20%), while a high percentage of relapsing patients were spared a useless mutilation. However, the percentage of patients developing distant spread remained

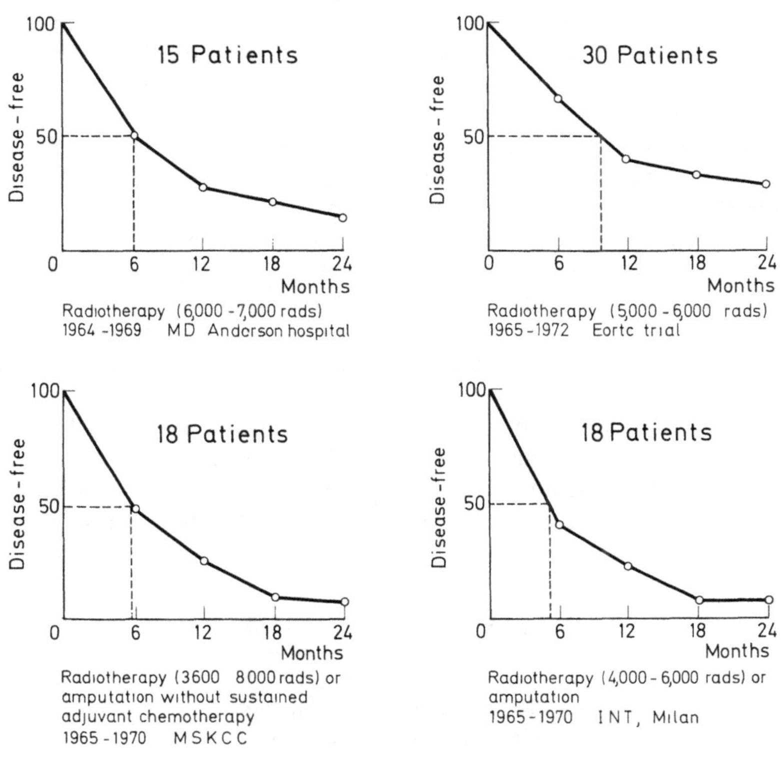

Fig. 1. Localized Ewing's sarcoma: disease-free survival with local treatment modality

very high, and radiotherapy also failed to eradicate the primary tumor in 20%–40%. In several reported series the median disease-free survival ranged between 6 and 10 months (Fig. 1) [3, 4, 14, 16]. Once metastases were clinically evident, patients showed only a moderate and transient benefit from optimal chemotherapy, which was able to induce remission and to prolong survival but not to save a consistent number of patients.

In the last 5–7 years, the radiotherapy technique has been improved and chemotherapy utilized early in the course of the disease, i.e., when only a single bone lesion was clinically evident to achieve better local control of the tumor and a high percentage of disease-free survivors. The aim of this paper is to review current concepts and recent results in the field of the combined treatment modality for localized Ewing's sarcoma and to focus on current problems raised by this therapeutic approach.

Radiation Therapy

Ewing's sarcoma is a radiosensitive neoplasm, and both pain relief and shrinkage of the tumor mass is almost invariably achieved at the level of the primary lesion. Doses ranging 3500–5000 rad may be able to destroy all malignant cells locally. However, local relapse may occur, sometimes after very high doses (> 6000 rad), and there is evidence that the incidence of local failure after radiotherapy is inversely proportional to the dose delivered [2]. Better results are being obtained with the administration of at least 6000 rad to the bulky site of the tumor area, using high-energy radiotherapy (Table 1). Due to the intramedullary extension of the tumor, radiation fields are shaped to include all involved bone, delivering dose of 4000 rad. The remaining dose is given with smaller fields only to the tumor area. The fraction is that of 800–1000 rad per week. Special care must be observed to spare as much normal surrounding soft tissue as possible to avoid the development of severe soft tissue fibrosis and the blockage of lymphatic drainage. This means that radiation treatment should be individualized as far as the shape of the radiation fields is concerned.

It is difficult to evaluate the role of recent radiation technique in the achievement of the current results with combined treatment approach (radiotherapy plus chemotherapy) for Ewing's sarcoma. However, the incidence of local failure seems to be decreased [2, 8, 11], and this is an important factor in the achievement of a prolonged disease-free status. Historical controls who showed a high local recurrence rate were treated with less adequate radiation modalities. Therefore, a comparative evaluation is difficult.

It is also important to point out that local control at the level of the primary site is often associated with severe morbidity, especially if the patient is young and the tumor is located in the lower limbs. The long-term functional results may be quite unsatisfactory, and it is not rare for amputation to be required subsequently to correct severe diasabling sequelae [13, 15]. The

Table 1. Localized Ewing's sarcoma: technique of radiotherapy

Energy	Megavoltage (CO 60 or higher)
Dose	4000–5000 rad to entire bearing bone
	1000–2000 additional rad to tumor site
Fraction	200 rad daily, 5 fractions per week
Shield	As much normal peripheral soft tissue as possible

irradiation program outlined cannot be utilized for all primary bone sites. For instance, in the presence of pelvic or vertebral lesions, high doses of irradiation are usually not well tolerated by the normal adjacent viscera. Therefore, radiotherapy has to be administered in lower doses.

Chemotherapy

Treatment plans currently under evaluation combine radiotherapy with chemotherapy. While different regimens and schedules of chemotherapy are being employed, two basic rules can be identified in all ongoing treatment protocols: (1) use of drugs proven to be effective in metastatic Ewing's sarcoma, i.e., vincristine (VCR), cyclophosphamide (CTX), adriamycin (ADM), and actinomycin D (Act. D) (Table 2) and (2) pulse-cyclic administration of two or more agents.

Tables 3 and 4 summarize the salient points and results of the most recent published studies [5, 6, 10, 13]. In our institute, treatment starts with radiation therapy to the primary tumor, and chemotherapy is administered when a total dose of 2500–3000 rad has been delivered.

Table 2. Single agents with established activity in metastatic Ewing's sarcoma

Drugs	Response rate (%)
Cyclophosphamide (CTX)	50–60
Actinomycin (Act. D)	60
Adriamycin (ADM)	35–70
Vincristine (VCR)	20

Table 3. Examples of recently combined treatment programs

Institution	Local treatment	Systemic treatment	Treatment duration
Milan [5]	RT 4500–7000	CTX-VCR-ADM	18 mo
Memorial Hospital [13]	Surgery or RT 5000–7000	CTX-VCR-ADM-Act. D	18–20 mo
Sidney Farber [6]	RT 5500–6000	CTX-VCR-Act. D	24 mo
Intergroup [10]	RT 5500–6500	CTX-VCR-ADM-Act. D *vs* CTX-VCR-Act. D *vs* CTX-VCR-Act. D + RT to lungs	20 mo

Table 4. Results of combined treatment programs

Institutions	Patients df/total	Follow-up	Disease-free survival	Local control (%)
Milan [5]	18/24	8–48 mo	68% at 2 yr	92
Memorial Hospital [13]	15/20	31–82 mo	75% at 3 yr	90
Sidney Farber [6]	7/9	28–78 mo	77% at 3 yr	100
Intergroup [10]	110/187	24 mo (median)	61% *vs* 31% *vs* 57% at 2 yr	87

df disease-free.

This sequence was decided upon to avoid skin and/or soft tissue reaction to ADM, which could prevent optimal completion of the radiation therapy. ADM (60 mg/m^2) + VCR (1.4 mg/m^2 given on the same day as ADM and 8 days later) were alternated monthly with CTX (1000 mg/m^2) + VCR for a total of 18 months. The total dose of ADM was planned not to exceed 600 mg/m^2. All 24 consecutive patients who entered the protocol underwent complete clinical remission, with disappearance both of pain and of clinical and radioisotopic evidence of tumor. The actuarial survival curve shows that 68% of patients are disease-free at 24 months from starting treatment. In our approach, surgery was seldom employed as primary treatment of the tumor. Only one patient had the tumor located in the mandible completely resected. In four patients partial resection was followed by radiotherapy, in accordance with the technique previously described. At present, two of six relapsed patients showed evidence of tumor reactivation at the primary site only after distant metastases had occurred. None of the five patients who underwent partial or complete resection of the primary tumor developed local or distant recurrence. In nine patients the planned radiotherapy program could not be followed for a number of reasons, and treatment was not considered to be optimum, either because the total cumulative dose administered was less than 6000 rad or because the duration was longer than 6 weeks. Table 5 shows that local and/or distant spread may be correlated with the adequacy of initial radiotherapy. Similar observations were made by the Intergroup Ewing's Sarcoma Study in the United States, who recorded a high number of failures in patients initially treated with suboptimal doses of radiotherapy (Table 6) [11]. This study followed a three-group randomized protocol designed to evaluate whether ADM or prophylactic lung irradiation could improve the results obtained with VCR + Act. D + CTX after local radiotherapy. The recently published results seem to indicate that radiotherapy followed by ADM + VCR + CTX + Act. D produced the

Table 5. Localized Ewing's sarcoma treated with combined modality: adequacy of RT ralated to relapse [5]

RT	Reasons	No. relapsed	
Optimal		1/14	(7%)
Nonoptimal	Decreased dose Increased time	5/9	(55%)

Table 6. Correlation of dose of RT with number of patients with distant metastases

Dose of RT	Relapse	
3000–< 4000	2/3	(67%)
4000–< 5000	9/24	(38%)
5000–< 6000	30/62	(48%)
> 6000	6/21	(29%)

Adapted from Intergroup, 1977 [11].

best results, with 61% of the patients remaining disease-free after 2 years. With this treatment regimen, local failure occurred in 6%, as against about 16% [10]. The Memorial Hospital group in New York utilized the T2 protocol (ADM + Act.D + VCR + CTX) as adjuvant treatment after surgery of radiotherapy and have recently updated their preliminary results [14]. The initially encouraging results were confirmed only in the subgroup with localized Ewing's sarcoma. In fact, 75% of 20 patients survived disease-free for more than 3 years from the beginning of treatment. Two patients showed local recurrence [13].
These above-mentioned results indicate that the combined treatment approach with radiotherapy plus chemotherapy is able to achieve a prolonged disease-free status and to decrease the incidence of tumor recurrence at the primary site.

Other Treatment Approaches

Immunotherapy has not yet been consistently evaluated in Ewing's sarcoma. Some authors have employed total body irradiation (TBI) [9], but the number of treated patients was too small to draw significant conclusions. There is evidence that TBI can induce clinical remission in some patients with metastatic Ewing's sarcoma. However, this technique does not seem advisable as an adjuvant treatment, especially because it is often associated with early and delayed toxicity. In our opinion, TBI has first to be adequately tested in disseminated disease to assess its effectiveness and morbidity. The CNS prophylaxis advised by some authors [7], either with brain irradiation or with intrathecal methotrexate, does not seem to be necessary in the adjuvant treatment of this malignant tumor. In our experience and in that of other clinical investigators [13], CNS involvement is rare at the first manifestation of relapse, and the risks of CNS prophylaxis do not justifiy its routine use in the adjuvant setting. The observation that the lung is the first site of metastasis in 50%–60% of patients in whom treatment fails led prophylactic lung radiotherapy to be considered in the early management of localized Ewing's sarcoma. The recent results of the Intergroup Ewing's Sarcoma Study showed that the combination of this treatment with chemotherapy did not improve the percentage of disease-free survivors [10]. Furthermore, the irradiation of the cardiac area may enhance the cardiotoxic potential of some drugs (ADM, CTX).

Conclusions

The chemotherapy-radiotherapy program in the management of clinically localized Ewing's sarcoma has resulted in a decreased incidence of local relapse as well as in prolonged disease-free status. However, despite intensive systemic treatment and optimal local irradiation, a percentage of patients develop local tumor recurrence, which is generally followed by subsequent distant spread. Furthermore, severe long-term disabling sequelae requiring corrective surgical procedures are being reported with high frequency. For these reasons, surgery has to be reconsidered in the initial approach to localized Ewing's sarcoma. In fact, surgery provides definitive control of the tumor at the primary site, and the consequent mutilation can be balanced against the risks of local relapse and the long-term morbidity following radiotherapy. Surgery may be the treatment of choice, especially in children, when tumor is located in the lower limbs and when the risks of growth impairment due to radiotherapy are high. In adolescent or adult patients, or when the tumor is located in sites that prevent the administration of high doses of radiotherapy, surgery may be associated with radiotherapy. Treatment can be individualized, with partial resection of the involved bone or excision of the primary tumor after chemotherapy and/or low dose radiotherapy.

It must be kept in mind that there is some evidence that distant spread may be correlated with suboptimal radiotherapy at the level of the primary tumor. Persistence of microscopic residual malignant cells at this site could be the source for distant metastases even in the absence of both clinical and radiologic signs of local recurrence.

All these facts show that a changing attitude toward the management of localized Ewing's sarcoma is emerging. Concern about the delayed effects of radiotherapy and of chemotherapy is based on the assumption that the probability of cure is being increased for this disease. In fact, the prognosis in Ewing's sarcoma has changed dramatically in recent years, and the outlook seems more favorable. However, a longer follow-up is required before it can be stated whether the cure rate has definitely been improved. In the historical control series, the survival curve shows a plateau only after 5 years from treatment onset [12]. The increased disease-free survival does not necessarily mean that an increase in the cure rate was obtained. Systemic chemotherapy could just delay the development of metastases. It seems important, however, that these patients be treated in the knowledge that cure is now possible in a more consistent number of patients. For this reason, there is much concern about the potential chronic toxicity of chemotherapy, and long-term morbidity from the chemotherapeutic agents is therefore under continuous evaluation. About 70% of patients with Ewing's sarcoma are only in their 2nd decade at the time of initial diagnosis, and "cured patients" will have most of their lives to live. Treatment must not only assure the best chance for cure but also optimal quality of life.

References

1. Boyer, C. W. (Jr.), Brickner, T. J. (Jr.), Perry, R. H.: Ewing's sarcoma. Case against surgery. Cancer *20,* 1602–1606 (1967)
2. Chabora, B. McC., Rosen, G., Cham, W., D'Angio, G. J., Tefft, M.: Radiotherapy of Ewing's sarcoma. Radiology *120,* 667–671 (1976)
3. Fernandez, C. H., Lindberg, R. D., Sutow, W. W., Samuels, M. L.: Localized Ewing's sarcoma. Treatment and results. Cancer *34,* 143–148 (1974)
4. Gasparini, M., Barni, S., Lattuada, A., Musumeci, R., Bonadonna, G., Fossati Bellani, F.: Ten year experience with Ewing's sarcoma. Tumori *63,* 77–89 (1977)
5. Gasparini, M., Fossati Bellani, F., Lombardi, F., Pilotti, S.: Sequential adjuvant combination chemotherapy in Ewing's sarcoma. Proceedings ASCO *19,* Abs. C-228 (1978)
6. Jaffe, N., Traggis, D., Salian, S., Cassady, J. R.: Improved outlook for Ewing's sarcoma with combination chemotherapy (vincristine, actinomycin D, and cyclophosphamide) and radiation therapy. Cancer *38,* 1925–1930 (1976)

7. Johnson, R. E., Pomeroy, T. C.: Integrated therapy for Ewing's sarcoma. Am. J. Roentgenol. *123,* 583–587 (1975)
8. Macintosh, D. J., Price, C. H. G., Jeffree, G. M.: Ewing's tumor. J. Bone Joint Surg. *57-B,* 331–340 (1975)
9. Millburn, L. F., O'Grady, L., Hendrickson, F. R.: Radical radiation therapy and total body irradiation in the treatment of Ewing's sarcoma. Cancer *22,* 919–925 (1968)
10. Nesbit, M., Vietti, T., Burgert, O., Tefft, M., Gehan, E., Perez, C., Razek, A., Kissane, J.: Intergroup Ewing's sarcoma study (IESS): results of three different treatment regimens. Proceedings AACR, Abs. 323 (1978)
11. Perez, C. A., Razek, A., Tefft, M., Nesbit, M., Burgert, E. O., Jr., Kissane, J., Vietti, T., Gehan, E. A.: Analysis of local tumor control in Ewing's sarcoma. Cancer *40,* 2864–2873 (1977)
12. Pritchard, D. J., Dahlin, D. C., Dauphine, R. T., Taylor, W. F., Beabout, J. W.: Ewing's sarcoma. A clinico-pathological and statistical analysis of patients surviving five years or longer. J. Bone Joint Surg. *57-A,* 10–16 (1975)
13. Rosen, G., Caparros, B., Mosende, C., McCormick, B., Huvos, A. G., Marcove, R. C.: Curability of Ewing's sarcoma and considerations for future therapeutic trials. Cancer *41,* 888–899 (1978)
14. Rosen, G., Wollner, N., Tan, C., Wu, S. J., Hajdu, S. I., Cham, W., D'Angio, G. J., Murphy, M. L.: Disease-free survival in children with Ewing's sarcoma treated with radiation therapy and adjuvant four-drug sequential chemotherapy. Cancer *33,* 384–393 (1974)
15. Tefft, M., Chabora, B. McC., Rosen, G.: Radiation in bone sarcomas. Cancer *39,* 806–816 (1977)
16. Zucker, J. M., Henry-Amar, M.: Therapeutic controlled trial in Ewing's sarcoma. Eur. J. Cancer *13,* 1019–1023 (1977)

EORTC/GTO Adjuvant Chemotherapy Program for Primary Ewing's Sarcoma: Results at 5 Years

B. P. Le Mevel, B. Hoerni, D. Durant, C. Kenesi, M. Salle, A. Trifaud, D. Liegey-Bagari, J. V. Bainvel, J. M. Rogez, P. Fumoleau, A. Mazabraud, J. Dumont, B. Tomend, E. Brossel, M. Garetta, D. Guerrin, C. Jasmin, H. Sancho-Garnier, and M. Gimenez

Introduction

Ewing's sarcoma is classically linked with a very poor prognosis after a local surgical treatment and/or radiotherapy: 5-year survival is less than 15% [1]. The recent progress made in chemotherapy had led to effective treatment of metastatic patients [10, 16–19]. The rapid appearance of these metastases after local control alone (more than 75% within 2 years) [1, 3, 5, 9] and the possibility of an effective systemic approach to these lesions had led to the concept of adjuvant chemotherapy after local treatment of Ewing's sarcoma. In 1973, after the encouraging results obtained by JOHNSON [6], HUSTU [5], and ROSEN [13, 14], the EORTC osteosarcoma working party started a therapeutic trial of adjuvant chemotherapy for primary Ewing's sarcoma.

Material and Methods

The local treatment consisted of radiation therapy of 4500 rad to the entire involved bone, plus 1500 rad to the tumor, in 6 weeks. An adjuvant chemotherapy was then given for several

- VINCRISTINE (VCR)
  1,5 mg/m^2 I.V. day 1, 10 and 20
- CYCLOPHOSPHAMIDE (CPM)
  1 g/m^2 I.V. or I.M. day 2, 11, and 21
- ADRIAMYCIN (ADM)
  60 mg/m^2 I.V. day 35 and 50
- PROCARBAZINE (PCB)
  200 mg/m^2 per os, day 70 at 80
  Free interval : 20 days
  For 18 months

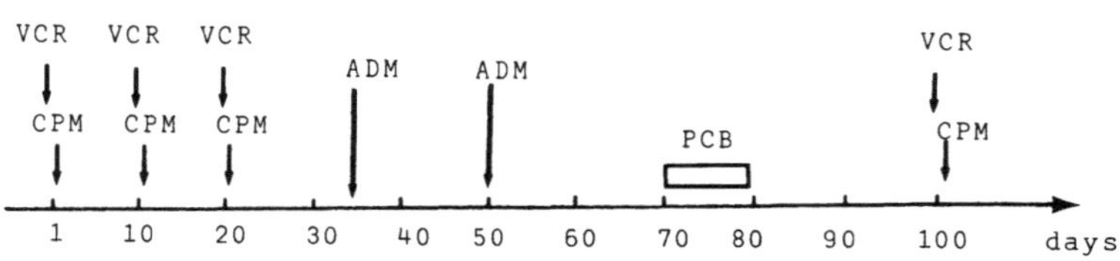

Fig. 1. E_3 protocol of adjuvant chemotherapy for primary Ewing's sarcoma

months. At the beginning of the trial, this adjuvant treatment was the E_3 protocol of the International Society of Pediatric Oncology (SIOP), given for 18 months. Figure 1 shows this protocol: after radiotherapy, a combination of vincristine and cyclophosphamide (three times at 10-day intervals), then adriamycin (twice at 15-day intervals), then procarbazine for 10 days is given in 80 days. This 3-month cycle is continued for 18 months.

In 1976, we decided to randomize our patients between this E_3 protocol and a new protocol $E_{76\text{-}5\text{-}170}$, shown in Figs. 2 and 3. Chemotherapy is started early along with radiotherapy but without adriamycin (to avoid the complications of this combination). The protocol consists of two phases: an attack phase of heavy treatment for 9–12 months combining adriamycin, vincristine, cyclophosphamide, and actinomycin D (Fig. 2). This is followed by a maintenance phase of lighter treatment combining cyclophosphamide alternatively with procarbazine and methotrexate for 12–18 months (Fig. 3).

Since 1973, 28 previously untreated patients with primary Ewing's sarcoma entered our trial. Five were excluded for varying reasons (metastatic patients, incorrect diagnosis, no available follow-up); 12 were treated under E_3 protocol and 11 under protocol E_{76}. The distribution of the 23 eligible patients with regard to their age, sex, or sites of primary tumor is very similar in both groups, as seen in Tables 1 and 2. The median age is 16 years with a range of 7 to 37

Starting with radiotherapy :

- VINCRISTINE
  1,5 mg/m^2 I.V. day 1
- CYCLOPHOSPHAMIDE
  300 mg/m^2 I.V. or I.M. day 2, 3, 4 and 5

Free interval : 3 weeks

After radiotherapy :

- ADRIAMYCIN
  300 mg/m^2 I.V. day 1 and 2
- VINCRISTINE
  1,5 mg/m^2 I.V. day 3
- CYCLOPHOSPHAMIDE
  300 mg/m^2 I.V. } day 4 and 5
- ACTINOMYCIN D (Act D)
  0,3 mg/m^2 I.V. } day 4 and 5

Free interval : 3 weeks

9 cycles

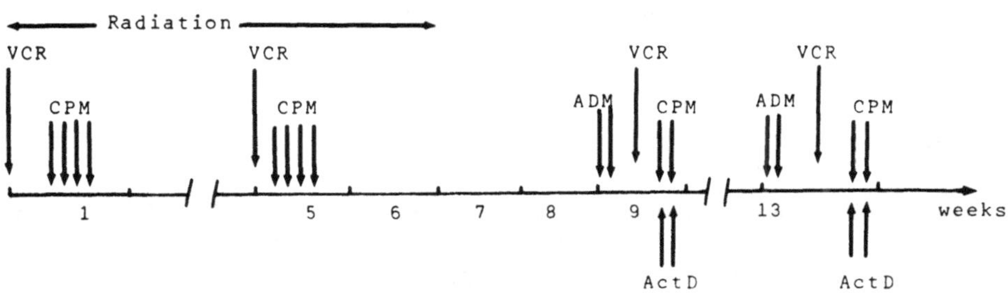

Fig. 2. $E_{76\text{-}5\text{-}170}$ protocol of adjuvant chemotherapy for primary Ewing's sarcoma

Maintenance chemotherapy

- METHOTREXATE (MTX)

  20 mg/m^2 I.M. q/2 weeks

- CYCLOPHOSPHAMIDE

  150 mg/m^2/day, per os, 7 days - q/4 weeks

  and after one week of free interval

- PROCARBAZINE

  200 mg/m^2/day, per os, 7 days - q/4 weeks

  For 18 months

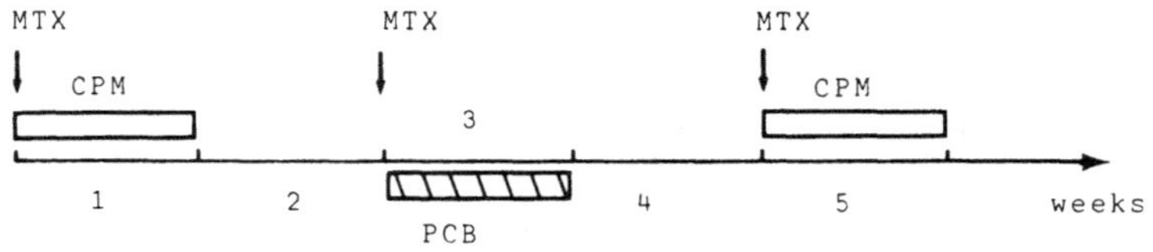

Fig. 3. $E_{76\text{-}5\text{-}170}$ protocol of adjuvant chemotherapy for primary Ewing's sarcoma: maintenance therapy

Table 1. Age and sex distribution of patients under E_3 and E_{76} adjuvant protocols

	Protocol E_3 (12 patients)	Protocol E_{76} (11 patients)	Total (23 patients)
Age (years)			
Range	7–37	8–37	7–37
Mean	17.6	17.09	17.13
Median	16.5	16	16
Sex			
Male	8	9	17
Female	4	2	6

years. There are more male than female patients (17 against 6). as to the site, it is noticeable that the number of tumors with relatively bad prognosis (nine pelvis, seven femurs) is high in both groups. This has to be taken into account in the evaluation of the survival and for comparison with other trials.

Results

The results of the trial are seen in Table 3. The 12 patients who entered the E_3 protocol were followed for a period ranging 10–64 months; seven remained free of disease for a median of 39 months; five relapsed after 7, 8, 16, 20, and 22 months; three died at 8, 26, and 31 months. The length of the follow-up period of the 11 patients who entered the other protocol is very

Table 2. Site of primary tumor of patients under E_3 and E_{76} adjuvant protocols

	Protocol E_3 (12 patients)	Protocol E_{76} (11 patients)	Total (23 patients)
Trunk			
Pelvis	5	4	9
Rib	1	–	1
Vertebrae	1	–	1
Proximal long bones			
Femur	4	3	7
Humerus	–	2	2
Distal long bones			
Tibia	1	1	2
Calcaneum	–	1	1

Table 3. Follow-up of patients under E_3 and E_{76} adjuvant protocols

Protocol E_3: 12 patients	Protocol E_{76}: 11 patients
Length of follow-up	Length of follow-up
Range: 10+ to 64+ months Mean: 36+ months	Range: 2+ to 24+ months Mean: 8+ months
Free of disease: 7	Free of disease: 11
Range: 17+ to 64+ months Mean: 39+ months	Range: 2+ to 24+ months Mean: 8+ months
Number of relapses: 5	Number of relapses: 0
At 7, 8, 16, 20, and 22 months	
Number of deaths: 3	Number of deaths: 0
At 8, 26, and 31 months	

short with a mean of 8 months; there was no relapse and no death occurred during this period ranging 2–24 months. Although the number of patients is small and the follow-up period is still short, curves representing first remission and overall survival have been drawn following the method of Kaplan and Meier [8], mainly for the patients who entered the E_3 protocol as seen in Figs. 4 and 5. A *56%* disease-free survival is observed at 3 years and remains the same at 5 years (Fig. 4). The overall survival at 5 years is *63%* (Fig. 5). Obviously, no comparison is yet available with patients of protocol $E_{76\text{-}5\text{-}170}$.

The five relapses observed are analyzed in Table 4: two pulmonary and three osseous metastases; there was no local relapse and no CNS involvement. It may be noteworthy to remark that all these five patients were male, with primary tumor of the pelvis or the femur.

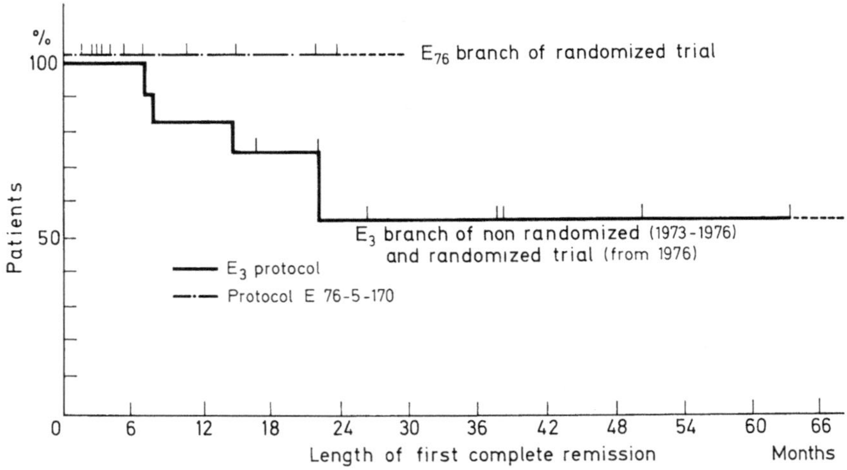

Fig. 4. Disease-free survival of primary Ewing's sarcoma patients under E_3 and $E_{76\text{-}5\text{-}170}$ adjuvant protocols (following the method of KAPLAN and MEIER [8])

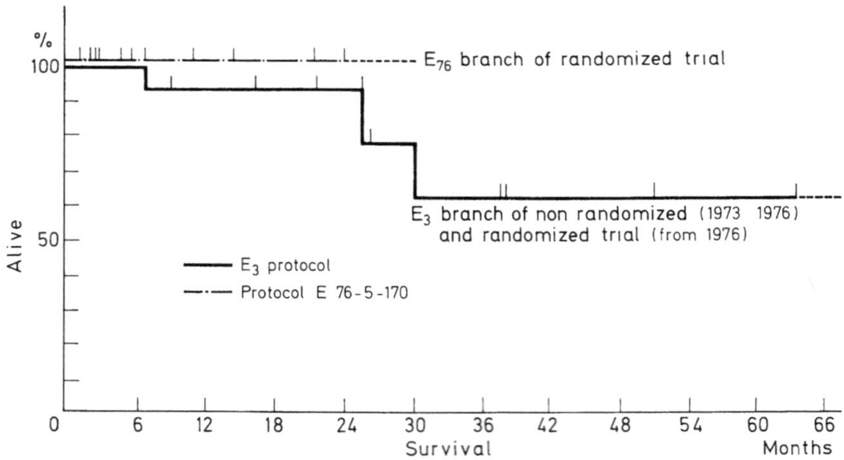

Fig. 5. Overall survival of primary Ewing's sarcoma patients under E_3 and $E_{76\text{-}5\text{-}170}$ adjuvant protocols (following the method of KAPLAN and MEIER [8])

The time between first clinical sign and diagnosis was often long and consequently the size of the tumor large; three of these relapses occurred very shortly after completing of the treatment.

Discussion

The results of our therapeutic trial are very encouraging: a 5-year survival may be anticipated for 63% of our patients with the E_3 protocol (by comparison to less than 15% classically). Those results are very similar to those recently obtained by other groups: FERNANDEZ [2],

Table 4. Relapses of patients under E_3 adjuvant protocol

	Sex	Delay between first sign and diagnosis (months)	Site of primary tumor	Size of primary tumor (cm)	Site of relapse[a]	Time of relapse (months)	Time of death (months)	Comments
TES..	♂	9	Femur	9/3	Lung	22	26	Delay and dose reduction in chemotherapy due to hematologic and digestive toxicity
GEO..	♂	6	Pelvis	8/8	Vertebrae	16	31	
DEV..	♂	3	Femur	17/8	Lung	7	8	Huge tumor (17 × 8 cm)
GER..	♂	3	Sacrum	7/4	Rib	22	—	Delay in chemotherapy due to patient
FEV..	♂	1	Femur	6/4.5	Tibia	8	—	No violation of protocol

[a] No local relapse and no CNS involvement.

Pomeroy [11], Zucker [20], Rosen [15], Gasparini [4], and Razek [12], ranging 55%–70%. This confirms clearly that the treatment of primary Ewing's sarcoma must be a multidisciplinary approach.

The five relapses observed occurred mainly shortly after completion of the E_3 adjuvant program. Furthermore, patients who remained free of disease for more than 2 years did not relapse afterward, as also observed by Rosen [15]. It is our feeling that avoidance of these

relapses might be possible by the use of an earlier and more aggressive combination therapy (as in protocol $E_{76\text{-}5\text{-}170}$, for example).
No local relapses nor severe functional failures were observed after the combination of 6000 rad and four-drug chemotherapy. This is very different from some other reports of more than 25% serious functional failures, and we do not intend to follow the plan for primary amputation in young patients with lesions in the knee area, as recently proposed [15]. We prefer to reserve it for eventual failures after conservative treatment.
We did not observe any CNS relapses. It seems that sanctuary meningeal disease does not occur very frequently in Ewing's sarcoma, and we do not intend to incorporate prophylactic CNS treatment as proposed by other investigators [7] because of its uncertain future risks.

Conclusion

In conclusion, our first results of the combination of adjuvant chemotherapy with local treatment of primary Ewing's sarcoma seem to clearly confirm that great progress has been made with this approach. However, this disease is a rare and we would like to stress that these patients should be entered in trials which will allow us to draw definite conclusions in the future. It seems possible to say at present that the treatment of Ewing's sarcoma must be a multidisciplinary treatment, for which we have still to define the best therapy.

References

1. Falk, S., Alpert, M.: Five years survival of patients with Ewing's sarcoma. Surg. Gynecol. Obstet. *124,* 319–324 (1967)
2. Fernandez, C. H., Lindberg, R. D., Sutow, W. W., Samuels, M. L.: Localised Ewing's sarcoma. Treatment and results. Cancer *34,* 143–148 (1974)
3. Gasparini, M., Barni, J., Lattuada, A., Musumeci, R., Bonadonna, G., Fossati-Belloni, F.: Ten years experience with Ewing's sarcoma. Tumori *63,* 77–90 (1977)
4. Gasparini, M., Fossati-Belloni, F., Lombardi, F., Pilotti, S.: Sequential adjuvant combination chemotherapy in Ewing's sarcoma. Proceedings of the 14th Annual Meeting of the American Society of Clinical Oncology. (Washington) *19,* (Abs. C. 228) (1978)
5. Hustu, H. D., Pinkel, D., Pratt, C. B.: Treatment of clinically localized Ewing's sarcoma with radiotherapy and combination chemotherapy. Cancer *30,* 1522–1527 (1972)
6. Johnson, R. E., Pomeroy, T. C.: Integrated therapy for Ewing's sarcoma. Am. J. Roentgenol. *114,* 532–535 (1972)
7. Johnson, R. E., Pomeroy, T. C.: Evaluation of therapeutic results in Ewing's sarcoma. Am. J. Roentgenol. *123,* 583–587 (1975)
8. Kaplan, E. L., Meier, P.: Non parametric estimation from imcomplete observations. J. Am. Statistics. Assoc. 455–481 (1958)
9. Macintosh, D. J., Price, Chg., Jeffree, G. M.: Ewing's tumor. A study of behaviour and treatment in forty-seven cases. J. Bone Joint Surg. B *57,* 331–340 (1975)
10. Oldham, R. K., Pomeroy, T. C.: Treatment of Ewing's sarcoma with actinomycin (NSC-123 127). Cancer Chemother. Rep. *56,* 635–639 (1972)
11. Pomeroy, T. C., Johnson, R. E.: Combined modality therapy of Ewing's sarcoma. Cancer *35,* 36–41 (1975)

12. Razek, A., Perez, C., Tefft, M., Vietti, T., Burgert, O., Gehan, E., Nesbit, M.: Local control related to radiation dose volume and site of primary lesion in Ewing's sarcoma. Proceedings of the 69th Annual Meeting of the American Association for Cancer Research. (Washington) *19*, (Abs. 672) (1978)
13. Rosen, G., Wollner, N., Wu, S. J., Hajdu, S. I., Cham, W., Murphy, M. L.: Prolonged disease free survival in children with Ewing's sarcoma treated with radiation therapy and adjuvant 4 drug sequential chemotherapy. Proceedings of the James Ewing Society *59*, (Abs. 23) 1973
14. Rosen, G., Wollner, N., Tan, C., Wu, S. J., Hajdu, S. I., Cham, W., D'Angio, G. J., Murphy, M. L.: Disease-free survival in children with Ewing's sarcoma treated with radiation therapy and adjuvant four drug sequential chemotherapy. Cancer *33*, 384–393 (1974)
15. Rosen, G., Caparros, B., Mosende, C., McCornick, B., Huvos, A. G., Marcove, R.: Curability of Ewing's sarcoma and considerations for future therapeutic trials. Cancer *41*, 888–899 (1978)
16. Senyszyn, J. J., Johnson, R. E., Curran, R. E.: Treatment of metastatic Ewing's sarcoma with actinomycin D (NSC-3053). Cancer Chemother. Rep. *54*, 103–107 (1970)
17. Sutow, W. W.: Vincristine (NSC-67574) therapy for malignant solid tumors in children (except wilm's tumor). Cancer Chemother. Rep. *52*, 485–487 (1968)
18. Sutow, W. W., Sullivan, M. P.: Cyclophosphamide therapy in children with Ewing's sarcoma. Cancer Chemother. Rep. *23*, 55–60 (1962)
19. Tan, C., Etcubanas, E., Wollner, N., Rosen, G., Murphy, M. L., Krakoff, I. H.: Adriamycin in children with acute leukemia and other neoplastic diseases. International Symposium on Adriamycin. Carter, S. K., Di Marco, A., Chione, M., Frakoff, I. H., Hethe, G. (eds.), pp. 204–212. Berlin: Springer 1972
20. Zucker, J. M., Henry-Amar: Therapeutic controlled trial in Ewing's sarcoma. Report of the results of a trial by the clinical Cooperation Group on Radio and Chemotherapy of the EORTC. Eur. J. Cancer *13*, 1019–1023 (1973)

Adjuvant Treatment of Soft Tissue Sarcoma in Children and Adults

V. H. C. Bramwell, P. A. Voûte, S. A. Rosenberg, and H. M. Pinedo

Introduction

Soft tissue sarcomas are a rare group of tumours comprising approximately 1% of all malignant tumours. Conventional management has relied heavily on surgery, but the inadequacy of this approach is reflected by local recurrence rates of 40% – 80% in adult sarcomas and as high as 90% in childhood sarcomas. CANTIN [3] in a review of 784 patients found that 382 had died of sarcoma and 65% had developed metastases concomitantly with local recurrence. The high local relapse rate is due to absence of encapsulation of the tumour, which spreads along fascial planes and nerve trunks and possibly also to a multifocal origin. Thus, more adequate methods of local control and prevention of dissemination are required and these include radiotherapy, chemotherapy and immunotherapy.

Although there is animal data to suggest that the proliferative kinetics of malignant cells in large tumour masses differ considerably from those in small tumours [27], this data has yet to be confirmed for human tumours and it seems sensible, therefore, to use chemotherapy known to be effective in advanced disease.

Whilst some histological types of sarcoma seem to carry a worse prognosis (e. g. rhabdomyosarcomas, leiomyosarcoma), other factors may be more important. SUIT et al. [30] treating 100 patients with localised soft tissue sarcoma using limited surgery and high dose radiation therapy made the following observations:

1. Histological grade affected prognosis (disease-free survivals of 86% for grade I tumours compared to 17% for grade III);
2. size of the primary tumour determined the subsequent local recurrence rate (18% for tumours > 5 cm compared to 8% for those < 5 cm);
3. site of primary tumour was important (local recurrence rate 33% for a proximal site compared with 5% for a distal site).

Therefore, accurate staging is important in sarcomas, both in deciding the most appropriate treatment strategy and in assessing results. A staging system for adult sarcomas has been proposed by RUSSEL et al (26) using the TMN system with the addition of histological grade G, giving four stages (Table 1) that correlate well with survival in 1,215 cases of 13 types of sarcoma (Fig. I). The staging of childhood rhabdomyosarcomas takes into account the resectability of the tumour and the presence or absence of bone marrow involvement (Table 2).

Although bone marrow involvement is said to be rare in adult sarcomas, this may be because it is not looked for. Over the last 18 months, bone marrow aspirates and trephines have been carried out on all patients with locally advanced or metastatic soft tissue sarcoma seen at the Christie Hospital, Manchester, and so far 2 of 23 have been positive – in one pleomorphic rhabdomyosarcoma and in one angiosarcoma of the breast.

Table 1. Staging of adult soft tissue sarcomas

T	Primary tumor	T_1	5 cm
		T_2	5 cm
		T_3	Any size invading bone, major vessel or nerve
N	Regional nodes	N_0	Not involved
		N_1	Histologically verified involved
M	Distant metastases	M_0	No distant metastases
		M_1	Distant metastases
G	Histological grading	G_1	Low
		G_2	Moderate
		G_3	High

Stage I	Grade I tumour with no nodal or distant metastases
	Ia < 5 cm
	Ib > 5 cm
Stage II	Grade 2 tumour with no nodal or distant metastases
	IIa < 5 cm
	IIb > 5 cm
Stage III	Grade 3 tumour with no nodal or distant metastases
	IIIa < 5 cm
	IIIb > 5 cm
	IIIc Tumour of any grade or size with regional lymph nodes involved but without distant metastases
Stage IV	IVa Tumour of any grade grossly invading bone, major vessel or major nerve with or without nodal metastases but without distant metastases.
	IVb Tumour with distant metastases

Adapted from Russel et al., Cancer *40*, 1562–1570 (1977).

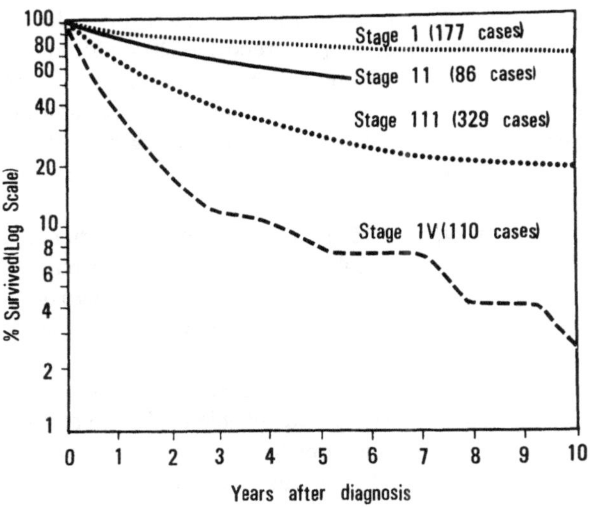

Fig. 1. Survival curves by steps for 702 cases with complete information for staging: 423 cases with slide review and 279 without. The curve for stage II was not plotted beyond 5 years since at that point the standard error was 5% or higher. Russel et al., Cancer *40*, 1562–1570 (1970)

Table 2. Staging of childhood rhabdomyosarcoma

Stage I	Localised disease
Stage II	Regional disease
Stage IIA	Completely resectable
Stage IIB	Non-resectable or only partially resectable
Stage III	Generalised disease
Stage IIIA	Distant metastases with normal bone marrow
Stage IIIB	Distant metastases with bone marrow containing rhabdomyoblasts

Source: Malpas et al. B. M. J. **1**, 247–249 (1976).

Childhood Soft Tissue Sarcoma

Rhabdomyosarcomas are the commonest group of soft tissue sarcomas occurring in childhood. These are usually of the embryonal or botryoid type, which tend to occur before the age of 6 years, but occasionally may be alveolar or pleomorphic in type, occurring in an older age group (12–16 years) and having a poorer prognosis. Other sarcomas are rare, including fibrosarcoma, liposarcoma, synovial sarcoma and undifferentiated sarcoma, but seem to have a better prognosis. For example, CHUNG and ENZINGER [4] reviewed 48 cases of infantile fibrosarcoma treated mainly by surgery alone and found 31 (65%) were disease-free and only four (8.3%) had died of disease 5 months – 21 years after treatment.

Poor overall survival rates (in the order of 10%–30%) have been reported for rhabdomyosarcoma treated by surgery or radiotherapy alone [7, 14, 29, 31]. However, the addition of adjuvant chemotherapy to primary surgery or radiotherapy has led to considerable improvement in both complete remission rate and disease-free survival. Vincristine, cyclophosphamide and actinomycin D have all been shown to be active as single agents [22, 32, 33] although reponses are often transient with rapid emergence of drug resistance. Combination chemotherapy with these three agents in advanced disease has produced superior results in terms of both remission rate and duration [23].

In 1972, PRATT et al. [24] reported 20 children with rhabdomyosarcoma treated with a coordinated programme combining surgery, radiotherapy and combination chemotherapy (Table 3). Eleven of 14 patients with localised tumours achieved a complete remission, seven continuing for 2–39 months from the start of chemotherapy. There were four temporary complete remissions and one partial remission in the six patients with metastatic disease.

DONALDSON, et al. [5] reported a 74% (14 patients) survival for a minimum of 2 years and 89% (17 patients) local control in 19 evaluable patients with rhabdomyosarcoma of the head and neck treated by local excision or biopsy, high dose radiotherapy – 6000 rad in 6 weeks – and combination chemotherapy with VAC (Table 3). Complications, however, were severe and included:

1. One death due to unexplained renal failure during chemotherapy.
2. Five patients with ocular problems. Three required exenteration of the orbit, one as the primary procedure, one for residual disease and the other for radiation keratitis, iritis and conjunctivitis. There was one asymptomatic radiation-induced cataract occurring 27

Table 3. Chemotherapy regimes for paediatric sarcomas

Pratt			
Vinc	1.5 mg/m^2	IV weekly × 6 concurrent with XRT (Vinc, Act D, Cyclo)	Vinc, Cyclo: Every 2 weeks for 6 months (for localised disease) or 12 months (regional or metastatic disease)
Act D	0.4 mg/m^2		
Cyclo	300 mg/m^2		
Donaldson			
Vinc	2 mg/m^2 IV weekly × 12		Starting concurrently with XRT
Act D	0.075 mg/kg IV for 5–8 days Courses repeated every 3 months to a total of 5		
Cyclo	2.5 mg/kg/day orally continuously for 2 years		
Heyn			
Chemotherapy commencing immediately after completion of XRT			
Act D	0.015 mg/kg/day IV × 5 days 0.075 mg/kg/week IV × 6 doses starting on day 21		Repeated every 9 weeks for 1 year
Malpas			
Vinc	1.5 mg/m^2	IV weekly × 6 concurrent with XRT (Vinc, Act D, Cyclo)	Then all three drugs every 2–3 weeks for 1 years
Act D	0.06 mg/m^2		
Cyclo	300 mg/m^2		
Voute			
Vinc	2 mg/m^2 IV every 2 weeks		
Act D	15 μg/kg IV days 1–5 every 12 weeks		
Cyclo	200 mg/m^2 days 1–5 every 6 weeks		

months after therapy and another patient suffered mild superficial keratitis with early corneal stippling year post therapy.

3. Most patients suffered severe mucositis, often requiring nasogastric feeding or intravenous fluids;
4. There was one case with probable osteonecrosis of the mandible and another with atrophy of the zygoma.
5. Severe dental decay occurred in two patients;
6. Seven episodes of ear infection occurred and one patient required a simple mastoidectomy;
7. Moderate bone marrows suppression was frequent.

Most of these complications could be attributed to the high dosages of radiation used, sometimes aggravated by actinomycin D.

In 1974, Heyn et al. [13] described a randomised study in 32 patients with rhabdomyosarcoma of all sites. Patients were eligible if the tumour had been completely removed surgically and there was no evidence of metastatic disease. All patients had post-operative radiotherapy to the tumour bed and were then randomised to receive either chemotherapy (Table 3) or no further treatment. An additional group of 11 patients with residual microscopic disease received post-operative radiotherapy and the same chemotherapy. Fifty-three percent (8/15) of the control group subsequently developed metastatic disease 3–30 months from diagnosis of whom six died. In the comparable treated group, only 17.6% (3/17) developed metastases with one death. The use of adjuvant combination chemotherapy in those patients rendered free of macroscopic tumour by surgery and radiotherapy produced a 2-year disease-free survival of 85.7% (24/28).

Some tumour sites, however, preclude radical surgery. MALPAS et al. [15] treated 11 patients with regional disease primarily with radiotherapy supplemented by adjuvant chemotherapy. After biopsy, radiotherapy (4000–6000 rad over 4–6 weeks) was administered using generous fields to include any local extension and the lymphatic drainage of the tumour. Concurrent weekly chemotherapy (Table 3) was followed by further courses of VAC at 2–3 weekly intervals for 1 year. Occasionally radiotherapy was preceded by several courses of chemotherapy if the tumour was very extensive. All 11 patients achieved a complete remission and in four who were submitted to 'second look surgery' for suspected recurrence or residual disease, there was no evidence of viable tumour. Three patients subsequently relapsed and died at 15, 16 and 26 months but the rest were disease-free 4–29 months from the start of treatment, and the median survival for the group has not been reached. A historical control group of 17 patients of similar stage treated by radiotherapy and surgery alone had only one survivor at 18 months and the median survival was 10 months. Analysis in January 1978 showed that no further relapses had occurred, an additional 11 patients had been treated, the total group having disease-free survivals ranging 3–67 months (personal communication).

An alternative approach to management of these tumours is primary chemotherapy, supplemented by adjuvant surgery or radiotherapy. This has the potential advantage that extensive and mutilating surgical procedures may be avoided. Similarly, as marginal recurrence is common, wide radiation fields may be needed to encompass local tissue infiltration, thus limiting the total radiation dose and producing late complications due to local growth retardation. Shrinkage of the tumour by chemotherapy may avoid the necessity for extensive fields and allow local high dose radiotherapy or limited surgery to be used.

The Amsterdam Study Group on Childhood Tumours conducted a study of this type between 1971 and 1975 [21], admitting 18 evaluable patients with tumours occurring in the urogenital tract (8 patients) and ENT region (10 patients). All patients were treated with initial chemo-

Table 4. Rhabdomyosarcoma of the ENT and urogenital tracted treated in Amsterdam with chemotherapy and limited adjuvant treatment (October 1972 – November 1975)

Patients entered	26
Previous treatment with surgery or radiotherapy	8
Patients evaluable	18
NED after chemotherapy alone	7
NED after chemotherapy and limited surgery	5
DWD (local recurrence)	3
DWC (local control but cerebral metastases)	3

NED No evidence of disease.
DWD Died with disease.

therapy (Table 3), which was administered over an 18-month period with frequent reassessment of the need for additional surgery or radiotherapy. Results of treatment are shown in Table 4. Seven patients had no evidence of disease after chemotherapy alone 24–26 months from the commencement of treatment (Table 5). Five patients required local treatment for residual disease during chemotherapy and are disease-free 24–60 months later (Table 6). Six patients died with disease. One patient with a bladder tumour completed 18 months chemotherapy but developed a vaginal recurrence 2 months later and succumbed despite further surgery and radiotherapy. There were two local recurrences during chemotherapy in a nasopharyngeal and a maxillary tumour, both of which proved to be resistant to radiotherapy. Three patients with tumours of the maxillary sinus, tonsil and pterygoid fossa all died of cerebral metastases but autopsy in each case showed local tumour control and in one case, resolution off lung metastases.

Although overall survival was not particularly good in this study, quality of life was considered to be important and 12 of the 18 children were spared mutilating treatment. Three children died of cerebral metastasis – a site notoriously resistant to these chemotherapeutic agents. These results have encouraged the International Society of Paediatric Oncology to initiate a European trial starting in October 1975, comparing chemotherapy and chemoradiotherapy in the treatment of rhabdomyosarcomas, additional limited surgery being possible in both groups. Chemotherapy is the VAC regime with the addition of adriamycin during the 10th week, actinomycin D and cyclophosphamide being given every 8 weeks.

Table 5. Rhabdomyosarcoma of ENT and urogenital tract treated in Amsterdam. Patients treated with chemotherapy alone who remain disease free

Primary tumour site	Survival (months from diagnosis)
Palate invading left pteryoid process	60
Tonsillar fossa	39
Bladder with local extension and lung metastases	31
Vagina	27
Paratesticular with local extension	60
Bladder	24
Parotid	36

Table 6. Rhabdomyosarcoma in urogenital tract and ENT region treated in Amsterdam. Patients treated with chemotherapy and surgery, disease-free

Primary tumour site	Type of surgery
Vagina: labia	Labiectomy
Oral tumour – local recurrence in cheek	Excision of cheek recurrence
Bladder: prostate	Hemi-prostatectomy
Bladder with lung metastases	Two pulmonary resections, partial bladder resection
Parotid	Parotidectomy

Adult Soft Tissue Sarcoma

Radiotherapy

The place of radiotherapy as an adjunct to surgery in soft tissue sarcomas is disputed. The degree of radioresponsiveness of soft tissue sarcomas has first to be established. Initial reports often described the use of orthovoltage irradiation in widely varying doses and schedules, usually on large inoperable tumours. Not surprisingly, responses were few and unpredictable and local tissue damage could be severe. Nevertheless, McNeer, et al. [16], in a review of 653 patients with soft tissue sarcomas of all types treated 1935–1959, reported 58 evaluable patients who had been treated by radiotherapy, alone or pre-operatively. Response (defined at greater than 25% regression) occurred in 42 (72%) and 33% showed histological or biological (i.e. no recurrence on follow-up of more than 5 years) sterilisation of the tumour. These patients were treated with a wide range of doses utilising a variety of techniques and types of equipment. However, Windeyer [36] treated 22 fibrosarcomas by radiotherapy alone with the object of cure. Most patients received 6000–8500 rad on megavoltage equipment over 6–8 weeks. Fourteen showed complete regression and five partial regression. Six of those with complete responses had a subsequent recurrence but 6/8 given radiotherapy to the primary tumour and 6/10 treated for tumours recurrent after previous surgery were disease-free at 5 years. As there are limitations to the volume of tissue that can be treated with a radical dose of radiation, size of the primary tumour is an important factor when making comparisons between studies. Thus, it seems that soft tissue sarcomas are responsive to radiation but high doses (≥ 6000 rad in 6 weeks) are needed and some histological types (e.g. liposarcomas) are more responsive than others (e.g. pleomorphic rhabdomyosarcomas) [16, 18].
Atkinson et al. [1] advocated pre-operative radiotherapy – 4500 rad over 4–5 weeks preceding surgery by 4–6 weeks – quoting 15 patients treated in this way with only one local recurrence and no metastases with an average follow-up of 40 months. Forty patients having no pre-operative irradiation experienced 40 episodes of recurrence following 54 local surgical procedures and seven patients developed metastases. However, this latter group was not strictly comparable as surgery was usually carried out at referring institutions and only selected high risk cases may have been referred for further management.
Adjuvant radiotherapy is most frequently administered post-operatively. Suit et al. [30] using high radiation doses (≥ 6000 rad in 6 weeks) in combination with surgery in 71 primary and 29 recurrent soft tissue sarcomas, achieved local control in 87% with follow-up of 2–12 years. Seventy-five percent of the 89 patients with extremity lesions retained a useful limb that was free from pain and oedema. Despite this, the 2-year survival rate was only 50% with the majority of patients dying of metastatic disease. Thus, although good local control may be achieved with radiation therapy, patients still succumb to metastatic disease.
Hellman, et al. [12] added razoxane (ICRF 159), an antimitotic drug that seems to potentiate the effects of radiation, to radiotherapy given with curative intent in a group of inoperable or incompletely excised sarcomas and showed a significant difference in the recurrence rate (26% cf. 64%) in favour of the razoxane-treated group. However, this trial has serious defects in that it was non-random, the numbers evaluable were small [33], the initial size of the tumour was not stated and there were major discrepancies in the histological type and primary site between the two groups.

Chemotherapy

There have been few studies of the use of adjuvant chemotherapy in adult soft tissue sarcoma. TOWNSEND et al. [35] reported 35 patients with localised sarcomas, 16 of whom received adjuvant chemotherapy post-operatively with high dose methotrexate and adriamycin. Eleven (68%) were disease-free at the time of analysis (with mean follow-up of 9.3 months) whereas 14 of 19 patients (77%) treated by surgery alone had developed metastases (mean time to recurrence 7.3 months). However, this study is difficult to interpret as it was non-random, included bone and soft tissue sarcomas and gave no indication of tumour type, size or grade. The same group in Los Angeles [17] used adjuvant therapy in 19 patients with extremity soft tissue sarcoma with the aim of avoiding amputation and retaining a functional pain-free limb. Five patients were submitted to wide excision followed by post-operative irradiation (6000 rad in 6–7 weeks) and there were no recurrences. Six patients had pre-operative perfusion of the limb with intra-arterial adriamycin followed 3 weeks later by radical surgery. In five of the six there was insufficient tumour regression to allow local excision, and amputation was necessary. Eight patients were treated with pre-operative radiotherapy and chemotherapy ± immunotherapy (Table 7). Local surgery was possible in

Table 7. Adjuvant therapy for sarcomas of an extremity

Day 1	Adriamycin 30 mg/m^2/day IA × 3
Day 4	XRT 3500 rad over 10 days
Day 21	Surgery
Day 29	Commencement post-operative chemotherapy Vincristine 1.5 mg/m^2 IV followed 1 h later by Methotrexate 100 mg/kg as 4-h infusion 4 h after completion of infusion – 'rescue' with IV Leucovorin 12 mg every 6 h for 3 days supplemented if methotrexate serum level at 4, 6, 12, 24 or 48 h exceeded 1×10^{-6} *M*
Day 43	Adriamycin 45 mg/m^2/day IV bolus × 2 These cycles are repeated every 2 weeks to maximum cumulative dose of adriamycin, 500 mg/m^2 when discontinued. Methotrexate given every 4 weeks for a further year. Immunotherapy given as below:

Adjuvant immunotherapy of localised soft tissue sarcoma[a]

5×10^8 viable organisms Tice BCG ID. Tine method, both axillae, both groins every week for 3 months, then every 2 weeks for 2 years. Tissue culture vaccine 1×10^8 sarcoma cells, total dose, ID both axillae, both groins and region of primary tumour site on same schedule.

Source: Morton et al., Ann. Surgery *184*, 268 (1976).
[a] Morton, J.A.M.A. *236*, 2187 (1976).

Table 8. Alomad

Day 1	Vincristine	1	mg/m² IV
	Methotrexate	250	mg/m² IV infusion over 24 h
Day 2	Leucovorin	50	mg/m² } IV
	Adriamycin	40	mg/m² } IV
	DTIC	500	mg/m² } IV
	Leucovorin	5	mg/m² orally every 8 h × 12
Days 15–29 and 57–71	Chlorambucil	6	mg/m²/day orally × 14
Days 22 and 64	Actinomycin D	1.2	mg/m² IV
Day 43	Adriamycin	50	mg/m² IV

seven and all were free of disease 4–34 months later. Of the 17 patients (including four chondrosarcomas) treated by wide excision alone, 11 had recurred within 2 years.

Sordillo et al. [28] used a complex adjuvant regime ALOMAD (Table 8) in 73 patients following surgery for soft tissue sarcoma. Sixty-one patients were evaluable and were divided into five groups. Group I consisted of 19 patients given adjuvant therapy following removal of a primary tumour and there had been one local recurrence, 18 patients having no evidence of disease 3–34 months (median 15) from surgery. Group II comprised eight patients treated for locally recurrent tumour and there had been one local recurrence and one patient had developed distant metastases, the rest having no evidence of disease 4–33 months (median 16) from surgery. The remaining three groups included patients given post-operative radiotherapy because of inadequate surgical margins (III), pre-operative radiotherapy and adriamycin for large tumours (IV) and chemotherapy administered after resection of pulmonary metastases (V). Taking these three groups together there had been 13 recurrences in 34 patients.

These studies also suffer from the defects that they were non-randomised, numbers in each treatment group were small and in Townsend's study, the control group were treated inadequately and consequently had a high rate of recurrence. The value of adjuvant radiotherapy and chemotherapy in allowing preservation of a limb can only be assessed by comparison of the disease-free intervals, and survivals of a group given adjuvant treatment with those of a concurrent randomised group treated by radical surgery alone, which in most cases would involve an amputation.

A randomised study comparing amputation with limb-sparing surgery and post-operative radiotherapy, both groups having adjuvant chemotherapy ± immunotherapy (Table 9) has been conducted by Rosenberg et al. [25] at the NCI May 1975 – June 1977. The value of adjuvant chemotherapy was assessed by comparison to a historical control group of 66 patients treated at the NCI by radical surgery alone. Forty-nine evaluable patients were entered – 23 with lesions of the head, neck and trunk, 26 with extremity tumours – and results of treatment are shown in Table 10. Follow-up ranges from 5–30 months with a median of 16 months. Actuarial analysis of all protocol patients compared with historical controls reveals improvement in disease-free interval ($P < 0.001$) as well as survival ($P < 0.001$) (Figs. 2 and 3). Toxic effects were few. Thirty-four of 49 patients received the maximum permitted escalation of chemotherapy. Three patients refused chemotherapy after 50 mg/m², 160 mg/m² and 210 mg/m² of adriamycin. Two were lost to follow-up 121 days and 114 days after

Table 9. Adjuvant chemotherapy used by ROSENBERG et al.

Chemotherapy started when surgical wound healed, the first dose being given 3 days prior to ensuing radiation.

Adriamycin	50 mg/m^2 IV escalating to 70 mg/m^2 depending on toxicity
Cyclophosphamide	500 mg/m^2 IV escalating 700 mg/m^2

Courses repeated at 4-weekly intervals until maximum cumulative dose of adriamycin reached, 550 mg/m^2. Patient then switched to high dose methotrexate.

Methotrexate	50 mg/kg by 6 h infusion followed 2 h after completion by 'rescue'
Leucovorin	15 mg/m^2 IV every 6 h × 8 doses

Hydration and alkalinisation carried out. Additional leucovorin given if 48 h serum level methotrexate 4×10^{-7} *M*.

Courses repeated every 28 days × 6 with escalation by 50 mg/kg to maximum 250 mg/kg if no toxicity with previous course.

Table 10. Results of protocol treatment[a]

Extremity	No. of patients	No. recurred	Site of initial recurrence	No. dead
Radical surgery	10	1[b]	Lungs	1
Limited surgery + radiotherapy	9	1	Lung	0
Limited surgery + radiotherapy + immunotherapy	7	1	Local	1
Historical control	46	26	–	23
Head, neck and trunk				
Surgery + radiotherapy	11	1	Lungs	0
Surgery + radiotherapy + immunotherapy	12	1[c]	Local	0
Historical control	20	10	–	6

[a] All patients received chemotherapy with adriamycin, cyclophosphamide and methotrexate.
[b] Left protocol after third adriamycin dose. Recurred 1 year later.
[c] Recurred at local site during radiotherapy and underwent local resection. Patient is disease-free at day 372.

randomisation and were disease-free. The third patient relapsed with pulmonary metastases 1 year later.

Although the use of historical controls is a criticism of this study, the 5-year survival of the control group parallels the survival curves of 1215 cases from ten institutions reviewed by the Task Force on Soft Tissue Sarcoma of the American Joint Committee for Cancer Staging and

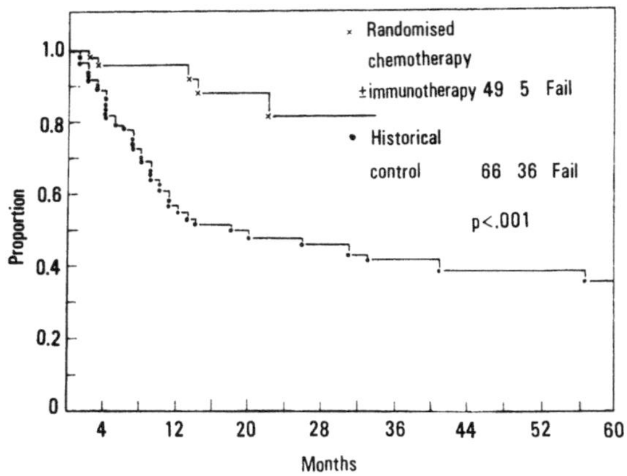

Fig. 2. Soft tissue sarcoma – adjuvant study by ROSENBERG et al. Actuarial analysis of time to first recurrence

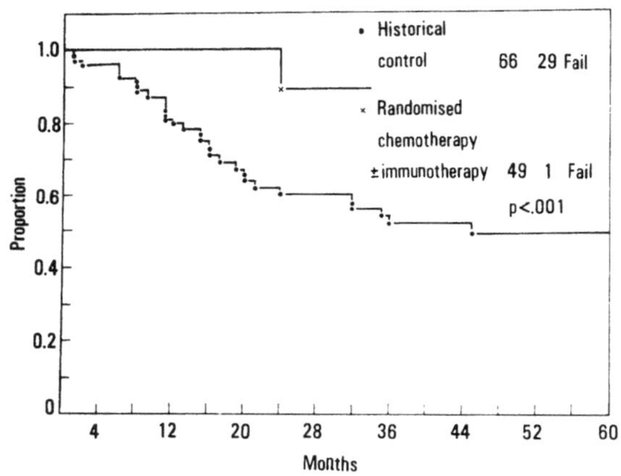

Fig. 3. Soft tissue sarcoma – adjuvant study by ROSENBERG et al. Actuarial analysis of survival

End Results [26] and should therefore be representative of surgical results. Nevertheless, there may be important differences between protocol patients and historical control groups. For example, the difficulty of establishing accurately the size of lesions in historical control patients as well as time from onset of symptoms to surgery and the changing pattern of referral of patients to the NCI may all influence the comparison of current protocol patients with historical patients. However, the differences between the two groups in terms of time to first recurrence and survival are both highly significant and the tentative conclusion that adjuvant chemotherapy delays or prevents dissemination of soft tissue sarcomas is possible. Clearly, longer follow-up is needed and randomised prospective trials comparing adjuvant chemotherapy with a control group treated by surgery alone are essential and both the NCI and the EORTC are initiating such trials.

Immunotherapy has been used in many types of tumour and the demonstration of tumour-associated antigens [6] prompted TOWNSEND et al. [34] to study the role of adjuvant immunotherapy with BCG and tumour cell vaccine in sarcomas. Eighteen patients with localised primary or locally recurrent soft tissue sarcomas were submitted to wide resection removing macroscopic tumour. Three to six weeks following operation, they were commenced on immunotherapy (Table 7). This group was compared with 15 patients treated simultaneously by surgery alone because they had refused immunotherapy. Eleven of 18 (61%) receiving immunotherapy remained free of disease compared with 5/15 (33%) having surgery alone. However, ten recurrences (66%) in the control group within 2 years seems rather high for localised disease, for although CANTIN et al. [3] report a 59% recurrence rate in 784 patients seen at the Memorial Hospital, there was only a 29% recurrence rate when the primary treatment was carried out at Memorial. As this was a non-randomised study involving few patients, the value of immunotherapy remains to be proven.

It would seem logical in an adjuvant trial to use chemotherapy that has been proven to be effective in metastatic disease. Recent studies have shown that several drugs have activity against soft tissue sarcoma. Adriamycin is the most potent drug and GOTTLIEB [9] reviewing the world literature found 96 of 357 responses (27%) although there was a wide variation between individual studies. Response to DTIC seems to be in the order of 16% [11] but there is very little data on other single agent chemotherapy in adult sarcomas. Synergism has been noted in experimental animal models between adriamycin and DTIC [8] and the clinical combination of these two agents appears to be superior to adriamycin alone, both in terms of remission rate and survival [10]. Cyclophosphamide and vincristine have been added to this combination because of their efficacy in childhood sarcomas, although few patients with adult sarcomas have received these drugs as single agents. The combination of these four agents (CYVADIC) has been used in a large number of patients by the South West Oncology Group with an overall response rate of 59% in one trial, and of 52% in a subsequent trial in which a slightly modified version was used [9]. Replacing either DTIC [2] or vincristine [19] by actinomycin D produced increased toxicity and an inferior response. The EORTC is currently conducting a trial in metastatic disease [20] comparing two schedules of CYVADIC. The S_1 regime (Table 11) using all four drugs concurrently but modified to give the same total dose of DTIC over 3 days instead of 5 (Table 11) forms the basis of an adjuvant trial recently initiated by the EORTC (May 1978). This trial will include all patients aged 20–70 with a proven histological diagnosis of soft tissue sarcoma (Table 12) who have had complete macroscopic removal of their tumour less than 13 weeks before entry and have no evidence of metastases. Post-operative radiotherapy, minimum dose 5000 rad in 4 weeks will be given to those cases where there is microscopic residual disease, there are inadequate surgical margins or the tumour has recurred locally. Patients will then be randomised into two groups, one receiving eight cycles of chemotherapy at monthly intervals and a control group receiving no further treatment. The disease-free interval and survival of the two groups will be compared.

Table 11. CYVADIC S_1 regime used in EORTC trial of therapy of metastatic soft tissue sarcoma.

Adriamycin	50 mg/m²	IV day 1
Cyclophosphamide	500 mg/m²	IV day 1
Vincristine	1.5 mg/m²	IV day 1
DTIC	250 mg/m²	IV days 1-5 repeated every 4 weeks

Modified CYVADIC S_1 regime used in EORTC adjuvant trial

Adriamycin	50 mg/m²	IV day 1
Cyclophosphamide	500 mg/m²	IV day 1
Vincristine	1.5 mg/m²	IV day 1
DTIC	400 mg/m²	IV days 1–3 repeated every 4 weeks for 8 cycles

Table 12. Histologic types of soft tissue sarcomas eligible for EORTC adjuvant trial

Fibrosarcoma
Liposarcoma
Leiomyosarcoma
Rhabdomyosarcoma
Malignant haemangioendothelioma (angiosarcoma)
Malignant lymphangiopericytoma
Malignant lymphangioendothelioma (lymphangiosarcoma)
Malignant synovioma
Malignant schwannoma (neurofibrosarcoma)
Malignant mesenchymoma
Alveolar soft parts sarcoma
Malignant granular cell tumour
Chondrosarcoma of soft parts
Osteosarcoma of soft parts
Malignant giant cell tumour of soft parts
Malignant fibroxanthoma
Clear cell sarcoma of tendons and aponeuroses

N.B. Cases of fibromatosis and well-differentiated liposarcomas are excluded.

Summary and Conclusions

As sarcomas of soft tissues are unusual tumours with widely ranging natural histories, there has been considerable controversy surrounding their management. The desire to avoid mutilating surgery must be balanced against the known frequency of local recurrence that may be accompanied by dissemination, and past experience has shown that the sole use of even extensive surgery may be inadequate. Several problems still remain to be answered:

1. Will *radiotherapy* eradicate microscopic residual disease and can wide local excision with pre- or post-operative radiotherapy ± chemoimmunotherapy replace amputation in extremity sarcomas? Although there is suggestive evidence from several studies that this may be so, the numbers of patients treated in this way have been small, duration of follow-up short and no prospective randomised controlled trials have been carried out comparing a group given adjuvant treatment with a group managed by radical surgery alone, and this should be rectified.
2. What *dosage of radiation* should be employed and are the results of radiotherapy or chemotherapy affected by the histological type? High radiation doses (≥ 6000 rad in 6 weeks) have been recommended by most authors, lower doses producing less consistent effects. There does not seem to be any statistically significant difference in the response of various histological types of soft tissue sarcoma to combination chemotherapy or radiotherapy, although some authors have commented on the relative radioresponsiveness of myxoliposarcoma.
3. Which *characteristics of the primary tumour* most influence prognosis? The chances of local recurrence and metastasis seem to depend less on histological type than on initial size, site and grade of the tumour and these factors must be carefully controlled when comparing results of treatment.
4. What is the *most appropriate combination of drugs* and the optimum scheduling and duration of adjuvant chemotherapy? Although adriamycin is undoubtedly effective in adult

sarcomas, adequate phase II studies have not been performed for cyclophosphamide and high dose methotrexate. Many of the studies of adjuvant chemotherapy discussed in this article used drugs and regimes of unproven value in adult soft tissue sarcoma and the use in adjuvant trials of the CYVADIC regime that has been extensively studied in metastatic disease seems more logical. Meanwhile, more thorough investigation of cyclophosphamide, high dose methotrexate and actinomycin D as single agents would be valuable, and phase II trials of newer agents such as cis-platinum are required.
The rarity of soft tissue sarcomas means that despite their inherent problems, large multicentre collaborative trials will be necessary to accrue sufficient patients to produce reliable information on the efficacy of adjuvant therapy. However, despite the many difficulties, sarcomas seem to be a group of tumours that are responsive to chemotherapy and there is every reason to hope that adjuvant therapy will be of considerable value.

References

1. Atkinson, L., Garvan, J. M., Newton, N. C.: Behaviour and management of soft connective tissue sarcomas. Cancer *16,* 1552–1562 (1963)
2. Benjamin, R. S., Gottlieb, J. A., Baker, L. O., Sinkovics, J. G.: Cyvadic vs. Cyvadact: a randomised trial of Cyclophosphamide, Vincristine and Adriamycin + DTIC or Actinomycin D in metastatic sarcomas. Proc. Am. Ass. Cancer Res. *17,* 256 (1976)
3. Cantin, J., McNeer, G. P., Chu, F. C., Booher, R. J.: The problem of local recurrence after treatment of soft tissue sarcoma. Ann. Surg. *168,* 47–53 (1968)
4. Chung, E. B., Enzinger, F. M.: Infantile fibrosarcoma. Cancer *38,* 729–739 (1976)
5. Donaldson, S. S., Castro, J. R., Wilbur, J. R., Jesse, R. H.: Rhabdomyosarcoma of head and neck in children – combination treatment by surgery, irradiation and chemotherapy. Cancer *31,* 26–35 (1973)
6. Filber, F. R., Morton, D. L.: Sarcoma specific antigens: detection by complement fixation with serum from sarcoma patients. J. Natl. Cancer Inst. *44,* 651–656 (1970)
7. Enzinger, F. M., Shiraki, M.: Alveolar rhabdomyosarcoma. Cancer *24,* 18–31 (1969)
8. Griswold, D. F., Laster, W. R., Schabel, F. M.: Therapeutic potentiation by Adriamycin and DTIC against B16 melanoma, C3H breast carcinoma, Lewis lung carcinoma and Leukaemia L1210. Proc. Am. Ass. Cancer Res. *14,* 15 (1973)
9. Gottlieb, J. A., Baker, L. J., O'Bryan, R. M., Sinkovics, J. G., Hoogstraten, B., Quagliana, J. M., Rivkin, S. E., Bodey, G. P., Rodriguez, V. T., Blumenschein, G. R., Saiki, J. H., Coltman, C., Burgess, M. A., Sullivan, P., Thigpen, T., Bottomley, R., Balcerzak, S., Moon, T. E.: Adriamycin (NSC-123127) used alone and in combination for soft tissue and bone sarcoma. Cancer Chemother. Rep. (Part. 3) *6,* 271–282 (1975)
10. Gottlieb, J. A., O'Bryan, R. M., Moon, T. E., Bodey, G. P., Sinkovics, T., Thigpen, T., Rivkin, S. E.: Improved survival with Adriamycin combinations vs. Adriamycin alone in patients with metastatic sarcoma. Proc. Am. Soc. Clin. Oncol. *16,* 238 (1975)
11. Gottlieb, J. A., Benjamin, R. S., Baker, L. H., O'Bryan, R. M., Sinkovics, J. G., Hoogstraten, B., Quagliana, J. M., Rivkin, S. E., Bodey, G. P., Rodriquez, V., Blumenschein, G. R., Saiki, J. H., Coltman, C., Burgess, M., A., Sullivan, P., Thigpen, T., Bottomley, R., Balcerzak, S., Moon, T. E.: Role of DTIC (NSC-45388) in the chemotherapy of sarcomas. Cancer Treat. Rep. *60,* 199–203 (1976)
12. Hellman, K., Ryall, R. D. H., Macdonald, E., Newton, K. A., James, S. E., Jones, S.: Comparison of radiotherapy with and without Razoxane (ICRF 159) in the treatment of soft tissue sarcomas. Cancer *41,* 100–107 (1978)
13. Heyn, R. M., Holland, R., Newton, H. A., Teft, M., Breslow, N., Hartmann, J. R.: The role of combined treatment of rhabdomyosarcoma in children. Cancer *34,* 2128–2142 (1974)

14. Horn, R. C., Enterline, H. T.: Rhabdomyosarcoma: a clinicopathological study and classification of 39 cases. Cancer *11,* 181–199 (1958)
15. Malpas, J. S., Freeman, J. E., Paxton, A., Walker-Smith, J., Stansfield, A. G., Wood, B. B. S.: Radiotherapy and adjuvant combination chemotherapy for childhood rhabdomyosarcoma. B. M. J. *1,* 247–249 (1976)
16. McNeer, G. P., Cantin, J., Chu, F., Nickson, J. J.: Effectiveness of radiation therapy in the management of sarcoma of the soft somaticissues. Cancer *22,* 391–397 (1968)
17. Morton, D. L., Filber, F. R., Townsend, C. M., Grant, T. T., Mirra, J., Weisenburger, T. H.: Limb salvage from a multidisciplinary approach for skeletal and soft tissue sarcoma of the extremity. Ann. Surg. *184,* 268–278 (1976)
18. Perry, H., Chu, C. H.: Radiation therapy in the palliative management of soft tissue sarcomas. Cancer *15,* 179–183 (1962)
19. Pilot Study EORTC (unpublished)
20. Pinedo, H. M., Vendrick, C. P. J., Staquet, M., Kenis, Y., Sylvester, R.: EORTC randomised trial for therapy of metastatic soft tissue sarcoma, Protocol 62761. March 1977. Eur. J. Cancer. (in press) (1978)
21. Pinedo, H. M., Voûte, P. A.: Combination chemotherapy in soft tissue sarcoma. In: Recent advances in cancer treatment. Tagnon, H. J., Staquet, M. J., (eds.). New York: Raven Press 1977
22. Pinkel, D.: Cyclophosphamide in children with cancer. Cancer *15,* 42–49 (1962)
23. Pratt, C. B., James, D. H., Holton, C. P., Pinkel, C.: Combination therapy including Vincristine for malignant solid tumours in children. Cancer Chemother. Rep. *52,* 489–495 (1968)
24. Pratt, C. B., Hustu, H. O., Fleming, I. D., Pinkel, D.: Coordinated treatment of childhood rhabdomyosarcoma with surgery, radiotherapy and combination chemotherapy. Cancer Res. *32,* 606–610 (1972)
25. Rosenberg, S. A., Kent, H., Costa, J., Webber, B. L., Young, R., Chabner, B., Baker, A. R., Brennan, M. F., Chretien, P. B., Cohen, M. H., Demoss, E. V., Sears, H. F., Seidp, C., Simon, R.: Prospective randomised evaluation of the role of limb sparing surgery, radiation therapy and adjuvant chemotherapy in the treatment of adult soft tissue sarcomas. Surgery. July 1978
26. Russel, W. O., Cohen, J., Enzinger, F., Hadju, S. I., Heise, H., Martin, R. G., Meissner, W., Miller, W. T., Schmitz, R. L., Suit, H. D.: A clinical and pathological staging system for soft tissue sarcomas. Cancer *40,* 1562–1570 (1977)
27. Skipper, H. E.: Adjuvant chemotherapy. Cancer *41,* 936–940 (1978)
28. Sordillo, P., Magill, G. B., Howard, J., Golbey, R. B.: Adjuvant chemotherapy of adult soft part sarcomas with 'ALOMAD'. Proc. Am. Soc. Clin. Oncol. *19,* 353 (1978)
29. Stobbe, G. D., Dargeon, H. W.: Embryonal rhabdomyosarcoma of the head and neck in children and adolescents. Cancer *3,* 826–836 (1950)
30. Suit, H. D., Russel, W. O., Martin, R. G.: Sarcoma of soft tissue: clinical and histopathological parameters and response to treatment. Cancer *35,* 1478–1483 (1975)
31. Sutow, W. W., Sullivan, M. P., Ried, H. L., Taylor, H. G., Griffith, K. M.: Prognosis in childhood rhabdomyosarcoma. Cancer *25,* 1384–1390 (1970)
32. Sutow, W. W., Berry, D. H., Haddy, T. B., Sullivan, M. P., Watkins, W. L. Windmiller, J.: Vincristine sulfate therapy inn children with metastatic soft tissue sarcoma. Paediatrics *38,* 465–472 (1966)
33. Tan, C. T. C., Dargeon, H. W., Burchenall, J. H.: Effect of Actinomycin D on cancer in childhood. Paediatrics *24,* 544–561 (1959)
34. Townsend, C. M., Eilber, F. R., Morton, D. L.: Skeletal and soft tissue sarcoma: Results of treatment with adjuvant immunotherapy J.A.M.A. *236,* 2187–2189 (1976)
35. Townsend, C. M., Eilber, F. R., Morton, D. L.: Skeletal and soft tissue sarcomas: results of surgical adjuvant chemotherapy. Proc. Am. Ass. Cancer Res. *17,* 265 (1976)
36. Windeyer, B., Dische, S., Mansfield, C. M.: The place of radiotherapy in the management of fibrosarcoma of soft tissues. Clin. Radiol. *17,* 32–40 (1966)

C. Breast Carcinoma

Place and Role of Radiotherapy After Surgery for Breast Cancer

K. E. Halnan

Introduction

Adjuvant X-ray therapy after surgery for breast cancer is at present unfashionable, partly because of the glamour of adjuvant chemotherapy, but more because of the stated lack of any beneficial effect of radiotherapy on survival and of even an alleged harmful effect, said to be caused by immunosuppression. This opinion was first put forward by Bond [5] after study of retrospective Birmingham cancer registration data, but groups compared were not randomly selected and some of those selected for radiotherapy may well have been allocated radiotherapy because of adverse prognostic features. The first Manchester trials [11] are frequently quoted but have been widely misinterpreted – they compared immediate with delayed radiotherapy rather than with no X-ray therapy at all. After numbers of other trials, Stjernswärd [17] advocated these views even more strongly, analysing the main large trials then published (in none of which were there significant differences in survival), including those from Copenhagen, Edinburgh, and the United States, and added them up, suggesting that significant differences in survival could be obtained by combining insignificant differences from quite different trials.

I suggest that abandonment of postoperative radiotherapy because of alleged harmful effect on survival is an emotional 'blanket' decision, which ignores three important points:

1. Analysis of the effect of radiation dose, techniques and anatomical fields (as compared with the analysis of different surgical techniques such as local excision, simple mastectomy, radical mastectomy and extended radical mastectomy);
2. Significant benefit may be demonstrated from radiotherapy in selected subsets of breast cancer, analysed for factors such as site, stage, grade, menopausal status and oestrogen receptor status;
3. Quality of life, related especially to local activity of breast cancer.

Analysis of Current Evidence

Effect on Survival and Quality of Life

Many large and important treatment trials are now being reported. One of the major ones in Britain has been the Cancer Research Campaign multicentre trial [19]. The latest (January

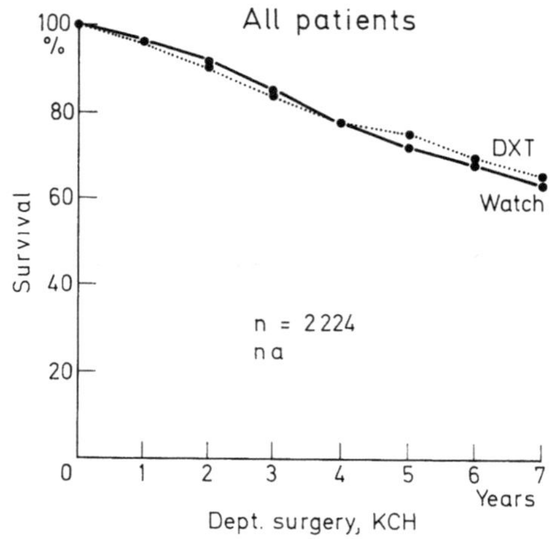

Fig. 1. Life table survival curves for 2224 patients with stages I and II breast cancer treated by simple mastectomy, followed by radiotherapy (DXT) or watched in the Cancer Research Campaign Breast Study

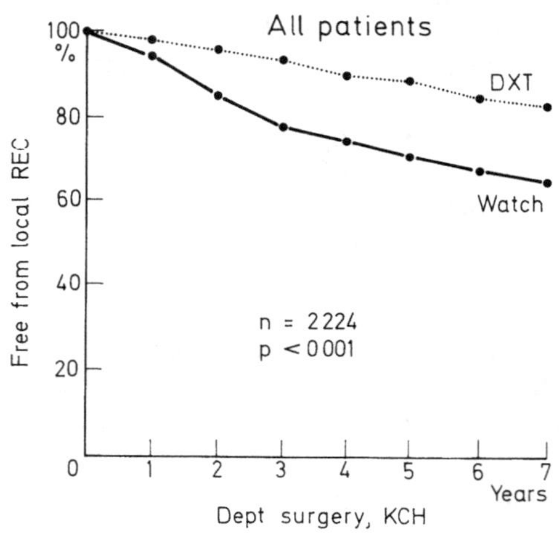

Fig. 2. Life table analysis of freedom from local recurrence in the Cancer Research Campaign Breast Study

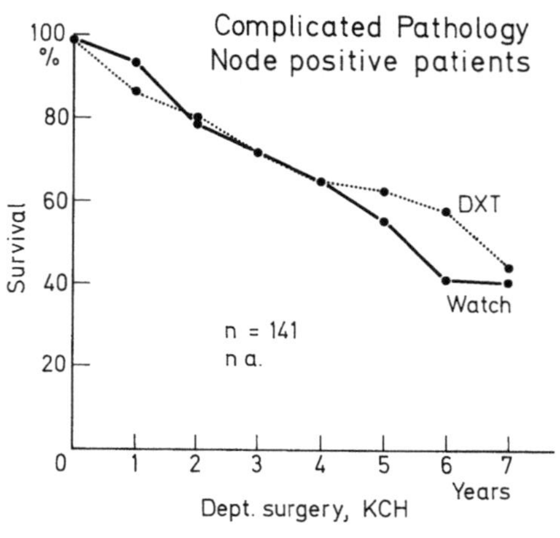

Fig. 3. Life table survival for 141 node-positive patients in the Cancer Research Campaign Breast Study

1978) unpublished results analyse 2224 stage I and II cases; there is no significant difference in survival up to 7 years (Fig. 1) but a highly significant difference in local recurrence (about 84% compared with 67% recurrence-free at 7 years) (Fig. 2). The survival curve for the 141 node-positive patients shows no difference for either treatment policy and the suggestion [9] made earlier that radiotherapy was harmful in this group has *not* been substantiated (Fig. 3). A large new Manchester trial has also now been published [8]; this has included 1020 patients with stages I and II cancer, treated by simple mastectomy, alone or followed by X-ray therapy. Again there has been no significant difference in the *overall* survival, but the value of radiotherapy was greater and more significant when neoplasms were more than 2 cm diameter, when patients were premenopausal and for medial tumours. KAAE and JOHANSEN [7] have also reported up-to-date results from Copenhagen, showing that there is no significant difference in either crude or recurrence-free survival at any period up to 15 years between simple mastectomy and irradiation compared with extended radical mastectomy, but that the morbidity after treatment (oedema and weakness of the arm) was greater after extended radical mastectomy. Controlled study of both preoperative and postoperative irradiation in Stockholm [18] shows slightly better survival after preoperative radiotherapy, not of statistical significance. Combination of overall results of all these trials, if this were scientifically valid, would *not* show any harm from radiotherapy.

Immunology

A circular argument has crept into the literature. When it was first alleged that radiotherapy was harmful it was suggested that this was because of immunosuppression. This is now put the other way round – it is alleged that radiotherapy is bound to be harmful (whether or not this can be proved) because of immunosuppression, caused by irradiation of lymph nodes especially.

If immunological defenses were really of great value spontaneous remission would be familiar in breast cancer, in fact it is rare; although some tumours are relatively slow to grow, untreated patients all die [4]. It has been shown in my own institute that there is peripheral lymphocyte depletion immediately after radiotherapy, and that there is significant lymphopenia even 2 years later [2]. This lymphopenia is, however, mainly of T cells. Patients with breast cancer in advanced stages, ill with distant metastases especially, do have highly deficient immune responses but this is *irrespective* of their primary treatment and seems related more to B cells than to T cells [14, 16]. There is no good evidence that any treatment – surgery, radiotherapy or chemotherapy – is harmful.

Benefits from Local Irradiation

Survival and recurrence have been discussed already. Radiotherapy can be shown to have a local effect on visible deposits of breast cancer – this effect is dose related and, like chemotherapy, also related inversely to the number of tumour cells. 'Conservative' treatment has long been practised in France [3] and is highly effective, high dose protracted treatment after local excision, or even no more than biopsy for small tumours, with the major part of the breast remaining. This kind of treatment has never received assessment in controlled trials because of prejudice towards mastectomy, but uncontrolled selected series are beginning to be reported now from Britain [15] and North America [12, 13].

The importance of technique and dosage seems to be shown most clearly by HØST and

BRENNHOVD [6] who report successive controlled trials of two different techniques. The first, used in 1964–1967, was relatively conventional using 250 kV X-rays, treating the internal mammary, axillary and supraclavicular regions to 3600 rad and the chest wall to 2500–3100 rad over 4 weeks. After 1967 cobalt 60 γ-rays were used, the chest wall was not irradiated at all but the lymph node regions were treated to 5700 rad skin dose in 4 weeks. There was no difference in survival of the two control groups, treated by radical mastectomy and ovarian irradiation, but there was a dramatic difference in the cobalt 60-treated group in which there was highly significant improvement in survival in stage II, especially in patients with medial tumours or with four or more involved axillary nodes.

It is foolish either to advocate or to condemn 'postoperative radiotherapy' in a general blanket kind of way without considering dose, technique or anatomical areas treated; it is as unwise as discussing all kinds of surgery together, combining all techniques from local resection to supra- or extended radical mastectomy. We must pay careful attention to the details of treatment. Similarly, as has already been indicated, we must analyse subsets of patients, not only for size and site of the primary tumour, but also for other factors – menopausal status, grade, hormone receptors, bone scan findings and so on.

Future Trials

If radiotherapy has a place then, as it should, in future trials it will need combining with chemotherapy and with hormone treatment. Two good examples can be quoted of what might be assessed in early and in more advanced breast cancer. MONTAGUE [10] from the M.D. Anderson Hospital gives chemotherapy first to stage III tumours (three to four courses of vincristine, adriamycin, cyclophosphamide). If there is complete remission X-ray therapy (5000 rad in 5 weeks) is then given, followed by 'CMF' adjuvant chemotherapy; but if there is only partial remission an extended simple mastectomy is performed before the X-ray therapy. This seems to be a very promising approach to deal with locally advanced tumours. At the Mayo Clinic more conventional random controlled trials are going on for stage I and II tumours, comparing adjuvant chemotherapy with or without radiation, after radical mastectomy [1]. It is too early for good assessment but so far the group with radiation is achieving good results and it will be possible later to assess whether radiation enhances the effectiveness of combination chemotherapy.

Conclusions

Thus, use of radiotherapy in breast cancer is no simple matter, we cannot say that 'radiotherapy' (unqualified) is a good or bad addition to surgery, let alone to other treatments. At least the following conclusions are worth serious consideration:

1. Adjuvant radiotherapy needs careful planning and dosage, using megavoltage X-rays, or cobalt 60 γ-rays, considering separately the primary tumour, the chest wall, clavicular, axillary and internal mammary lymphatic regions;
2. There is no good evidence that radiotherapy impairs survival;
3. Local and regional recurrence can be very significantly reduced by radiotherapy;
4. Survival may be improved by appropriate radiotherapy in subgroups such as stage II tumours arising medially, or with four or more involved lymph nodes.
5. Adjuvant ovarian irradiation may be beneficial in premenopausal and menopausal patients;

6. Adjuvant radiotherapy may allow surgery to be limited to excision biopsy in suitable patients;
7. The place of adjuvant radiotherapy needs continued evaluation in large random controlled trials, in combination with chemotherapy and endocrine therapy and after limited as well as after classical surgery. These trials must allow analysis according to factors such as primary size and site, node status, menopause, hormone receptors, bone scanning, tumour markers (if good ones be found) and tumour grade.

References

1. Ahmann, D. L., Payne, W. S., Scanlon, P. W. et al.: Repeated adjuvant chemotherapy with phenylalanine mustard or 5-fluouracil, cyclophosphamide and prednisone with or without radiation, after mastectomy for breast cancer. Lancet *1978 I,* 893–896
2. Anderson, J. M., Campbell, J. B., Wood, S. E., Boyd, J. E., Kelly, F.: Clin. Oncol. *1,* 201–206 (1975)
3. Baclesse, F.: Roentgen therapy as the sole method of treatment of cancer of the breast. Am. J. Roentgenol. *62,* 311–319 (1949)
4. Bloom, H. J. G.: Survival of women with untreated breast cancer: past and present. In: Prognostic factors in breast cancer. Forrest, A. P. M., Kunkler, P. B. (eds.), pp. 3–19. Edinburgh, London: Livingstone 1968
5. Bond, W. H.: In: Treatment of carcinoma of the breast. Jarrett, A. S. (ed.). pp. 24–39. Amsterdam: Excerpta Medica Foundation 1968
6. Høst, H., Brennhovd, I. O: The effect of postoperative radiotherapy in breast cancer. Int. J. Radiat. Oncol. Biol. Phys. *2,* 1061–1067 (1977)
7. Kaae, S., Johansen, H.: Does simple mastectomy followed by irradiation offer survival comparable to radical procedures. Int. J. Radiat. Oncol. Biol. Phys. *2,* 1163–1166 (1977)
8. Lythgoe, J. P., Leck, I., Swindell, R.: Manchester regional breast study. Lancet *1978 I,* 744–747
9. McDonald, A. M., Simpson, J. S., MacIntyre, J.: Treatment of early cancer of the breast. Histological staging and role of radiotherapy. Lancet *1976 I,* 1098–1100
10. Montague, E. D.: Radiation management of advanced breast cancer. Int. J. Radiat. Oncol. Biol. Phys. *4,* 305–307 (1978)
11. Paterson, R., Russell, M. H.: Clinical trials in malignant disease. III. Breast cancer: evaluation of post-operative radiotherapy. J. Faculty Radiologists *10,* 175–180 (1959)
12. Peters, M. V.: Cutting the 'Gordian' knot in early breast cancer. Am. R. Coll. Phys. Surg. Can. *8,* 186–192 (1975)
13. Prosnitz, L. R., Goldenberg, I. S., Packard, R. A., Levene, M. B., Harris, J., Hellman, S., Wallner, P. E., Brady, L. W., Mansfield, C. M., Kramer, S.: Radiation therapy as initial treatment for early stage cancer of the breast without mastectomy. Cancer *39,* 917–923 (1977)
14. Roberts, M. M., Jones-Williams, W.: The delayed hypersensitivity reaction in breast cancer. Br. J. Surg. *61,* 549–552 (1974)
15. Snelling, M. D.: Radiotherapy. In: Treatment of breast cancer. Atkins, H. (ed.), pp. 67–86. London: M.T.P. 1974
16. Stein, J. A., Adler, A., Efraim, S. B., Maor, J.: Immunocompetence, immunosuppression, and human breast cancer. Cancer *38,* 1171–1187 (1976)
17. Stjernswärd, J.: Decreased survival correlated to local irradiation in "early" operable breast cancer. Lancet *1974 II,* 1285–1286
18. Wallgren, A.: A controlled study: preoperative versus postoperative irradiation. Int. J. Radiat. Oncol. Biol. Phys. *2,* 1167–1169 (1977)
19. Working Party of the Cancer Research Campaign: Management of early cancer of the breast. Br. Med. J. *1976 I,* 1035–1039

Combined Modality Management of Operable Breast Cancer[1]

A. Rossi, P. Valagussa, and G. Bonadonna

Once combined modality therapy of solid tumors had been revitalized on the basis of new biologic and clinical concepts [13], breast cancer was deemed to be one of the signal tumors to test the new strategic approach, in view of its frequency, the high recurrence rate after local-regional treatment, and its responsiveness to various anticancer drugs. The experimental and clinical principles for adjuvant chemotherapy of resectable cancer have been thoroughly reviewed and discussed in recent years [7, 14, 15, 43, 56]. According to the new proposed strategy, the local-regional modality (surgery and/or radiotherapy) removes the bulk of the tumor, whereas systemic treatment (chemotherapy, hormone therapy, and/or immunotherapy) is applied with the specific intention of destroying disseminated micrometastases, which are thought to be responsible for primary treatment failure.

The preliminary results of new adjuvant trials with cyclic chemotherapy were reported after 18 [23] and 27 months [4] of follow-up, respectively, with the intention of informing the medical profession that a new perspective was opening up for improving the cure rate of breast cancer. However, evaluation of the new preliminary findings also generated considerable emotion, at both professional and public levels [18, 33, 35, 51, 54]. Discussion and even polemics simply testify to the relevance of the problem. However, clinical decisions and further research should be based on sound evaluation of results derived from continuous updating of ongoing clinical trials.

The scope of this paper is to review the available results on current combined modalities for early breast cancer and to delineate some future perspectives in this controversial field.

Local Modalities

The clinical basis for the use of adjuvant systemic therapy derives from the observation that surgery and/or radiotherapy alone are curative in only a limited fraction of patients with localized disease. When derived from prospective trials with accurate initial staging and adequate follow-up observation, long-term results of local-regional modalities appear strikingly comparable in various case series [27, 63]. Table 1 reports the 5- and 10-year disease-free survival related to the status of axillary nodes and menopause in women with operable breast cancer treated with radical mastectomy at institutions affiliated to the National Surgical Adjuvant Breast Project (NSABP) in the United States and at the Istituto Nazionale Tumori, Milan, Italy. It appears evident that to a great extent prognosis is related to the precence of axillary metastases, whereas menopausal status does not exert any influence on disease-free survival.

In operable patients, radiotherapy has been employed as an adjunct to surgery for many years. An exhaustive review of published studies on postoperative irradiation is beyond the scope of this paper and was recently carried out by Stjernswärd [61]. In short, radiotherapy

1 Supported in part by contract No. 1-CM-33714 with DCT, NCI, NIH.

Table 1. 5- and 10-year disease-free survival in patients with operable breast cancer (percentages)

	NSABP series 409 patients		Milan series 716 patients	
	5 years	10 years	5 years	10 years
All patients	60.3	50.5	56.1	47.1
N–	82.3	75.9	79.0	72.1
N+	34.9	23.9	36.4	24.5
Premenopausal				
N–	78.8	74.5	76.2	69.2
N+	30.0	23.7	36.3	24.5
Postmenopausal				
N–	83.6	76.4	80.6	73.6
N+	37.5	24.0	36.4	24.4

failed to improve the overall survival, though it did reduce the incidence of local-regional recurrence. In some studies [26] the disease-free survival was also not significantly affected by postoperative radiation (Table 2). The practical conclusion to be drawn is that, at present, there seems to be no place for the routine use of radiotherapy *alone* to improve long-term results in breast cancer.

In the combined modality approach, the role of surgery is, besides accurate staging, removal of the bulk of detectable tumor. In this perspective, a modification of the standard radical treatment, i.e., radical mastectomy, could be conceivable at least for selected subsets of women. A less mutilating local procedure is desirable only if comparable effective control of local-regional disease can be assured. Interesting results are being obtained in this field [24, 31, 40, 64]. However, the crucial problem in the cure of breast cancer is still the control of distant micrometastases. From the strategic point of view, only the adjunct of an effective systemic and prolonged treatment seems to be able to achieve this scope.

Table 2. Comparative disease-free survival at 5 years with and without postoperative radiotherapy on operable breast cancer

	Radical mastectomy alone		Radical mastectomy plus radiotherapy	
	No.	%	No.	%
Total	117	49.6	180	50.6
N–	52	71.2	56	78.6
N+	65	32.3	124	37.9
1–3	33	42.4	57	49.1
> 3	32	21.9	67	28.4

Adapted from Fisher et al. [26].

Adjuvant Chemotherapy

In the past, short-term single-agent chemotherapy was used as an adjuvant on the basis of time-honored concepts about the mode of spread of solid tumors and cell kill by drugs. The results of these studies have been critically reviewed [7, 62]. Briefly, the incorrect study design and the short-term chemotherapy program were considered to be the major reason for the negative or inconclusive results.

The new generation of adjuvant trials applied chemotherapy in accordance with the following principles [7, 56]:

1. drug(s) known to be effective in clinically advanced disease were thought to be even more active in the presence of micrometastases. Therefore, they were selected and employed at the optimal dose level and through intermittent schedules to minimize host toxicity;
2. treatment was started as soon as possible after radical mastectomy, usually within 4 weeks, i.e., while residual tumor burden was minimal;
3. treatment must be prolonged to assure maximum cell kill by cytotoxic drugs. In fact, the duration of adjuvant therapy must encompass the tumor cell doubling time.

Table 3. Outline of some adjuvant regimens

Acronym	Drug(s)	Dose schedule	Route	Duration of therapy
(23)	L-PAM	0.15 mg/kg, days 1–5	PO	q. 6 weeks for 2 years
CMF (4)	CTX	100 mg/m^2, days 1–14	PO	q. 4 weeks for 1 year
	MTX	40 mg/m^2, days 1, 8	IV	
	FU	600 mg/m^2, days 1, 8	IV	
FAC (10)	FU	400 mg/m^2, days 1, 8	IV	q. 4 weeks for 2 years
	ADM[a]	40 mg/m^2, days 1	IV	
	CTX	400 mg/m^2, days 1	IV	
LMF (P) (58)	CLB	4 mg/m^2, days 1–14	PO	q. 4 weeks for 6 months
	MTX	5–7.5 mg, days 1–3 and 8–10	PO	
	FU	500–700 mg days 1, 8	PO	
	PRED[b]	50–75 mg days 1–14 tapered to 10–15 after 1st cycle	PO	
CVFM (48)	CTX	300 mg, days 1, 8	IV	q. 4 weeks for 6 months
	VCR	0.65 mg, days 1, 8	IV	
	FU	500 mg, days 1	IV	
	MTX	37.5 mg, days 8	IV	
AC (30)	ADM	30 mg/m^2, day 1	IV	q. 3 weeks for 8 cycles
	CTX	150 mg/m^2, days 3–6	PO	
CFP (1)	CTX	150 mg/m^2, days 1–5	IV	q. 6 weeks for 10 cycles
	FU	300 mg/m^2, days 1–5	IV	
	PRED	30 mg, days 1–7	PO	

[a] Replaced by MTX after total dose of 300 mg/m^2.
[b] Only in the first 120 patients.

Table 3 shows the outline of some adjuvant regimens being evaluated in the adjuvant setting. Only melphalan (L-PAM) was employed singly, whereas cyclophosphamide (CTX), methotrexate (MTX), fluorouracil (FU), adriamycin (ADM), chlorambucil or Leukeran (CLB), vincristine (VCR), and prednisone (PRED), were included in different combination regimens. In most studies treatment was started 2–4 weeks postoperatively, while in some trials a delay up to 10 weeks was allowed. The duration of chemotherapy ranged from a minimum of 6 months to a maximum of 2 years.

Selection of Patients and Study Design

Common characteristics of recent adjuvant studies have been the use of prospective controlled clinical trials, fairly uniform patient selection at least as far as the axillary node status was concerned (N+), follow-up studies, and statistical analysis of the results. Table 4 summarizes some essential data concerning adjuvant trials, including an untreated control group. Patients were assigned randomly to the different groups in all studies except in the trials of the M.D. Anderson Hospital [10, 11] and the University of Arizona [30] where patients were consecutively treated with adjuvant chemo- or chemoimmunotherapy, and the results compared with those of a historical control group.

The presence of histologically positive axillary nodes was considered the main condition for inclusion into all current trials. Patients had localized breast cancer that was potentially curable with local modalities (T1, T2, or T3 according to the international UICC classification). However, nearly 40% of the patients in the M.D. Anderson series had resectable stage III breast cancer [10, 11]. Furthermore, the extent of the primary tumor was not clearly specified in the study conducted by the Multicenter Breast Cancer Chemotherapy Group (MBCCG) [48].

Table 4. Prospective surgical adjuvant trials with an untreated control group

Study group	No. of patients	Status of N	Local modality	Drug regimen	Control group		Time of analysis
NSABP [25]	348	N+	RM	L-PAM	R	1972–1975[a]	24 months
Milan [8]	386	N+	RM	CMF	R	1973–1975	48 months
MDAH [9, 11]	131	N+	RM + RT	FAC–BCG	H	1974–1976	24 months
University of Arizona [30, 34]	32 77	N– N+	RM + RT	AC	H	1974[b]	17–21 months
Osako [57, 58]	125 115	N– N+	RM	LMF–BCG	R	1974–1977[a]	24 months
MBCCG [21, 48]	253	N+, N–	"Conventional"	CVFM	R	1974–1977[a]	24 months

R Randomized; *H* Historical.

[a] Cooperative series.

[b] Ongoing.

Radical mastectomy (RM) was employed as the surgical procedure in four studies. In the MBCCG trial the type of local therapy, including different extents of surgery and radiotherapy according to the "conventional treatment" applied in that country, was left to the decision of participating investigators. Local radiotherapy (RT) was given in 16% of patients at the M.D. Anderson Hospital, whereas in the prospective study designed at the University of Arizona, RT was given in half the patients with medial tumors, larger tumors (> 4 cm in diameter) and/or one to three positive axillary nodes, and in all patients with more than four positive nodes.

Axillary node involvement was demonstrated by lymph node dissection, except in the MBCCG study, in which only a lymph node biopsy was performed in most patients. Furthermore, in this study a small (as yet unknow) fraction of patients had negative nodes or had no axillary biopsy. In the Ostschweizerische Arbeitsgemeinschaft für Klinische Onkologie (OSAKO) [58] and in the University of Arizona study, N-patients were also included into the study, but the results were analyzed separately. It is worth emphasizing that the rationale for starting an adjuvant trial in N- women in the OSAKO group was based on the observation of Mutzner [49] that in Switzerland a high incidence of recurrence was documented in patients staged as having negative axillary nodes. In two studies [10, 11, 58] immunotherapy was added to chemotherapy. The M.D. Anderson group administered BCG by scarification between two cycles of chemotherapy for 2 consecutive years, whereas in the OSAKO trial BCG was given monthly by scarification after completion of chemotherapy and continued for 2 years.

Table 5 shows the outline of other ongoing adjuvant chemotherapy trials in which there is no untreated control group. These studies were started even more recently, and median follow-up ranges from 10 to 24 months. The trial in progress at the University of California at Los Angeles [32, 60] compares a modified schedule of the original CMF (12 cycles given in 64 weeks) to the same treatment plus active immunotherapy with BCG (given by multiple-

Table 5. Other ongoing surgical adjuvant trials with no untreated control group

Study group	Evaluable patients	Status of N	Local modality	Adjuvant therapy	Median follow-up
UCLA [59, 60]	121	N+	RM ± RT	CMF ± BCG ± TCV[a]	21–24 months
Mayo Clinic [1]	166	N+	RM	L-PAM vs. CFP ± RT[a]	24 months
Bowman Gray School of Medicine [17]	87	N+	RM	L-PAM ± RT vs. CMF ± RT	16 months
Central Pennsylvania Oncology Group [42]	91	N+	RM ± RT	L-PAM vs. LMFP[a]	10 months
Milan [8]	275[b]	N+	RM	CMF 6 vs. 12 cycles	15 months

TCV Tumor cell vaccine.
[a] Random allocation to treatments.
[b] Premenopausal patients only.

puncture technique) alone or associated with tumor cell vaccine (TCV). The trials in progress at the Mayo Clinic [1], the Bowman Gray School of Medicine [17] and the Central Pennsylvania Oncology Group [42] compare single-agent (L-PAM) chemotherapy with various types of combination chemotherapy. CMF and LMFP (CLB 8 mg PO, MTX 5 mg PO and PRED 60 mg PO on days 1–5, FU 15 mg/kg PO each week; repeat every 4 weeks) are given for 2 years. Furthermore, in two studies [1, 17] the contribution of radiation therapy is also being evaluated. Finally, the second CMF program started at the Istituto Nazionale Tumori, Milan, after patient accrual in the first CMF trial was completed in September 1975, compares a shorter treatment (CMF for six cycles) with the conventional 12 cycles of CMF. From September 1975 to December 1976 both pre- and postmenopausal women were included into this comparative study. Since January 1, 1977 the trial has continued only in premenopausal women, in view of the updated results of the first CMF program [5], which showed different efficacy of CMF in pre- and postmenopausal women. A preliminary evaluation was conducted on 275 premenopausal women, with a median follow-up of 15 months [8].

Results

The results of the first CMF program were recently updated after a 4-year follow-up [8]. Table 6 shows the incidence and first site of treatment failure related to menopausal status and to overall survival. The 4-year analysis essentially confirmed the 3-year results [6]. Twelve cycles of adjuvant CMF markedly reduced the cumulative relapse rate only in premenopausal women (25% vs. 59.2%). Postmenopausal patients derived no appreciable benefit from adjuvant treatment (CMF 43.8%, control 47.6%). In both pre- and postmenopausal women, treatment failure was more frequently due to recurrence in distant sites. Cancer in the

Table 6. CMF program: 4-year relapse rate (actuarial analysis)

	Controls (179 patients) %	CMF (207 patients) %	*P* value
Total failure	52.7	34.4	<0.0001
Local-regional	11.9	7.3	
Distant[a]	40.8	27.1	
Total survival	73.6	83.0	0.05
Premenopause	59.2	25.0	0.00001
Local-regional	10.8	4.9	
Distant[a]	48.4	20.1	
Total survival	70.6	89.6	0.02
Postmenopause	47.6	43.8	0.25
Local-regional	9.5	8.4	
Distant[a]	38.1	35.4	
Total survival	75.4	76.5	0.60

[a] ± Local-regional.

Table 7. CMF program: 4-year relapse rate related to drug-induced amenorrhea

Age group	With amenorrhea	Without amenorrhea	*P* value
Total	17.9	37.8	0.10
⩽ 40 years[a]	18.0	37.9	
> 40 years[b]	14.3	11.7	

Reversible: [a] 63%; [b] 4%.

contralateral breast with no concomitant metastasis at other sites was observed in a total of seven women who were classified as primary treatment failures (control four, CMF three). Radical mastectomy was performed in four patients (control three, CMF one). Three women (control one, CMF two) had subsequent recurrences at distant sites within 7–15 months. The overall survival was significantly improved only in premenopausal patients given CMF, 89.6% being alive at 4 years as against 70.6% of control patients ($P = 0.02$). The incidence of relapse was also compared in premenopausal patients who did or did not become amenorrheic during CMF (Table 7). The presence of amenorrhea was correlated with a lower incidence of relapse only in women younger than 40 years, but the difference was not statistically significant. It should be noted, however, that in this group of patients amenorrhea was transient in more than 60% of women.

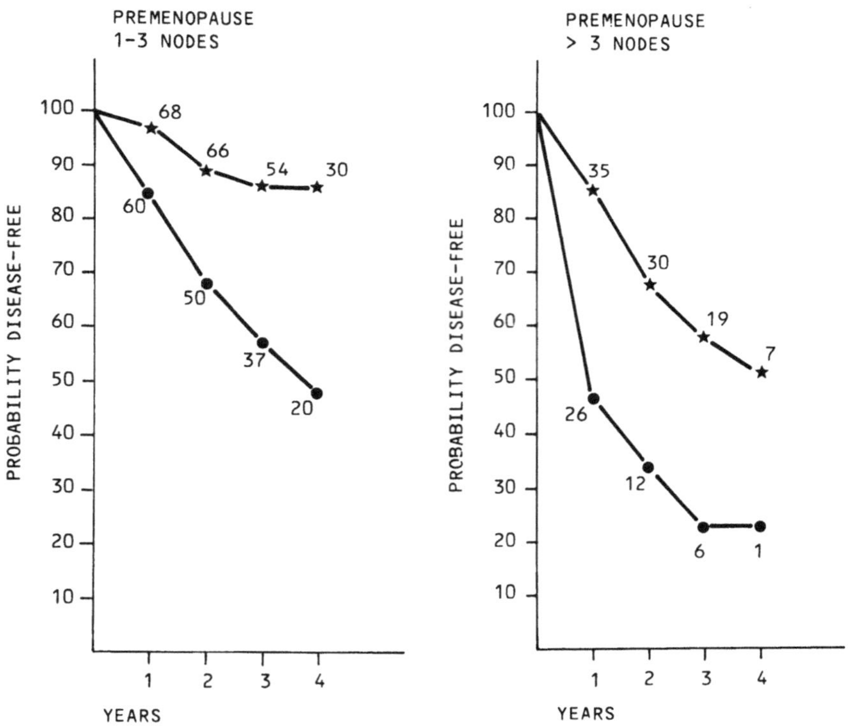

Fig. 1. CMF program. Premenopausal patients: disease-free survival related to number of positive axillary nodes. ●——●: RM; ★——★: RM + CMF

Figures 1 and 2 show the disease-free survival in control and CMF patients, related to menopausal status and extent of axillary nodal involvement. Premenopausal patients treated with CMF had a significantly higher probability of being disease-free in both nodal subgroups throughout the observation period.

A comparison of the results of the Milan CMF program and those of other studies can be attempted, but at present the comparison is limited to the 24-month relapse rate. The comparison is also somewhat limited by the fact that only in the CMF program are all patients at risk for the entire examination period. The comparative findings are reported in Table 8. In all studies, women given adjuvant chemotherapy had a lower recurrence rate than controls, although the advantage was not always statistically significant. If the data are broken down between pre- and postmenopausal patients, it appears evident that only premenopausal women with limited nodal involvement (N+ 1–3) benefited from L-PAM treatment [25], whereas some benefit was derived in all premenopausal nodal subgroups given CMF. The low incidence of relapse regardless of the menopausal status reported by the M.D. Anderson group [9, 10, 11] after chemoimmunotherapy appears promising, but findings need to be confirmed by subsequent analysis. On the other hand, the OSAKO trial [57, 58] reported a difference, though not significant, in favor of postmenopausal patients treated with LMF-BCG compared with controls. It should be recalled that the Swiss investigators found a significant improvement in the disease-free survival after LMF plus BCG in both pre- and postmenopausal women with negative nodes, statistical significance being reached only in postmenopausal patients ($P = 0.02$). Again, these results need a further observation time to

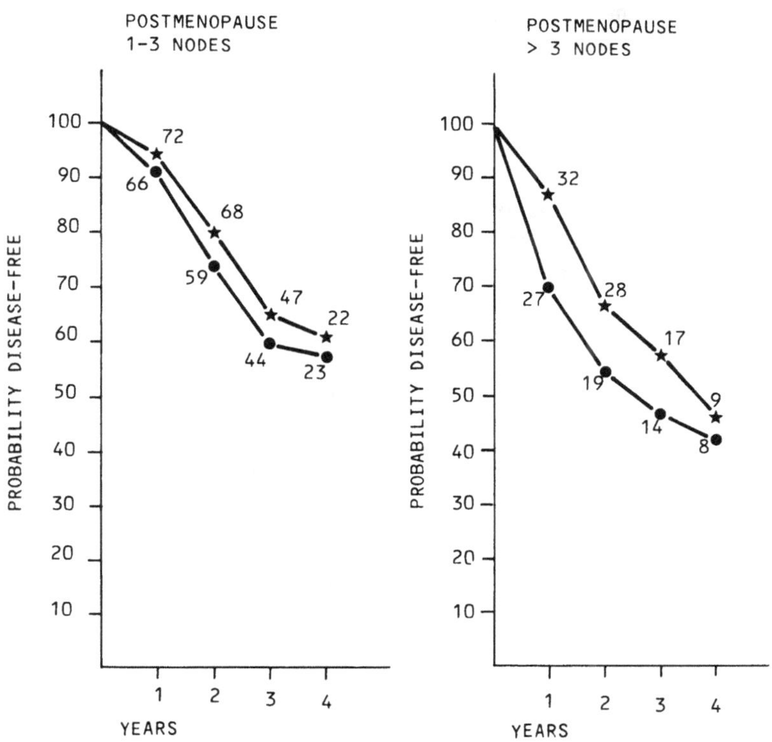

Fig. 2. CMF program. Postmenopausal patients: disease-free survival related to number of positive axillary nodes. ●——●: RM; ★——★: RM + CMF

be fully interpreted. The data of the MBCCG study [21, 48] are not entirely comparable with those of other trials because there are too many variables concerning primary treatment and because of the very short median follow-up (nearly 15 months). Although all studies reported an improvement in total survival, figures were stated to be statistically significant in the FAC-BCG trial, which used a historical control group. At 2 years, 94% of women given chemoimmunotherapy were alive, as against 85% of control patients ($P = 0.01$). These data are comparable to the 2-year overall survival in the CMF programm (CMF 94.7%, control 90.5%).

The results of more recent trials must be considered as very preliminary, due to the small number of patients in the study and the short follow-up. However, available data will be briefly reviewed, as they provide further evidence of the usefulness of adjuvant systemic therapy. At the University of Arizona [30, 34], 7% of 77 evaluable patients followed up for a median of 17—21 months have relapsed so far. In the UCLA series [32, 59, 60], no patient given CMF alone showed treatment failure. In contrast, patients treated with CMF plus immunotherapy had a total relapse rate of 23% after a mean follow-up of 21—24 months. The investigators of the Mayo Clinic [1] have recently reported the following treatment failure rates in the three, treatment groups, after a median follow-up of about 24 months: L-PAM: 31%, CFP: 21%, CFP plus RT: 16%. These data and the findings of the Central Pennsylvania Oncology Group [42] seem to be in favor of multiple-agent therapy as against single-agent chemotherapy. The cooperative group, in fact, reported a relapse rate of 13% after therapy with LMFP, compared with 22% after PAM. If the results of the Mayo Clinic study were analyzed according to menopausal status, only in premenopausal women was adjuvant treatment the only factor significantly associated with an improved disease-free interval, regardless of nodal

Table 8. Comparative 2-year recurrence rate in some adjuvant trials for operable breast cancer with positive nodes

Therapy	No. of patients	Total failure	Premenopausal			Postmenopausal		
			Total	N+1–3	≥4	Total	N+1–3	≥4
Control vs.	169	31.4	36.7	25.8[a]	48.3	28.4	16.1	41.5
L-PAM [25]	179	23.5	22.0	6.5[a]	40.7	24.2	13.8	36.4
Control vs.	179	36.5[a]	42.2[a]	32.1[a]	65.4[a]	31.3	25.8	44.4
CMF[b] [8]	207	21.3[a]	17.4[a]	10.2[a]	29.4[a]	21.9	20.8	34.4
Control[c] vs.	151	35.0[a]	–	30.0	60.0[a]	–	22.0[b]	38.0[a]
FAC + BCG [9, 11]	131	12.0[a]	–	15.0	23.0[a]	–	0[a]	12.0[a]
Control vs.	57	33.3	35.5	–	–	30.8	–	–
LMF + BCG [75, 58]	58	22.4	31.0	–	–	13.8	–	–
Control vs.	128	39.9	43.2	–	–	38.1	–	–
CVFM [21, 48]	125	22.5	40.2	–	–	9.1	–	–

[a] Indicates significant difference.
[b] Median follow-up: 40 months.
[c] Historical.

involvement and primary tumor size ($P = 0.03$). A similar trend was reported by the Bowman Gray School of Medicine study, in which more favorable results were obtained in pre- than in postmenopausal women treated with chemotherapy alone [17]. In contrast, premenopausal patients had a higher incidence of early relapse than postmenopausal women in the University of Arizona trial (pre-: 17.4%; post-: 3.7%) and the UCLA trial (pre-: 30%, post-: 16%). The results of the second CMF program were recently analyzed for premenopausal women at the Istituto Nazionale Tumori, Milan. Due to the limited number of patients evaluable in the different subsets, no statistical difference was detectable between short-term and long-term therapy. The actuarial analysis at 2 years from surgery showed a 12.4% relapse rate for premenopausal patients given 12 cycles, compared with 19.2% for those treated with six cycles.

Toxicity

Toxic manifestations secondary to different adjuvant regimens are reported in Table 9. Combination chemotherapy induced numerous acute side-effects, but they were moderate and, with the exception of amenorrhea, always reversible. Myelosuppression was a very common finding, but it was never associated with serious complications. Therapy was followed by various degrees of nausea and vomiting in most patients. Gastrointestinal symptoms together with hair loss represented the most disturbing side-effect from the patient's point of view. However, only a minority of patients refused to complete the planned treatment program.

The occurrence of amenorrhea during chemotherapy is of great importance, not only from the toxicologic point of view but because of the endocrine implications of this finding. Cessation of menses was interpreted as evidence of ovarian suppression, probably induced by alkylating

Table 9. Comparative percentage of toxic manifestations after some adjuvant regimens

	L-PAM	CMF	FAC	LMF	CVFM	AC	CFP
Nausea, vomiting	30	90	93	20	26	67	59
Leukopenia	60	78	–[a]	50	–	50	90
Thrombocytopenia	–	79	–[a]	50	–	0	22
Hair loss	–	69	97	0	8	98	71
Amenorrhea	–	78	71	–	–	64	25
Stomatitis	–	19	1	–	1.5	–	–
Diarrhea	–	–	–	–	–	–	51
Cystitis	–	30	–	–	–	–	–
Conjunctivitis	–	32	–	–	–	–	–
Skin reactions	–	–	1	–	–	3	–
Cardiomyopathy	–	–	0	–	–	0	–
Infections	0	0	3	0.004	–	0	–
Bleeding	–	–	–	–	–	–	–
Refused therapy	–	11	–	1	15	–	–

[a] Myelosuppression was expressed as median count at nadir. Granulocytes: 2400 per mm^3; platelets 260,000 per mm^3.

agents. Furthermore, some authors [51] attributed the efficacy of chemotherapy in premenopausal women to "chemical castration". The study of Rose and Davis [55] demonstrated that the plasma levels of estradiol plus estrone and androstenedione were markedly reduced in premenopausal women after 6 months of adjuvant chemotherapy (L-PAM or CMFV). Furthermore, follicle-stimulating hormone (FSH) and luteinizing hormone (LH) levels were increased. Koyama et al. [37] measured urinary estrogen and serum progesterone levels weekly for approximately 6 months postoperatively in six patients receiving adjuvant treatment with cyclophosphamide. At the onset of amenorrhea, the levels of both hormones ceased to show their normal cyclic changes and remained persistently low. Meanwhile, serum FSH and LH were markedly elevated. Furthermore, no ovarian follicles were histologically found in three amenorrheic women who underwent therapeutic oophorectomy after cyclophosphamide therapy. The above-mentioned biochemical findings were confirmed in a preliminary hormonal evaluation performed at the Istituto Nazionale Tumori of Milan on 15 women aged 37–48 years (median 42), who had been given CMF for 6–12 cycles and had drug-induced amenorrhea (reversible in 3/15 patients). The median time from onset of amenorrhea to the endocrine evaluation was 14 months. LH, thyroid-stimulating hormone (TSH), prolactin, and 17-β estradiol levels were comparable to those observed in a group of postmenopausal women with early breast cancer not treated with adjuvant chemotherapy [52]. That amenorrhea does not necessarily mean permanent castration was demonstrated by the histologic results of a retrospective study carried out at the Istituto Nazionale Tumori of Milan [8]. In 20 premenopausal breast cancer patients aged 28–45 years (median 40.5 years), a therapeutic oophorectomy was performed after treatment with combination chemotherapy including CMF. Of these patients, 40% had become amenorrheic during treatment. In these patients, oophorectomy was performed not later than 1 year from the last menstruation. Histologic examination of the ovaries revealed that follicles were present in 55% of all patients. Absence of ovarian follicles was demonstrated in only 62.5% of amenorrheic women, but also in 37.5% of women who continued to menstruate regularly during chemotherapy. Furthermore, no difference in the thickness of ovarian cortex was evident in patients given cytotoxic drugs and

Table 10. Second primary tumors other than breast adenocarcinoma in patients given adjuvant CMF compared to controls

Controls (197 patients)[a]			CMF (207 patients)[a]		
No.	Tumor	months post RM	No.	Tumor	months post RM
1	Cervix ca (in situ)	3	1	Gastric ca[b]	37
1	Melanoma	20	1	Cystosarcoma phyllodes	40
1	Leiomyoblastoma[c] of uterus	40			
3/179	(1.7%)		2/207	(1%)	

[a] Median follow-up: 40 months (range: 29–57 months).
[b] Only three cycles of adjuvant CMF were given.
[c] Twelve months after 12 cycles of CMF for recurrence.

an age-matched control group of patients not treated with chemotherapy before oophorectomy (1.0 mm vs. 0.9 mm).

Another aspect of long-term toxicity, namely possible carcinogenesis, is a cause of concern to many clinicians. Current adjuvant chemotherapy trials have so far not reported an incidence of second neoplasms that is higher in treated than in control patients. Table 10 reports in detail both incidence and type of second tumors other than breast adenocarcinoma as detected in control and CMF patients in the Milan study. So far, the incidence of second tumors is comparable in the two groups. In particular, no patient developed acute leukemia in the group treated with chemotherapy. The NSABP study has not revealed any difference in the incidence of second primary non-breast cancer so far. In fact, the incidence of new neoplasms was 3.3% in patients treated with L-PAM, as against 1.2% for the control group [22]. Acute myelogenous leukemia was an incidental autopsy finding in a 77-year-old woman treated with L-PAM who died of metastatic disease.

Adjuvant Hormone Therapy

As breast cancer is an endocrine-responsive tumor, it appears logical to consider hormone therapy also as systemic adjuvant treatment. However, the use of this modality has been limited in the past by the fact that only about 30% of patients have hormone-responsive tumors, as indicated by the response rate to hormonal manipulations in unselected women with advanced disease. Prophylactic castration was the endocrine procedure most commonly used in premenopausal patients. The results of adjuvant castration versus adjuvant CMF have recently been reviewed [3]. In short, patient selection and study design in most trials were far from being impeccable and any benefit of treatment was limited to a prolongation of the disease-free interval. The results reported by MEAKIN et al. [46] deserve a separate comment. Following mastectomy and local-regional radiation therapy, 705 patients were randomized to no further therapy, ovarian irradiation with a dose of up to 2000 rad in 5 days, or ovarian irradiation in the same dosage plus prednisone for 5 years. At 10 years, in premenopausal women aged 45 years or more and with positive nodes, ovarian irradiation plus prednisone resulted in a significant delay in recurrence ($P = 0.03$) and a prolongation of survival ($P = 0.06$). However, even though surgical or radiologic castration is still supported by some centers, adjuvant castration has been abandoned in most institutions as an unproven therapeutic method. As far as other endocrine manipulations are concerned, the value of adjuvant bilateral adrenalectomy was reported by DAO [19] who recently confirmed [20] the beneficial effect of this procedure in 17 postmenopausal women with more than three positive lymph nodes. In fact, at 10 years from mastectomy plus ablative endocrine surgery, 72% of patients were alive and disease-free. The relevance of this interesting finding was limited, however, by the small number of patients in the study.

Recent developments in tumor cell biochemistry, such as estrogen receptor (ER) determination, by allowing a more rational use of hormonal manipulation, made all data from previous trials practically obsolete and prompted a reappraisal of endocrine therapy on a new basis. ER assay in breast cancer tissue was in fact demonstrated to be an indicator for more selective use of hormone therapy, a higher ER content being correlated to a higher probability of response to endocrine therapy in advanced disease [44, 45]. These data, as well as recent findings on adjuvant chemotherapy favoring premenopausal women, suggested the opportunity for a reassessment of the role of hormone therapy in the management of primary breast cancer.

Perspectives

The results derived from the updating of current adjuvant chemotherapy trials demonstrate that the strategy of a combined modality approach for high-risk patients with primary breast cancer is correct and should continue to be further evaluated. In fact, all patients treated postoperatively with cytotoxic drugs showed at least some improvement in the early disease-free survival. Data concerning patients with a longer follow-up period are available at present only for the CMF program, where at 4 years from mastectomy both disease-free and overall survival were significantly prolonged as a consequence of adjuvant chemotherapy. However, in most studies favorable results were limited to premenopausal women. The opposite result reported by the M.D. Anderson Hospital, the University of California, and the University of Arizona requires a longer follow-up analysis to confirm the usefulness of adjuvant therapy also in postmenopausal women. The toxicity from drug treatment was acceptable in the hands of experienced oncologists and, so far, no increased incidence of second cancers has been demonstrated in patients receiving prolonged multidrug programs. As far as endocrine therapy is concerned, only new prospective trials taking ER into consideration will allow a better definition of the usefulness of adjuvant hormone therapy.

Despite early and intermediate favorable results, the problem of optimal curative treatment for operable breast cancer is far from being solved. The main problems are presently related to: (1) further definition of new factors influencing prognosis, (2) correlation between menopausal status and responsiveness to adjuvant therapy, (3) long-term survival versus chronic toxicity. At present, this latter point is particularly relevant for premenopausal women, since for postmenopausal patients an effective adjuvant treatment remains to be clearly defined.

Prognostic Factors

The status of the axillary nodes at mastectomy has so far been the best indicator of which patients are candidates for additional treatment. However, patients with negative nodes show recurrence within 10 years. Nime et al. [50] found in a small series that patients having negative axillary nodes and intramammary lymphatic tumor emboli have a higher relapse rate, especially in distant sites, compared to those without this finding (43% vs. 4%). These data, if confirmed in larger series, could signify an improvement of the cure rate even in this group of patients with apparently limited disease.

ER content has been recently reported to have a relevant significance in predicting the prognosis in operable breast cancer. Walt [65] found a high incidence of visceral metastasis and a short survival in patients categorized as ER–. Subsequently, Knight et al. [36] confirmed that ER– patients have a higher recurrence rate at 20 months and a shorter survival, regardless of primary size and location of the tumor, age, and status of involved axillary nodes. Lippmann et al. [41] retrospectively evaluated the influence of ER on response to cytotoxic chemotherapy in 70 patients with metastatic or surgically unresectable primary breast cancer. Of 45 patients with low or absent ER values, 34 (76%) responded to chemotherapy as against 3 of 25 (12%) patients with higher values. The response was independent of other known variables. The authors concluded that ER values were an important predictor of response to cytotoxic chemotherapy in metastatic breast cancer. In contrast, Frenning et al. [28] observed that ER+ patients showed a higher response rate to chemotherapy than ER–

patients (80% vs. 37%) and also a longer duration of response (18 vs. 8 months). However, in this series, ER+ women were older, had a longer disease-free interval, and had chemotherapy initiated at a longer interval after the first recurrence than ER− patients. Furthermore, MEYER et al. [47], who studied both ER content and thymidine labeling index (TLI), found a significant association between high TLI and absence of ER. The authors concluded that this finding was an expression of redifferentiation and that breast tumors with these biologic characteristics included the highest proportion of tumors unresponsive to hormonal therapy. A more definitive interpretation of all reported data can be provided only by prospective controlled trials.

Hormonal Effect of Chemotherapy

On the basis of the above considerations, the current data suggesting that premenopausal women benefit more from adjuvant chemotherapy may find a more convincing interpretation than the hypothesis of chemical castration by cytotoxic drugs [51, 55]. In fact, the different benefit from chemotherapy related to menopausal status may only reflect a different proportion of ER− tumors in pre- versus postmenopausal women. Younger women bearing tumors with low or negative ER content would be more responsive to chemotherapeutic agents [41]. The finding that ER− premenopausal patients treated with CMF have the same incidence of recurrence as ER+ patients at 2 years (ER−: 27%; ER+: 11.7%) may support this hypothesis [8]. Future adjuvant trials will yield more convincing data only if stratification parameters also include ER assay on the primary tumor.

Carcinogenesis Secondary to Chemotherapy

Prolonged chemotherapy may produce long-term toxicity, including an increased incidence of second tumors. Drug-induced carcinogenesis, especially acute nonlymphocytic leukemia, has been reported after intensive or prolonged therapy for Hodgkin's disease, multiple myeloma, and ovarian cancer [2, 12, 29, 53, 66]. In Hodgkin's disease and ovarian cancer, second tumors occurred when combined radiation and cytotoxic therapy with alkylating agents were employed. As far as breast cancer is concerned, only one report showed a marked increase of second neoplasms. LERNER [38] observed 3 of 13 (23%) cases of acute myeloblastic leukemia after chemotherapy with chlorambucil. This finding can be conceivably attributed to the excessively long duration of therapy (5—7 years) with an alkylating agent. The same author [39] reported new solid tumors in 2 of 37 (5%) women treated with adjuvant L-PAM. On the other hand, CHAN [16] found no difference in the incidence of new cancers in a large series of patients treated postoperatively with thiotepa with or without radiotherapy. An interesting finding is that the frequency of second malignancies was found to be in direct proportion to the cumulative dose of thiotepa. At present, no adjuvant treatment is administered for longer than 2 years. However, the above considerations suggest once again that the use of cytotoxic adjuvant therapy should be limited to groups who are at high risk of early recurrence to prevent overtreatment and potential risk to women who are cured by a local modality alone.

References

1. Ahmann, D. L., Payne, W. S., Scanlon, P. W., O'Fallon, J. R., Bisel, H. F., Hahn, R. G., Edmonson, J. H., Ingle, J. N., Frytak, S., O'Connell, M. J., Rubin, J.: Repeated adjuvant chemotherapy with phenylalanine mustard or 5-fluorouracil, cyclophosphamide, and prednisone with or without radiation, after mastectomy for breast cancer. Lancet *1978 I,* 893–896
2. Arseneau, J. C., Sponzo, R. W., Levin, D. L., Schnipper, L. E., Bonner, H., Young, R. C., Canellos, G. P., Johnson, R. E., De Vita, V. T.: Non-lymphomatous malignant tumors complicating Hodgkin's disease: possible association with intensive therapy. N. Engl. J. Med. *287,* 1119–1122 (1972)
3. Bonadonna, G.: Adjuvant castration versus adjuvant chemotherapy. Int. J. Radiat. Oncol. Biol. Phys. (in press) (1978)
4. Bonadonna, G., Brusamolino, E., Valagussa, P., Rossi, A., Brugnatelli, L., Brambilla, C., De Lena, M., Tancini, G., Bajetta, E., Musumeci, R., Veronesi, U.: Combination chemotherapy as an adjuvant treatment in operable breast cancer. N. Engl. J. Med. *294,* 405–410 (1976)
5. Bonadonna, G., Rossi, A., Valagussa, P., Banfi, A., Veronesi, U.: The CMF program for operable breast cancer with positive axillary nodes: updated analysis on the disease-free interval, site of relapse and drug tolerance. Cancer *39,* 2904–2915 (1977)
6. Bonadonna, G., Rossi, A., Valagussa, P., Banfi, A., Veronesi, U.: Adjuvant chemotherapy with CMF in breast cancer with positive axillary nodes. In: Adjuvant therapy of cancer. Salmon, S. E., Jones, S. E. (eds.), p. 83. Amsterdam: North Holland 1977
7. Bonadonna, G., Tancini, G., Rossi, A., Gasparini, M.: Chemotherapy in the prevention of the recurrence of resectable cancer. Ann. Rev. Med. *29,* 149–175 (1978)
8. Bonadonna, G., Valagussa, P., Rossi, A., Zucali, R., Tancini, G., Bajetta, E., Brambilla, C., De Lena, M., Di Fronzo, G., Banfi, A., Rilke, F., Veronesi, U.: Are surgical adjuvant trials altering the course of breast cancer? Semin. Oncol. (in press) (1978)
9. Buzdar, A. V.: personal communication
10. Buzdar, A. V., Blumenschein, G. R., Guttermann, J. U., Tashima, C. K., Hortobagyi, G. N., Wheeler, W., Gehan, E., Freireich, E. J., Hersh, E.: Adjuvant chemoimmunotherapy following regional therapy in breast cancer. In: Adjuvant therapy of cancer. Salmon, S. E., Jones, S. E. (eds.), p. 139. Amsterdam: North Holland 1977
11. Buzdar, A. V., Guttermann, J. U., Blumenschein, G. R., Hortobagyi, G. N., Tashima, C. K., Smith, T. L., Hersh, E. M., Freireich, E. J., Gehan, E. A.: Intensive postoperative chemoimmunotherapy for patients with stage II and stage III breast cancer. Cancer *41,* 1064–1075 (1978)
12. Canellos, G. P., De Vita, V. T., Arseneau, J. C., Wang-Peng, J., Johnson, R. E. C.: Second malignancies complicating Hodgkin's disease in remission. Lancet *1975 I,* 947–949
13. Carbone, P. P.: Systemic treatment of breast cancer: past, present and future. Int. J. Radiat. Oncol. Biol. Phys. *1,* 759–767 (1976)
14. Carter, S. K.: Integration of chemotherapy into combined modality treatment of solid tumors. VII Adenocarcinoma of the breast. Cancer Treat. Rev. *3,* 141–174 (1976)
15. Carter, S. K.: The adjunctive use of chemotherapy. Current concepts and unresolved problems. (in press) (1978)
16. Chan, P. Y. M., Sadoff, L., Winkley, J. H.: Second malignancies following first breast cancer in prolonged Thiotepa adjuvant chemotherapy. In: Adjuvant therapy of cancer. Salmon, S. E., Jones, S. E. (eds.), p. 597. Amsterdam: North Holland 1977
17. Cooper, R., Muss, H., Richards, F., II, Stuart, J., White, D., Raben, M., Spurr, C.: A randomized clinical trial of l-phenilalanine mustard (L-PAM) and cyclophosphamide, methotrexate, and fluorouracil (CMF) with and without radiation therapy (R.T.) for adjuvant therapy of breast cancer. Proc. Am. Soc. Clin. Oncol. *19,* 337 (1978)
18. Culliton, B. J.: Breast cancer: reports of new therapy are greatly exaggerated. Science *191,* 1029–1031 (1976)

19. Dao, T. L., Nemoto, T., Chamberlain, A., Bross, I.: Adrenalectomy with radical mastectomy in the treatment of high-risk breast cancer. Cancer *35*, 478–482 (1975)
20. Dao, T. L.: Endocrine surgery as adjuvant therapy in breast cancer. In: Hormone deprivation in breast cancer. Mayer, M., Saez, S., Stoll, B. A. (eds.). Proceedings of the International Symposium. Lyon, 2–3 June 1977
21. Edelstyn, G. A.: personal communication
22. Fisher, B.: personal communication
23. Fisher, B., Carbone, P., Economou, S. G., Frelick, R., Glass, A., Lerner, H., Redmond, C., Zelen, M., Band, P., Katrych, D. L., Wolmark, N., Fisher, E. R., and Other Cooperative Investigators: L-phenylalanine mustard (L-PAM) in the management of primary breast cancer. A report of early findings. N. Engl. J. Med. *292*, 117–122 (1975)
24. Fisher, B., Montague, E., Redmond, C., Barton, B., Borland, D., Fisher, E. R., Deutsch, M., Schwarz, G., Margolese, R., Donegan, W., Volk, H., Konvolinka, C., Gardner, B., Cohn, I., Lesnick, G., Cruz, A. B., Lawrence, W., Nealon, T., Butcher, H., Lawton, R.: Comparison of radical mastectomy with alternative treatments for primary breast cancer: a first report of results from a prospective randomized clinical trial. Cancer *39*, 2827–2839 (1977)
25. Fisher, B., Redmond, C., and Participating NSABP Investigators: Studies of the national surgical adjuvant breast project (NSABP). In: Adjuvant therapy of cancer. Salmon, S. E., Jones, S. E. (eds.), p. 67. Amsterdam: North Holland 1977
26. Fisher, B., Slack, N. H., Cavanaugh, P. J., Gardner, B., Ravdin, R. G., and Cooperating Investigators: Postoperative radiotherapy in the treatment of breast cancer: results of the NSABP clinical trial. Ann. Surg. *172*, 711–732 (1970)
27. Fisher, B., Slack, N., Katrych, D., Wolmark, N.: Ten year follow-up results of patients with carcinoma of the breast in a co-operative clinical trial evaluating surgical adjuvant chemotherapy. Surg. Gynecol. Obstet. *140*, 528–534 (1975)
28. Frenning, D. H., Kennedy, B. J., Vosika, G. J., Kiang, D. T.: Correlation of estrogens receptors and response to chemotherapy in advanced breast cancer. Proc. Am. Soc. Clin. Oncol. *19*, 347 (1978)
29. Gonzales, F., Trujillo, J. M., Alexanian, R.: Acute leukemia in multiple myeloma. Ann. Int. Med. *86*, 440–443 (1977)
30. Hammond, N., Jones, S. E., Salmon, S. E., Giordano, G., Jackson, R., Miller, R., Heusinkveld, R.: Adjuvant treatment of breast cancer with adriamycin-cyclophosphamide with or without radiation therapy. In: Adjuvant therapy of cancer. Salmon, S. E., Jones, S. E. (eds.), p. 153. Amsterdam: North Holland 1977
31. Harris, J. R., Levene, M. B., Hellman, S., Weber, E.: Definitive radiation therapy for stage I and II carcinoma of the breast. Proc. Am. Soc. Clin. Oncol. *19*, 314 (1978)
32. Haskell, C. M., Sparks, F. C., Graze, P. R., Korenmann, S. G.: Systemic therapy for metastatic breast cancer. Ann. Int. Med. *86*, 68–80 (1977)
33. Holland, J. F.: Major advance in breast cancer therapy. N. Engl. J. Med. *294*, 440–441 (1976)
34. Jones, S. E.: personal communication
35. Karim, A. B. M. F.: Radiotherapy and chemotherapy in early breast cancer. Lancet *1976 II*, 36
36. Knight, W. A., III, Livingston, R. B., Gregory, E. J., Walder, A. I., McGuire, W. L.: Absent estrogen receptor and decreased survival in human breast cancer. Proc. Am. Soc. Clin. Oncol. *19*, 392 (1978)
37. Koyama, H., Wada, T., Nishizawa, Y., Imanaga, T., Aori, Y., Terasawa, T., Kosaki, G., Yamamoto, T., Wada, A.: Cyclphosphamide-induced ovarian failure and its therapeutic significance in patients with breast cancer. Cancer *39*, 1403–1409 (1977)
38. Lerner, H.: Acute myelogenous leukemia in patients receiving chlorambucil as a long term therapy in breast cancer at the Pennsylvania Hospital. Proc. Am. Assoc. Cancer Res. *18*, 170 (1977)

39. Lerner, H.: Second malignancies diagnosed in breast cancer patients while receiving adjuvant chemotherapy at the Pennsylvania Hospital. Proc. Am. Soc. Clin. Oncol. *18,* 340 (1977)
40. Levene, M. B., Harris, J. R., Hellman, S.: Treatment of carcinoma of the breast by radiation therapy. Cancer *39,* 2840–2845 (1977)
41. Lippman, M. E., Allegra, J. C., Thompson, E. B., Simon, R., Barlock, A., Green, L., Huff, K. K., Do, H. M. T., Aitken, S. C., Warren, R.: The relation between estrogen receptors and response rate to cytotoxic chemotherapy in metastatic breast cancer. N. Engl. J. Med. *298,* 1223–1228 (1978)
42. Lipton, A., Antle, C., Demuth, W., Dixon, R., Gottlieb, R., Heckard, R., Kane, R., Kukrika, M., Moquin, R., Nahrwold, D., Patterson, L., Ricci, J., Shaver, W., Stryker, J., Ward, S., White, D., Harvey, H., Badder, E.: L-phenylalanine mustard (L-PAM) vs. combination chemotherapy as adjuvant therapy in operable breast cancer. In: Adjuvant therapy of cancer. Salmon, S. E., Jones, S. E. (eds.), p. 123. Amsterdam: North Holland 1977
43. Martin, D. S., Fugman, R. A., Stolfi, R. L., Hayworth, P. E.: Solid tumor animal model therapeutically predictive for human breast cancer. Cancer Chemother. Rep. *5,* 89–109 (1975)
44. McGuire, W. L., Horwitz, K. B., Pearson, O. H., Segaloff, A.: Current status of estrogen and progesterone receptors in breast cancer. Cancer *39,* 2934–2947 (1977)
45. McGuire, W. L.: Hormone receptors: their role in predicting prognosis and response to endocrine therapy. Semin. Oncol. (in press) (1978)
46. Meakin, J. W., Allt, W. E. C., Beale, F. A., Brown, T. C., Bush, R. S., Clark, R. M., Fitzpatrick, P. J., Hawkins, N. V., Jenkin, R. D. T., Pringle, J. F., Rider, W. D., Hayward, J. L., Bulbrook, R. D.: Ovarian irradiation and prednisone following surgery for carcinoma of the breast. In: Adjuvant therapy of cancer. Salmon, S. E., Jones, S. E. (eds.), p. 95. Amsterdam: North Holland 1977
47. Meyer, J. S., Rao, B. R., Stevens, S. C., White, W. L.: Low incidence of estrogen receptor in breast carcinomas with rapid rates of cellular replication. Cancer *40,* 2290–2298, (1977)
48. Multicentre Breast Cancer Chemotherapy Group: Multimodal therapy for histological stage II breast cancer. Lancet *1977 II,* 396–397
49. Mutzner, F., Amgwerd, R., Gessner, U.: Prognose des lokalen primären Mammakarcinoms unter der bisherigen Therapie. Schweiz. Med. Wochenschr. *107,* 992–994 (1977)
50. Nime, F. A., Rosen, P. P., Thaler, H. T., Ashikari, R., Urban, J. A.: Prognostic significance of tumor emboli in intramammary lymphatics in patients with mammary carcinoma. Am. J. Surg. Pathol. *1,* 25–30 (1977)
51. Pourquier, H.: Adjuvant chemotherapy of breast cancer: is it a direct cytotoxic or has it an indirect hormone effect? Int. J. Radiat. Oncol. Biol. Phys. (in press) (1978)
52. Recchione, C., Rossi, A.: Unpublished data
53. Reimer, R. R., Hoover, R., Fraumeni, J. F., Jr., Young, R. C.: Acute leukemia after alkylating agent therapy of ovarian cancer. N. Engl. J. Med. *297,* 177–181 (1977)
54. Rodriguez-Antunez, A.: The triumphalistic oncology. Surg. Gynecol. Obstet. *146,* 617–618 (1978)
55. Rose, D. P., Davis, T. E.: Ovarian function in patients receiving adjuvant chemotherapy for breast cancer. Lancet *1977 I,* 1174–1176
56. Schabel, F. M.: Rationale for adjuvant chemotherapy. Cancer *39,* 2875–2882 (1977)
57. Senn, H. J.: personal communication
58. Senn, H. J., Jungi, W. F., Amgwerd, R., Sprenger, F., Hochveli, R., Engelhart, G., Heinz, C., Wick, A., Enderlin, F., Creux, G. S., Meon, B., Lanz, R., Bigler, R.: Adjuvant chemoimmunotherapy with LMF+BCG in node-negative and node-positive breast cancer patients. Antibiot. Chemother. *24,* 213–228 (1978)
59. Sparks, F. C.: personal communication
60. Sparks, F. C., Meyerowitz, B. E., Ramming, K. P., Wolk, R. W., Goldsmith, M. H., Lemkin, R. S. R., Spears, I. K., Morton, D. L.: Adjuvant chemotherapy and chemoimmunotherapy for breast

cancer. In: Adjuvant therapy of cancer. Salmon, S. E., Jones, S. E. (eds.), p. 109. Amsterdam: North Holland 1977

61. Stjernswärd, J.: Adjuvant radiotherapy trials in breast cancer. Cancer *39,* 2846–2867 (1977)
62. Tormey, D. C.: Combined chemotherapy and surgery in breast cancer: a review. Cancer **36,** 881–892 (1975)
63. Valagussa, P., Bonadonna, G., Veronesi, U.: Patterns of relapse and survival following radical mastectomy. Cancer *41,* 1170–1178 (1978)
64. Veronesi, U., Banfi, A., Saccozzi, R., Salvadori, B., Zucali, R., Uslenghi, C., Greco, M., Luini, A., Rilke, F., Sultan, L.: Conservative treatment of breast cancer: a trial in progress at the Cancer Institute of Milan. Cancer *39,* 2822–2826 (1977)
65. Walt, A. J., Singhakowinta, A., Brooks, S. C., Cortez, A.: The surgical implications of estrophile protein estimations in carcinoma of the breast. Surgery *80,* 506–512 (1976)
66. Williams, C. J., Coleman, C. N., Glatstein, E. J., Rosenberg, S. A., Kaplan, H. S.: Hematological malignancies in remission of Hodgkin's disease. Proc. Am. Soc. Clin. Oncol. *18,* 288 (1977)

Treatment of Early Breast Cancer With Adriamycin-Cyclophosphamide With or Without Radiation Therapy: Initial Results of a Brief and Effective Adjuvant Program

S. E. Salmon, A. Wendt, S. E. Jones, R. Jackson, G. Giordano, R. Miller, R. Heusinkveld, and T. E. Moon

Introduction

We initiated study of the combination of adriamycin and cyclophosphamide (A–C) for advanced breast cancer at the University of Arizona in 1973 [12]. That study was based on evidence that both agents were quite active individually, had different mechanisms of action, and were useful in relatively low growth fraction solid tumors. Results of our initial study plus those obtained simultaneously by workers at the Southern Research Institute [4] suggested that the A–C combination was synergistic or potentiating. We observed an overall objective response rate of 78% in 51 patients with advanced breast cancer who had not recceived prior chemotherapy [12]. A number of subsequent trails in advanced breast cancer using A–C plus other drugs (e.g., 5-fluorouracil) have yielded almost identical results [2, 8], suggesting that A–C is the active component of these regimens. The high response rate, acceptable toxicity, and ease of administration to advanced breast cancer patients encouraged us to initiate a surgical adjuvant breast cancer program with this regimen. We reasoned that a relatively brief adjuvant program could be formulated with both drugs administered intensively to eradicate a minimum number of occult micrometastases. Furthermore, we believed that the duration of therapy could be related to the tumor stage as defined by pathologic staging (e.g., more treatment for more advanced stages). The kinetic considerations applied in design of this trial are summarized elsewhere [15]. Thus, in mid-1974 we initiated the Arizona Breast Cancer Adjuvant Program [9, 11, 14]. This report summarizes the updated preliminary results as of May 1978.

Methods

Since July 1974, patients undergoing recent surgery for breast cancer who were potentially eligible for adjuvant treatment have been referred for possible inclusion in the program. After referral, patients are evaluated for evidence of metastatic disease by means of a careful physical examination, routine laboratory work, chest radiograph, and bone scan. If the bone scan is abnormal, appropriate X-rays are obtained. Unless the X-rays confirm overt metastatic disease, patients are eligible for adjuvant treatment. Additional laboratory, radiographic, or nuclear medicine studies are performed when clinically indicated. Patients also have baseline cardiac examination plus serial examination with several noninvasive tests of ventricular function (e.g., systolic time intervals, echocardiography) [5].

The eligibility criteria for this study include initiation of chemotherapy within 2 months after surgery for infiltrating ductal adenocarcinoma of pathologic stage I, II, or III extent, no evidence of overt metastases, no prior breast cancer or heart disease, and informed written consent in accord with University of Arizona guidelines for protection of human subjects. The assignment of treatment depends on assessment of the potential risk of relapse, which, in turn, is predicated on knowledge of the stage of disease and nodal status (Table 1).

Table 1. Arizona breast cancer adjuvant program: treatment plan based on pathologic stage of disease

Stage of disease	Treatment plan
Stage I (negative nodes, tumor < 2 cm)	3 courses of A–C
Stage II (positive nodes, tumor < 5 cm)	8 courses of A–C ± radiation therapy
Stage III (tumor > 5 cm, fixed nodes, supraclavicular nodes)	8 courses of A–C ± radiation therapy

Table 2. Arizona breast cancer adjuvant program: drug doses and schedule of chemotherapy[a]

Drug	Dose					
	Day 1	2	3	4	5	6
Adriamycin (mg/M^2 IV)	30	–	–	–	–	–
Cyclophosphamide (mg/M^2 p.o.)	–	–	150	150	150	150

[a] Administered every 3 weeks (3 cycles for stage I; 8 cycles for stages II, III).

The schedule of chemotherapy used for all patients is summarized in Table 2. The individual doses employed in the adjuvant trial are 75% of the "full" doses originally employed in advanced breast cancer. This change was made to minimize acute gastrointestinal side-effects. However, the interval between treatments was reduced from every 4 weeks (in advanced disease) to every 3 weeks in the adjuvant program. Thus, the effective dose rate was the same in our adjuvant and advanced breast cancer protocols. Patients with stage I breast cancer were eligible for our program, but received only three cycles of treatment over 9 weeks based on a presumed minimum number of micrometastases. Patients with stage II breast cancer received eight cycles of A–C over 24 weeks, after which all treatment is discontinued. A subset of stage II patients (particularly those with four or more positive nodes) received regional radiotherapy after the first two cycles of A–C.

Radiotherapy was administered at least 1 week after the second dose of adriamycin, and was delivered to a dose of 4400 rad by linear accelerator to the chest wall, supraclavicular, axillary, and internal mammary nodes [9]. Within 1–2 weeks after completion of radiotherapy, chemotherapy was reinitiated and continued without interruption for the remaining six cycles. Patients with pathologic stage III breast cancer all received eight courses of A–C 11/20 (55%) also received as described above.

Following completion of the adjuvant treatment as described, patients were followed off all therapy. Careful clinical and laboratory reexamination was carried out every 3 months. Repeat bone scans were obtained at 6-month intervals for the Ist year and annually thereafter unless the scan was initially abnormal or had changed with time, in which circumstance more frequent scans were obtained. Relapse was confirmed radiographically in all cases and histologically when possible. Survival and relapse-free survival were calculated by the method of Kaplan and Meier [13] and differences evaluated by the method of Gehan [7].

Results

Between June 1974 and May 1978, 131 eligible patients were entered on this ongoing adjuvant trial. Surgical therapy for stage I and II patients consisted of either a modified radical mastectomy (67%) or radical mastectomy (33%). A few of the stage III patients had a simple mastectomy. The distribution of major prognostic factors for the 79 patients with stage II breast cancer is summarized in Table 3 and is quite comparable to that of patients in other ongoing trials [1, 8]. All patients began chemotherapy within 2 months of surgery. Radiation therapy was administered after two cycles of chemotherapy to 36% of the stage II patients and 55% of the stage III patients. Adjuvant chemotherapy with A–C was quite well tolerated (Table 4). Alopecia was the most common side-effect. Myelosuppression was mild and was essentially limited to leukopenia. Dose reductions were required in only 23% of patients. There were no episodes of sepsis or bacterial infection and severe thrombocytopenia was not observed. Nausea or anorexia with oral cyclophosphamide was reported by about 50% of patients. Cessation of menses and/or hot flashes occurred in 67% of premenopausal patients. Serial studies of cardiac function have not shown evidence of decline in ventricular function.

Therapeutic results for all patients are summarized in Tables 5 and 6. Of 32 stage I patients, none have relapsed, with a median follow-up of 18 months. Of 79 stage II patients, seven have relapsed, with a median follow-up of 22 months. Of 79 stage II patients, seven have relapsed, with a median follow-up of 22 months. Only 2 of the 45 stage IIA patients have relapsed (one premenopausal, one postmenopausal), whereas 5 of 34 stage IIB patients have relapsed (three premenopausal, two postmenopausal). Statistical comparison between the actuarial curves of time to relapse shows advantage for stage IIA patients ($P = 0.04$). Of the 45 stage IIA patients, ten received radiotherapy and have not relapsed. Of the 35 patients who did not receive radiotherapy, two have relapsed. In the stage IIB category only 3 of 25 patients who received radiotherapy have relapsed while 2 of 9 patients who did not receive radiotherapy have relapsed. There is currently no statistical difference between the curves of time to relapse between stage II patients (or stage IIA and IIB subclasses) in relation to whether they received

Table 3. Prognostic factors of 79 stage II breast cancer patients entered on the Arizona adjuvant program

Feature	Percent of patients
Menopausal status	
Premenopausal	29
Postmenopausal	71
Size of primary tumor	
< 2 cm	16
2–5 cm	84
Number of pathologically involved axillary lymph nodes	
1–3 (stage IIA)	57
4 or more (stage IIB)	43
Regional radiotherapy	44

Table 4. Side-effects of A–C adjuvant chemotherapy for stage II breast cancer

Side-effect	Percent
Bacterial infections	0
Overt cardiac toxicity	0
Myelosuppression	
Anemia (requiring transfusion)	0
Thrombocytopenia (platelets < 100,000)	0
Leukopenia	
WBC 2500–4000/mm^3	40
WBC < 2500/mm^3	10
Nausea	67
Alopecia	98
Cessation of menses/hot flashes (in premenopausal patients)	64

Table 5. Arizona breast cancer adjuvant program: preliminary results (July 1974–May 1978)

Tumor stage	Number of patients	Number of relapses (%)	Median follow-up (months)
I	32	0 (0)	18
II	79	7 (9)	22
III	20	11 (55)	29
Total	131		

Table 6. Arizona breast cancer adjuvant program: relation of risk factors to relapse in stage II and III patients (No. of relapses/No. treated [%])

Stage (median follow-up)	Total	Premeno-pausal	Postmeno-pausal	A–C	AC + XRT
IIA[a] (18 mos)	2/45 (4%)	1/11 (9%)	1/34 (3%)	2/35 (6%)	0/10 (0%)
IIB[a] (22 mos)	5/34 (14%)	3/12 (25%)	2/22 (6%)	2/9 (22%)	3/25 (12%)
III (29 mos)	11/20 (55%)	4/9 (44%)	7/11 (64%)	4/9 (44%)	7/11 (64%)

[a] Stage IIA = 1–3 positive nodes; IIB = 4 or more positive axillary lymph nodes.

radiotherapy in addition to chemotherapy ($P = > 0.9$). In the stage III category, 11 of 20 patients have relapsed (55%) with a median follow-up of 29 months. Seven of the 11 stage III relapses were in postmenopausal patients. Relapses occurred in 7 of the 11 stage III patients who received radiotherapy and in 4 of 9 who did not. In view of the relatively high relapse rate in the stage III category, this trial was closed to new entry in July 1977, and a new protocol incorporating tamoxifen along with A–C and radiotherapy was opened.

Discussion

This report provides initial evidence of efficacy of a brief and intensive program of adriamycin-cyclophosphamide therapy for surgical adjuvant therapy of stage II breast cancer. The results indicate lack of early toxicity plus efficacy, which is at least equal and possibly superior to adjuvant trials with melphalan [6] and CMF [1]. The results with our 6-month treatment program are quite similar to those recently presented by BUZDAR et al. [3] who used 2 years of treatment with 5-fluorouracil-adriamycin-cyclophosphamide (FAC) plus BCG. Both studies indicate eqivalent benefit in pre- and postmenopausal patients, suggesting that direct cytocidal effects against breast cancer rather than ovarian suppression account for the results. It is our belief that early use of adriamycin is the major difference between these programs and those of FISHER [6] and BONADONNA [1], which did not include this agent.

We are very much encouraged by the findings that only 7 of 79 of our stage II patients have relapsed thus far with a median follow-up of almost 2 years, with about 75% of the patients off treatment. The finding that four of the seven relapses occurred within 1 year after discontinuation of chemotherapy suggests that with an apparent break in the early relapse curve of our study, this may be the time of greatest risk of recurrence. While we have not yet seen clear evidence of additive efficacy of regional radiotherapy to A–C chemotherapy, additional pathents with substages IIA and IIB will have to be accrued on both the chemotherapy alone and chemotherapy plus radiotherapy arms to reach a definite conclusion on this question. It is too early to make any definite comment on the therapeutic effects of A–C in the stage I patients that we have treated. However, it is encouraging that no relapses have been observed as patients within this group who harbor occult micrometastases after surgery would be predicted to have a very small tumor burden that potentially could be eliminated with a very brief course of treatment. On the other hand, the program of 6 months of A–C plus radiotherapy has proven inadequate in intensity to have major effect on the residual tumor burden and early relapse rate in stage III patients. In fact, 4 of the 11 stage III relapses occurred during adjuvant treatment. For that reason we have sought to intensify treatment with the addition of the cytotoxic antiestrogen tamoxifen [17] for this group of very high risk patients.

To minimize the potential of late cardiax toxicity due to adriamycin, we have limited the total dose to 90 mgm/M^2 in stage I patients and 240 mgm/M^2 in stages II and III breast cancer. However, it is clear that many years of careful surveillance will be required to evaluate potential delayed effects such as subclinical cardiac toxicity and induction of second malignancies by the therapeutic agents utilized. These points are particularly germane to our program for stage I breast cancer patients.

We plan to continue case accrual in our stage I and II patients without modification of the protocol, as large numbers of patients will be the key to the ultimate analysis that will be made in comparison to our own local historical controls as well as the control and treated groups in the other major clinical trials.

One of the additional factors that we have been evaluating in the Arizona adjuvant program has been the diagnostic value of baseline and serial bone scanning for detecting otherwise occult disease at the time of surgery or evidence of early recurrence on serial scans. However, bone scan data alone has not been used to identify patients who relapsed in our study. In our initial analysis recently reported by HAMMOND et al. [10], serial bone scans proved useful in identifying adjuvant patients who subsequently had overt relapse. Our major experience with this phenomenon has been in the 35 stage II and III patients who underwent serial scans. In general, changes in serial scans were predictive of relapse whether the change was one of normalization of an initially equivocal or abnormal scan or development of abnormalities in a previously normal or equivocal scan. In the case of normalization, the change appears likely to reflect tumor mass reduction with A–C of relatively large burdens of otherwise occult disease, whereas the serial development of definite abnormalities was direct evidence of recurrence as could be demonstrated radiologically or by biopsy. Stable bone scans on serial observation were associated with a reduced risk of recurrence (no recurrence among 20 patients followed for a mean time of 20 months after mastectomy). In comparison, 6 patients among 16 patients followed for a mean of 23 months who had serial changes in the appearance of their bone scans have developed overt relapse ($P = 0.01$). Serial use of bone scans should enable us to select a subgroup of patients at high risk of overt recurrence who might benefit from a more intensive or prolonged duration of chemotherapy.

Acknowledgements

The authors wish to thank ELLEN CHASE for editing and data collection and many Tucson surgeons and medical oncologists for their participation in this program. This work was supported in part by a research grant (CA-17094) from the National Cancer Institute, National Institutes of Health, Department of Health, Education, and Welfare.

References

1. Bonadonna, G., Rossi, A., Valagussa, P. et al.: Adjuvant chemotherapy with CMF in breast cancer with positive axillary nodes. In: Adjuvant therapy of cancer. Salmon, S., Jones, S. (eds.), pp. 83–94. Amsterdam: Elsevier/North Holland 1977
2. Bull, J. M., Tormey, D. C., Li, S-H et al.: A randomized comparative trial of Adriamycin versus Methotrexate in combination drug therapy. Cancer *41*, 1649–1657 (1978)
3. Buzdar, A. U., Gutterman, J. V., Blumenschein, G. R. et al.: Intensive postoperative chemoimmunotherapy for patients with stage II and stage III breast cancer. Cancer *41*, 1064–1075 (1978)
4. Corbett, T., Griswold, D., Mayo, J. et al.: Cyclophosphamide-adriamycin combination chemotherapy of transplantable Murine tumors. Cancer Res. *35*, 1568–1573 (1975)
5. Ewy, G., Jones, S., Groves, B.: Adriamycin heart disease. Ariz. Med. *33*, 274–278 (1976)
6. Fisher, B. et al.: L-Phenylalanine Mustard (L-PAM) in the management of primary breast cancer: A report of early findings. New Engl. J. Med. *292*, 117–122 (1975)
7. Gehan, E.: A generalized Wilcoxon test for comparing arbitrarily singly-censored samples. Biometrika *52*, 203–223 (1965)
8. Gutterman, J. V., Cardenas, J. O., Blumenschein, G. R. et al.: Chemoimmunotherapy of advanced breast cancer: Prolongation of remission and survival with BCG. Br. Med. J. *1976 II*, 1222–1225

9. Hammond, N., Jones, S., Salmon, S. et al.: Adjuvant treatment of breast cancer with Adriamycin-Cyclophosphamide with or without radiation therapy. In: Adjuvant therapy of cancer. Salmon, S., Jones, S. (eds.), pp. 153–160. Amsterdam: Elsevier/North Holland 1977
10. Hammond, N., Jones, S., Salmon, S. et al.: Predictive value of bone scans in an adjuvant breast cancer program. Cancer *41,* 138–142 (1978)
11. Jones, S.: Clinical oncology in Arizona. Chemotherapy of breast cancer – investigational treatment. Ariz. Med. *31,* 197–198 (1974)
12. Jones, S., Durie, B., Salmon, S.: Combination chemotherapy with Adriamycin and Cyclophosphamide for advanced breast cancer. Cancer *36,* 90–97 (1975)
13. Kaplan, E., Meier, P.: Non-parametric estimations from incomplete observations. J. Am. Stat. Assoc. *53,* 457–481 (1958)
14. Salmon, S. E.: Progress in adjuvant chemotherapy in early breast cancer. Ariz. Med. *32,* 108–109 (1975)
15. Salmon, S. E.: Kinetic rationale for adjuvant chemotherapy of cancer. In: adjuvant therapy of cancer. Salmon, S., Jones, S. (eds.), pp. 3–14. Amsterdam: Elsevier/North Holland 1977
16. Salmon, S. E.: Kinetics of minimal residual disease. In: Adjuvant Therapies and Markers of Post-Surgical Minimal Residual Disease I. Bonadonna, G., Mathé, G., Salmon, S. E. (eds.), RRCR *67,* pp. 5–15. Berlin, Heidelberg, New York: Springer 1979
17. Tormey, D. C., Simon, R. C., Lippman, M. E. et al.: Evaluation of Tamoxifen dose in advanced breast cancer: a progress report. Cancer Treat. Rep. *60,* 1451–1459 (1976)

Results of a Randomized Trial of Prophylactic Chemotherapy in T_3-T_4 Breast Cancer Patients Previously Treated by Radiotherapy

B. Serrou, H. Sancho-Garnier, P. Cappelaere, R. Plagne, R. Metz, M. Schneider, P. Chollet, M. Namer, H. Pujol, J. Gary-Bobo, G. Meyer, and G. Mathé

Introduction

The goal of this study was to evaluate results obtained with complementary chemotherapy administered to women with locally evolved breast cancer compared with those obtained in patients receiving simple immunotherapy or no complementary treatment. This study was undertaken in April 1975, before the first results of FISHER [4, 5] and BONADONNA [1] were published. The focus of this study is based on the choice of local treatment i.e., radiotherapy. In addition, the study includes a group undergoing no complementary treatment (for at least part of this study) and 75 patients in menopause. The results, although early, favor the use of complementary chemotherapy.

Patients, Material, and Methods

Participating Centers

Five anti-cancer centers participated in this trial: Clermont-Ferrand (12 patients), Lille (30 patients), Montpellier (19 patients), Nancy (10 patients), and Nice (9 patients).

Choice of Patients

The patients chosen were T3 and T4 (TNM classification) breast tumor-bearing women without regard to lymph node involvement. They were less than 70 years old and had not received any previous treatment; 59 patients were classified as having adenocarcinoma, as having 6 undifferentiated tumors, 1 atypical case, 7 with positive cytology and 1 with epithelioma of unspecified origin. No significant difference could be shown among the three randomized groups. Tumors in 47 patients were grade T3 and in 32 were grade T4: no significant difference was observed among the three randomized groups.

Primary Lesion Treatment

All patients in this trial were submitted to radiotherapy following a protocol prepared by each center. Surgery, when necessary, was a function of the residual mass and was untertaken as follows: in the first group without complementary treatment (22 patients), two axillary lymph node excisions, two mastectomies, and six mastectomies associated with lymph node dissection; in the group receiving chemotherapy (29 patients), one axillary lymph node dissection and ten mastectomies associated with lymph node dissection; and in the immunotherapy group (29 patients), eight mastectomies associated with lymph node dissection. No statistically significant difference could be established among these groups.

Randomization

Following locoregional treatment, the patients were randomized into three groups. The first group received no complementary treatment. The second group was submitted to adjuvant chemotherapy, i.e., vincristine (1 mg/m^2 IV) on days 1 and 2, cyclophosphamide (300 mg/m^2 IV), and 5-fluorouracil (400 mg/m^2 IV) on days 3, 4, 5, and 6. This cyclic chemotherapy was repeated once a month over a 12-month period. The third group was submitted to immunotherapy (150 mg fresh BCG from the Institut Pasteur) administered once a week either by scarification or by the heaf-gun technique. In addition, 150 mg BCG was given PO. Immunotherapy was maintained for 1 year. In all cases, the complementary treatment was initiated 4 weeks after the end of radiotherapy.

Evaluation Criteria

The following criteria were employed: the number of relapses, the number of metastases, length of disease-free interval, toxicity, and survival time.

Patient Distribution by Menopausal Status

Of 80 patients, 20 were premenopausal, with no significant difference among the three groups; 60 patients were in a natural or artificial postmenopausal state. No significant difference was noted among the three groups.

Follow-up

All patients were followed for at least 1 year.

Results (Fig. 1)

Eighty-two patients were randomized into three groups: 22 patients in the abstention group and 29 patients in each of the chemotherapy and immunotherapy groups. The smallest number of patients was in the abstention group because this group was halted in 1976 after review of the results presented by Bonadonna [1]. Two patients were excluded from the study: one patient because she was treated by chemotherapy after 3 months of immunotherapy; and one patient from the abstention group who was mistakely treated by chemotherapy at 3 months.

Among the patients actually undergoing treatment, in the immunotherapy group (29 patients), two refused treatment. For these two patients no evolution was noted at 14 and 18 months, respectively. In the chemotherapy group (29 patients), two refused treatment after two cycles: one is in an evolutionary period after 15 months and one is nonevolutionary at 19 months; two patients died without relapse, one in acute respiratory failure and one of a cerebrovascular accident. These patients were not excluded from the analysis.

In the abstention group, 9 of 22 patients are in evolution after 1 year (i.e., 41%). In the immunotherapy group, 12 of 29 patients are in evolution (i.e., 41%). In the chemotherapy

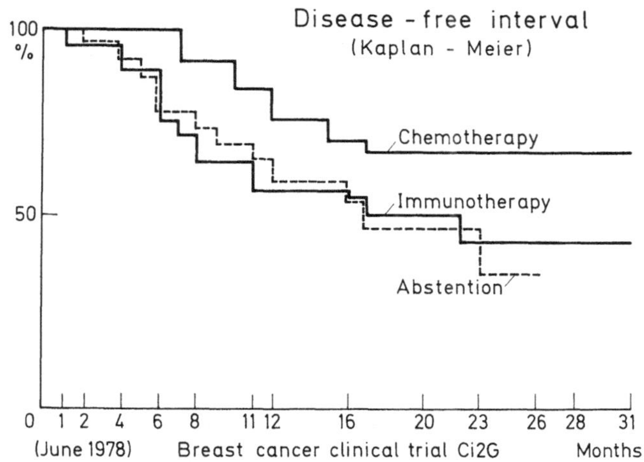

Fig. 1. Results of breast cancer clinical trial

group, 5 of 26 patients are in evolution after 1 year (i.e., 19%); two patients died within 6 months due to intercurrent causes. The difference between the chemotherapy group and the abstention and immunotherapy groups is significant ($P < 0.05$ and $P > 0.03$). Nevertheless, if the entire curve is considered, the values are not significantly different at 36 months, but it is noted that only 36% of the abstention group are free of relapse compared to 68% in the chemotherapy group. No major toxicity was noted for any patient in the study.

Discussion

This study demonstrates the value of adjuvant chemotherapy for patients with evolutionary breast tumors in stages T3 and T4 after previous treatment by locoregional irradiation. However, the results do not yet affirm whether this is a temporary retardation or a long-lasting effect on survival time. These results are very similar to those recently presented in the literature concerning therapy following locoregional surgical treatment [1–5, Chapts. 31 and 37 this book]. This is the first published trial showing any value of chemotherapy following radiotherapy in the treatment of breast cancer patients with no metastases. In addition, 75% of the patients treated were menopausal (natural or artificial). Our results support those of Fisher [4, 5] and Bonadonna [1] at 1 year for postmenopausal women. One important question remains to be dealt with i.e., whether our results will decrease over time. The results at 36 months, although not yet significant, still leave room for future confirmation.
BCG immunotherapy was completely ineffective in this group of patients. Even so, BCG did not make the prognosis worse than that of the abstention group. The inefficacy of BCG can possibly be explained by the fact that the disease remaining after radiotherapy is too extensive to judge the effectiveness of this therapy [6]. In addition, due to the size of tumor mass these patients are immunodepressed and should probably be restored to immunologic competence before being stimulated. The recent results of Rojas et al. [7], using levamisole after radiotherapy for the same tumor stage, supports this argument. All these hypotheses could explain the effectiveness of a complementary chemoimmunotherapy 3 and Chapt. 37 this book.

In summary, adjuvant chemotherapy of evolved breast tumors (T3 and T4) previously treated by radiotherapy appears to yield encouraging results significant after 1 year, which is our minimum observation time for all the patients. Only a longer follow-up will allow us to confirm or reject these promising preliminary results.

References

1. Bonadonna, G., Rossi, A., Valagussa, P., Banfi, A., Veronesi, U.: The CMF program for operable breast cancer with positive axillary nodes. Cancer *39,* 2904–2915 (1977)
2. Bonadonna, G., Valagussa, P., Rossi, A., Veronesi, U.: Improvement of disease-free and overall survival by adjuvant CMF in operable breast cancer. Proc. AACR *19,* 215 (1978) (Abs. 860)
3. Buzdar, A. U., Gutterman, J. U., Blumenschein, G. R., Hortobagyi, G. N., Tashima, C. K., Smith, T. L., Hersh, E. M., Freireich, E. J., Gehan, E. A.: Intensive post-operative chemoimmunotherapy for patients with stage II and stage III breast cancer. Cancer *41,* 1064–1075 (1978)
4. Fisher, B., Slack, N., Katrych, D., Wolmark, N.: Ten year follow-up results of patients with carcinoma of the breast in a co-operative clinical trial evaluating surgical adjuvant chemotherapy. Surg. Gynecol. Obstet. *140,* 529–534 (1975)
5. Fisher, B., Carbone, P., Economov, S. G., Frelick, R., Glass, A., Lerner, H., Redmond, C., Zelen, M., Band, P., Katrych, D. L., Wolmark, N., Fisher, E. R.: L-phenylalanine mustard in the management of primary breast cancer. N. Engl. J. Med. *292,* 117–126 (1975)
6. Mathé, G.: Cancer active immunotherapy. Recent Results Cancer Res. (1976)
7. Rojas, A. J., Feierstein, J. N., Glait, H. M., Oliveri, A. J.: Levamisole action in breast cancer stage III. In: Immunotherapy of cancer: present status of trials in man. Terry, W. D., Windhorst, D. (eds.), p. 635. New York: Raven Press 1977

Four Drug Combination Cytotoxic Chemotherapy Following Surgery for Breast Cancer

G. A. Edelstyn, I. S. Bates, D. Brinkley, K. D. MacRae, H. Spittle, and T. Wheeler

Introduction

There have been many studies designed to lead to an improvement in the prognosis for patients with breast cancer. Every branch of therapeutics has been investigated including surgical techniques, post- and pre-operative radiotherapy, oophorectomy, other endocrine procedures both ablative and additive, non-specific immunostimulation and the addition of systemic cytoxic drugs. The Multicentre Cancer Chemotherapy Group present the following data in a series of 247 patients treated with vincristine, cyclophosphamide, methotrexate and 5-fluorouracil.

Method

A prospective randomized clinical trial was started in 1975 in which 247 patients from 18 hospitals were entered. All patients had stage II adenocarcinoma of the breast with histologically proven metastases in the axillary nodes. Clinically the patients were T1 or T2, N1A or N1B, Mo. None of the patients were older than 70 years. All patients admitted to the trial had primary treatment that was intended to be curative in conventional terms. The surgery was either a simple mastectomy with axillary node sampling or modified radical mastectomy. Most patients had post-operative radiotherapy. The data on the value of post-operative irradiation will be available later. The work at the Mayo Clinic suggests that radiation still has a place of importance in reducing local recurrence of disease even when chemotherapy is given [2].
Each referring hospital was issued with a set of random allocation envelopes, the subsequent data was collected, stored and analysed centrally by the Secretariat in Belfast and statistical examination was performed by one member of the group (Mac Rae). Random allocation to receive chemotherapy or to be a control was made at the completion of primary treatment.
The chemotherapy that was given had been designed in a series of earlier studies in advanced disease [4, 5] and is listed in Table 1. Treatment was given by rapid intravenous injection. If

Table 1. Chemotherapy regimen

Cyclophosphamide	300 mg
Vincristine	0.65 mg
5-Fluorouracil	500 mg
4–6 clear days later	
Cyclophosphamide	300 mg
Vincristine	0.65 mg
Methotrexate	37.5 mg

the patient weighed less than 54 kg the dose of cyclophosphamide was reduced to 200 mg and methotrexate to 25 mg. The first injection of cytotoxic drugs was given within 10 weeks of operation. The paired injections were given each month for 6 months.

Results

The early results are given in Tables 2 and 3, 2 years after multi-modal therapy for stage II breast cancer. Of those given chemotherapy, 77.5% were alive and free from recurrence compared to 60% of the controls. Six of the 247 patients have died from breast cancer, four had had chemotherapy and two were controls.

These results are early and the unique demonstration of apparent success in the post-menopausal patients may disappear in line with the findings of BONADONNA et al. [3] and FISHER et al. [6] and AHMANN et al. [2].

Table 2. Survival free from recurrence (%) (as of 31. 1. 78), age up to 49 years

Months	Chemotherapy (51)	SE	Control (42)	SE
6	96	2.8	87.5	5.2
12	89.3	4.5	66.7	7.6
18	79.6	6.7	66.7	7.6
24	59.8	11.4	56.8	9.1

Table 3. Survival free from recurrence (%) (as of 31. 1. 78), age 50–70 years

Months	Chemotherapy (73)	SE	Control (81)	SE
6	97.2	2.0	96.3	2.1
12	90.9	3.6	74.0	5.2
18	90.9	3.6	65.6	6.1
24	90.9	3.6	61.9	6.8

Toxicity

In general the treatment was well-tolerated by the patients, 11 of whom did not complete six courses. In no patient did the haemaglobin fall below 10 G, the WBC fell below 2.4×10^9/liter in one, and the platelets below 100×10^9/liter in one other. The recorded toxic symptoms in the 124 patients given chemotherapy are shown in Table 4.

In 4 of the 11 patients who did not have 6 months treatment it was because of complications, severe neuropathy, stomatitis and severe nausea. Two patients refused treatment after one and two courses, respectively. In one patient treatment was stopped because of intercurrent disease. In four the information is not available. The toxic effects of treatment are in accord with the findings of AHMANN [2], BONADONNA [3] and FISHER [6].

Table 4. Toxic symptoms in 124 patients given

VCF/VCM symptom	No. of patients
Severe nausea	11
Nausea	32
Mild stomatitis	3
Severe diarrhoea	1
Severe neurological symptoms	1
Some neuropathy	4
Slight hair loss	7
Complete hair loss	3

Discussion

The best adjuvant therapy is not necessarily the most effective but the one that most patients can accept and is effective. Treatment is still directed towards patients with a large residual tumour burden after surgery and is therefore only relatively effective. Four in this series of 124 patients given chemotherapy have died within 2 years of diagnosis from uncontrolled disease. Bonadonna [3] has suggested increasing the treatment to be given to postmenopausal patients.

The Multicentre group has plans to increase the number of courses of treatment to be given and to re-design the form of treatment in line with the suggestions of Norton and Simon [7]. The aim will be to maintain the level of toxicity to the present standard but to test the theoretical improvement in tumour cell killing by re-scheduling the prescription of the standard drugs with a boost in dose at the end of the cycle. There is no question about this; adjuvant cytotoxic chemotherapy is toxic, but almost any effective medical treatment carries a risk of side-effects. Vomiting, anorexia and epilation are seriously resented for themselves and because the symptoms recur and are aggravated by each course of treatment.

Endocrine treatment will be added to post-operative chemotherapy in certain subsets of patients. Currently the Multicentre Group has a sequential study with tamoxifen after cytotoxics. The question of the cytotoxic effects on the ovary accounting for the preferential effect in premenopausal patients must be resolved. In Cambridge we are measuring the effect of this form of cytotoxic treatment on the levels of serum luteinising hormone (LH) and follicular stimulating hormone (FSH) and the urine oestrogens excretion, to re-examine more critically the studies by Rose and Davis [8]. This data will be available shortly.

Finally, regarding the question of controlled trials, with the relative ineffectiveness of current cytotoxic therapy, it is important to assess the treatment of relapse in the context of those patients who have already been exposed to these drugs as an adjuvant programme. The Mayo Clinic has already recorded its findings that early introduction of cytotoxic drugs in the management of advanced disease in premenopausal patients after oophorectomy was advantageous. Delaying the use of chemotherapy led to a worse prognosis [1].

If the early introduction of cytotoxics denies stage II patients the benefits of intensive treatment in relapse, this very important factor will have to be assessed by further detailed trials to devise worthwhile primary treatment. The first steps in the treatment of residual disease after surgery for breast cancer have been made but there are many more studies to be investigated.

Summary

A prospective randomized clinical trial of treatment with vincristine, cyclophosphamide, methotrexate and 5-fluorouracil after conventional curative treatment for stage II breast cancer is described. The results at 2 years are recorded together with details of toxicity. Future plans are discussed briefly.

Acknowledgement

We wish to acknowledge the participation of all the collaborators in this study, the co-ordinator Dr. Erica Mansbacher and the support of Action Cancer in Belfast.

References

1. Ahmann, D. L., O'Connell, M. J., Hahn, R. G., Bisel, H. F., Lee, R. A., Edmonson, J. H.: An evaluation of early or delayed adjuvant chemotherapy in premenopausel patients with advanced breast cancer undergoing oophorectomy. New Engl. J. Med. *297,* 356–360 (1977)
2. Ahmann, D. L., Scanlon, P. W., Bisel, H. F., Edmonson, J. H., Frytak, S., Payne, W. S., O'Fallon, J. R., Hahn, R. J., Ingle, J. N., O'Connell, M. J., Rubin, J.: Repeated adjuvant chemotherapy with Phenyl-alanine mustard, or 5-Fluorouracil, Cyclophosphamide and Prednisone with or without radiation after mastectomy for breast cancer. Lancet *1978/I,* 893–896
3. Bonadonna, G., Rossi, A., Valagussa, P., Banfi, A., Veronesi, U.: The CMF program for operable breast cancer with positive axillary nodes. Cancer *39,* 2904–2915 (1977)
4. Edelstyn, G. A., Bates, T. S., Brinkley, D., Macrae, K. D., Spittle, M., Wheeler, T.: Comparison of 5-day, 1-day and 2-day cyclical combination chemotherapy in advanced breast cancer. Lancet *1975/II,* 209–211
5. Edelstyn, G. A., Bates, T. S., Brinkley, D., Macrae, K. D., Spittle, M., Wheeler, T.: Short-course cyclical chemotherapy in advanced breast cancer. Lancet *1977/I,* 592
6. Fisher, B., Glass, A., Redmond, C., Fisher, E. R., Barton, B., Such, E., Carbone, P., Economou, S., Foster, R., Frelick, R., Lerner, H., Levitt, M., Margolese, R., Mac Farlane, J., Plotkin, D., Shibata, H., Volk, H.: L Phenyalanine mustard (L-PAM) in the management of primary breast cancer. Cancer *39,* 2883–2903 (1977)
7. Norton, L., Simon, R.: Tumour size and sensitivity to therapy and design of treatment schedules. Cancer Treat. Rep. *61,* 1307–1317 (1977)
8. Rose, D. P., Davis, T. E.: Ovarian function in patients receiving adjuvant chemotherapy for breast cancer. Lancet *1977/I,* 1174–1176

Pilot Study on Adjuvant Chemotherapy and Hormonal Therapy for Irradiated Inoperable Breast Cancer

C. Schaake, E. Engelsman, and E. Hamersma

Introduction

Adjuvant therapy for breast cancer has produced encouraging preliminary results in recent years [1, 2, 5]. Inoperable patients having a very poor prognosis were selected for a pilot study employing intensive chemotherapy. Inoperability has been well-defined in our institute since 1956 [3, 6]. Patients with inoperable breast cancer treated by locoregional irradiation show a 10-year survival of less than 5%. Distant metastasis is generally the cause of death. This group of patients seemed highly eligible for adjuvant systemic treatment since virtually all patients have occult metastatic disease. It might be expected that improvement both of the relapse-free interval and the overall survival should be apparent rather quickly. The pilot study was started in 1975.

Patients and Methods

All patients in this study had inoperable breast cancer without evidence of generalized disease. Screening procedures included physical examination, blood tests, X-ray mammography, chest X-ray, and bone scan. The conclusion of inoperability rested on either of two reasons:

1. Inoperability because of local criteria [6];
2. Inoperability because of a positive apical axillary lymph node biopsy [3].

In both groups local tumor control was achieved for the majority of patients by megavoltage radiotherapy. The breast and regional lymph nodes were irradiated. The applied dose was 4000 rad in 3 weeks, followed by a booster of 1500 rad in five fractions. With this treatment schedule the 2½-year survival is 50%; 20% will survive 5 years. The 10-year survival is less than 5% due to generalized disease. Because of this poor prognosis, it seemed justified to apply intensive chemotherapy as an adjuvant treatment for 1 year. Cycling intermittent chemotherapy as an adjuvant treatment for 1 year. Cycling intermittent chemotherapy consisting of CMF and ADM-VCR combinations given alternatingly plus tamoxifen was effective in about 70% of patients with disseminated breast cancer (EORTC protocol 10741) [4]. Table 1 shows the applied doses in the pilot study. If necessary individual adjustments were made. Patients had to be in a good general condition and had to be less than 68 years of age. Adriamycin applied shortly after radiotherapy raised toxicity problems in almost all patients. There was a relapse of the radiation reaction of the skin. More severe fibrosis of the subcutaneous tissues and the pectoral muscles was seen. Rib fractures were frequent. We did not see cardiotoxicity nor severe radiation pneumonia. Because of the complications, adriamycin and vincristine were dropped after 1 year. We continued to give CMF monthly plus tamoxifen.

Table 1. Dose schedule for the pilot study. (28-day cycle)

Regimen	Dose
Adriamycin	60 mg/m^2 on day 1
Vincristine	1.4 mg/m^2 on days 1 and 8
Cyclophosphamide	100 mg/m^2 on days 1–14
Methotrexate	15 mg/m^2 on days 1 and 8
5-Fluorouracil	400 mg/m^2 on days 1 and 8
Tamoxifen	30 mg daily

Table 2. Classification of the treated and control groups according to age and menopausal status

	Treated group	Control group
Number	59	53
Age (mean)	52	66
Premenopausal	27	5
Postmenopausal	32	48

Meanwhile the radiotherapy was changed 4000 rad in 4 weeks instead of 3; the booster was reduced to 5–7 × 200 rad. Special attention was paid to the overlapping areas of the fields. After 2 years the pilot study was closed. Fifty-nine patients had been admitted for treatment. A "control" group was formed by 53 patients irradiated in about the same period. They did not receive adjuvant therapy either because of their age or general condition, because they lived too far away, or because of social or psychologic reasons, or refusal. This group was treated with relevant therapy when metastases appeared.

A summary of findings concerning age and menopausal status is presented in Table 2. The pilot study has the following drawbacks limiting definite conclusions:

1. Different treatment schedules in the treated group (code name ACTAL)
2. A questionable control group (nonrandomized)

Patients were seen for follow-up every 3 months after treatment. Physical examination and blood tests were done every 3 months, bone scan and chest X-ray every 6 months. Once a year mammography was performed. CEA levels were monitored.

Results and Discussion

Actuarially expressed, the results as of May 1978 are illustrated in Figs. 1–4. The number of premenopausal patients without evidence of disease is significantly higher in the treated group ($P = 0.0016$) (Fig. 1). The number of recurrence-free postmenopausal patients is not significantly higher than in the control group ($P = 0.10$) (Fig. 2). After correction for the small

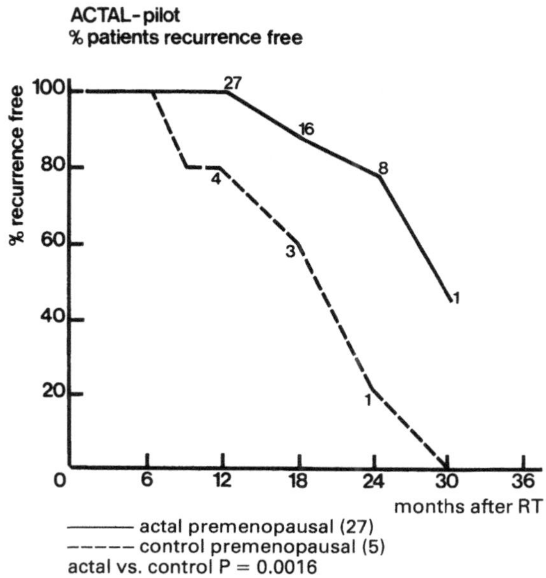

Fig. 1. Actuarial curves of recurrence-free interval in premenopausal inoperable irradiated breast cancer patients; adjuvant therapy (Actal) vs. control

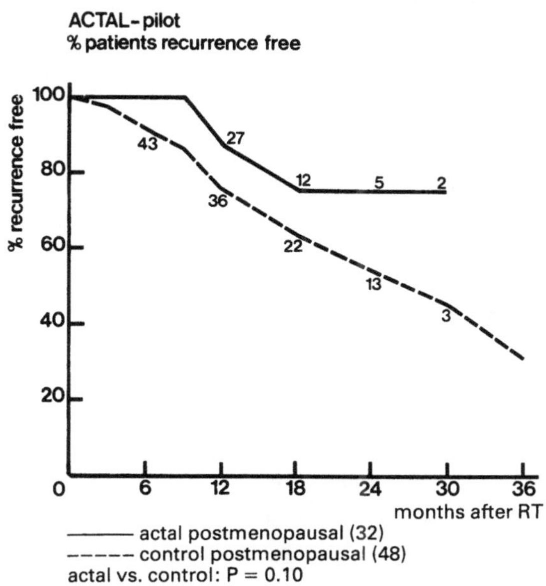

Fig. 2. Actuarial curves of recurrence-free interval in postmenopausal inoperable irradiated breast cancer patients; adjuvant therapy (ACTAL) vs. control

number of premenopausal patients in the control group, the proportion of recurrence-free patients is significantly higher for the treated group as a whole than in the untreated group ($P = 0.0040$). So far there is no significant difference in survival between the treated and the untreated groups ($P = 0.30$ after correction for the small number of premenopausal patients in the control group). There seems to be a suggestion of a plateau phase for the treated groups (Figs. 3 and 4).

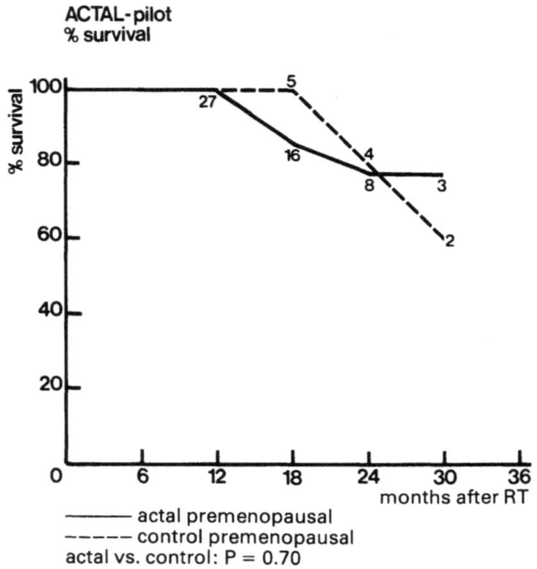

Fig. 3. Actuarial curves of survival in premenopausal inoperable irradiated breast cancer patients; adjuvant therapy (ACTAL) vs. control

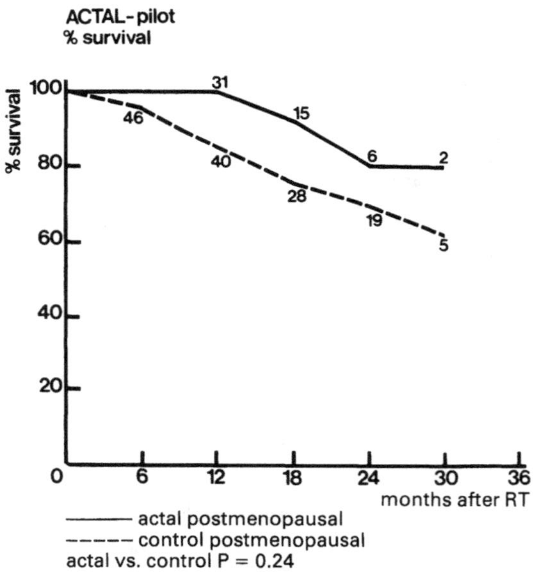

Fig. 4. Actuarial curves of survival in postmenopausal inoperable irradiated breast cancer patients; adjuvant therapy (ACTAL) vs. control

Treating inoperable breast cancer patients with adjuvant therapy has no risk of overtreatment. On the other hand, a number of these patients will have so great a tumor load that they will reveal metastases during treatment or soon afterward. The absence of improvement in survival might be due to the fact that we found it very difficult if not impossible to select adequate therapy for the pilot study patients after relapse. It is possible that improvement in the survival will become evident when the relapse-free survival continues to be longer. Monitoring CEA levels proved useful in predicting generalized disease: a steady increase in CEA levels was sometimes seen 6 months before metastasis could be detected.

Table 3. Randomized controlled clinical trial of adjuvant therapy for inoperable breast cancer

Group 1:	Radiotherapy
Group 2:	Radiotherapy + CMF + tamoxifen for 1 year
Group 3:	ADR | VCR || CMF – 2 cycles – radiotherapy – ADR | VCR || CMF – 4 cycles + tamoxifen from the beginning of treatment

In July 1977, we started a randomized controlled clinical trial with three groups (Table 3). The dose of adriamycin is reduced in the first and second cycle after radiotherapy. The radiation dose is limited to 4000 rad in 4 weeks without booster; no bolus is used. No severe complications have been seen until now in the 30 patients entered in the trial.

Summary

A pilot study of adjuvant chemotherapy and hormonal therapy for inoperable breast cancer was performed. The patients were known to have a bad prognosis because of occult generalized disease. At the time of first treatment, the patients selected showed no signs of systemic disease. Local control of the breast and regional lymph nodes was achieved by radiotherapy. Adjuvant therapy consisted of alternating chemotherapy and tamoxifen. Adriamycin was dropped from the treatment schedule after 1 year because of enhanced radiation side-effects. Meanwhile the radiotherapy schedule was changed. A questionable control group was formed by patients radiated in the same period who failed to meet the entry criteria for various reasons.

At presents, patients in the treated group show a better relapse-free survival than patients in the control group. The difference is statistically significant for premenopausal women. There is no significant difference in the overall survival between the treated group and the control group after an average follow-up of 2 years. After 2 years, the pilot study was closed. A randomized controlled clinical trial was started. In one group of this trial intensive chemotherapy is the first treatment employed.

References

1. Bonadonna, G., Brusamolino, Valagussa, P. et al.: Combination chemotherapy as an adjuvant treatment in operable breast cancer. N. Engl. J. Med. *294*, 405–410 (1976)
2. Bonadonna, J. et al.: The CMF program for operable breast cancer with positive axillary nodes. Cancer *39*, 2904–2915 (1977)
3. van Dongen, J. A.: Subclavicular biopsy as a guideline for the treatment of breast cancer. World J. Surg. *1*, 306–308 (1977)
4. Engelsman, E.: Current EORTC trials. In: Breast cancer: Trends in research and treatment. pp. 217–223. New York: Raven Press 1976
5. Fisher, B., Carbone, P., Economov, S. J. et al.: [-Phenylalanine mustard (L-PAM)] in the management of primary breast cancer: A report of early findings. N. Engl. J. Med. *292*, 117–122 (1975)
6. Haagensen, C. D.: Diseases of the breast. Philadelphia: W. B. Saunders 1971

Ovarian Irradiation and Prednisone Following Surgery and Radiotherapy for Carcinoma of the Breast

J. W. Meakin, W. E. C. Allt, F. A. Beale, R. S. Bush, R. M. Clark, P. J. Fitzpatrick, N. V. Hawkins, R. D. T. Jenkin, J. F. Pringle, J. G. Reid, and W. D. Rider

Introduction

Because some recurrent breast cancers regress following therapeutic castration, several clinical trials have been carried out to test the value of prophylactic ovarian ablation as part of primary treatment. In the Manchester Trial, [2] ovarian irradiation (450 rad in one fraction), in premenopausal patients with histologically negative and positive axillary nodes, delayed the appearance of distant metastases ($P = 0.04$) but did not significantly prolong survival ($P =$ 0.07 at 10 years. In the Oslo Trial, [5] ovarian irradiation (1000 rad in six daily fractions), in premenopausal (histologically positive axillary nodes) and postmenopausal (histologically negative and positive axillary nodes) patients, delayed recurrence and also prolonged survival at 7 years but the differences were small. In the Trial of the National Surgical Adjuvant Breast Group, [6] oophorectomy did not result in a significant delay in recurrence nor prolongation in survival during 3–5 years of follow-up in premenopausal patients who had either histologically negative or positive axillary nodes. Because of the ambiguity resulting from these trials, the following study was begun in 1965 to test the hypothesis that prophylactic ovarian irradiation, with or without prednisone, could not only delay recurrence but also prolong survival.

Materials and Methods

From 1965 to 1972, following mastectomy, premenopausal and postmenopausal patients, aged 35–70 years, with or without histologically positive axillary nodes, received irradiation to the chest wall and regional nodal areas. They were then randomized to receive no further treatment (NT), or ovarian irradiation to a dose of 2000 rad in 5 days (R), or (if 45 years or more) ovarian irradiation in the same dosage plus prednisone, 7.5 mg daily (R + P) for up to 5 years. Patients, entered on study, have been followed for up to 10 years. Patients were considered premenopausal if their last menses had occurred within 6 months of the date of surgery. Patients who had had a hysterectomy, but not an oophorectomy, were considered premenopausal up to the age of 50 years. The generalized Wilcoxan test [4] has been used to determine the significance of differences in the results.

Results

Of 779 randomized patients 23 were ineligible by protocol and are omitted from all analyses. An additional 51 patients were eligible by protocol but did not receive the randomly assigned treatment; analyses of the data with or without these patients included has not affected the results. Therefore, the following data relate to 705 randomized patients who were eligible by protocol and did receive the assigned treatment as of May 1977.

For reporting the data, the patients are divided into three groups: (a) premenopausal less than 45 years of age, (b) premenopausal 45 years or more in age, and (c) postmenopausal.

Premenopausal Patients Less Than 45 Years of Age

In this group (35—44 years), clinical stages (TNM) I, II, and III were entered and were randomized only between NT and R. The two groups were comparable for age and stage. Histologically positive axillary lymph nodes were identified in 83% of the NT group and in 91% of the R group.

In Figures 1 and 2 the recurrence-free and survival curves (actuarial) are presented. Numbers of patients followed to specific times are recorded on the graphs. While there is a persistent

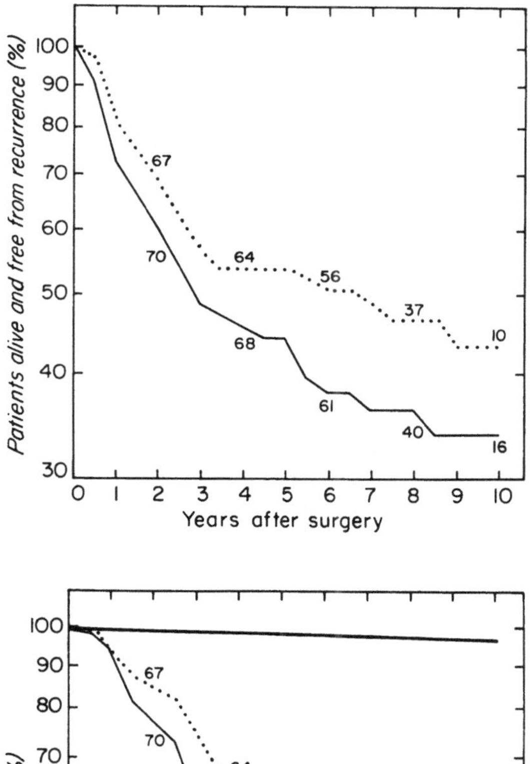

Fig. 1. Premenopausal patients less than 45 years. NT (70 patients) ———; R (67 patients) · · · · ·; (NT *vs* R; $P = 0.13$). No. of patients followed to specific times are recorded on the graphs

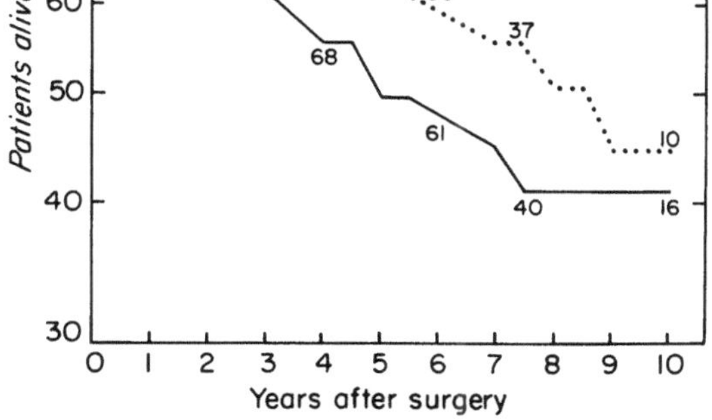

Fig. 2. Premenopausal patients less than 45 years. NT (70 patients) ———; R (67 patients) · · · · ·; (NT *vs* R; $P = 0.19$). Natural survival for age range shown in heavy line at top. No. of patients followed to specific times are recorded on the graphs

delay in recurrence and prolongation of survival, the differences are not statistically significant ($P = 0.13$ for Fig. 1 and $P = 0.19$ for Fig. 2). Separate analyses of the histologically node-positive patients only from Figs. 1 and 2 reveals a similar degree of delay in recurrence and improvement in survival between the NT and R groups as follows: (a) Fig. 1, $P = 0.12$; (b) Fig. 2, $P = 0.17$.

Premenopausal Patients 45 Years or More

In this group clinical stages (TNM) I, II, and III were randomized between NT, R, or R + P. The three groups were comparable for age and stage. Histologically positive axillary nodes

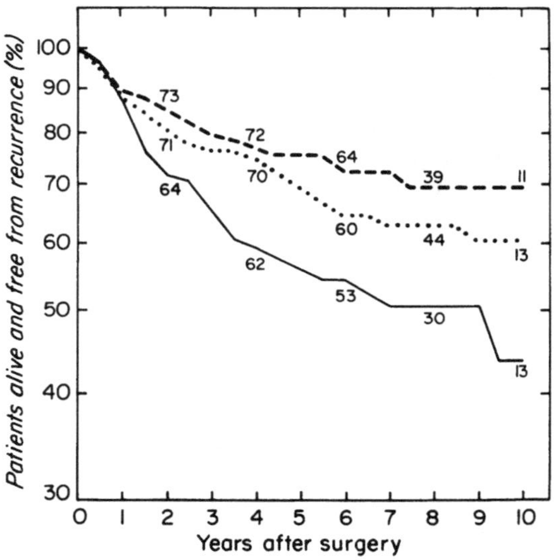

Fig. 3. Premenopausal patients 45 years or more. NT (64 patients) ——; R (71 patients) ·····; R + P (73 patients) – – – –; (NT *vs* R; $P = 0.18$; NT *vs* R + P; $P = 0.02$; R *vs* R + P; $P = 0.31$). No. of patients followed to specific times are recorded on the graphs

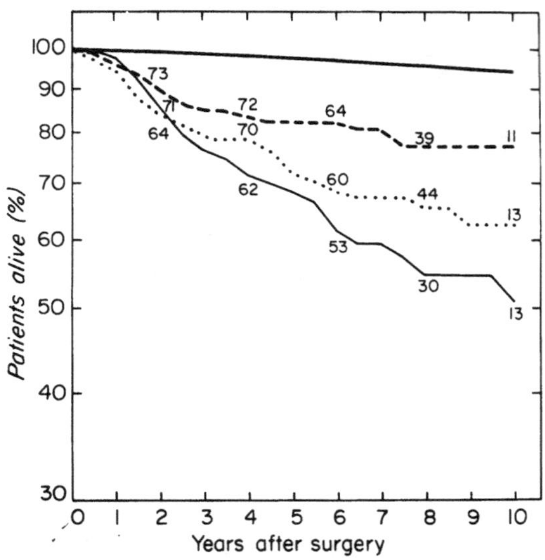

Fig. 4. Premenopausal patients 45 years or more. NT (64 patients) ——; R (71 patients) ·····; R + P (73 patients) – – – –; (NT *vs* R; $P = 0.44$; NT *vs* R + P; $P = 0.02$; R *vs* R + P; $P = 0.11$). Natural survival for age range shown in heavy line at top. No. of patients followed to specific times are recorded on the graphs

were identified as follows: NT, 69%; R, 66%; R + P, 71%. The actuarial recurrence-free and survival curves are shown in Figs. 3 and 4. Numbers of patients, followed to specific times, are recorded on the graphs. In Fig. 3 while R and R + P delay recurrence, only R + P does so to a statistically significant degree (NT versus R + P, $P = 0.02$). In Fig. 4 R and R + P prolong survival, but only R + P does so significantly over the NT group ($P = 0.02$). If only the patients with histologically positive axillary nodes from Figs. 3 and 4 are analyzed, the significance of the differences between the NT and R + P groups decreases to: (a) Fig. 3, $P = 0.04$; (b) Fig. 4, $P = 0.06$.

Postmenopausal Patients

No differences in time to recurrence nor in survival could be demonstrated between the NT, R, and R + P groups.

Discussion

These data are in agreement with the Manchester [2] and Oslo [5] Trials in demonstrating an apparent delay in recurrence and prolongation of survival after adjuvant ovarian irradiation alone, but were not statistically significant in this study. The lack of agreement with the results of the NSABP [6] Trial of prophylactic oophorectomy is possibly the effect of chance or that an irradiated ovary may result in a different physiologic state from that after a surgical oophorectomy. Alternatively, further follow-up data from the NSABP [6] Trial may demonstrate some value for surgical oophorectomy, for it may be noted that the effect of ovarian ablation in our study did not become firm until after 3–5 years of follow-up.

However, the data of this study indicate that the addition of small doses of prednisone to ovarian irradiation produces significant delay in recurrence and prolongation in survival in premenopausal patients. Whether the prednisone produced its effect by suppressing estrogen of adrenal origin or by some other mechanism is not known. Other possible mechanisms include a reduction in prolactin secretion (perhaps mediated by reduced estrogen production), immunologic factors, or direct antitumor effects. Again it is emphasized that the effect of ovarian irradiation plus prednisone did not become definite until after 3 years of follow-up.

One of the important features of these data is that ovarian ablation and prednisone were effective in premenopausal patients with histologically positive axillary nodes to a degree comparable to the published data for adjuvant melphalan [3] and CMF [1] (cyclophosphamide, methotrexate, 5-fluorouracil) in premenopausal patients. Thus, it would seem rational in future studies to examine the role of adjuvant hormonal therapy, both as a complement to and as an alternative to adjuvant chemotherapy.

Summary

Following surgery and regional radiotherapy for operable carcinoma of the breast in premenopausal women, ovarian irradiation (2000 rad in five daily fractions) plus prednisone (7.5 mg per day) results in delayed recurrence and prolonged survival.

Acknowledgement

We are indebted to the many surgeons who agreed to the entry of their patients into this study, to Drs. A. Phillips, A. Sellers, and G. DeBoer for their biostatistical help, to Drs. A. Alaton and the late Dr. E. Kruyff for their assistance in the clinical assessment of patients, and to the clinical trial secretaries who helped monitor the study. This study was supported by the Ontario Cancer Treatment and Research Foundation and the Imperial Cancer Research Fund.

References

1. Bonadonna, G., Rossi, A., Valagussa, A. et al.: Adjuvant chemotherapy with CMF in breast cancer with positive axillary nodes. In: Adjuvant therapy of cancer. Salmon, S. E., Jones, S. E. (eds.), pp. 83–94. Amsterdam: North-Holland 1977
2. Cole, M. P.: Suppression of ovarian function in primary breast cancer. In: Prognostic factors in breast cancer. Forrest, A. P. M., Kunkler, P. B. (eds.), pp. 146–156. Edinburg: Livingstone 1968
3. Fisher, B., Redmond, C.: Studies of the National Surgical Adjuvant Breast Project (NSABP). In: Adjuvant therapy of cancer. Salmon, S. E., Jones, S. E. (eds.), pp. 67–81. Amsterdam: North-Holland 1977
4. Gehan, E. A.: A generalized Wilcoxon test for comparing arbitrarily singly-sensored samples. Biometrika *52,* 203–223 (1965)
5. Nissen-Meyer, R.: Suppression of ovarian function in primary breast cancer. In: Prognostic factors in breast cancer. Forrest, A. P. M., Kunkler, P. B. (eds.), pp. 139–145. Edinburgh: Livingstone 1968
6. Ravdin, R. G., Lewison, E. F., Slack, N. H. et al.: Results of a clinical trial concerning the worth of prophylactic oophorectomy for breast cancer. Surg. Gynecol. Obstet. *131,* 1055–1064 (1970)

Adjuvant Therapy of Stage II, III Breast Cancer

A. V. Buzdar, J. U. Gutterman, G. R. Blumenschein, Ch. K. Tashima,
G. N. Hortobágyi, H. Y. Yap, E. M. Hersh, and E. A. Gehan

Introduction

Combination chemotherapy has significantly improved the response rate in the treatment of advanced breast cancer, and the adriamycin-containing regimens have been shown to be superior to non-adriamycin-containing combinations in the treatment of advanced disease [1, 4, 9, 11]. A combination of adriamycin, 5-fluorouracil, and cyclophosphamide (FAC) was reported by us to produce 75% remission in stage IV breast cancer [1]. Addition of nonspecific immunotherapy with BCG (FAC-BCG) to that regimen prolonged the duration of remission and survival [8]. From January 1974, all patients with stage II or III breast cancer following regional therapy were treated with a similar FAC-BCG regimen. The preliminary result of this study has been previously reported [5, 6]. The updated results reported in this paper show that this combination is effective in prolonging the disease-free interval and survival of stage II, III breast cancer.

Materials and Methods

From January 1974 to October 1976, 131 patients with stage II or III breast cancer following regional therapy were entered into the FAC-BCG study. Chemoimmunotherapy regimen as shown in Table 1 was started within 8–10 weeks of radiation and mastectomy. Except for 21

Table 1.

Adjuvant FAC-BCG regimen		
5-fluorouracil	400 mg/m^2 IV day 1 and 8	
Adriamycin	40 mg/m^2 IV day 1	
Cyclophosphamide	400 mg/m^2 IV day 1	q 28 days
BCG (6 × 10^8 organisms by scarification)	Days 9, 16, and 23	cycle
Maximum dose of adriamycin	300 mg/m^2	
Maintenance regimen		
5-fluorouracil	500 mg/m^2 day 1 and 8 (PO in 4 divided doses)	
Methotrexate	30 mg/m^2 IM day 1 and 8	q 28 days
Cyclophosphamide	500 mg/m^2 day 2 (PO in 4 divided doses)	cycle
BCG (6 × 10^8 organisms by scarification)	Days 9, 16, and 23	

patients in the FAC-BCG group, all of the patients received routine postoperative radiation therapy in the FAC-BCG group. Adriamycin was discontinued at a total dose of 300 mg/m^2, and the patients were switched to maintenance therapy as shown in Table 1. Chemoimmunotherapy was discontinued at the end of 2 years. The details of the experimental design, treatment, statistical methods and comparability of the two groups have been previously reported [8]. The disease-free interval and the survival of the FAC-BCG group was compared to a group of historical control patients. The historical control group consisted of all the patients with a diagnosis of breast cancer who were admitted to M. D. Anderson Hospital between January 1972 and December 1973. These patients have stage II or stage III disease (according to UICC classifications). This group comprised 151 patients. Patients receiving FAB-BCG were followed with weekly blood counts, but SMA-100, E, and urinalysis were performed before each cyle of therapy. Chest X-ray, bone scan, liver scan, and skeletal survey were done every 4 months or earlier if indicated by clinical course. Mammograms on the remaining breast were done every year. The patients in the control group were examined for evidence of recurrent disease at least every 4 months and had SMA-100, chest X-ray, skeletal survey, and yearly mammograms. Bone scan and liver scans were only done if indicated by clinical course. Evidence of tumor was confirmed by biopsy when possible or by clinical, pathologic, radiologic, or radioisotopic studies.

Results

Figure 1 shows the overall disease-free interval of two groups. In the FAC-BCG group, the longest follow-up was 48 months (median follow-up 28 months). Only 30 patients at the time of this analysis had less than a 2-year follow-up. Eighty-eight percent of the FAC-BCG patients were free of disease compared to 65% of control patients ($P < 0.01$). Table 2 shows the percentage disease-free by various patient characteristics. In the FAC-BCG group irrespective of menopausal status, number of involved nodes, or stage of disease, there was a significantly higher proportion of patients free of disease, except for premenopausal patients with one to three nodes. It is possible that with longer follow-up this group could demonstrate

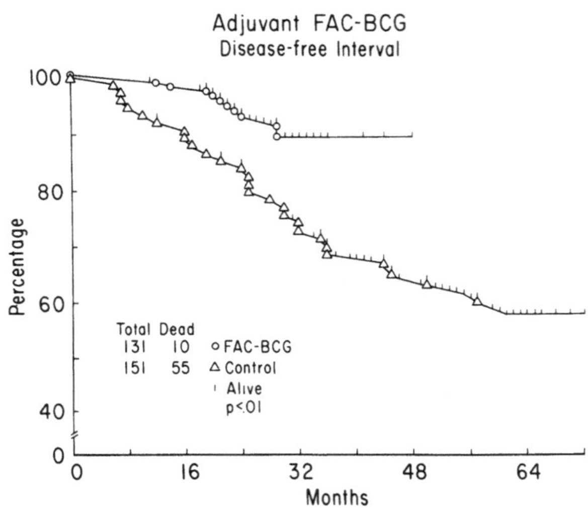

Fig. 1. Overall disease interval

Table 2. Percentage disease-free at median follow-up of 28 months

Characteristics	Controls		FAC-BCG		P value one tail
	No. of patients	Percent disease-free	No. of patients	Percent disease-free	
All patients	151	65	131	88	< 0.01
Stage[a]					
II	91	70	98	92	< 0.01
III	60	56	33	76	0.01
Premenopausal[b]					
1–3 nodes	14	70	20	85	0.16
≥ 4 nodes	24	40	35	77	< 0.01
Postmenopausal					
1–3 nodes	46	78	25	100	0.01
≥ 4 nodes	67	62	50	88	< 0.01

[a] According to UICC classification.

[b] One male patient was included in FAC-BCG group and was disease-free at this analysis.

better disease-free survival. Figure 2 illustrates the disease-free interval of postmenopausal women. In patients with one to three positive nodes in the FAC-BCG group, all the patients were free of disease compared to 78% in the control group, and these differences were significant ($P = 0.01$). In the group with more than four positive nodes, 88% of the FAC-BCG patients were free of disease compared to 62% in the control group, and these differences were highly significant ($P < 0.01$). Figure 3 shows the overall survival of patients. Ninty-four percent of the FAC-BCG patients were alive compared to 85% of the control patients at 28

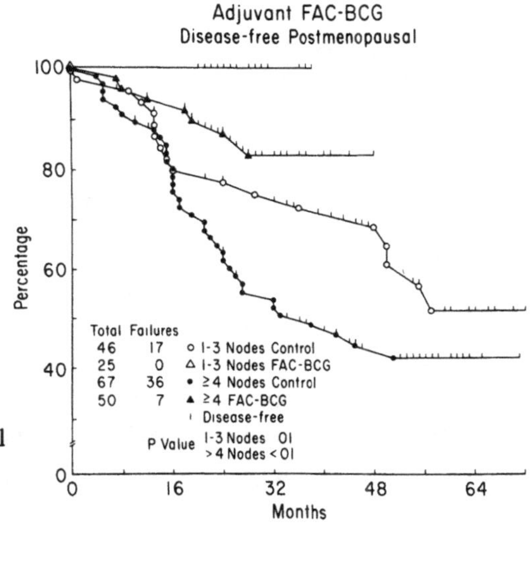

Fig. 2. Disease-free interval of postmenopausal patients

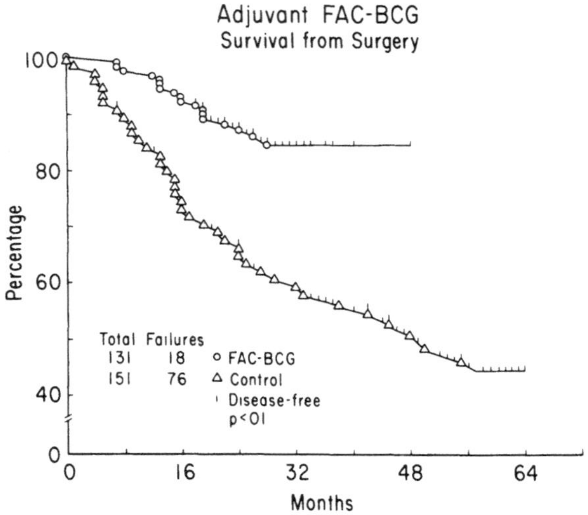

Fig. 3. Overall survival

months. These differences were highly significant ($P < 0.01$). The detailed toxicity of this treatment has been previously reported [8]; since that report, two patients have developed congestive cardiac failure, possibly related to adriamycin. One patient has improved after digitalization, but other patients continued to require supportive therapy.

Discussion

This treatment has been effective in prolonging the disease-free interval and survival of stage II and stage III breast cancer patients irrespective of menopausal status or number of involved nodes, and as shown in the Table 3 these results compare favorably to the previous reports with L-PAM [7] or CMF [3]. The L-PAM study had no significant impact on the disease-free survival of postmenopausal women. However, the CMF study had success in prolonging the

Table 3. Comparison of disease-free interval of L-PAM, CMF, and FAC-BCG studies (estimated percent disease-free at 24 months)

Characteristics	L-PAM		CMF		FAC-BCG	
	Control	Treatment	Control	Treatment	Control	Treatment
< 50 years						
1–3 nodes	70.9	96.9	70	96	71	85
≥ 4 nodes	48.9	55.5	20	64	42	77
> 50 years						
1–3 nodes	86	88.2	80	78	77	100
≥ 4 nodes	61.5	59.7	60	67	64	88
Total	68.4	76.2	64	80	64	88

disease-free interval of postmenopausal women in an earlier report [2], but on a follow-up report at the median follow-up of 17 months of study there were no significant differences in the relapse rate between the treated and the control group [3]. Our chemoimmunotherapy regimen has been effective in prolonging the disease-free interval of pre-as well as postmenopausal women. In postmenopausal patients with one to three positive nodes, there has been no recurrence up to the present time, and in four or more positive nodes, 88% of FAC-BCG patients were free of disease beyond 2 years. As shown in Table 3, the relapse rate in the control group between the three studies is comparable in each subgroup, except in premenopausal patients with more than four positive nodes in the CMF study. L-PAM and CMF studies utilize the concurrent controls, and in the FAC-BCG the historical controls were used. From this data it is obvious that in comparable risk groups the relapse rate has remained uniform and little has changed in the natural history of breast cancer. The possible reason this regimen was more effective than L-PAM or CMF may be due to the fact that an adriamycin-containing combination regimen was used, as adriamycin-containing combinations have been shown to be superior to non-adriamycin-containing treatments [4, 11]. The results of this study are consistent with animal experimental data that show that effective treatments for advanced disease are likely to be effective as an adjuvant for micrometastases [4]. It is difficult to determine the role of the postoperative irradiation and immunotherapy from this study. Currently, we are studying the role of radiotherapy and nonspecific immunotherapy (BCG) in a prospective randomized trial.

Acknowledgement

The authors would like to thank Gay Canavan for her help in the preparation of this manuscript.

References

1. Blumenschein, G. R., Cardenas, J. O., Freireich, E. J. et al.: FAC chemotherapy for breast cancer. Proc. Am. Soc. Clin. Oncol. March, 1974
2. Bonadonna, G., Brusamolino, E., Valagussa, P. et al.: Combination chemotherapy as an adjuvant treatment in operable breast cancer. N. Engl. J. Med. *294*, 405–410 (1976)
3. Bonadonna, G., Rossi, A., Valagussa, B. S. et al.: The CMF program for operable breast cancer with positive axillary nodes; updated analysis with disease-free interval and site of relapse and recurrence. Cancer *39*, 2904–2915 (1977)
4. Bull, J. M., Tormey, D. C., Li, S. S., Carbon, T. P. et al.: A randomized comparative trial of Adriamycin vs. Methotrexate in combination drug therapy. Cancer *41* (5), 1649–1657 (1978)
5. Buzdar, A. U., Blumenschein, G. R., Gutterman, J. U. et al.: Adjuvant chemoimmunotherapy following regional therapy in breast cancer. In: Adjuvant therapy of cancer. Salmon, S. E., Jones, S. E. (eds.), pp. 139–146. Amsterdam: Elsevier/North-Holland 1977
6. Buzdar, A. U., Gutterman, J. U., Blumenschein, G. R.: Intensive postoperative chemoimmunotherapy of patients with stage II and stage III breast cancer. Cancer *4*, 1064–1075 (1978)
7. Fisher, B., Glass, A., Redmond, C. et al.: L-phenylalanine mustard (L-PAM) in the management of primary breast cancer – an update of earlier findings and a comparison with those utilizing L-PAM plus 5-fluorouracil (5-FU). Cancer *39*, 2883–2903 (1977)

8. Gutterman, J. U., Cardenas, J. O., Blumenschein, G. R. et al.: Chemoimmunotherapy of disseminated breast cancer prolongation of remission and survival. Br. Med. J. *1976 II,* 122–125
9. Jones, S. E., Durie, D. G., Salmon, S. E.: Combination chemotherapy with Adriamycin and Cyclophosphamide for advanced breast cancer. Cancer *36,* 90–97 (1975)
10. Schable, F. M. (Jr.): Experimental basis for adjuvant chemotherapy. In: Adjuvant therapy of cancer. Salmon, S. E., Jones, S. E. (eds.), pp. 3–14. Amsterdam: Elsevier/North Holland 1977
11. Smalley, R. V., Carpenter, J., Bartolucci, A. et al.: A comparison of cyclophosphamide, adriamycin, 5-fluorouracil and cyclophosphamide and methotrexate, 5-fluorouracil, vincristine, prednisone (CMFVP) in patients with metastatic breast cancer: A Southwestern Cancer Study Group Project. Cancer *40* (2), 625–632 (1977)

Randomized Trial With Poly A-Poly U as Adjuvant Therapy Complementing Surgery in Patients With Breast Cancer: In Vitro Study of Cellular Immunity

F. Lacour, G. Delage, A. Spira, E. Nahon-Merlin, J. Lacour, A. M. Michelson, and S. Bayet

Introduction

Poly A-poly U is known to be potent in stimulating cellular and humoral immunity [4, 8]. The observation that its use, following surgery, had a definite inhibitory effect on tumor growth of spontaneous mammary adenocarcinoma in mice without any toxicity [19, 21] prompted the initiation of a therapeutic trial with the polyribonucleotide complex.

Although numerous attempts to stimulate the host immune responses by nonspecific agents have been made during the last years, these studies have been difficult to evaluate, since most of them lacked adequate comparability of the groups. It is only with randomized controlled studies that the role of adjuvant therapy can be evaluated. Therefore, the first randomized trial using poly A-poly U as an adjuvant therapy complementing surgery in patients with breast cancer was started in November 1972 at the Institut Gustave-Roussy, France [22, 23]. Thus far, the results on 229 patients are available. Of these, one group of 113 patients was given conventional therapy and the second group of 116 patients was given treatment with poly A-poly U in addition to the conventional therapy. The leukocyte migration inhibition test (LMIT) was used to estimate the cellular immune response. Tumor tissue obtained at surgery, and serum and leukocytes collected periodically, were assayed. Each assay was performed in the presence of: (1) *autologous* tumor extract (T), (2) *autologous* serum (S), and (3) a combination of both autologous tumor extract and serum (T+S). The present report describes the results obtained for those patients who have been followed for more than year.

Material and Methods

Selection of Patients

Patients were selected according to the UICC classification, using the TNM system. Patients with tumors of small size, namely T1 N0 or N1 M0, were excluded since their prognosis is generally favorable and it would be difficult to identify clearly the effects of poly A-poly U treatment. Patients with tumors larger than 7 cm at their greatest diameter were also excluded, since they are routinely treated in our institute with preoperative radiotherapy followed by modified radical mastectomy. Patients corresponding to category T2 and part of T3 N0 N1 M0 were selected for trial if the tumor was an infiltrating carcinoma of 2–7 cm at its greatest diameter, without skin involvement or complete fixation to the pectoralis major, without palpable nodes (or with palpable but moveable nodes), and without any detectable metastasis. These patients were randomized into two groups as follows.

Conventional Treatment Group (CT)

Patients were submitted to either radical mastectomy or modified radical mastectomy without any additional treatment if the nodes were free of cancer. If the nodes were metastatic, postoperative radiotherapy was employed and a radiotherapeutic castration was performed if the women were still menstruating or were within 2 years of the menopause.

Conventional Treatment + Poly A-Poly U Group (CT+Poly A-Poly U)

These patients were treated exactly as those in the CT group, but they also received 30 mg of poly A-poly U injected intravenously once a week for 6 weeks, beginning 7 days after surgery. In the CT group, patients received the same amount of saline. The preparation of poly A-poly U and of the complex [12] and tumor extracts, serum, and leukocytes [29] were described previously.

Leukocyte Migration Inhibition Test (LMIT)

The LMIT was modified from the technique originally described by Soborg and Bendixen [30] and performed as previously described [29]. Four series of tests were performed at the same time, each of them in quadriplicate in an autologous system.

1. T = 10% colt serum + tumor extract 200 μg/ml proteins;
2. S = 10% patient serum;
3. T + S = 10% patient serum + tumor extract;
4. Control = 10% colt serum.

The migration index of autologous lymphocytes is given by the formula:

$$MI = \frac{\text{Mean of migration of 4 replicates in the presence of T or S or T + S}}{\text{Mean of migration of 4 replicates in the absence of T or S or T + S}} .$$

A migration index of 0.80 or below can be considered, in first approximation, as an inhibition of migration [14, 26]. We verified that is was the lower limit of the 5% confidence interval of mean migration index of the controls.

To eliminate the possibility that prolonged storage might have resulted in toxicity of extracts, control tests with leukocytes from healthy donors were performed with those extracts that had been positive when tested initially with autologous leukocytes. No toxicity was noted since only 3 out of 30 showed an inhibitory effect. Comparison of the groups was performed using the chi square test.

Results

Leukocyte Migration Inhibition

Horizontal studies of migration of leukocytes in the presence of (1) autologous tumor extract, (2) autologous serum, and (3) autologous tumor extract in conjunction with autologous serum were performed in a group of 159 of the breast cancer patients in the trial. Seventy-five of these patients belong to the CT group and 84 to the CT + poly A-poly U group. Tests were performed 7 days, 2 months, 4 months, and 1 year after the operation.

Table 1 summarizes results of tests with this material that were perfomed at the same time at each period.

Table 1. Effect of autologous tumor extract (T), autologous serum (S), and autologous tumor extract plus serum (T + S) on the migration of leukocytes of breast cancer patients

Leukocyte (postop)	Test material added	Conventional treatment (CT)		CT + poly A-poly U	
		Pos/total (LMIT)	% pos (LMIT)	Pos/total	% pos
7 days	T	30/75	40 (1)[a]	31/84	37 (2)[2]
	S	22/75	29 (3)	30/85	35 (4)
	T + S	30/67	45 (5)	40/81	49 (6)
2 months	T	25/55	45 (1)	24/80	30 (2)
	S	21/56	38 (3)	43/83	52 (4)
	T + S	34/51	67 (5)	49/78	63 (6)
4 months	T	33/58	57 (1)	36/68	53 (2)
	S	26/60	43 (3)	19/69	28 (4)
	T + S	36/56	64 (5)	36/63	57 (6)
1 year	T	31/48	65 (1)	29/45	64 (2)
	S	30/50	60 (3)	27/50	54 (4)
	T + S	33/45	73 (5)	31/43	72 (6)

[a] No significant difference was found between CT and CT + poly A-poly U groups of patients. (1) $P \leqslant 0.05$; (2) $P \leqslant 0.001$; (3) $P \leqslant 0.01$; (4) $P \leqslant 0.01$; (5) $P \leqslant 0.05$; (6) $P \leqslant 0.10$ NS.

Inhibition in the Presence of Autologous Tumor Extracts

With autologous tumor extract from patients, an inhibition activity in the CT group generally increased regularly and significantly ($P \leqslant 0.05$) with time and rose from 40% when tested 7 days after the operation to 65% when tested 1 year after surgery. Similar patterns were observed in the CT + poly A-poly U group; 37% of the LMITs were positive on the 7th day after the operation and 64% 1 year after surgery ($P \leqslant 0.001$). However, the difference between the two groups is not significant ($P > 0.10$). In a previous study, control tests were performed with 17 autologous normal tissue extracts (muscle or breast). No inhibition was found [29].

Inhibition by Autologous Sera

The migration of leukocytes in medium supplemented with 10% autologous serum was compared with migration in medium supplemented by 10% colt serum. The first test on each patient was performed with autologous serum separated from blood taken 7 days previously, shortly before, or during the operation. Autologous serum caused inhibition of leukocyte migration in the CT group (29%) and in the CT + poly A-poly U group (35%); the difference between the two groups is not significant. The number of patients with a positive LMIT increased significantly with time after surgery in both groups ($P \leqslant 0.01$ in each group) except in the third test in the CT + poly A-poly U group. Decomplemented and fresh sera were found to have the same effect indicating that the serum-mediated inhibition is not complement dependent [20].

Inhibition by Autologous Tumor Extract and Autologous Serum

The percentagee of positive-LMIT patients was always higher in both groups when extract was used in conjunction with autologous serum than the percentage obtained by tumor extract alone or by serum alone. This percentage also increased with time in both groups. The results of the present study confirm and extend our earlier finding in which we noted a synergistic effect of the serum [20]. From the date in Table 2, concerning patients who had complete sets of tests, it can be seen that in the CT group, the LMIT was positive in the presence of the combination of tumor extract and serum in 7 out of 77 patients, while neither tumor extract nor the serum used separately showed inhibitory effects. In two patients, increased inhibition of migration, i.e., a reduction of more than 20% below that produced by serum alone or tumor extract alone, occurred. In 9 out of the 77 patients (12%), a synergistic effect was noted. Similar results were found in the CT + poly A-poly U group. In 9 out of the 78 patients (12%), no effect was found with serum or tumor extract alone and inhibition was only observed when they were used in combination.

Table 2. Effects of tumor extract (T) and of serum (S), compared to the effects of tumor extract in conjunction with serum (T + S), on the migration of autologous leukocytes of 18 patients, showing the presence of a serum synergistic factor (SSF)

CT group (patient)	Migration index of leukocytes			
	T	S	T + S	
1	0.83	0.83	0.28	
2	0.99	1.08	0.69	[a] 9/77 12%
3	1.21	0.99	0.69	
4	0.86	0.81	0.59	
5	0.93	0.85	0.55	
6	1.00	1.10	0.78	
7	0.69	0.68	0.44	
8	0.86	0.58	0.31	
9	1.06	1.59	0.62	
CT + poly A-poly U group (patient)	**T**	**S**	**T + S**	
1	0.98	1.21	0.70	
2	0.78	1.05	0.51	[a] 9/78 12%
3	1.01	1.17	0.77	
4	0.89	0.76	0.43	
5	1.11	1.06	0.75	
6	1.02	1.08	0.75	
7	1.08	1.20	0.60	
8	0.95	0.90	0.64	
9	1.14	1.02	0.52	

[a] Number of patients who had a complete set of tests (T, S, and T + S).

The results of the LMIT were analyzed to determine whether there might be a possible relationship between such findings and the prognosis, since the status of axillary lymph nodes constitutes an important prognostic factor. Table 3 shows data on N+ and N-patients. The percentages of those with a positive LMIT in the presence of T, S, and T + S in the CT and CT + poly A-poly U groups were similar.

Most of the N+ patients received complementary radiotherapy but as shown in Table 4, this additional treatment did not appear to influence the results of the LMIT. The only factor that seemed to be correlated with this prognosis was the SS factor. Clinical and histologic findings

Table 3. Percentage of patients with positive LMIT as related to the status of axillary lymph nodes

		N	%	N +	%
7 days	T	20/46	43	41/113	36
	S	18/46	39	34/114	30
	T + S	24/43	56	46/105	44
2 months	T	18/42	43	31/93	33
	S	20/42	48	44/97	45
	T + S	24/39	62	59/90	66
4 months	T	22/40	55	47/86	55
	S	12/40	30	33/89	37
	T + S	22/36	61	50/83	60
1 year	T	20/25	80	40/68	59
	S	14/27	52	43/73	59
	T + S	18/24	75	46/64	72

No significant difference was found between N – and N +.

Table 4. Percentage of patients with positive LMIT as related to post operative irradiation

		Not irradiated postop	%	Irradiated postop	%
2 months	T	18/45	40	31/89	35
	S	23/45	51	40/93	43
	T + S	27/42	64	55/86	64
4 months	T	22/43	51	46/82	56
	S	15/44	34	30/84	36
	T + S	24/40	60	47/78	60
1 year	T	22/28	79	38/65	58
	S	15/30	50	42/70	60
	T + S	20/27	74	44/61	72

No significant difference was found between nonirradiated and irradiated groups.

Table 5. Clinical and histologic findings in 18 patients with synergistic factor

Conventional treatment (CT)		CT + poly A-poly U	Total No.
No. of patients	9	9	18
Axil. N +	8	7	15 (83%)
Axil. N −	1	2	3
Bloom III	3	3	6
Metastasis	6	2	8 (44%)

for 18 patients possessing the synergistic serum factor are shown in Table 5. These patients were equally distributed in both categories of treatment: nine patients in each. The two subgroups are comparable with regard to age (mean age 54 years), tumor extension (expressed by the TNM of the UICC classification), histologic grading following Bloom and Richardson [2], and percentage of N+ patients. They differ, however, with regard to the number of patients with metastases (Table 5). In this same group of patients selected because their serum contained SS factor, both the incidence of nodal involvement (83% compared to 68% among those patients who had no SS factor) and the percentage of patients with metastases (44% compared to 21%) were higher. Thus, in contrast to a previous report concerning a rather small number of patients [20], these results suggest that the presence of SS factor may have a bad prognostic significance.

The second observation concerns the number of metastases in the two subgroups of patients: six out of nine in the CT group (66%) versus two out of nine in the CT + poly A-poly U group (22%). The same trend between the two therapeutic categories was observed in the whole population of the trial. When we looked for more details of the N+ patients of both subgroups with SS factor, it was observed that in the CT subgroup with SS factor there were two patients with one single involved node who did well, three patients with two involved nodes who developed metastasis, and three patients with three or more involved nodes who all had metastases. In the CT + poly A-poly U subgroup, four patients had two involved nodes and none of them had any treatment failure; of the three patients with three or more involved nodes, only two developed metastases.

Discussion

Poly A-poly U decreases the incidence of metastases and increases the survival from mammary tumors in C3H/He mice when used as an adjunct to surgical removal of the primary cancer. The effect on metastases was even more striking in a transplantable melanoma in hamsters [21]. It has also been demonstrated that it retards tumor growth in mice bearing transplantable leukemia [27]. A prophylactic effect on leukemia on mammary tumors in mice was also described [10, 18]. There is little information on poly A-poly U in cancer in man. Wanebo et al. [31] described only paradoxic immunologic effects of this complex in a limited series of cancer patients.

The present sequential study of cell-mediated immunity in breast cancer patients did not show any statistically significant difference in the immune reactions tested by the LMIT between the two groups of patients: CT and CT + poly A-poly U. However, there is something to be learned from the cumulative data of both groups. The results of the LMIT in 159 patients with breast cancer confirm previous findings that cell-mediated immunity can be detected in such patients [29]. The use of autologous material eliminates the problems of allogenic recognition. The reactivity of leukocytes against autologous tumor antigens regularly increased with time. Our results differ from those obtained by Jones et al. [15] who tested the leukocytic reactivity of 107 patients with breast cancer stage I and II at 7 days, 2 months, 6 months, and 1 year after surgery. In their randomized trial, patients were treated differently from those of our own series: they were submitted to a simple mastectomy with nodal biopsies, with or without postsurgical radiotherapy and only tumor tissue was tested. They observed a decrease in the proportion of positive LMIT patients from the first to the second test and an increase from the third to the fourth. It is possible that the difference between the observations of Jones et al. and ours may be due, partially at least, to the difference in therapeutic methods.

In our series we also observed an increase with time of the activity of autologous serum that was previously shown to have an inhibitory effect on leukocyte migration [5, 6, 20]. The effect of serum in addition to tumor extracts was also tested to investigate whether sera from breast cancer patients could abolish the inhibitory action of autologous tumor extracts on leukocyte migration. Autologous serum did not reverse the leukocyte migration inhibition, and a blocking effect [11, 13] was noted in two cases. To the contrary, serum enhanced the tumor inhibition effect on leukocyte migration, confirming our earlier observation [20] which has also subsequently been confirmed by Cochran et al. [6]. It was not possible to detect any significant difference between the activity of tumor extracts on leukocytes from patients with or without positive axillary lymph nodes (the involvement of which are known to indicate a bad prognosis (Table 3)).

The LMIT with tumor extract has been frequently used for the study of cellular immunity in breast cancer patients [1, 3, 7, 9, 16, 17, 20, 24, 25, 28, 29, 32]. Most of these studies were performed with homologous extracts and did not provide convincing data in favor of the prognostic value of the test. Using both autologous tumor extract and autologous serum to test the reactivity of leukocytes, we have shown the presence of a synergistic serum factor. The presence of this synergistic factor seems to be correlated with a poor prognosis. The nature of this factor still remains to be determined. It should be emphasized that the incidence of metastases was much higher in the CT subgroup than in the CT + poly A-poly U subgroup. The same trend was also observed in the whole series of patients.

However, these figures are still not large enough to permit any definitive statistical conclusion. More firm data will emerge as the number of patients in the trial increases. A longer period of observation is mandatory before a new appraisal is done. All patients will then have been followed for 3 years at least, at which time it may be possible to determine both whether poly A-poly U is beneficial and whether the presence of the synergistic serum factor can be of prognostic value. We also do not know whether or not patients with a progressive increase of LMIT postivity have a better host defense. Perhaps with a longer clinical follow-up, this question will be answered.

Summary

The immunologic reactivity of patients with initially operable breast cancer was measured by the leukocyte migration inhibition test using *autologous* tumor extract (T), *autologous* serum (S), and a combination of both (T+S). These patients formed part of a randomized clinical

trial comparing, on the one hand, conventional treatment and, on the other, conventional treatment complemented by injections of poly A-poly U.
A sequential study was carried out on 159 patients, testing them 7 days, 2 months, 4 months, and 1 year after the operation. Statistical comparisons revealed no significant difference in the reaction of the two groups. In addition, no significant differences were found between those with lymph node involvement and those without. Radiotherapy given to those with lymph node involvement did not significantly change their reactions.
We were able to show that the percentage of patients with a positive leukocyte migration inhibition test (LMIT) increases regularly and significantly with time. This study confirmed the presence in some autologous serum of a synergistic factor (SS factor) which increased the inhibition of migration of leukocytes by autologous tumor extract. This factor was found in 18 patients, equally divided between both therapeutic groups. In the group with SS factor, the percentage with lymph node involvement appeared greater (83% compared with 68% among those patients who had no SS factor), and the incidence of metastases was also increased (44% compared with 21%). This factor seemed to indicate a bad prognosis. However, there was a difference in the results between the two therapeutic groups in patients with the synergistic factor. Of nine patients undergoing conventional treatment, six had developed metastases, whereas only two out of the nine patients who also poly A-poly U developed metastases. The same trend was observed in the whole trial population.

Acknowledgement

We thank Mrs J. Viguier for her excellent assistance. This investigation was supported by the Cancer Research Institute (New York), CNRS, and INSERM.

References

1. Andersen, V., Bendixen, G., Schiødt, T.: An in vitro demonstration of cellular immunity against autologous mammary carcinoma in man. Acta Med. Scand. *186,* 101–103 (1969)
2. Bloom, H. J. G., Richardson, W. W.: Histological grading and prognosis in breast cancer. A study of 1409 cases of which 359 have been followed for 15 years. Br. J. Cancer *11,* 359–377 (1957)
3. Brandes, L. J., Goldenberg, G. J.: Peripheral leukocyte migration inhibition reactivity to breast cancer antigens in Patients with breast cancer and in normal Controls. Cancer Res. *36,* 3707–3710 (1976)
4. Braun, W., Nakano, M.: Antibody formation: Stimulation by polyadenylic and polycytidylic acids. Science *157,* 819–821 (1967)
5. Bruley-Rosset, M., Botto, H. G., Goutner, A.: Serum migration inhibitory activity in patients with infectious diseases and various neoplasia. Eur. J. Cancer *13,* 325–327 (1977)
6. Cochran, A. J., Mackie, R. M., Ross, C. E., Ogg, L. J., Jackson, A. M.: Leukocyte migration inhibition by cancer patients' sera. Int. J. Cancer *18,* 274–281 (1976)
7. Cochran, A. J., Mackie, R. M., Thomas, C. E., Grant, R. M., Cameron-Mowat, D. E., Spilg, W. G. S.: Cellular immunity to breast carcinoma and malignant melanoma. Br. J. Cancer *28* [Suppl I], 77–82 (1973)
8. Cone, R. E., Johnson, A. G.: Regulation of the immune system by synthetic polynucleotides. III Action on antigen-reactive cells of thymic origin. J. Exp. Med. *133,* 665–676 (1971)

9. Dean, J. H., McCoy, J. L., Cannon, G. B., Leonard, C. M., Perlin, E., Kreutner, A., Oldham, R. K., Herberman, R. B.: Cell-mediated immune responses of breast cancer Patients to autologous tumor-associated antigens. J. Natl. Cancer Inst. *58*, 549–555 (1977)

10. Drake, W. P., Cimino, E. F., Mardiney, M. R. (Jr.), Sutherland, J. C.: Prophylactic therapy of spontaneous leukemia in AKR mice by polyadenylic-polyuridylic acid. J. Natl. Cancer. Inst. *52*, 941–944 (1974)

11. Falk, R. E., Mann, P., Langer, B.: Cell-mediated immunity to human tumors. Arch. Surg. *107*, 261–265 (1973)

12. Fenster, E. D., Lacour, F., Harel, J.: Nuclear penetration and stimulation of nucleic acids synthesis by Poly A. poly U in mammalian cells. Exp. Cell Res. *94*, 315–320 (1975)

13. Guillou, P. J., Giles, G. R.: Inhibition of leukocyte migration by tumour-associated antigens of the colon and rectum. Gut *14*, 733–738 (1973)

14. Jones, B. M.: Mechanisms of leukocyte migration inhibition by breast tumour cell fractions. Br. J. Cancer *34*, 14–19 (1976)

15. Jones, B. M., Connolly, C. E., Isaacson, P., Turner, D. T. L., Turnbull, A. R.: Tumour-directed leucocyte migration inhibition in operable breast cancer: Additional clinical corelations. Br. J. Cancer *34*, 94–96 (1976)

16. Jones, B. M., Turnbull, A. R.: Horizontal studies of cell mediated immune reactions to autologous tumour antigens in patients with operable mammary carcinoma. Br. J. Cancer *32*, 339–344 (1975)

17. Kadish, A. S., Marcus, D. M., Bloom, B. R.: Inhibition of leukocyte migration by human breast-cancer-associated antigens. Int. J. Cancer *18*, 581–586 (1976)

18. Lacour, F., Delage, G., Chianale, C.: Reduced incidence of spontaneous mammary tumors in C_3H/He mice after treatment with polyadenylate-polyuridylate. Science *187*, 256–257 (1975)

19. Lacour, F., Delage, G., Fenster, E., Harel, J.: Inhibitory action of Poly A. poly U on tumor growth: enhancement of host immune response? In: Fundamental aspects of neoplasia. Gottlieb, A. A., Plescia, O. J., Bishop, D. H. L. (eds.), pp. 123–138. New York: Springer 1975

20. Lacour, F., Lacour, J., Spira, A., Bayet, S.: Effect of autologous serum on in vitro inhibition of leukocyte migration by autochthonous tumor extracts from human patients. In: Recent results in cancer research. Mathé, G., Weiner, R. (eds.), Vol. 47, pp. 129–132. Berlin, Heidelberg, New York: Springer 1974

21. Lacour, F., Spira, A., Lacour, J., Prade, M.: Polyadenylic-polyuridylic acid, an adjunct to surgery in the treatment of spontaneous mammary tumors in C_3H/He mice and transplantable melanoma in the hamster. Cancer Res. *32*, 648–649 (1972)

22. Lacour, J.: Trials with Poly A. poly U as adjuvant therapy complementing surgery in randomized Patients with breast cancer. In: Fundamental aspects of neoplasia. Gottlieb, A. A., Plescia, O. J., Bishop, D. H. L. (eds.), pp. 229–232. New York: Springer 1975

23. Lacour, J., Lacour, F., Spira, A., Delage, G., Michelson, A. M.: An immunotherapeutic trial of Poly A. poly U adjuvant in the management of breast cancer. Bull. Cancer *61*, 275–280 (1974)

24. McCoy, J. L., Jerome, L. F., Anderson, C., Cannon, G. B., Alford, T. C., Connor, R. J., Oldham, R. K., Herberman, R. B.: Leukocyte migration inhibition by soluble extracts of MCF-7 tissue culture cell line derived from breast carcinoma. J. Natl. Cancer Inst. *57*, 1045–1049 (1976)

25. McCoy, J. L., Jerome, L. F., Dean, J. H., Cannon, G. B., Alford, T. C., Doering, T., Herberman, R. B.: Inhibition of leukocyte migration by tumor-associated antigens in soluble extracts of human breast carcinoma. J. Natl. Cancer Inst. *53*, 11–17 (1974)

26. Morris, J. A., Stevens, A. E., Hebert, C. N.: An evaluation of the methods available for analysing results from migration inhibitory factor (MIF) test. J. Immunol. Methods *12*, 275–283 (1976)

27. Pendergrast, W. J. (Jr.), Drake, W. P., Mardiney, M. R. (Jr.): The dependence of successful immunotherapy on adequate tumor burden as shown by the treatment of AKR leukemia with Poly A. poly U. J. Natl. Cancer Inst. *55,* 1223–1225 (1975)
28. Rieche, K., Arndt, A., Pasternak, G.: Cellular immunity in mammary cancer patients as measured by the leukocyte migration test (LMT). A follow-up study. Int. J. Cancer *17,* 212–218 (1976)
29. Segall, A., Weiler, O., Genin, J., Lacour, J., Lacour, F.: In vitro study of cellular immunity against autochthonous human cancer. Int. J. Cancer *9,* 417–425 (1972)
30. Søborg, M., Bendixen, G.: Human lymphocytes migration as a parameter of hypersensitivity. Acta Med. Scand. *181,* 247–265 (1967)
31. Wanebo, H. J., Kemeny, M., Pinsky, C. M., Hirshaut, Y., Oettgen, H. F.: Influence of Poly A. poly U on immune response in cancer patients. Ann. N.Y. Acad. Sci. *277,* 288–298 (1976)
32. Wolberg, W. H.: Inhibition of migration of human autogenous and allogeneic leukocytes by extracts of Patients' cancers. Cancer Res., *31,* 798–802 (1971)

Levamisole: As Adjuvant to Cyclic Chemotherapy in Breast Cancer

E. J. W. Stephens, H. F. Wood, and B. Mason

Selection of Patients

Sixty women under the age of 65 attending the Clinical Oncology Unit at Auckland Hospital, Auckland, New Zealand and who had symptomatic end-stage mammary carcinoma were invited to participate in this study after its nature and aims had been explained to them. Fifty-five patients were postmenopausal by natural or artificial means. Fifty-four of these women had failed to achieve a remission or had achieved and then lost a remission by a variety of hormonal manipulations both additive and ablative. A further six women were incorporated into this study as primary therapy because of the known absence of cellular oestrogen receptors or because of rapidly progressive visceral disease without knowledge of oestrogen receptor status. The 60 patients were treated between September 1975 and December 1976, the minimum follow-up being 15 months and the maximum 27 months at the time of reporting.

Method

All patients received a regimen of combination cytotoxic therapy involving cyclophosphamide, adriamycin and 5-flourouracil, as indicated in Table 1. All injections were given by rapid intravenous injection, as day stay patients, into a paediatric vein seeker unit attached to a fast running intravenous infusion.

A philosophy of remission induction (6 × 28-day courses) and remission maintenance (12 × 56-day courses) was embarked upon. In addition, patients were randomised in double-blind fashion to receive either 150 mg/day levamisole in divided doses on days 15, 16 and 17 and 22, 23 and 24 of each cycle or identical placebo tablets. Treatment was terminated upon reaching an adriamycin ceiling of 550 mg/m^2 (if no prior mediastinum or left chest irradiation) or 450 mg/m^2 (with prior irradiation) regardless of the disease status. However, patients continued on levamisole or placebo beyond this time until analysis.

At the time of relapse patients were treated on symptomatic grounds utilising radiation therapy or other ancillary means. If chemotherapy remained the treatment of choice a back-

Table 1. FAC regime

Drug	Dose	Route	Days
5-Flourouracil	500 mg/m^2	IV	1 and 8
Adriamycin	50 mg/m^2	IV	1
Cyclophosphamide	500 mg/m^2	IV	1

Table 2. MMF regime

Drug	Dose	Route	Days
Melphalan	30–40 mg/m^2	IV	1
Methotrexate	40 mg/m^2	IV	4 and 7
5-Flourouracil	600 mg/m^2	IV	4 and 7

up regime of methotrexate, melphalan and 5-flourouracil was used until further relapse (Table 2). In addition, at relapse some patients were entered in a separate trial of medical adrenalectomy by means of 6-aminoglutethimide (reported separately) [6]. However, the constant variable in all patients remained the presence or absence of levamisole as adjuvant to cyclic chemotherapy as the initial intensive therapeutic manoeuvre.

No patients are lost to follow-up. The principal end point for analysis has been survival. However, response to chemotherapy and duration of remission are also reported.

Results

Two patients have been omitted from analysis. One died before receiving the trial preparation, the other had the trial medication accidentally omitted during the first cycle. Thirty-one patients were randomized to receive levamisole and 29 to receive placebo; both dropouts had been allotted to the levamisole group. Therefore, after these exclusions, 29 patients are evaluable in each group.

Remission Rate

No patient achieved a sustained complete remission according to the criteria of remission employed (ECOG). However, the partial remission rate (50% or greater reduction in measurable metastases for a minimum of 3 months) of 43% is in accordance with similar studies; 64% of the total group showed static disease or remissions. However, the partial remission

Table 3. Remission rates with FAC chemotherapy

	Result of FAC treatment[a]			
	Partial remission	Static disease	Progressive	Levamisole vs. placebo
Levamisole group (n = 29)	17	6	6	$P^b = 0.0042$
Placebo group (n = 29)	8	6	15	

[a] There were no complete remissions.
[b] Mann-Whitney *U* test.

rate was higher in the levamisole-treated patients than the control group. Equal numbers showed no real alteration in their assessable parameters, while a larger proportion of placebo-treated patients showed progression of their disease. The difference between these groups is significant (Table 3).

Duration of Remission

This information is not readily extractable as, in effect, there were two end points. A negative one – progression of disease – and a positive one – when a patient attained their adriamycin ceiling. Nevertheless, it was possible to identify patients who had a sustained partial remission or where there was no evidence of disease progression over a 6-month period. There were 32 such patients, 21 of whom had received levamisole and the remaining 11 belonged to the placebo group. This difference fails to reach statistical significance.

Survival

Levamisole-treated patients survived longer than placebo controls, the median survival time being prolonged by 7 months. As of now, the optimum dosage and frequency of administration of levamisole is unclear. However, the effect is dose dependent, and the maximum effect is probably present at a dosage of 2–4 mg/kg for 2 or 3 days each 2nd week (Fig. 1). In this study a fixed dosage was used and patients whose weight greatly exceeded 70 kg were probably underdosed.

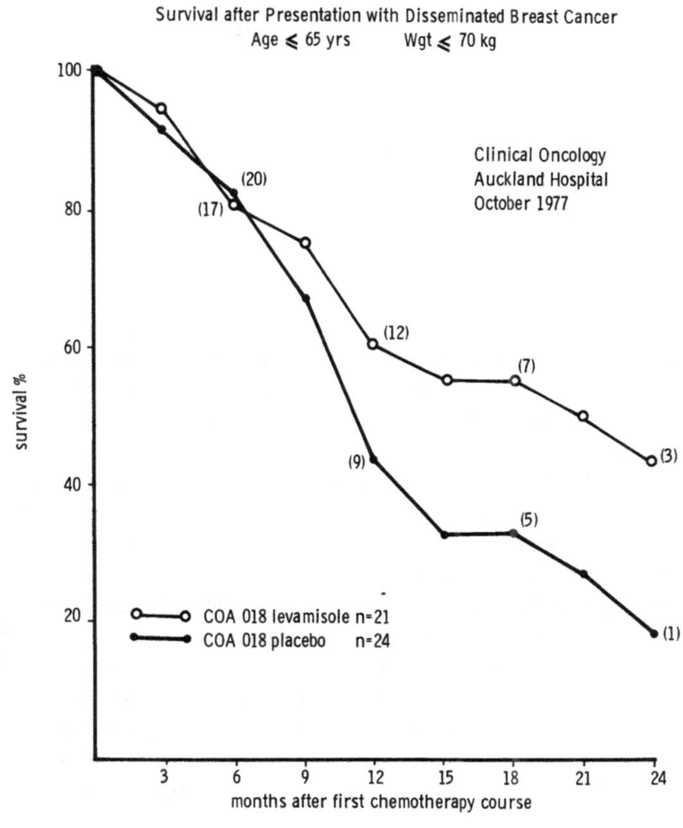

Fig. 1. Survival of patients 70 kg body weight or less

Table 4. Mean survival with and without levamisole

	Mean survival	
	Levamisole	Placebo
Patients CR + static disease at 6 months	22 months[a]	12 months
Patients with progressive disease	7 months[b]	5 months

[a] Significant, students t-test, $P < 0.05$.
[b] Not significant.

Table 5. Patient distribution of the two groups

	Levamisole group (n = 29)	Placebo group (n = 29)	Total population n = 58)
Age (years) Median (+ range)	50 (32–63)	52 (30–65)	51 (30–65)
Weight (kg) Median (+ range)	60 (43–102)	61 (45–116)	60 (43–116)
Menopausal status			
Natural menopause	13	19	32
Menopause induced by surgery or radiation	13	8	21
Premenopausal	3	2	5

This prolongation of survival occurs in fact only in those patients who achieved remission or disease stabilisation with FAC chemotherapy. When the total group is broken down into responders and nonresponders and reevaluated, it is clear that a significant levamisole-associated increase in survival is found in responders but not in nonresponders (Table 4).

The unexpected improvement in survival has prompted us to perform a further analysis of the individual patient profiles and also to look in depth at the toxicity suffered by these patients, as on first impressions it did seem that the levamisole-treated patients received more chemotherapy and tolerated it better that controls.

The two patient groups were remarkably well matched in age, weight and menopausal status (Table 5). In addition the disease profile as shown by site of dominant metastatic disease, and the disease tempo, as illustrated by the "disease-free interval" differed little between the groups (Tables 6 and 7). It has been reported [7] that levamisole favours more rapid bone marrow recovery if given between chemotherapy cycles. In addition it could be assumed that an agent enhancing a depressed immune response may offer some protection against therapy-associated infective episodes and general well-being. Several additional aspects were therefore

Table 6. Disease profile according to dominant metastatic disease

Dominant disease site	Levamisole group	Placebo group	Total population
Skeletal metastases	12	11	33
Soft tissue/chest wall	7	8	15
Visceral			
Lung nodular and effusions	5	3	22
Lung, lymphatic infiltration	3	2	
Liver	3	2	
Other: CNS, intra-abdominal	1	3	

Table 7. Disease profile according to disease tempo

	Duration of disease-free interval
Levamisole group	31 months
Placebo group	29 months
Total population	30 months

analysed to identify if and then why treatment was better tolerated in the levamisole group.

1. *Calculation of the time* taken to complete the initial six courses of FAC chemotherapy. This is an indirect measure of the time necessary for marrow recovery between treatment cycles. The minimum theoretical time would be 5 × 28, i.e., 140 days from the first injection of the first cycle to the first injection of the sixth cycle. The mean time was 152 days in the levamisole and 1 week longer (159 days) in the control group;
2. *Calculation of the total dose* of cytotoxics given during the first six cycles as a percentage of the total calculated dose based on an "ideal" dose of cytotoxics according to surface area per cycle. The actual figures were 92% for levamisole and 88.2% for the control group. Therefore, in summary, the levamisole patients received on average more chemotherapy (i.e., higher doses) in a shorter time period than those not receiving this drug and, as indicated previously, a better response rate, and as detailed next, less specific and nonspecific morbidity;
3. *Calculation of weight loss* during the first six cycles of therapy. Weight changes were expressed as the percentage change at 6 months as compared to the pretreatment weight. The weight of the levamisole-treated patients *increased* by a mean of 1.7% of body weight, while the placebo group *lost* an average of 3.4% of body weight.
   Additionally, the transfusion rate was lower in the levamisole-treated group versus controls (six control patients and one levamisole patient required blood transfusion in the first 6 months), while two control patients and two levamisole patients suffered major infective episodes during this period. No drug-induced deaths were seen in either patient group during this period.

Discussion

Numerous studies have failed to show a direct antitumor effect of levamisole in either animal or human subjects. However, previous investigations have indicated that the addition of levamisole in an adjunctive manner to surgery [1] or radiation therapy [9] in various malignancies does increase the disease-free interval and possibly ultimate survival. Similar studies using levamisole as adjunct to cyclic chemotherapy [2, 5] have also shown increased survival in treated groups, although in the former report [5] an improved response rate was not seen. However, in that study the response rate in the control arm was substantially higher than in our trial, leaving little room for improvement.

The published data both in animals [9] and humans [2, 5, 9] do suggest that in some way levamisole does enhance or maintain the antitumor effects of conventional therapy in responding patients. But, there is little effect in those patients where substantial cell kill, and therefore prolonged remission, is not obtained. How this can occur is not clear, and the continual uncertainty about the mechanism of action of levamisole at a cellular level does little but allow for speculation. It could be that the results of this study allow one to speculate on two hypotheses to explain the positive effect.

Firstly, there seems little doubt that in vivo and in vitro levamisole exerts and enhances an effect on some end results of the immune response when this is impaired. Current thought presumes that this effect is consequent upon interaction between levamisole and the macrophage input to T cell and probably B cell replication. Experimentally it has been found [8] that preexistent suppression of host immune responses does decrease the therapeutic effect of both cyclophosphamide and melphalan in mouse mammary carcinoma. It is conceivable that the reversal of depressed cellular immunity that has been identified as being present [3], and related to prognosis [4], and reversible [10], in human subjects with neoplastic disease, can result in an enhanced response to cytostatic chemotherapy. This enhanced cell kill should bear some direct relationship to survival.

Conversely, levamisole may be exerting some as yet unknown influence on the host's ability to restore cell numbers in normal replicating tissues, such as the bone marrow and gastrointestinal tract, allowing more rapid recovery after each therapeutic cycle, the end result being an ameliorated tolerance to this therapy in levamisole-treated patients. Our data, when patients gained weight and suffered less morbid events than controls, while receiving higher drug doses in a shorter time than controls, would tend to support this suggestion. Conversely, which came first — a more robust patient, living longer because enhancement of cellular immunity allowed a greater cell kill, or a similar patient whose positive response was merely the reflection of more treatment?

Whatever the answer, the levamisole story remains inconclusive and all the more fascinating. But, with the advantage of levamisole being a chemically reproducible small molecule and a pharmaceutical preparation of low toxicity in comparison to most weapons in the medical oncologists armamentarium, one can anticipate that even modest improvements in survival will be sufficient to have practitioners in this field look past nematodes and towards macrophages.

Summary

The addition of levamisole, administered in adjunctive manner between the cycles of conventional high dose chemotherapy in patients with hormone resistant end stage breast cancer substantially improved the survival of treated patients. Analysis of this double-blind study in 60 such patients suggests that improvement in remission status and survival is related to better tolerability of such cytotoxic therapy as regards both specific and nonspecific cytotoxicity. This improved tolerability enabled patients to receive higher doses of cytotoxic drugs over a shorter time period resulting in an improved remission rate and ultimate survival.

References

1. Amery, W. K.: Overview of other controlled clinical data; an attempt at defining the future position of Levamisole in cancer therapy. Symposium of Immunotherapy of Malignant Disease. Vienna, 9–10 November 1976
2. Hall, S. W. et al.: In: Control of neoplasia by modulation of the immune system. Chirigos, M. A. (ed.). New York: Raven Press 1976
3. Hersh, E. M., Mavlight, G. M., Gutterman, J.: Immunodeficiency in cancer and the importance of immune evaluation of the cancer patient. Med. Clin. North Am. *603*, 623 (1976)
4. Hersh, E. M. et al.: Immunocompetence, immunodeficiency and prognosis in cancer. Ann. N.Y. Acad. Sci. *276*, 386 (1976)
5. Hortobagyi, G. N. et al.: In: Control of neoplasia by modulation of the immune system. Chirigos, M. A. (ed.). New York: Raven Press 1976
6. Koelmeyer, T. D., Stephens, E. J. W.: Aminogluthethimide in end stage breast cancer. Clin. Oncol. (1978) (to be published)
7. Lods, J. C. et al.: Levamisole and bone marrow restoration after chemotherapy. Lancet *1976/I*, 548
8. Radov, L. A. et al.: Int. J. Cancer *17*, 773 (1976)
9. Rojas, A. F. et al.: Levamisole in advanced human breast cancer. Lancet *1976/I*, 211
10. Watkins, S. M.: Effects of surgery on lymphocyte transformation in patients with cancer. Clin. Exp. Immunol. *14*, 69 (1973)

D. Ovary, Uterus and Testis Cancer

Laparoscopy and Peritoneal Cytology as Markers in the Follow-Up of Ovarian Epithelial Tumors

C. Mangioni, G. Bolis, M. D. Incalci, P. Molteni, and L. Morasca

Introduction

In a large percentage of ovarian cancer patients, primary surgical treatment leaves a situation of clinically non-followable tumor. The spread of ovarian cancer is, however, usually confined initially to the peritoneal cavity, but in view of the size and number of the sites, early diagnosis of relapse becomes even more difficult than primary diagnosis. Biochemical markers such as α fetoprotein, CEA, or βHCG, found to be specific for monitoring infrequent special tumors of the ovary [11, 14, 15], have not yet been shown to be of value in detecting the early phases of relapse in the epithelial types [3–10].

Laparoscopy, first introduced in 1973 for restaging of ovarian cancer patients, proved to be a means of finding diaphragmatic implantations not detected at laparotomy [1]. This minor surgery rapidly became the "new deal" for accurate post-therapy evaluation of response [9], and in several situations it replaced major surgery in the second-look procedure [13]. We used it as a systematic monitoring approach in ovarian cancer [5].

Peritoneal cytology, already developed in the past as a fine cytochemical method of staging [6], also proved to be correlated with prognosis [2] and appeared to us as an obvious complement of laparoscopic examination. This presentation discusses data on the systematic monitoring of patients with ovarian epithelial tumors, during the clinically non-followable phase leading to cure or to relapse.

Selection of Patients

The data reported were collected in 93 consecutive patients with "no evidence of disease" (NED) admitted to this department from October 1975 to April 1978. Thirty-four were assumed to have "no residual tumor" (NRT) and 38 "minimal residual tumor" (MRT), not followable by physical roentgenography or laboratory evaluation. Among these, 17 were included because of positive cytology only (ten stage IC, three stage IIC, and four stage III). The last 21 patients included were late stage III, becoming NED after chemotherapy. Intensive [7] staging during primary surgery, or laparoscopic restaging, gave a distribution of 36 stage I, 14 stage II, and 43 stage III patients in the population studied. All the patients entered a chemotherapeutic protocol for at least 12 months.

Method

Laparoscopy was performed under local or general anesthesia in ward patients with a Palmer Jacobs Operative 10-mm peritoneoscope equipped with standard 170° and angular 130° lenses (R. Wolff, W. Germany). The standard two-puncture method was applied. During laparoscopy all free fluid found in the Douglas or paracolic spaces was collected. Independently of any free fluid collected, the peritoneal cavity was also washed with 500 ml of saline solution and the washings were retrieved. Each sample was then submitted for cytologic examination.

Criteria for Utilization

Laparoscopic restaging was performed in 33 patients referred from other hospitals within 30 days of primary surgery, while in the 60 patients who had undergone surgery in our service, staging was performed during laparatomy always supported by peritoneal cytology and attentive diaphragm examination. Follow-up was started after 4—6 months of therapy in patients with positive cytology at stage I and in patients with stage IIB, IIC, and III. It was repeated every 6 months in NED patients with laparoscopic residual tumor. This policy enabled us to check the response to treatment and to switch to alternative therapies in due time. Second-look laparoscopy was systematically performed after 1 year in patients under precautional therapy but was left to the end of treatment in other patients. Third-look laparoscopy was limited to stage III to check on cure in NRT patients. It was performed about 1 year after withdrawal of therapy.

Results

In stage I patients, 41 laparoscopies were performed and no positive histologic samples were obtained; cytology was positive in 4 of 18 restagings and in 2 of 5 follow-up samples. All the patients with NED are alive at this time (Table 1). Of 14 stage II patients, only one gave positive cytology with histologically positive tumor during laparoscopic monitoring at the second look. This patient died about 2 years after initial therapy, while the other 13 with NED are still alive (Table 2).

Table 1. Results of 41 laparoscopies in 36[a] consecutive ovarian epithelial cancer patients — at stage I[b] after primary surgery, between Oct. 1975 and April 1978

Indication for laparoscopy	No. of laparoscopies	With positive cytology	With positive histology
Restaging	18	4	0
Follow-up during chemotherapy	5	2	0
Second-look after 1 year	18	0	0

[a] 36/36 NED at April 1978.
[b] Stage IA = 22 patients; IB = 4 patients; IC = 10 patients.

Table 2. Results of 17 laparoscopies in 14[a] consecutive ovarian epithelial cancer patients at stage II[b] after primary surgery, between Oct. 1975 and April 1978

Indication for laparoscopy	No. of laparoscopies	With positive cytology	With positive histology
Restaging	2	0	0
Follow-up during chemotherapy	4	0	0
Second look after 1 year chemotherapy	8	1	1
Third look 1 year after withdrawal of chemotherapy	3	0	0

[a] 13/14 NED at April 1978.
[b] Stage IIA = 6 patients; IIB = 2 patients; IIC = 6 patients.

Table 3. Results of 57 laparoscopies in 43[a] consecutive ovarian epithelial cancer patients at stage III[b] after primary surgery, between Oct. 1975 and April 1978

Indication for laparoscopy	No. of laparoscopies	With positive cytology		With positive histology	
early		NRD and early	Late	NRD and early	Late
Restaging	10	4	1	0	3
Follow-up during chemotherapy	25	0	4	0	14
Second look after 1 year chemotherapy	15	0	1	0	4
Third look 1 year after withdrawal of chemotherapy	7	0	2	0	1

[a] No residual disease = 6 patients; early = 16 patients; late = 21 patients.
[b] Surviving at April 1978: 36/43; no clinical or laparoscopic evidence of disease: 27/36.

Table 4. Relapses after primary treatment and course of peritoneal cytology in 52 ovarian epithelial cancer patients followed up for more than 1 year

Cytologic course	Follow-up	Second look	Third look
40 positive patients			
No cytologic change	6/7 (86%)	5/9 (56%)	2/3 (67%)
Cytologic remission	1/9[a] (11%)	3/14 (21%)	1/6 (17%)
12 negative patients			
Persistent negative	2/6 (33%)	0/8	0/1

[a] $P < 0.01$.

Stage III patients (NED at the time of laparoscopy) have an higher incidence of positive cytologic and histologic findings (Table 3); of these, the 21 late stage III patients who gave a complete response during chemotherapy, represented our high risk population. Seven of these patients died of neoplasia, three are still alive with progression, and four are controlled by other therapies after relapse; of the other 22 patients (early stage III and NR) listed in this group, only four contributed positive cytology and histology findings. Two of four relapsed cases, all still alive, are controlled; the other two are progressing.

The relationship between cytologic findings and relapses is assessed in Table 4; positive patients with cytologic remission had the lowest percentage of relapses. In contrast, persistent positives had the highest percentage of relapses. Among negative patients, the percentage of relapses was between these two, limited to follow-up. Operative implications connected with the laparoscopic procedure were very few: in one patient perforation of the large bowel, due to extensive adhesion from previous surgery, required a laparotomy. Two other patients had fever for 1 day. These were the only pathologic indices in over 250 laparoscopies performed in the period indicated.

Discussion

Information obtained by laparoscopy in stage I seems to add little to clinical evaluation when our results are considered. However, the population defined as stage I by laparoscopic examination is truly stage I since unrecognized stages II and III have already been excluded from the group. In fact, 5 of 23 patients (22%) in stage I became stage III after intensive combined restaging (anatomic, radiologic, and surgical procedures) and were not included in the stage I population. When stage II patients are considered in function of laparoscopic findings, the same considerations can be made on the usefulness of this procedure in upstaging three of five referred cases. On the other hand, laparoscopy was specifically indicated in stage I and II patients to detect early diaphragmatic leaves [1]. In view of this indication, we carefully explored the diaphragmatic surface in all the 238 laparoscopies performed in the period indicated and found 20 patients with positive nodules in the diaphragmatic area. In four cases the positive patients were diagnosed during restaging and had additional sites, and in the other 16 cases diaphragmatic leaves were associated with abdominal relapses. In stage I and II patients with localized ovarian cancer, no diaphragmatic metastases were found. This observation is in full agreement with the data of Piver et al. [8].

While the stage I and II population were carefully kept free from contaminating upstaged patients, in stage III, two populations with different risks were considered together. "No residual" and "early" stage III patients have in fact a more favorable prognosis than "late" stage III patients who became "NED" because of response to chemotherapy. On the other hand, the no residual and early categories include patients who entered this stage after surgery. It was thus difficult to decide which patients should be excluded and it was also evident that laparoscopy was indicated because of clinically non-followable disease regardless of the therapeutic means used to reach this stage.

It seems to us that clinically non-followable stage III patients obtain greatest advantage from laparoscopic follow-up repeated approximately every 6 months, this being a means of monitoring the response, the stabilization, and slow progression to continue, withdraw, or adapt therapy.

Second-look laparoscopy avoids major surgery in about 30% of patients, but negative findings still call for laparotomic look. In fact, in 5 of 11 major surgery cases performed after negative second-look laparoscopy, positive localizations were found, three in retroperitoneal lymph nodes and three in the omentum. Third-look laparoscopy is limited to cases with persistent complete clinical remission for 1 year after withdrawal of chemotherapy. This is to permit early diagnosis of late relapses. Among second-look negative patients, 16 (23%) have in fact been reported by other authors as dying from tumor [4, 12].

Laparoscopy may acquire prognostic value when combined with cytologic examination. Large series of cytologic findings showed a significant difference of survival between positive and negative cytology patients. These data were consistent both at first-look and at second-look laparotomy [2]. Our data also suggest that patients undergoing cytologic remission at follow-up have a significantly lower risk of relapse than no change patients and also seem in some way at a still lower risk than persistently negative patients. Data on this last point, however, is too limited to be statistically significant. At second and third look, however, the difference fades out, suggesting that early cytologic remission is more valuable for prognostic purposes than later remission. At this stage, laparoscopy seems to offer several practical advantages over laparotomic procedures, mainly the low risk and frequent repeatibility of a low cost procedure that does not preclude major surgery. This suggests the technique might usefully be included in the general strategy for long-term treatment of ovarian cancer. The approaches we follow today are:

1. Laparoscopy and cytology are two of the basic procedures for intensive restaging in all referred patients within 30 days of surgery performed in another hospital.
2. Follow-up during chemotherapy is systematic within 6 months of primary surgery in stage IA cured by single ovariectomy and in all other stages up to late III of NED patients. In late III NED patients, the laparoscopic procedure is repeated more frequently, to a custom-tailored schedule, depending on the chemotherapy already given and the drugs still available to control the disease.
3. At second-look monitoring, laparoscopy is widely accepted as a means of avoiding major surgery in a worthwhile proportion of patients and is routinely by us. It is also indicated after 1 year precautional chemotherapy in stage IA, IB, IC, and IIA patients without imploying in this case major surgery for negative subjects. In IIB and IIC patients, the indication for major surgery in laparoscopically negative cases is maintained. In stage III cases, persistent clinical remission after chemotherapy is monitored laparascopically and second look is updated at 24 months.
4. Third look, up to stage IIB, 1 year after withdrawal of therapy in patients with no clinical evidence of diseases, is regularly performed to detect early relapses in these high risk patients.

Acknowledgement

This work was partially supported by a generous donation from Mrs. Masella Russo, Milan, Italy.

References

1. Bagley, C. M. (Jr.), Young, R. C., Schein, P. S., Chabner, B. A., De Vita, V. T.: Ovarian carcinoma metastatic to the diaphragm: Frequently undiagnosed at laparotomy. A preliminary report. Am. J. Obstet. Gynecol. *116*, 397 (1973)

2. Creasman, W. T., Rutledge, F.: The prognostic value of peritoneal cytology in gynecologic malignant disease. Am. J. Obstet. Gynecol. *110,* 773 (1971)
3. DiSaia, P. J., Morrow, C. P., Haverback, B. J., Dyce, B. J.: Carcinoembryonic antigen in cancer of the female reproductive system. Serial plasma value correlated with disease state. Cancer *39,* 2365 (1977)
4. Mangioni, C., Bolis, G., Natale, N.: Terapia sequenziale dei tumori epiteliali dell'ovaio. L'utilità del second-look. Ann. Ostet. Ginecol. *97,* 205 (1976)
5. Mangioni, C., Bolis, G., Molteni, P.: Advantages and limits of laparoscopy in ovarian cancer. Gynecol. Oncol. (in press) (1978)
6. McGowan, L.: Peritoneal fluid profiles. Symposium on Ovarian Carcinoma. NCI Monograph *42,* 75 (1975)
7. Musumeci, R., Banfi, A., Bolis, G., Candiani, G. B., De Palo, G., Di Re, F., Luciani, L., Lattuada, A., Mangioni, C., Mattioli, G., Natale, N.: Lymphangiography in patients with ovarian epithelial cancer. Cancer *40,* 1444 (1977)
8. Piver, M. S., Lopez, R. G., Xynos, F., Barlow, J. J.: Value of pre-therapy peritoneoscopy in localized ovarian cancer. Am. J. Obstet. Gynecol. *127,* 288 (1977)
9. Rosenoff, S. H., DeVita, V. T. (Jr.), Hubbard, S., Young, R. C.: Peritoneoscopy in the staging and follow-up of ovarian cancer. Semin. Oncol. *2,* 223 (1975)
10. Samaan, N. A., Smith, J. P., Rutledge, F. N., Schultz, P. N.: The significance of measurement of human placental lactogen, human chorionic gonadotrophin and carcinoembryonic antigen in patients with ovarian carcinoma. Am. J. Obstet. Gynecol. *126,* 186 (1976)
11. Sell, A., Søgaard, H., Nørgaard-Pedersen, B.: Serum alphafoetoprotein as a marker for the effect of post-operative radiation therapy and/or chemotherapy in eight cases of ovarian endodermal sinus tumour. Int. J. Cancer *18,* 574 (1976)
12. Smith, J. P., Delgado, G., Rutledge, F.: Second-look operation in ovarian carcinoma. Postchemotherapy. Cancer *38,* 1438 (1976)
13. Spinelli, P., Luini, A., Pizzetti, P., De Palo, G. M.: Laparoscopy in staging and restaging of 95 patients with ovarian carcinoma. Tumori *62,* 493 (1976)
14. Stone, M., Bagshawe, K. D., Kardana, A., Searle, F., Dent, J.: β-human chorionic gonadotrophin and carcino-embryonic antigen in the management of ovarian carcinoma. Br. J. Obstet. Gynecol. *84,* 375 (1977)
15. Talerman, A., Haije, W. G., Baggerman, L.: Allpha-1 antitrypsin (AAT) and alphafoetoprotein (AFP) in sera of patients with germ-cell neoplasm: value as tumour markers in patients with endodermal sinus tumour. (Yolk sac tumour). Int. J. Cancer *19,* 741 (1977)

Radiotherapy in Ovarian Cancer for Post-Surgical Minimal Residual Disease

D. Chassagne and J. P. Wolff

Introduction

In ovarian carcinomas more than in any other solid tumor, post-surgical minimal residual disease is difficult to define precisely and this definition may differ according to stage. In stage I (A, B, and C) there is a possibility of malignant cells being left behind in the peritoneal cavity. Centrifugation of the peritoneal washings during and at the end of surgery can show the presence of cancer cells in numerous cases [2—4], but this "positive" finding does not prove that a subsequent seeding of "cancer colonies" is inevitable. However, these facts explain at least partially a 20% incidence of failure in stage I and therefore may justify an additive therapy in stage I. In stage IIA or IIB, the above may apply, but there is also the possibility of microscopic residual disease, especially around the peritoneal suture line. In addition, for stage IIB the residual disease may range from an implant a few millimeters in size to a bulky unresectable tumor. The definition of minimal residual disease is, therefore, impossible to give precisely, unless a size of residual macrosopic disease is stated and widely accepted.

For stage III, the same remarks as in stage IIB can be developed, but one should mention the possibility of a "minimal stage III", defined by FIGO classification as proved microscopic implant either in the gut or in the omentum. Our experience has shown the reality of this concept: among 18 omentectomies we found six cases with microscopic metastases [19]. Recent papers emphasize the existence of tumor implants in the subdiaphragmatic area in all stages. These metastases can only be found by systematic peritoneoscopy either at the time of surgery or after. The reported incidence of these hidden metastases ranges from a few percent up to 50% [11, 14, 21, 22].

Systematic lymphangiography can also show a 10%—30% [11, 12] incidence of involvement in the para-aortic region, but interpretation of lymphangiograms is extremely difficult and should be done with reference to the pathologic findings. In addition, microscopic involvement of para-aortic nodes, which is not detectable by lymphangiography, is always possible. All these occult para-aortic lymph node and/or diaphragmatic metastases fall within the spectrum of post-surgical residual disease.

Significance of Residual Lesions

According to the literature, prognosis is closely related to the importance of residual disease: [3—5, 9, 16, 25]. For Fuks [12] the effectiveness of radiotherapy depend upon the size of residual tumor, whereas Underwood states that radiotherapy is only useful after complete removal of the lesions [26]. In stages IIB and III, the survival rate of Dargent's series was 37.6% after complete surgery and 18% after incomplete surgery [8]. The team working at the M.D. Anderson Hospital [9, 25] clearly states a relationship between prognosis and size of remaining lesions, concluding that radiotherapy is useful for tumors less than 2 cm in diameter but is of little or no value for tumors greater than 2 cm. The prognostic significance of residual disease after surgery makes clear the necessity of postsurgical adjuvant treatment. The place of radiotherapy in minimal post-surgical residual disease is still not clearly established [3, 4, 6].

Results of Radiotherapy

Historical series allow a comparison between surgery alone and surgery followed by various types of radiotherapy; FUKS [12] has provided an excellent review of these data (Table 1). Although the range of 5-year cure rates varies considerably (from 55% to 88% in stage I and from 0% to 11% in stage III with surgery alone), there is no clear evidence of any benefit from radiotherapy in either stage I or stage III (survival at 5 years varies, from 40% to 82% in stage I and from 0% to 17% in stage III. The failure of radiotherapy to improve the 5-year cure rates *in stage I* may be explained by the following:

1. Some stage I cases were understaged due to lack of systematic exploration, for instance of para-aortic nodes or subdiaphragmatic regions.
2. Radiotherapy was mainly directed toward the pelvic region in these historical series and was therefore unable to cure tumor implants located outside the pelvis.

In stage III the reasons for radiation failure are clear. In many cases in these published series bulky tumor was left behind, and we have already considered the poor results of radiotherapy when the size of remaining tumor is greater than 2 cm [9]. In addition, whole abdomen irradiation (whatever technique is used) can only deliver a maximum dose of 3500–4000 rad to the upper abdomen. This dose is not sufficient by itself to destroy a macroscopic tumor implant. Furthermore, the liver and both kidneys must be shielded from radiation at the 2000-rad level, and consequently all remaining cancer cells located in front of the kidneys and liver receive only 2000 rad or less.

In contrast to stages I and III, the results considered by FUKS (Table 1) show an improvement for *stage II* when radiotherapy is added to surgery (without radiotherapy: 0% to 33%, with radiotherapy: 13% to 53%). There are two possible explanations for this benefit from radiotherapy:

1. Stage II is defined as disease located only in the pelvis.
2. Radiotherapy is able to deliver a tumoricidal dose of 5000–6000 rad to the whole pelvis.

No definitive conclusions can be drawn from these published series. However, none of them was randomized and too many discrepancies can alter the results of all data ever published [3]. Unfortunately, the same remarks apply to the systematic use of *radioactive colloids* in the postoperative recovery period. Very impressive results have been published with gold or phosphorus in stage I [1, 7, 20]. Despite the use of such techniques for more than 30 years, no definite proof of the effectiveness of this superficial betatherapy has been ever shown. A well-planned randomized trial is certainly needed in this field.

Few randomized series involving radiotherapy have been published; a brief review seems relevant:

1. FAZEKAS and MAIER compared the use of the *openfield and moving strip techniques* for whole abdomen irradiation: there are no difference at 5 years [10]. Despite this paper, there is still much controversy among radiotherapists about this technical problem. In our opinion the problem lies elsewhere.

Table 1. Published series (1960–1973) on treatment results in patients with carcinoma of the ovary

Author and reference	Surgery			Surgery and external irradiation		
	Stage I	Stage II	Stage III	Stage I	Stage II	Stage III
Kent (1960) [45]	48/86 (56%)	9/32 (28%)	6/55 (11%)	45/66 (68%)	19/36 (53%)	6/52 11%)
Rubin (1962) [17]	15/17 (88%)	–	1/33 (3%)	20/25 (80%)	3/13 (69%)	8/52 (15%)
Van Orden (1966) [46]	11/18 (61%)	2/8 (25%)	–	9/11 (82%)	8/22 (36%)	–
Ross (1966) [47]	36/44 (81%)	1/9 (11%)	1/14 (7%)	18/32 (56%)	5/23 (22%)	0/12 (0%)
Munnell (1968) [19]	92/118 (78%)	0/16 (0%)	1/84 (1%)	35/56 (62%)	9/29 (31%)	13/89 (15%)
Dalley (1969) [21]	11/20 (55%)	0/5 (0%)	0/5 (0%)	37/92 (40%)	7/51 (13%)	1/20 (5%)
Barr (1970) [48]	29/40 (72%)	9/27 (33%)	4/45 (9%)	11/17 (65%)	43/91 (47%)	14/80 (17%)
Kottmeier (1971) [24]	–	–	–	29/64 (45%)	23/97 (24%)	8/146 (5%)
Aure (1971) [23]	–	–	–	90/153 (59%)	32/122 (26%)	8/85 (9%)
Delclos (1973) [25]	–	–	–	27/40 (67%)	20/72 (28%)	13/93 (14%)
Clark (1973) [49]	28/46 (60%)	1/6 (17%)	1/44 (2%)	54/101 (53%)	16/51 (31%)	17/280 (6%)

From Fuks, Z. External radiotherapy of ovarian cancer. Standard approaches and new frontiers. Semin. Oncol. *2*, 253–266 (1975).

2. JOHNSON et al. [18] compared the results of *surgery plus cyclophosphamide to surgery plus whole abdomen irradiation* in 50 advanced ovarian cancers. There are no differences at 5 years, the results being equally poor with less than 10% survival in both groups.
3. SMITH et al. [25] reported the *M.D. Anderson Hospital trial* for all stages (with no ascites and no implants overlying liver or kidneys, and with residual masses smaller than 2 cm). This randomized trial compared whole abdomen radiotherapy plus pelvic boost with 12 cycles of melphalan, with 70 patients in the radiotherapy group and 79 in the chemotherapy group. Although there were no significant differences in histology, there was unfortunately a discrepancy in the stage distribution (32 stage IIB in the radiotherapy group versus 22 stage IIB in the chemotherapy group). The published results are preliminary, as few patients are at risk at 5 years. No difference can be seen in the survival of patients for all stages combined. The complications with irradiation seem to be more serious than the myelosuppression observed in the chemotherapy group.
4. The *American Gynecology Oncology Group* has initiated a trial with four groups [3, 17]. Preliminary results do not show any difference between radiotherapy alone, radiotherapy followed by melphalan, melphalan alone, and melphalan followed by radiotherapy. In stages IA and IB, the same group's results in a three-group trial do not show any differences between surgery alone, surgery and radiotherapy, and surgery plus melphalan.

No definite conclusions can be drawn from these randomized studies, except that the treatment of ovarian cancer is still a challenge to all therapists. Recently, the Stanford University group [12–14] has described a new technique of irradiation, by which a tumoricidal dose can be delivered to a specially shaped target volume including the diaphragmatic, para-aortic, and pelvic regions. At the same time, new proposals have been made by the radiochemotherapy and the ovarian EORTC groups to answer simple questions by simplified trials. For instance, is pelvic radiotherapy useful or not in the early stages after apparent complete removal of the cancer? Unless new weapons can be found, more progress will come only from careful, well-planned trials in which all possible parameters are taken into account [2–6, 23, 24].

In conclusion, we again stress that the challenge of ovarian cancer can only be solved by large series of patients and continuous cooperation of all specialists involved: surgeon, gynecologist, pathologist, medical oncologist, and radiotherapist. Radiotherapy certainly has a place in the treatment of post-surgical residual disease in ovarian cancer, but this place is not yet clearly established, especially as chemotherapy is growing in importance.

References

1. Aldermann, S. J., Dillon, T. F., Krummerman, M. S., Phillips, B. P., Chung, A. F.: Post-operative use of radioactive phosphorus in stage I ovarian carcinoma. Obstet. Gynecol. *49*, 659–662 (1977)
2. Barber, H. R., Kwon, T. H.: Current status of the treatment of gynecologic cancer by site-ovary. Cancer *38*, 610–619 (1976)
3. Brady, L. W.: Future prospect of radiotherapy in gynecologic oncology. Cancer [Suppl. 1] *38*, 553–565 (1976)
4. Brady, L. W.: Combined modality therapy of gynecologic cancer. Cancer *35*, 76–83 (1975)
5. Bush, R. S., Allt, W. E., Beale, F. A., Bean, H., Pringle, J. F.: Treatment of epithelial carcinoma of the ovary: operation, irradiation and chemotherapy. Am. J. Obstet. Gynecol. *127*, 692–704 (1977)

6. Chassagne, D.: Résultats et indications de la radiothérapie dans le cancer de l'ovaire. Louvain Med. *90*, 541–549 (1971)
7. Clark, D. G. C., Hilaris, B. S., Roussis, C. et al.: The role of radiation therapy (including isotopes) in the treatment of cancer of the ovary (results of 614 patients treated at Memorial Hospital New York. In: Clinical cancer. Ariel, I. M. (ed.), Vol. 5, pp. 227–235. New York: Grune and Stratton 1973
8. Dargent, M., Dargent, D., Lansac, J.: Traitement des tumeurs malignes primitives de l'ovaire. Etude rétrospective de 349 observations recueillies entre 1946 et 1966 au Centre Anti-Cencéreux de Lyon. J. Gynecol. Obstet. Biol. Reprod. (Paris) *2*, 421–431 (1972)
9. Delclos, L., Smith, J. P.: Ovarian cancer with special regards to types of radiotherapy. Natl. Cancer Inst. Monogr. *42*, 129–135 (1975)
10. Fazekas, V. T., Maier, V. G.: Irradiation of ovarian carcinomas. A prospective comparison of the open field and moving-strip techniques. Am. J. Roentgenol. *120*, 118–123 (1974)
11. Fisher, R. I., Young, R. C.: Advances in the staging and treatment of ovarian cancer. Cancer *39*, 967–972 (1977)
12. Fuks, Z.: External radiotherapy of ovarian cancer: standard approaches and new frontiers. Semin. Oncol. *2*, 253–266 (1975)
13. Fuks, Z.: The role of radiation therapy in the management of ovarian carcinoma. Jor. J. Med. Sci. *13*, 815–828 (1977)
14. Gladstein, E., Fuks, Z., Bagshaw, M. A.: Diaphragmatic treatment in ovarian carcinoma: a new radiotherapeutic technique. Int. J. Radiat. Oncol. Biol. Phys. *2*, 357–362 (1977)
15. Henderson, D.: Cancer of the ovary. Proceed. Annu. Clin. Conf. Cancer Ov. Windsor (Ontario), 1965. pp. 149–159
16. Hintz, B. L., Fuks, Z., Kempson, R. L., Eltringham, J., Zalovdek, C., Williamson, T. J., Bagshaw, M. A.: Results of post-operative megavoltage radiotherapy of malignant surface epithelial tumors of the ovary. Radiology *114*, 695–700 (1975)
17. Hreschchyshyn, M. M.: Results of gynecologic oncology group trials on ovarian cancer: Preliminary report. Natl. Cancer Inst. Monogr. *42*, 115–165 (1975)
18. Johnson, C. F., Decker, D. G., Van Herick, M. et al.: Advanced ovarian cancer: therapy with radiation and cyclophosphamide in a random series. Am. J. Roentgenol. *114*, 136–141 (1972)
19. Michel, G., Prade, M., Charpentier, P.: Intérêt de l'omentectomie systématique chez les malades porteuses de tumeurs malignes de l'ovaire. Gynecol. *27*, 455–457 (1976)
20. Muller, H. H.: Curative aim and results of routine intraperitoneal radio-colloid administration in the treatment of ovarian cancer. Am. J. Roentgenol. *89*, 533–540 (1963)
21. Piver, M. S., Lopez, R. G., Xynos, F., Barlow, J. J.: The value of pre-therapy peritoneoscopy in localized ovarian cancer. Am. J. Obstet. Gynecol. *127*, 288–290 (1977)
22. Rosenoff, S. H., De Vita, V. T., Hubbard, S., Young, R. C.: Peritoneoscopy in the staging and follow-up of ovarian cancer. Semin. Oncol. *2*, 223–228 (1975)
23. Rubin, P.: Understanding the problem of understaging in ovarian cancer. Semin. Oncol. *2*, 235–242 (1975)
24. Sack, H.: Die Strahlenbehandlung der Ovarialtumoren. Strahlentherapie *153*, 319–324 (1976)
25. Smith, J. P., Rutledge, F. N., Delclos, L.: Results of chemotherapy as an adjunct to surgery in patients with localized ovarian cancer. Semin. Oncol. *2*, 277–282 (1975)
26. Underwood, P. B., Merrit, J. O., Hitz, L. H., Wallence, K. H., Marks, R. D.: Carcinoma of the ovary: the adjunctive use of irradiation. Gynecol. Oncol. *3*, 298–307 (1976)
27. Wallner, P. E., Brady, L. W., Lewis, G. C. (Jr.), Nuss, R. C.: Post-operative pelvic irradiation of stage II ovarian carcinoma. Int. J. Radiat. Oncol. Biol. Phys. *2*, 281–288 (1977)
28. Wolff, J. P., Weill, S., Dergelet, L.: Cancer de l'ovaire. Etude clinique et pronostique. 6th International Congrěss of Gynecology and Obstetrics. New York, April 1970

Chemotherapeutic Sensitivity of Minimal Residual Disease Following Surgical Excision of Ovarian Carcinoma

J. H. Edmonson, T. R. Fleming, D. G. Decker, E. O. Jorgensen, G. D. Malkasian, J. A. Jefferies, L. K. Kvols, and M. J. Webb

Between mid-1974 and mid-1977, we simultaneously studied 82 patients with advanced evaluable ovarian carcinoma and 29 patients with minimal residual disease. These were randomized to receive either 1000 mg/m^2 of cyclophosphamide or 500 mg/m^2 of cyclophosphamide plus 40 mg/m^2 of adriamycin intravenously every 3—4 weeks. Our intent was to administer chemotherapy at 3-week intervals in the advanced cases and at 4-week intervals in the minimal residual cases. All patients in each of these studies had histologically proved epithelial-type ovarian carcinoma and all had adequate renal, hepatic, and bone marrow function as indicated by serum creatinine less than 1.5 mg/dl, the absence of direct reacting serum bilirubin, leukocyte counts greater than 4100/μl, and platelet counts greater than 130,000/μl. No bedridden cases or patients with active cardiac disease cases were accepted in either randomization, and the minimal residual disease cases were required to be fully ambulatory and could not have received any previous antitumor chemotherapy or radiotherapy.

Patients included in the minimal residual disease randomization had experienced surgical excision of all tumor masses greater than 2 cm in diameter at the time of total abdominal hysterectomy, bilateral salpingo-oophorectomy, and omentectomy within 1 month preceding accession to this study. Following surgery, they were categorized according to the distribution of residual disease in stages II and IIIA. We have arbitrarily defined IIIA disease as FIGO stage III with no postsurgical tumor masses greater than 2 cm in diameter. Those patients with stage IIIB, i.e., with larger residual postsurgical tumor masses, and with stage IV disease were included in the advanced category. The minimal residual disease patients were stratified by stage, extent of residual disease (i.e., grossly complete versus incomplete excision), and Broder's grade and histology, while those with advanced evaluable disease were stratified by type of previous treatment and performance status. Among the advanced evaluable disease cases, seven had previously received other chemotherapy and 11 had received some type of radiation treatment. Previously treated patients were equally balanced between the two regimens. Most of these advanced disease cases had at some time received significant debulking surgery prior to treatment except for 11 in whom only biopsy was performed at the time of the staging laparotomy.

In the advanced evaluable cases, the initially assigned treatment was continued until progression of disease was noted; however, crossover to the cyclophosphamide regimen occurred when, after approximately 10 months of treatment, a patient had received 520 mg/m^2 of adriamycin. At the time of progression, advanced evaluable patients then received the alternate of the two chemotherapeutic regimens.

For minimal residual disease cases, treatment was continued for 1 year on the initial chemotherapy regimen unless progression occurred earlier and, following 1 year of treatment, "second-look' surgery was recommended. Six patients receiving cyclophosphamide alone were eligible for second-look surgery following 1 year of treatment as were nine patients receiving the combination of cyclophosphamide plus adriamycin. In each treatment group, two patients among those eligible declined to accept this operation. Following secondary laparotomy, three of the four cyclophosphamide-treated patients began a 2nd year of chemotherapy while only two of the seven second-look patients initially receiving the combination did. All except one of these patients receiving further treatment after reexploration did so because of evidence of progression found at laparotomy. Patients with minimal residual disease who have later progressed have also been offered secondary treatment with either chemotherapy (with the alternate regimen if not already utilized) or occasionally intraperitoneal radioisotopes. We have attempted to repeatedly achieve disease-free status in as many of these minimal disease patients as possible in hope of achieving cure. After completing either of these two protocols, phase II new drug trials have been utilized without much apparent clinical benefit.

Among the 82 cases originally placed on the advanced evaluable disease protocol, two were ineligible respectively because of prior treatment with cyclophosphamide and because of abnormal renal function. Nine others apparently had been mistakenly staged according to the presurgical status instead of the postoperative condition and actually belonged in the minimal residual disease category. All 29 patients originally included in the minimal residual disease protocol were eligible, but one actually had advanced disease and had been erroneously placed in the minimal disease category. Thus, our primary analysis included 71 advanced evaluable patients and 28 patients with minimal residual disease. A secondary analysis then realigned these initially misstaged and misplaced cases so that the entire 109 eligible cases were able to be evaluated.

Twelve of the 35 patients with advanced evaluable disease initially treated with cyclophosphamide alone experienced partial regression of disease as did 13 of the 36 who initially received the combination regimen. Two of these 13 cases then went on to achieve complete tumor regression on the combination regimen. Time-to-progression curves were nearly identical for the two treatments in the advanced disease category. Similarly, survival curves for the two treatments also were nearly identical. Median survival for these advanced evaluable cases was approximately 12 months regardless of initial treatment. Among patients initially placed on the minimal residual disease protocol, median survival was approximately 21 months. These two populations were thus distinctly different. Among minimal disease patients, an apparent difference in time-to-progression favored the combination drug regimen ($P=0.06$; Cox covariate analysis). An analysis of survival curves revealed a similar trend again favoring the cyclophosphamide plus adriamycin regimen ($P=0.12$). When the nine patients previously misstaged were realigned with the minimal residual disease population, a treatment related time-to-progression difference was present as with the initial analysis ($P = 0.03$). Similarly, the secondary analysis for survival duration yielded a trend favoring the combination regimen ($P < 0.10$). Prognoses for survival and time-to-progression were better ($P = 0.03$) for patients with complete pretreatment excision of tumor than those with incomplete excision when all of the minimal residual disease patients were considered. Also noted among minimal disease patients was better prognosis for survival $P < 0.001$ and for time-to-progresssion ($P = 0.02$) among younger patients and longer time-to-progression intervals among those patients with lower grade tumors ($P = 0.03$).

Among advanced disease patients, we were not surprised to find that patients who had better ECOG (Eastern Cooperative Oncology Group) performance status prior to treatment survived longer than those with poor performance status ($P < 0.001$). Those whose previous treatment had been surgery alone also survived longer than did those who had received previous other treatments ($P = 0.04$). Most unexpected was the finding among these 72 advanced disease cases of an unequivocal survival ($P < 0.001$) and time-to-progression ($P < 0.01$) superiority favoring the older patients. This effect was apparent despite the less favorable performance status scores of the older patients. We have been unable to explain this powerful reversal of the expected age effect on survival by factors such as extent of pretreatment tumor burden or tumor grade. The presence of menstrual activity within 1 year preceding treatment was strongly correlated with this poorer prognosis in young women, and this could be true of course by natural coincidence. Among the 16 women in our study between 45–55 years of age, however, those eight who had ceased menstruating at least 1 year before beginning treatment had a median survival of approximately 12 months, which was twice that of the eight who still had ovarian endocrine activity at some time during the year prior to beginning treatment. Perhaps the presence of advanced disease allows the recognition of subtle growth-promoting effects that host resistance can overcome in cases with lesser tumor burdens. Myelosuppressive effects of the two drug regimens were moderate and equal. The combination regimen produced slightly more alopecia and mucositis.

Conclusions

1. Although no therapeutic differences were found between regimens containing cyclophosphamide alone and cyclophosphamide plus adriamycin in advanced ovarian carcinoma, the therapeutic index of the combination regimen was superior in patients with minimal residual disease.
2. Prognosis was clearly better regardless of treatment for patients with minimal residual disease, and within this category those who had grossly complete tumor excision prior to treatment survived longer than those with incomplete tumor excision.
3. Among patients with advanced disease, prognosis was better for older patients despite their generally less favorable performance status scores.

Chemoimmunotherapy for Advanced Ovarian Carcinoma With Adriamycin-Cyclophosphamide ± BCG: Early Report of a Southwest Oncology Group Study[1]

D. S. Alberts, S. E. Salmon, and T. E. Moon

Introduction

While ovarian carcinomas of the epithelial type are sensitive to a number of chemotherapeutic agents, treatment has not markedly increased the percentage of 5-year survivors having advanced disease at the time of diagnosis. Several groups, including our own, have previously shown that the combination of adriamycin and cyclophosphamide (A-C) induces a high percentage of partial remissions in patients with stages III and IV disease [5, 7]. Unfortunately, remission duration is still relatively short, and it is still too early to determine whether this combination therapy will have an important impact on the prolongation of survival.

One possible direction for the therapy of ovarian carcinoma is the use of nonspecific immunostimulants such as BCG or C. Parvum added to various chemotherapy regimens. In our own studies of tumor colony formation by ovarian carcinoma stem cells, we found that functioning peritoneal macrophages present within the tumor cell population are required for ovarian tumor colony growth [3]. The evidence for tumor-associated antigens in ovarian cancer [2], the recognized relationship of immunocompetence to survival in this disease [1, 4, 9], and the positive experimental evidence for curative immunotherapy in mouse ovarian tumor models [6] suggests that ovarian cancer may be amenable to the use of immunotherapeutic approaches.

Approximately 30 months ago, the Southwest Oncology Group initiated protocol 7524, a randomized study for the evaluation of BCG as an immune adjuvant to adriamycin-cyclophosphamide chemotherapy for patients with advanced ovarian cancers of the epithelial type. The preliminary results of this study will be the focus of this paper.

Methods

Starting in January 1976, patients with recurrent or stages III and IV ovarian cancer of the epithelial type who had measurable disease and had received no prior chemotherapy were entered into the Southwest Oncology Group study 7524. The study schema is summarized in Table 1.

Histopathologic review is conducted for all study cases. Patients with adequate bone marrow reserve receive 40 mg/m^2 of adriamycin intravenously and 200 mg/m^2 of cyclophosphamide daily for 4 days or a total dose of 800 mg/m^2 orally, beginning 2 days after adriamycin administration. Patients with impaired bone marrow receive adriamycin and cyclophosphamide at one-half the usual dosage with gradual escalation of dosages on subsequent therapy courses as tolerated. At the time of registration, half the patients are assigned to receive Pasteur Institute BCG, 6×10^8 viable organisms by scarification to rotating upper and

1 Supported by grants from the US Public Health Service (CA 16943, CA 12014, and CA 13612).

Table 1

Remission induction	NR off study (q 3–4 weeks × 12)	Maintenance (q 4 weeks)
Randomize	Restage	
Adriamycin 40 mg/m² IV D1 Cytoxan 200 mg/m²/day po D3–6	*Documented* CR *or* PR	Cytoxan 200 mg/m² po q day × 5 for 12 months
Adriamycin 40 mg/m² IV D1 Cytoxan 200 mg/m²/day po D 3–6 BCG (scarification) D 8 + 15	*Documented* CR *or* PR	Cytoxan 200 mg/m² po q day × 5 + BCG (scarification) D 15 only for 12 months

lower extremity sites on days 8 and 15 of each course of adriamycin-cyclophosphamide therapy. Courses of therapy are repeated at 3–4 week intervals depending upon tolerance to the myelosuppression caused by chemotherapy. The adriamycin dosage is not to exceed a total of 500 mg/m² body surface area, but the cyclophosphamide or cyclophosphamide + BCG therapy continues for a total 2 years for those patients showing complete or partial response, improvement, or stabilization of disease.

The prestudy evaluation includes routine hematologic tests and serum chemistries, as well as chest X-ray, sigmoidoscopy, barium enema, intravenous pyelography, and paracentesis and/or thoracentesis with cytologic evaluation when indicated. Where available, laparoscopy, abdominal and pelvic sonography, computed axial tomography, and whole body radionuclide scanning are recommended for initial tumor localization and follow-up evaluation. No patient is determined to be in complete remission unless a "second-look" exploratory laparotomy shows no evidence of residual disease. Patients classified as having a partial remission must have at least a 50% or greater decrease in tumor mass and/or complete disappearance of proven malignant effusions for greater than 1 month.

Results

At this time, available results are only preliminary. Eighty-seven patients from more than 20 Southwest Oncology Group institutions have been entered in the first 2 years of the study of which 66 are currently evaluable for response, having had at least two courses of therapy. Staging and prior therapy characteristics for the registered patients are included in Table 2. There were 43 A-C+BCG patients and 44 A-C patients. Over 90% of the A-C+BCG patients had not had prior radiation therapy as opposed to 84% of the A-C patients. Although there were more patients in the A-C+BCG group with stage III disease, there was an almost equal balance between the two therapy groups with respect to stage IV patients. Furthermore, there were more patients in the chemoimmunotherapy group of the study with liver involvement.

Table 2. Staging and prior therapy characteristics

	A-C + BCG	A-C
Number registered	43	44
Prior radiation Rx	4	7
No prior radiation Rx	39 (90.7%)	37 (84.1%)
Stage III	25 (58.1%)	20 (45.4%)
Stage IV	14 (32.6%)	16 (36.4%)
Lung involvement	6 (14.0%)	7 (15.9%)
Liver involvement	12 (27.9%)	10 (22.7%)
Recurrent disease	5	7
Performance status 60	2	4
Performance status 60	41	40

Table 3. Staging and prior therapy characteristics

	A-C + BCG	A-C
Cell type		
Serous	11	7
Mucinous	3	3
Endometrioid	3	2
Poorly differentiated	16	16
Unspecified	10	16

There was an almost identical number of patients in the two groups of the study who had a good performance status.

Table 3 summarizes the histologic types of epithelial ovarian carcinoma in the patient population as determined by each institution's pathologists. On the basis of this on-study data for this patient population, there appears to be an even balance of histologic types of ovarian cancer in each group of the study. There also appears to be a relatively large group of patients in each group with poorly differentiated tumors. Robert O'Toole of Ohio State University is conducting a pathologic review on biopsy material from all the ovarian cancer patients in this study, but this data is not currently available.

Approximately 65% of patients entered in each group of the study had only biopsy or relatively minor surgical procedures prior to the start of treatment, and the large percentage of patients in this study had far advanced cancer. A very small percentage of patients (< 2%) underwent minimal or major "debulking" surgical procedures.

Of the 34 fully evaluable patients in the A-C group of this study, only 11 (32%) had documented partial remissions (PRs), whereas seven additional patients have shown improvement (Table 4). To be categorized as having a partial response, a patient must have had a 50% or greater reduction in tumor mass for greater than 1 month or complete disappearance of malignant effusions for greater than 1 month. The partial plus improved patients comprise 53% of all those entered in the A-C group. There have been 16 partial remissions of the 32 patients entered in the A-C+BCG group of the study and one patient with improvement. Only two patients in the entire study were categorized as having had complete responses (CRs).

Table 4. Response data

	A-C + BCG	A-C
Evaluable	32	34
CR	2 (56%)	0 (32%)
PR[a]	16	11
Improved	1 (3%)	7 (21%)
No response	8	10
Increasing disease	2	5
Unknown	3	1
Died	7 (22%)	16 (47%)

[a] This category includes all patients in partial remission as well as those in clinical complete remissions who await exploratory laparotomy or laparoscopy to establish actual response status

Both patients had no evidence of disease at the time of second-look exploratory laparotomy and both had received A-C+BCG. No patient was considered to have had a complete response unless she had surgical documentation of complete disappearance of disease. The CR+PR rate for A-C+BCG patients of 56% at this time approaches statistical difference at the $P = 0.07$ level from the 32% CR+PR rate observed in the A-C group.
As of December 1977, 16 of 34 patients (47%) on A-C therapy have died versus seven (only 22%) of the A-C+BCG group (Table 4). This difference is significant at the $P < 0.05$ level. Figure 1 shows the actuarial survival curves for patients on A-C+BCG and A-C alone. Using

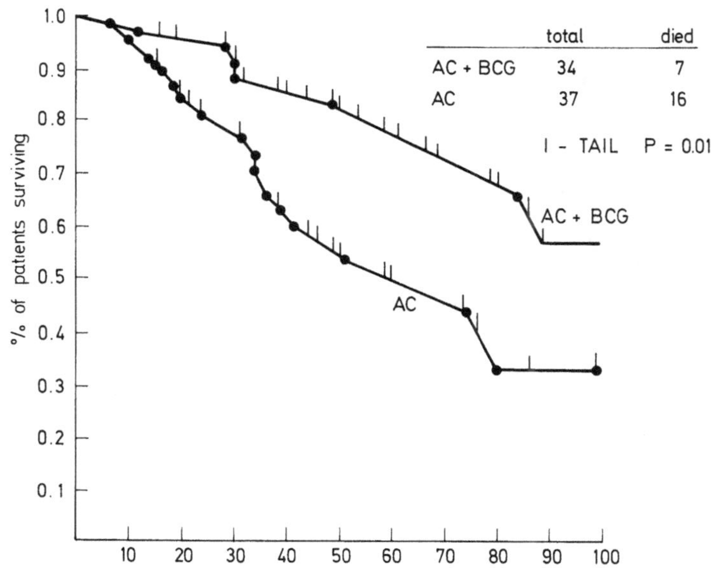

Fig. 1. Actuarial survival from onset of chemotherapy for 66 women with stage III to IV ovarian carcinoma randomized to SWOG trial 7524. The upper curve is for patients receiving A-C+BCG and the lower curve for patients receiving A-C chemotherapy alone. At the time of this analysis, survival with chemoimmunotherapy is superior to that with chemotherapy alone ($P = 0.01$)

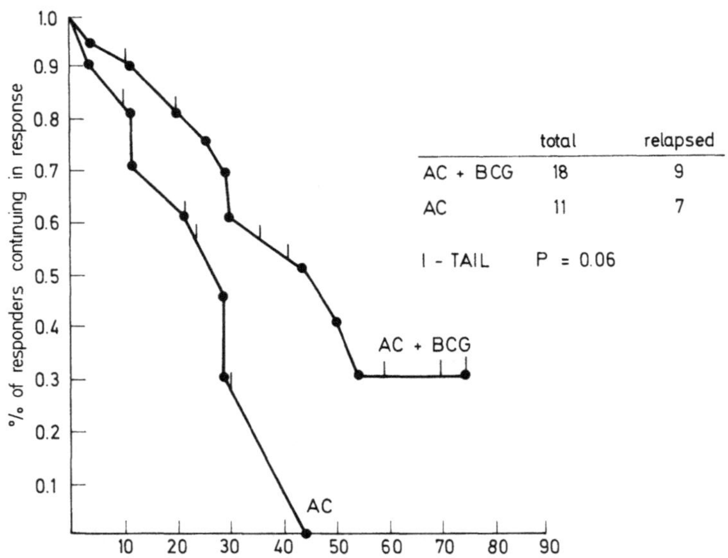

Fig. 2. Remission duration for 66 women with stage III to IV ovarian carcinoma randomized to SWOG trial 7524. The upper curve is for patients receiving A-C+BCG and the lower curve for patients receiving A-C chemotherapy alone. At the time of this analysis, remission duration for patients receiving chemoimmunotherapy appears to be better than that for patients with chemotherapy alone ($P = 0.06$); however, the effect of BCG on remission duration appears to be less marked than on overall survival as shown in Fig. 1

a one-tailed Wilcoxan test, survival duration for the A-C+BCG patients was statistically better than that of patients receiving only A-C ($P = 0.01$). The median survival from onset of chemotherapy was 93 weeks for the A-C+BCG patients and 59 weeks for the A-C group. The median duration of response (Fig. 2) was 45 weeks for the A-C+BCG group and 26 weeks for A-C patients ($P = 0.06$).

There were no therapy-associated deaths in either group of the study. Myelosuppression from both treatment programs was well-tolerated. The mean white blood count nadirs were 3000 and 3400/mm^3, respectively, for the A-C+BCG and A-C patients. Life-threatening leukopenia occurred in only two patients on A-C and one patient on A-C+BCG. Only three patients had either severe of life-threatening depressions of their platelet counts, and mean platelet count nadirs were 201,000 and 181,000/mm^3, respectively, for A-C+BCG versus A-C groups of the study.

BCG skin reactivity to scarification was considered to be optimal in the majority of treated patients. Twenty-three patients had skin reactivity reported between 2+ and 4+ at various times in their therapy. Only four patients were noted to have had no reaction to BCG. Of 29 patients with detailed protocol entries in this category, 22 experienced no BCG toxicity and none have 3+ or 4+ ratings. There were no drug-related deaths and no instances of liver disfunction related to BCG immunotherapy.

Discussion

The preliminary results of this Southwest Oncology Group study of chemotherapy versus chemotherapy + adjuvant BCG immunotherapy in advanced ovarian cancer patients suggests advantage for the A-C+BCG treatment with respect to the partial response rate, remission duration, and survival. The mechanism by which BCG apparently augments the effect of A-C remains obscure but conceivably could be a local or regional effect. Based on our in vitro studies [3, 8], we speculate that regional BCG scarification might alter the function of intraperitoneal macrophages and thereby reduce the proliferation of clonogenic tumor cells. Final validation of the efficacy of BCG immunotherapy in the setting of adriamycin-cyclophosphamide therapy will depend upon 1–2 more years of patient accrual and observation as well as complete histologic review of all pathologic specimens for patients entered on this trial. If this study remains positive, it will provide an important new approach to the treatment of patients with recurrent or stages III and IV disease. The addition of adjuvant nonspecific immunostimulant therapy to an effective combination chemotherapy regimen will hopefully offer the possibility of improved 5-year survival rates. This relatively well-tolerated chemoimmunotherapy regimen could be used to treat earlier stage disease where there is a high risk of relapse despite aggressive surgery and adjuvant radiation therapy and/or single agent chemotherapy.

References

1. Di Saia, P. J.: Overview of tumor immunology in gynecologic oncology. Cancer *38,* 566–580 (1976)
2. Gall, S. A., Walling, J., et al.: Demonstration of tumor-associated antigens in human gynecologic malignancies. Am. J. Obstet, Gynecol. *115,* 387–393 (1973)
3. Hamburger, A. W., Salmon, S. E. et al.: Direct cloning of human ovarian carcinoma cells in agar. Cancer Res. *38,* 3438–3444 (1978)
4. Khoo, S. K., McKay, E. V.: Immunologic reactivity of female patients with genital cancer: status in preinvasive, locally invasive, and disseminated disease. Am. J. Obstet. Gynecol. *119,* 1018–1025 (1974)
5. Lloyd, R. E., Jones, S. E. et al.: Combination chemotherapy with adriamycin (NSC-123127) and cyclophosphamide (NSC-26271) for solid tumors: a phase II trial. Cancer Treat. Rep. *60,* 77–83 (1976)
6. Order, S. E., Donahue, V., et al.: Immunotherapy of ovarian carcinoma, an experimental model. Cancer *32,* 573–579 (1973)
7. Parker, L. M., Lokich, J. J. et al.: Adriamycin-cyclophosphamide therapy in ovarian cancer. Proc. AACR and ASCO *16,* 263 (1975)
8. Salmon, S. E., Hamburger, A. W.: Immunoproliferation and cancer: a common macrophage-derived promoter substance. Lancet *I,* 1289–1290 (1978)
9. Wolff, J. P., DeOliveira, C. F.: Lymphocytes in patients with ovarian cancer. Obstet. Gynecol. *45,* 656–658 (1974)

Active Specific Immunotherapy in Ovarian Cancer

M. E. Crowther, L. Levin, T. A. Poulton, M. J. Saffrey, O. M. Curling, and C. N. Hudson

Introduction

The rationale of any programme of active specific immunotherapy depends on the demonstration of appropriate tumour-directed, cell-mediated immune responses, and agents designed to manipulate these immunological responses must be shown to have some therapeutic effect. In a pilot study on patients with ovarian carcinoma, Powles (personal communication, 1972) showed that the lymphocytes of patients with ovarian cancer would respond in vitro in a one-way mixed cell reaction to their autologous tumour cells. Subsequently, Levin [8] in this laboratory used a blastogenic assay system to show that patients with ovarian cancer could respond to a cell membrane extract of both autologous and certain allogeneic tumours. Lymphocytes from two-thirds of the patients in remission would in general respond, but much less so with relapsing disease, a well-recognised "blocking" phenomenon. Recent work has now shown a good correlation between circulating levels of immune complexes and the clinical state of patients with ovarian carcinoma [18], and there is evidence to suggest that "blocking factors" may be immune complexes of tumour-associated antigen and antibody.

The interpretation of in vitro tests of immune response is the subject of considerable debate, but additional evidence for a tumour-associated response comes from the demonstration in patients with ovarian cancer of a delayed hypersensitivity skin reaction to the injection of autologous tumour cell extract – in four of six patients in remission, such response was verified histologically by biopsy [9]. Controversial as these results may be, there was thought to be sufficient justification for an experimental immunotherapy programme, the protocol of which was based on the one in use in acute myeloid leukaemia [19], namely the monthly administration of allogeneic irradiated tumour cells and BCG.

Patients and Methods

Preparation of Cells for Immunotherapy

Ovarian tumours, fresh from theatre and in sterile containers, are manually disaggregated and gently homogenised, washed and filtered until a suspension of single cells or small clumps is obtained. Viability is assessed by trypan blue exclusion, and a viability of 30%–50% is regarded as good in these tumours. Because of their intra-abdominal site, these tumours are not bacterially contaminated. Only surface epithelial ovarian carcinomas are used, and serous papillary tumours have proved to be the easiest to prepare – mucinous tumours are not used because of cell trapping in mucin.

In a Planar freezer, 2×10^7 viable cells in 2 ml are cryopreserved in medium and 10% dimethylsulphoxide (DMSO), and the ampoules are stored in liquid nitrogen. Before cells are used, the donor patient is tested for Australia antigen and each batch of cells is subject to bacterial culture. Prior to immunotherapy, one ampoule per patient is rapidly thawed at 37° C, washed twice and made up to 0.4 ml in medium without antibiotic for immediate irradiation with 10,000 rad. Glaxo strain BCG is reconstituted to 1 ml, and 0.1 ml of a 1 in 40 dilution containing approximately 2×10^5 live organisms is added to the cells for final intradermal injection in four sites, either in the deltoid region or the thigh. Cells have been shown to be viable prior to irradiation as they can be grown in tissue culture and this ability is lost following irradiation.

Chemotherapy continues to be given, usually in a bolus midway between immunotherapy. Most patients are given 1 g of cyclophosphamide orally over 3 days, but patients in relapse are changed to intravenous chemotherapy with 40 mg/m² of adriamycin, 500 mg/m² of cyclophosphamide and 20 mg/m² of cis-platinum. Currently as part of the Medical Research Council Chemotherapy Study, intermittent and continuous oral therapy is being used.

Criteria for Entry and Protocol

This pilot study had one primary objective, i.e., to test the safety of the procedure, and for this reason it was set up in patients with disseminated disease beyond cure by surgery. Criteria for entry are that patients have primary surface epithelial ovarian carcinoma, excluding low-grade malignancy, in stage III or IV (FIGO classification) with incomplete initial surgery or, in a small number of patients, recurrent disease. Patients must show disease control by chemotherapy at 4 months following surgery. Unlike leukaemia there is no fine criterion of relapse and the term "disease stasis" covers the situation where there is no crude evidence of progressive disease as assessed by palpation or ultrasonic scan and no recrudescence of malignant effusions.

Side-Effects

Side-effects have been minimal, sometimes "flu-like" symptoms occur following the first course, lasting 24 h. We have seen no BCG granulomata, systemic infection [22] nor tumour deposits at the site of immunisation. Three patients have suffered from hyperimmunisation to BCG and the lesions took some months to heal. In such cases cells only are given for a few cycles and then BCG is reintroduced at lower concentration.

Early immunotherapy sites in patients resemble ordinary BCG inoculation sites. In patients in remission, further courses lead to flaring of previous sites, and cells alone have the capacity to cause this phenomenon. As patients pass into relapse, this ability to flare is lost and the BCG lesions become weaker and weaker – similar to the anergy seen in response to the Mantoux test in patients with fulminating tuberculosis.

Results

Figure 1 illustrates the actuarial survival of 17 patients, 15 of whom have been followed until dealth or for more than 2 years. A control group has been obtained by retrospective matching [7]. There was little difference between the two groups in terms of tumour histology and degree of differentiation. The actuarial survival curve calculated to 48 months shows that the median survival shifts from 12 months in the control group to 24 months in the immunother-

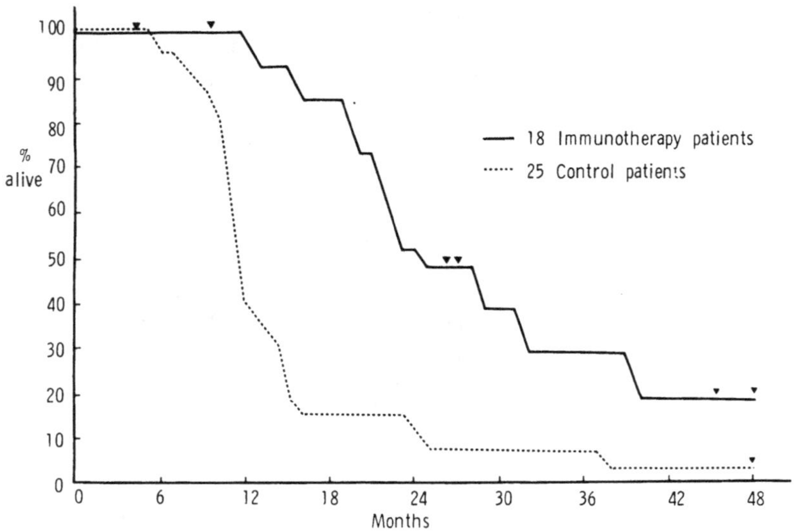

Fig. 1. Actuarial survival in patients with ovarian cancer treated with immunotherapy compared with patients treated with chemotherapy alone (N. E. Thames Series). ▼ represents patients who are still alive

apy group, but the downward trend is inevitable, a feature noted in the acute myeloid leukaemia trial [20]. At 48 months, survival for the immunotherapy group is calculated to be 19% compared with 4% for the control group ($P \leq 0.01$). The other noticeable feature is that immunotherapy appears to facilitate response to change in chemotherapy when patients relapse and that disease control may occur a number of times before final relapse. Similar findings have been noted by those concerned with acute myeloid leukaemia trials [4]. This pilot study is subject to all the valid criticisms of retrospective control analysis and to the other criticism that the reason for better survival in the immunotherapy patients was that they were seen more regularly and therefore relapse could be picked up earlier and treated more aggressively. Currently therefore, we have established a randomised prospective study using also the uniform induction chemotherapy protocol of the present Medical Research Council Chemotherapy Study.

Evidence for Immunostimulation

Twice weekly blastogenic responses of patients' lymphocytes to PPD and ovarian tumour cell membrane extract over each month of immunotherapy has been possible in some cases. Patient N.S. is a woman with stage III disease whose primary surgery was biopsy alone. Following dramatic regression of tumour on cyclophosphamide, she underwent "second-look" laparotomy for removal of uterus and ovaries; at that time numerous biopsies throughout the peritoneal cavity, liver and diaphragm could show no evidence of viable tumour. Her first course of immunotherapy was with BCG and allogeneic tumour cells. Lymphocyte responses over that month (Fig 2) show that baseline counts (unstimulated cells) alter in a manner consistent with in vivo activation of cells by BCG, i.e. they reflect the increased number of circulating "immunoblasts." In vitro this is displayed by an increase in the uptake

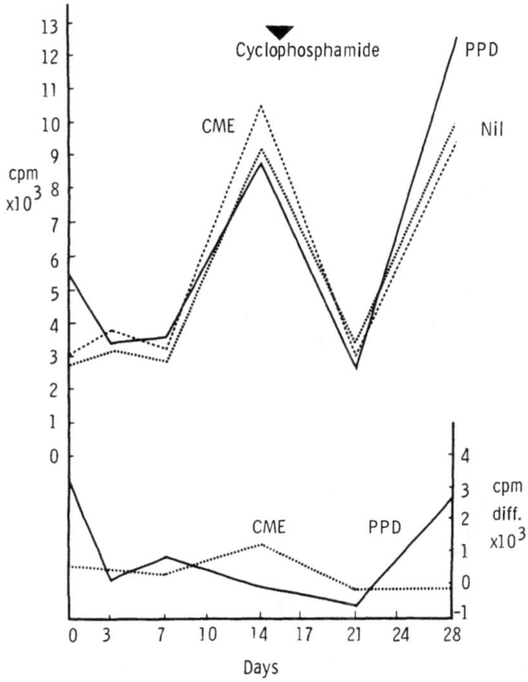

Fig. 2. Serial blastogenic responses during 1st. course of immunotherapy with BCG and cells (patient N.S.)

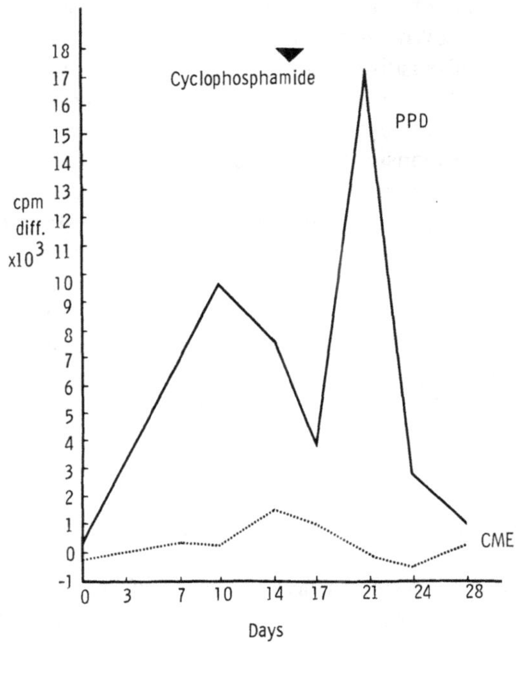

Fig. 3. Serial blastogenic responses during 2nd course of immunotherapy with BCG and cells (patient N.S.)

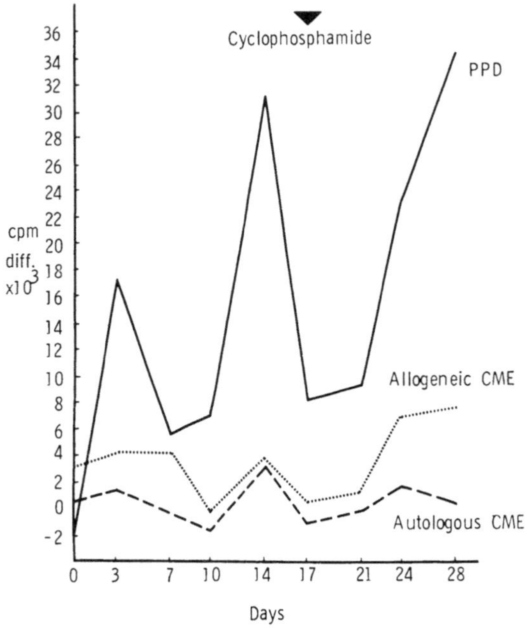

Fig. 4. Serial blastogenic responses during immunotherapy with autologous cells (patient M.T.) Disease static

of ^{125}IUDR into cells immediately following immunotherapy, a decrease that begins prior to chemotherapy and continues throughout, and then a restoration as part of the rebound phenomenon that normally follows the immunosuppression of pulsed chemotherapy [1]. If, however, counts per minute difference between stimulated cells (i.e. with PPD or cell membrane extract) and control cells are considered, there is little difference and certainly no discernible pattern.

The next month (Fig 3.), however, shows a marked change in this pattern. There is an initial boost following immunotherapy, a spontaneous fall that may reflect lymph node sequestration of sensitised immunoblasts [5] and a paradoxical and rapidly rebounding rise that begins while the patient is still taking her chemotherapy, and finally a fall. There is only a small change in response to cell membrane extract.

This responsiveness has also been seen following administration of cells alone, suggesting that there may be some cross reactivity between BCG and the tumour-associated antigen [13]. Likewise, in a patient who had clinically static but detectable stage III disease, there was a similar biphasic pattern and again a rebound phenomenon during and following cyclophosphamide (Fig 4). Analysis of T cell rosetting cells [25] in a small study of ovarian cancer patients with large tumour masses confirms reports by others that both the "active" (TE_a) and "total" (TE_t) populations of T cells are reduced. In ten immunotherapy patients, six of whom had large tumour loads at the time of assessment, we found that TE_a had risen to normal values, but that TE_t, although greater than values for patients in relapse, had not risen to normal values.

Discussion

Numerous studies have shown that chemoimmunotherapy prolongs survival when compared with chemotherapy alone [10, 19]. In contrast with this, McIllmurray [14] and his colleagues stopped an immunotherapy trial in patients with malignant melanoma in view of the alarming number of relapses in the "vaccinated" group compared with the control group. The problem with immunotherapy, as indeed with chemotherapy, is that work tends to be empirical since it is not always possible to use the results from animal experimentation in the human situation.

The two most obvious areas of dispute are the nature of the vaccine components and the use of chemotherapy. Animal experiments have suggested that the use of BCG with irradiated tumour cells is superior to either used alone as immunotherapeutic agents [15]. This would suggest that the specific effect of the tumour cells in activating sensitised lymphocytes is non-specifically amplified by the BCG. In humans, however, the results are conflicting. CURRIE [3] has shown that BCG alone has no effect on the level of serum inhibitory effects in patients with malignant melanoma, whereas the inclusion of irradiated allogeneic tumour cells in the mixture leads to a prompt fall. Clinically, POWLES [21] has shown that tumour cells mixed with BCG result in longer remission in acute myeloid leukaemia patients compared with those receiving tumour cells and BCG given at different sites.

The interspersal of chemotherapy with immunotherapy would also seem to be important and timing of this, to avoid the immunosuppressive effects of chemotherapy, is vital. CURRIE [2] showed that chemotherapy given prior to immunotherapy in a murine fibosarcoma model led to an increased anti-tumour effect and that the time interval between the two was important. On the other hand, MATHÉ [11] showed that BCG given before cyclophosphamide could reduce the effect of the drug and suggested that the BCG might be potentiating the immuno-suppressive effects of the cyclophosphamide [12].

Clearly for immunotherapy to be effective, chemotherapy must be used to maintain a small tumour load, but its timing must not be such that the stimulatory effects of immunotherapy are abrogated. Indeed, in our patients it appears as if immunotherapy offers some measure of protection from the immunosuppressive effects of chemotherapy. Certainly the white cell count does not drop as greatly in these patients compared with those on chemotherapy alone. It may be that BCG by its effect on bone marrow and haemopoietic stem cells has a protective effect [17] against the toxicity of chemotherapeutic agents.

The paradoxical rise in lymphocyte activity during and following chemotherapy is interesting and requires explanation. In animals, cyclophosphamide can be shown to destroy a population of suppressor T cells [23] and so reverse a state of immunological tolerance to dinitrophenols and lead to delayed hypersensitivity reactions to picryl chloride. Furthermore, the cyclophosphamide as well as reversing this state of tolerance was associated with the ability of T cells to proliferate in draining lymph nodes following sensitisation with picryl chloride [16]. It has since been shown that it suppresses B cells in preference to T cells and is selectively cytotoxic to short-lived cells that have a rapid turnover in peripheral blood [24].

Conclusion

It may very well be that BCG by its effects on bone marrow protects the host against the severely immunosuppressive effect of cyclophosphamide and also encourages the reestablishment of normal levels of active T-cells. Cyclophosphamide, on the other hand, may break the state of "immunological tolerance" that exists in relapse patients by actively destroying suppressor cells and allowing the release of sensitised cells from the lymph nodes draining the immunotherapy sites into the circulation. Further study on the subpopulations of cells to try to define more clearly the mechanism of immunotherapy needs to be done. This pilot study suggests that immunotherapy is a safe and possibly useful procedure in selected patients. The progress of the randomised prospective study will be followed with interest, because in so many other situations such studies are now failing to endorse earlier enthusiasm [6].

Acknowledgement

This study is supported by the Cancer Research Campaign, and the epidemiological study organised by the Association of Obstetricians and Gynaecologists of the N. E. THAMES Region has been supported by the Regional Research Funds, the Peel Medical Trust and the Charities Aid Foundation. The authors are grateful to clinicians who have allowed patients to be investigated and treated in this way. C.N.H. and L.L. were awarded the 1977 Edgar Gentilli Prize by the Royal College of Obstetricians and Gynaecologists. This study would never have been launched without the personal interest and assistance of the late GORDON HAMILTON FAIRLEY.

References

1. Cheema, A. R., Hersh, E. M.: Patient survival after chemotherapy and its relationship to in vitro lymphocyte blastogenesis. Cancer *28,* 851 (1971)
2. Currie, G. A., Bagshawe, K.: Active immunotherapy with Corynebacterium parvum and chemotherapy in murine fibrosarcomas. Br. Med. J. *1970 I,* 541
3. Currie, G. A., McElwain, T. J.: Active immunotherapy as an adjunct to chemotherapy in the treatment of disseminated malignant melanoma; a pilot study. Br. J. Cancer *31,* 143 (1975)
4. Freeman, C. B., Harris, R., Geary, C. G. et al.: Active immunotherapy used alone for maintenance of patients with acute myeloid leukaemia. Br. Med. J. *4,* 571 (1973)
5. Frost, P., Lance, E. H.: The cellular origin of the lymphocyte trap. Immunology *26,* 175–186 (1974)
6. Hedley, D. W., McElwain, T. J., Currie, G. A.: Specific active immunotherapy does not prolong survival in surgically treated patients with stage IIB malignant melanoma and may promote early recurrence. Br. J. Cancer *37,* 491 (1978)
7. Hudson, C. N., Levin, L., McHardy, J. E. et al.: Active specific immunotherapy for ovarian cancer Lancet *1976 II,* 877
8. Levin, L., McHardy, J. E., Curling, O. M., Hudson, C. N.: Tumour antigenicity in ovarian cancer. Br. J. Cancer *32,* 152 (1975)
9. Levin, L., McHardy, J. E., Poulton, T. A. et al.: Tumour associated immunity and immunocompetence in ovarian cancer. Br. J. Obstet. Gynaecol. *83,* 393 (1976)
10. Mathé, G., Amiel, J. L., Schwarzenberg, L. et al.: Active immunotherapy for acute lymphoblastic leukaemia. Lancet *1969 I,* 697
11. Mathé, G., Halle-Pannenko, O., Bourut, C.: Immune manipulation by BCG administered before or after Cyclophosphamide for chemo-immunotherapy of L1210 leukaemia. Eur. J. Cancer *10,* 661 (1974)
12. Mathé, G., Halle-Pannenko, O., Bourut, C.,: Potentiation of a cyclophosphamide-induced immuno-depression by the administration of BCG. Transplant Proc. *6,* 431 (1974)
13. Minden, P., McClatchy, J. K., Wainberg, M. et al.: Shared antigens between Mycobacterium Bovis (BCG) and neoplastic cells. J. Natl. Can. Inst. *53,* 1325 (1974)
14. McIllmurray, M. B., Embleton, M. J., Reeves, W. G. et al.: Controlled trial of active immunotherapy in management of Stage IIB malignant melanoma. Br. Med. J. *1977 I,* 540

15. Parr, L.: Response of syngeneic murine lymphomata to immunotherapy in relation to the antigenicity of the tumour. Br. J. Cancer *26,* 174 (1972)
16. Pomak, L., Turk, J. L.: Reversal of immunological tolerance by Cyclophosphamide through inhibition of suppressor cell activity. Nature *249,* 654 (1974)
17. Pouillart, P., Palangie, T., Schwarzenberg, L. et al.: Letter: effect of BCG on haemopoietic stem cells. Biomedicine [Express] *23,* 469 (1975)
18. Poulton, T., Crowther, M. E., Hay, F., Nineham, L.: Immune complexes in ovarian cancer. Lancet (in press) (1978)
19. Powles, R. L., Crowther, D., Bateman, C. J. T. et al.: Immunotherapy for acute myelogenous leukaemia. Br. J. Cancer *28,* 365 (1973)
20. Powles, R. L., Russell, J., Lister, T. A. et al.: Immunotherapy for acute myelogenous leukaemia: a controlled clinical study 2½ years after entry of the last patient. Br. J. Cancer *35,* 265 (1977)
21. Powles, R. L., Russell, J. A., Selby, P. J. et al.: Maintenance of remission in acute myelogenous mixture of BCG and irradiated leukaemia cells. Lancet *1977 II,* 1107
22. Sparks, F. C., Silverstein, M. J., Hunt, J. S. et al.: Complications of BCG immunotherapy in patients with cancer. New Engl. J. Med. *289,* 827 (1973)
23. Turk, J. L., Parker, D., Poulter, L. W.: Functional aspects of the selective depletion of lymphoid tissue by Cyclophosphamide. Immunology *23,* 493 (1972)
24. Turk, J. L., Poulter, L. W.: Selective depletion of lymphoid tissue by Cyclophosphamide. Clin. Exp. Immunol. *10,* 285 (1972)
25. Wybran, J., Fudenberg, H.: Rosette formation, a test for cellular immunity. Trans. Assoc. Am. Physicians *84,* 239 (1971)

Clinical Studies on PSK: Combination Therapy of PSK With Radiation in Cancer of the Uterine Cervix

T. Taguchi

Introduction

PSK is a polysaccharide preparation obtained from the mycelia of the CM-101 strain of Coriolus versicolor (Fr.) Quél in Basidiomycetes by hot-water extraction followed by sedimentation with ammonium sulfate saturation, dialysis, and drying. This preparation is a protein-bount polysaccharide containing about 38% protein, which consists of 18 kinds of amino acids such as aspartic acid, glutamic acid, etc. PSK possesses quite unique immunologic characteristics:

1. Helper T cell in vivo a) Restoration of depressed antibody-forming capacities to heterologous erythrocytes in tumor-bearing mice; b) Potentiation of antibody production when 1×10^7 sheep erythrocytes as an immunizing dose was used, but no difference when 4×10^8 sheep erythrocytes was used [15].
2. Delayed type hypersensitivity T cell in vivo a) Prevention of depressed delayed skin reaction against picryl chloride in tumor-bearing mice [13]; b) Potentiation of foot pad reaction against the tumor in tumor-bearing mice [4–6].
3. Effector T cell in vivo a) Potentiation of the cytotoxicity against the tumor in tumor-bearing mice; b) Restoration of depressed allograft rejection in tumor-bearing mice [8];
4. Suppressor T cell in vivo a) Restoration of enhanced suppressor T cell activity of antibody production to TNP-BSA in tumor-bearing mice [14].
5. Macrophage in vivo a) Restoration of the resistance against *Listeria monocytogenes* infection in tumor-bearing mice [9]; b) Potentiation of the phagocytic activity against *Candida tropicalis* in mice [3]; c) Potentiation of the phagocytic activity against sheep erythrocytes in mice [Ishida, N., 1977 unpublished]; d) Potentiation of in vivo chemotaxis to PHA in mice [10].

Clinical Studies

The combination effect of PSK with radiation therapy was first observed in the treatment of patients with uterine cervical cancer by Kasamatsu et al. (Fig. 1) [2]. He found a marked histologic improvement of the primary focus in the biopsy specimens obtained from patients with stage III uterine cervical cancer.

Stage III Uterine Cervical Cancer

Every day (5 days a week) 200 rad were irradiated with two sources at the front and back with a 6 Me V X-ray (using linear accelerator) on the whole pelvis of a stage III cervical cancer patient, for a total of 5000 rad. Before irradiation was started, 3 g/day or 6 g/day of PSK was

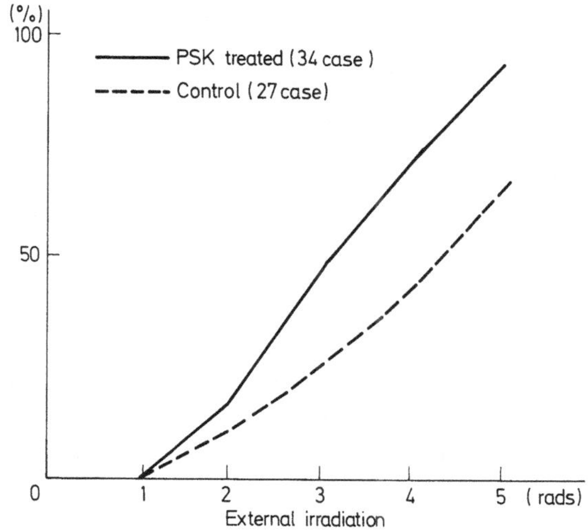

Fig. 1. Rate of grade III or IV in biopsy specimens under external irradiation

continuously administered orally. The test sample was obtained from the primary foci every 1000 rad (Fig. 1), and the irradiation effect was evaluated according to the Oboshi and Shimozato classification method.

Table 1 indicates the histologic gradings of cancerous tissue proposed by Oboshi and Shimosato in Japan. Using these gradings, the rate of appearance of grade III (IV) in Kasamatsu's study was 71% in PSK-treated and 44% in non-PSK-treated patients with 4000 rad irradiation and 94% in PSK-treated and 67% non-PSK-patients with 5000 rad showing a significant increase in effective cases.

After 2 or 3 years observation, a higher survival rate was found in the patients given PSK (Table 2).

Table 1. Histologic gradings

Grade I:	No morphologic change observed on tumor cells or only slight change so that clasmatosis of tumor cells was not apparent
Grade II:	Some fusion and necrosis observed; however, tumor cells considered viable remained
Grade III:	Tumor cells still remained; however, growth and recurrence not expected due to remarkable morphologic change
Grade IV:	No tumor cells remained at all

Table 2. Uterine cervical cancer (epidermoid cancer) stage III, survival rate

	Case	2-year survival rate	3-year survival rate
PSK + radiation	34	32/34 (94%)	29/34 (85%)
Radiation	27	20/27 (74%)	16/27 (59%)

Stage II Uterine Cervical Cancer

SONODA et al. [12] obtained results very similar to KASAMATSU's. After outer pelvic irradiation of patients with stage II uterine cervical cancer at 200 rad five times a week, biopsy of the primary focus was made at the time of total 1000, 2000, and 3000 rad irradiation, and the radiation effect was examined histopathologically. In his study, enhancement of histologic effect of PSK was observed in cases of 1000 or 2000 rad total irradiation (Fig. 2).

Uterine Cervical Cancer

KWAI et al. [1] also reported on telecobalt irradiation (Fig. 3) on the primary focus of patients with uterine cervical cancer; biopsy specimens were obtained 7 days after irradiation. After examining the radiosensitivity effect histopathologically, he found a significant increase in

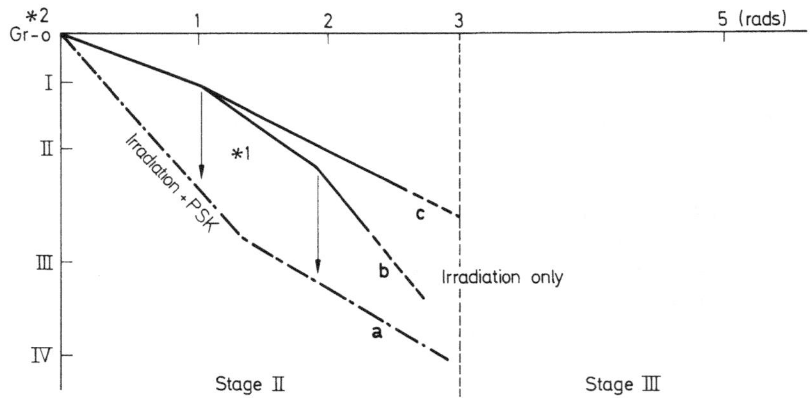

Fig. 2. Illustration of PSK effect in combined therapy with irradiation. 1: Arrow range indicates enhancement by PSK administration. 2: Gr. indicates "grade" (irradiation effect classified by Oboshi); (A): Stage II irradiation + PSK; (B): stage II irradiation only; (C): stage III irradiation only

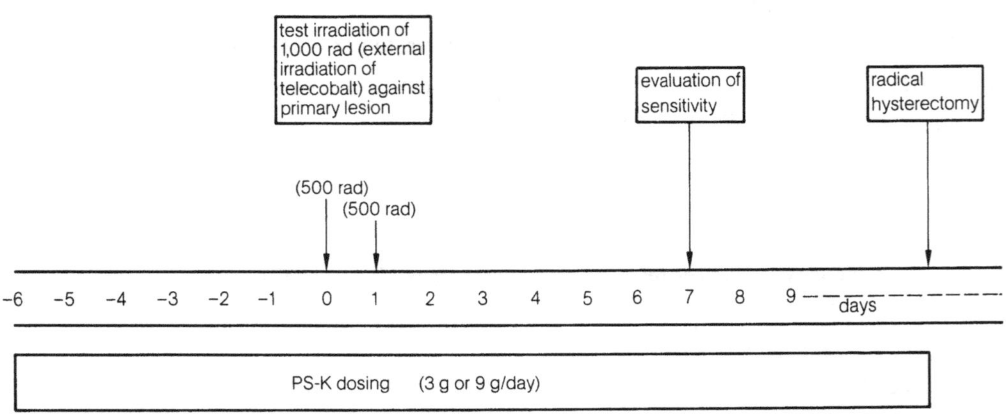

Fig. 3. Radiation system

Table 3. Comparison of radiosensitivity in each individual case

Treatment methods	No. of cases	Radiosensitivity		
		Good	Moderate	Poor
PSK + 100 rad radical hysterectomy	32	14 (43.8%)	11 (34.3%)	7 (21.9%)
Radical hysterectomy (1000 rad)	64	14 (21.9%)	24 (37.5%)	26 (40.6%)
PSK + 1000 rad radiation therapy	20	6 (30.0%)	9 (45.0%)	5 (25.0%)
Radiation therapy (1000 rad)	152	35 (23.0%)	54 (35.6%)	63 (41.4%)

effective cases by a combination of PSK with radiation in which better prognosis was reported (Table 3). In conclusion, PSK will be one of the preparations valuable in combination with radiation.

References

1. Kwai, S. et al.: 7th Asian Congress of Obstetrics and Gynecology. (1977)
2. Kasamatsu, T. et al.: Jpn. J. Cancer Clin. *22*, 1093 (1976)
3. Kamitsuka, A. et al.: 31th Annual Meeting of the Japanese Society for Medical Mycology. (1977)
4. Kimura, I. et al.: 36th Annual Meeting of the Japanese Cancer Association. (1977)
5. Kobayashi, H. et al.: Cancer Res *37*, 3042 (1977)
6. Mizuno, D. et al.: GANN *67*, 685 (1977)
7. Nomoto, K. et al.: GANN *66*, 365 (1975)
8. Nomoto, K. et al.: GANN *66*, 649 (1975)
9. Nomoto, K. et al.: 35th Annual Meeting of the Japanese Cancer Association. (1976)
10. Nomoto, K. et al.: 37th Annual Meeting of the Japanese Cancer Association. (1978)
11. Nomoto, K. et al.: 12th International Cancer Congress. (1978)
12. Sonoda, T.: Cancer Chemother. *2*, 1009 (1975)
13. Taguchi, T. et al.: Cancer Chemother. *2*, 13 (1975)
14. Taguchi, T. et al.: 12th International Cancer Congress. (1978)
15. Yamada, K. et al.: GANN *67*, 97 (1976

Irradiation as Adjuvant Therapy in the Management of Testicular Tumors

H. F. Hope-Stone

It has been accepted for the last 3 decades that many testicular tumors respond well to irradiation, that such adjuvant therapy will lead to almost a 100% cure rate in seminoma (in contrast to the 40% rate achieved prior to 1940 when irradiation was not given) and in some teratomata will achieve a very similar response.

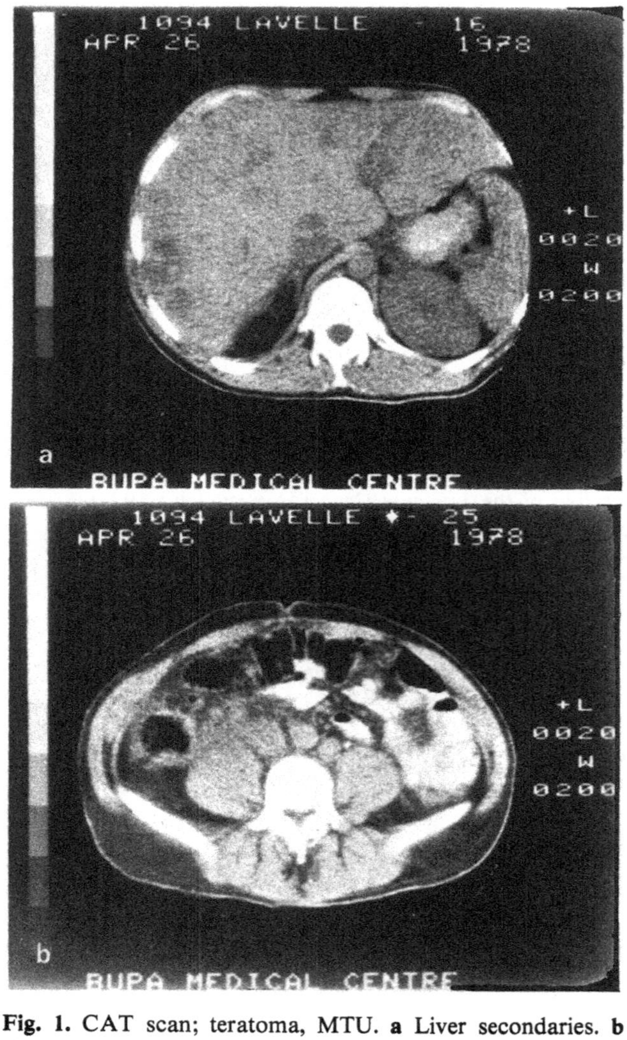

Fig. 1. CAT scan; teratoma, MTU. **a** Liver secondaries. **b** Para-aortic glands producing right obstructive uropathy

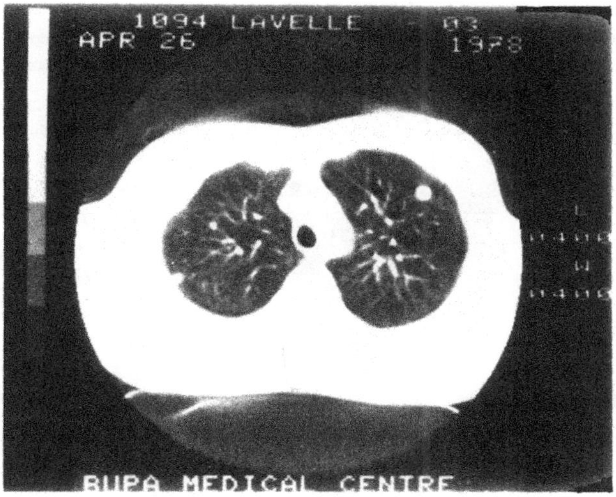

Fig. 2. CAT scan; teratoma, MTU; lung metastases

To decide the way these tumors should be irradiated, it is necessary to stage them. This can be done in a simple manner by clinical examination combined with chest X-ray, and more accurately by lymphangiography and whole lung tomography. With the former, the obvious metastases will be seen, but interpretation may be difficult, as the nodes can appear to be involved, but tomography of these nodes may show this to be untrue. An intravenous pyelogram (IVP) or even an inferior veno-cavogram may help. Computerised axial tomography (CAT) is a further advance, as can be seen in Fig. 1a and b. A chest X-ray will pick up gross metastases, but whole lung tomograms are better for showing up multiple small lesions. Similarly, CAT scanning of the lungs might indicate the presence of more than one lesion (Fig. 2).

At the London Hospital, staging has been as follows [1]:

Stage I: no definite tumor in the abdomen, but occult metastases are assumed to be present in the pelvic or para-aortic nodes

Stage II: definite abdominal lymph node metastases, but presumed occult metastases above the diaphragm

Stage IIIA: with supra-clavicular nodes or mediastinal lymph nodes and occult metastases below the diaphragm

Stage IIIB: with intrapulmonary metastases

Stage IIIC: with supra-clavicular and intrapulmonary metastases and abdominal glands.

The treatment policy is therefore based on the presence of these occult metastases. If we look at this policy stage by stage, we see that in stage I we are interested in the occult metastases in the pelvic and para-aortic lymph nodes, and it is these that we irradiate, using the classical T-shaped field and using an IVP to outline the position of the kidneys. The kidneys are not included in the direct radiation field, as irradiation nephritis may occur above a dose of 2250 rad [3].

It goes without saying that the orchidectomy must be carried out through the inguinal approach. Once the scrotum is incised, the groin lymph nodes and the scrotum itself may be contaminated, and the incidence of local recurrence is very high (Table 1), thus making the prognosis much worse. It would also be necessary to irradiate both these nodes and the

Table 1. Incidence of local recurrence with and without scrotal incision

Scrotal orchidectomy, biopsy, etc.	11 of 46 cases (24%)
No scrotal incision	3 of 329 cases (1%)

Table 2. Protocol for trial chemotherapy regime, the London Hospital and Institute of Urology, teratoma MTU, stage II and III

Platinum 20 mg/m^2	Days 1–5, 21–25
Vinblastine 0.2 mg/kg	Days 1, 2, 21, 22
Bleomycin 30 U (IV)	Days 2, 9, 16, 23, 30, 37

scrotum, and the patient will then become infertile. Normally the good testis is shielded, and measurements suggest that the latter will receive a dose of 50–150 rad, which will not cause sterility.

In seminoma, a tumor dose of 3000 rad in 20 daily fractions is given, with a pair of parallel and opposed megavoltage fields. For the teratomata, the dose is increased to 4000 rad in the same time. At these dose levels there is no danger of irradiation myelitis, small bowel fistula or stomach ulceration. The marrow is rarely severely affected.

In stage II seminoma, with known pelvic and para-aortic node involvement, these areas are irradiated first, although if the tumor is very extensive the whole abdomen is irradiated to 2250 rad and treatment then continued to the higher dose after shielding the kidneys. After a month's gap, prophylactic irradiation is given to the mediastinum and supra-clavicular nodes using a standard T-shaped field and shielding the lungs to prevent pneumonitis.

In teratomata, in the MTI group, irradiation is given as described for seminoma, but with a dose of 4000 rad. In the MTU group (embryonal carcinoma), it might be better to give chemotherapy first, using perhaps cis-platinum, vinblastine and bleomycin, and follow this later with irradiation to the site of the original bulk disease (Table 2).

Stage IIIA in seminoma and MTI teratoma with supra-clavicular and mediastinal gland involvement, these areas are irradiated in the first instance, and then subsequently prophylactic irradiation is given to the pelvic and para-aortic lymph nodes. Stage IIIB, in seminoma with lung involvement, irradiation is still the treatment of choice, taking the whole lungs to a dose of 2200 rad over 4 weeks; irradiation pneumonitis should not occur at this dose level.

In MTI teratoma, this may also be worth trying, as shown in the case of a patient who developed lung metastases 6 months after irradiation of the pelvic and para-aortic nodes. He was given 2200 rad and has survived for 8 years. In stage IIIA and IIIB MTU teratoma, there is certainly good reason to start with chemotherapy and only to give irradiation at a later date to the site of the original bulk disease.

In seminoma the results continue to be excellent (Table 3), although the poor survival in stage III is disquietening; however, in recent years (Fig. 3 and Table 4) even these groups have improved. In teratoma MTI it is now quite accepted – in the United Kingdom at least – that irradiation is the treatment of choice at least in the early stages, and there is now no place for retroperitoneal lymphadenectomy. In 1976 I reported the latest results for teratoma [2], and this favourable trend continues to the present time.

Table 3. Results of radiotherapy in seminoma of the testis treated by orchidectomy and irradiation (1960–1976)

Clinical stage	Years	1	2	3	4	5
I	No.	64	61	54	51	47
	Surv.	64	61	53[a]	50	46
	CSR %	100	100	98	98	98
II	No.	26	24	19	18	14
	Surv.	25	22	14	12	8
	CSR %	96	92	74	67	57
III	No.	7	7	7	5	5
	Surv.	4	2	2	1	0
	CSR %	57	29	29	20	0

[a] Coronary.
CSR% = Crude Survival Rate percentage.

Table 4. Results of radiotherapy in seminoma of the testis treated by orchidectomy and irradiation at the London Hospital (1970–1978)

Stage	Years	< 1	1	2	3	4	5
I	No.	31	28	25	23	17	14
	Surv.	31	28	25	23	17	14
	CSR %	100	100	100	100	100	100
II	No.	16	15	13	12	10	8
	Surv.	16	15	13	11[a]	9	7
	CSR %	100	100	100	92	90	88
III	No.	4	4	4	3	3	1
	Surv.	4	4	4	2[b]	2	1
	CSR %	100	100	100	67	67	100

[a] Leukaemia; PM no seminoma.
[b] Anaplastic and atypical metastases in vertebrate.

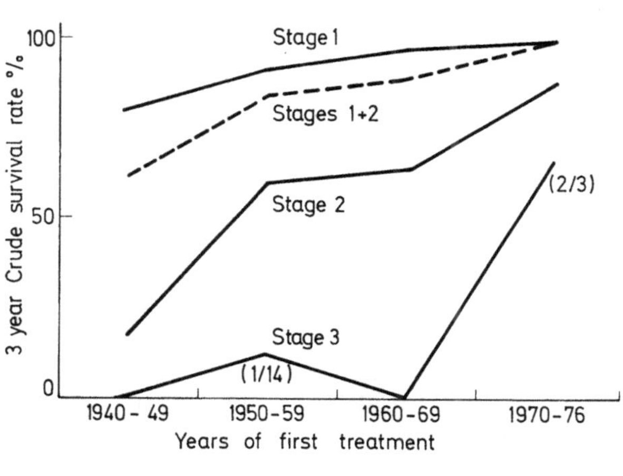

Fig. 3. Seminoma. Improvement of 3-year survival figures (1940–1976)

Table 5. Results of radiotherapy in teratoma (MTI) treated by orchidectomy and irradiation (1960–1976)

Clinical stage	Years	1	2	3	4	5
I	No.	28	28	27	24	24
	Surv.	28	27	26	23	23
	CSR %	100	96	96	96	96
II	No.	10	8	8	8	6
	Surv.	7	5	5	4	3
	CSR %	70	62	62	50	50
III	No.	8	6	6	6	3
	Surv.	2	1	1	1	0
	CSR %	25	17	17	17	0

Table 6. Results of radiotherapy in teratoma (MTI) treated by orchidectomy and irradiation in the London Hospital (1970–1978)

Stage	Years	< 1	1	2	3	4	5
I	No.	12	12	11	10	9	6
	Surv.	12	12	11	10	9	6
	CSR %	100	100	100	100	100	100
II	No.	8	8	7	5	5	3
	Surv.	8	7	6	4	3	1
	CSR %	100	87	86	80	60	33
III	No.	5	5	4	3	3	3
	Surv.	5	3	2	1	1	0
	CSR %	100	60	50	33	33	0

Table 7. MTU embryonal carcinoma (1960–1976)

Clinical stage	Years	1	2	3	4	5
I	No.	18	16	16	13	12
	Surv.	18	12	9	6	4
	CSR %	100	75	56	46	33
II	No.	17	16	11	10	4
	Surv.	12	8	4	3	1
	CSR %	71	50	36	30	25
III	No.	24	20	18	18	18
	Surv.	4	0	0	0	0
	CSR %	17	0	0	0	0

Table 5 shows the London Hospital results from 1960 through 1976. The stage II and III results are not so good (although there are very few cases in these categories). Certainly in stage I it is inconceivable that radical lymph node dissection could improve the results. The most recent results confirm this trend (Table 6).

In the MTU teratomata (embryonal carcinoma), the results from 1960 to 1976 are poor (Table 7), but looking at the more recent figures there has been quite marked improvement (Table 8), reflecting better irradiation techniques. A similar overall improvement is seen for all the teratomata at 2 years (Fig. 4 and Table 9).

Thus in stage I teratoma, MTI and MTU, Blandy and I would contend that there is no place for radical lymph node dissection that does nothing to improve survival, but certainly in the majority of cases, if carried out properly, will render the patient impotent.

It is interesting to see that at the Walter Reed General Hospital a randomized trial comparing irradiation alone with irradiation plus surgery has just been reported [4]. Ninety-one cases of stage I and II MTI and MTU teratoma were divided into two groups; one received 4000 rad to the pelvic and para-aortic nodes followed subsequently by irradiation to the mediastinum and supraclavicular nodes. The other group was given 3000 rad to the pelvic and para-aortic nodes, followed by retroperitoneal lymphadenectomy and post-operative irradiation (1500 rad) to the same region, and subsequently 4000 rad prophylactically to the mediastinum and supra-clavicular nodes. The results (Table 10) were not statistically different and were similar to a similar group of cases treated by irradiation alone at the London Hospital (Table 11). Despite this, at the 14th International Congress of Radiology in Rio de Janeiro, Maier still

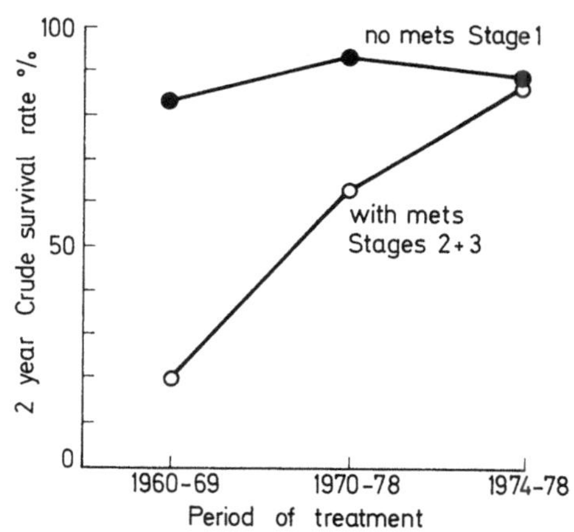

a

		no mets			with mets		
		surv.	no.	csr %	surv.	no.	csr %
1960	69	24	29	83	5	25	20
1970	78	18	19	94	21	33	64
1974	78	8	9	89	14	16	88

b

Fig. 4. The London-Hospital improved two-year survival rates for non-Seminomas (1960–1978). **a** Figures, **b** Graphs

Table 8. The London Hospital (1970–1978) malignant teratoma undifferentiated MTU

Stage	Years	< 1	1	2	3	4	5
I	No.	10	9	8	7	6	6
	Surv.	10	9	7[a]	6	5	5
	CSR %	100	100	88	86	83	83
II	No.	10	10	10	9	8	6
	Surv.	10	9	7	4	3	1
	CSR %	100	90	70	45	37	17
III	No.	13	13	12	7	6	6
	Surv.	13	8	6	1	0	0
	CSR %	100	62	50	14	0	0

[a] Ca bladder, aged 75.

Table 9. The London Hospital, 2-year crude survival rate for all teratomas

Period	Stage	MTI			MTU		
		S[a]	No.	CSR	S	No.	CSR
1960–1969	1	17	18	94%	7	11	64%
	2	2	4	50%	3	6	50%
	3	0	3	0%	0	12	0%
1970–1978	1	11	11	100%	7	8	88%
	2	6	7	86%	7	10	70%
	3	2	4	50%	6	12	50%
1974–1978	1	4	4	100%	4	5	80%
	2	5	5	100%	3	3	100%
	3	0	1	0%	6	7	86%

[a] S, survival.

Table 10. Randomized trial, Walter Reed General Hospital (1968–1973), embryonal carcinoma, teratoma, terato-carcinoma (MTU and MTI, stage I and II) (Maier, 1972)

	No. of cases	No. surviving 3 years	3-year survivors
DXT only	40	34	85%
DXT + radical lymphadenectomy + DXT	51	46	91%

Table 11. Results of radiotherapy at the London Hospital for teratoma of the testis, stages I and II (MTU and MTI)

No. of cases	No. surviving 3 years	3-year survivors
62	45	75%

advocated the combined surgical and radiotherapeutic approach. As there is little doubt that their patients are most likely to die from distant metastases, it would seem more sensible to try a different approach altogether. I would therefore advocate that in the MTU teratoma stage II and III and MTI stage III, chemotherapy should be given first, followed by irradiation of bulk disease. A trial of this method is now being undertaken at the London Hospital in conjunction with the Institute of Urology.

References

1. Blandy, J. P., Hope-Stone, H. F., Dayan, A. D.: Tumours of the Testicle. London: William Heinemann 1970
2. Hope-Stone, H. F.: Recent Results in Cancer Research. Vol. 60, pp. 250–257. Berlin, Heidelberg, New York: Springer 1977
3. Kunkler, P. B., Farr, R. F., Luxton, R. W.: The Limits of renal tolerance to x-rays. Br. J. Radiol. *25*, 190–221 (1952)
4. Maier, J. G.: Management of testicular carcinoma. Reported at the 14th Int. Congr. Radiology, Rio de Janeiro, 1977

Adjuvant Chemotherapy in Embryonal Carcinoma of the Testis

E. Pommatau, C. Ardiet, M. Brunat-Mentigny, J. L. Chassard, and M. Mayer

Introduction

There are only a few randomized studies on adjuvant chemotherapy in nonseminomatous germ cell testicular tumors. This is so because these tumors are rare (3.1 in every 100,000 in the United States) and because it is difficult to form a cooperative group among institutes that have differing ideas on the technique of lymphadenectomy, the value of irradiation, and the type of chemotherapy that must be used in testicular tumors. However, embryonal carcinoma of the testicles, which are very sensitive to chemotherapy, are a choice tumor for studying adjuvant chemotherapy.

In 1962 and 1963, we had the good fortune to see metastases regress in three patients receiving a combination (LI) of Actinomycin D, Cytoxan and Methotrexate. These three patients are still alive no evidence of disease. It was then that we thought of using adjuvant chemotherapy in operable testicular tumors. This treatment has been carried out systematically in our institute since 1965.

Material and Methods

Patients

Our series deals with 57 patients, all treated in Centre Léon Bérard between 1963 and June 1975 and bearing nonseminomatous germ cell testicular tumors (embryonal carcinoma, teratocarcinoma, choriocarcinoma). Pure seminoma or mature teratomas were excluded. The patients had stage I or II testicular tumors: 1. Stage I: disease only in the testicle 2. Stage II: retroperitoneal disease 3. Stage III: (disease above the diaphragm or visceral). Stage III patients have been excluded. Since we have only a small number of patients, we did not carry out a randomized trial. All patients treated during that period have been included in the study even if they did not receive the treatment as planned.

Treatment

Lymphadenectomy

Because of eventual sexual sequelae, we do not perform systematic bilateral lymphadenectomy. We remove the nodes high up, as high as the renal pedicle, and sometimes higher. We examine the contralateral nodes and remove only those considered likely to contain metastases.

Irradiation

If after surgery the nodes were not involved (N^-), irradiation was not given. If nodes were involved (N^+), irradiation was given, often limited to the remaining nodes or to the bed of the involved nodes. A few patients received extended irradiation including iliac, epigastric, and supraclavicular nodes.

Chemotherapy

All patients received a combination of drugs (LI): Actinomycin D: from day 1–5 and 11–15, Cytoxan from day 1–20, Methotrexate from day 1–20. If possible, the first course was given between orchidectomy and lymphadenectomy. Treatment was given over 1–2 years unless the patient refused it. The second course was given 1 month after lymphadenectomy and every 3 months thereafter. In the case of recurrence or metastasis, mithramycin and since 1973 bleomycin or V.A.B. was given. No patient received cis-platinum.

Biologic for Follow up Markers

α-Fetoprotein (α-FP)

Since 1970, α-fetoprotein has been measured, first using an immunoelectrophoretic method, and then since 1974 by radioimmunologic assay (Abbot then C.I.S.). Less than 20 ng/ml is considered quite a normal level.

HCG and LH

In the past, HCG and LH were detected by biologic and immunologic methods (in sera and urines). Today, we determine the quantity present of HCG K, HCG K1, and β-HCG (CIS) by radioimmunologic assays in sera.
The study of a new marker, β-S-P1 is already being carried out by Sizaret. We have also carried out plasmatic progesterone assays in some patients (by radioimmunologic assay).
Precise and quantitative studies were not carried out for our patients before 1970. We shall therefore have to separate the results: clinical results of patients receiving an adjuvant chemotherapy treated more than 3 years ago and results of patients with markers. Marker results are reported for patients treated less than 3 years.

Clinical Results of Adjuvant Chemotherapy

From the total of 57 patients (stage I and II) with or without surgery and irradiation have 8 died while 49 are alive and well (86%).
In the first series, 22 patients received only chemotherapy, after lymphadenectomy (N^-), of whom three received only one course and 19 received several courses over 1 or 2 years. Twenty-one of these patients are alive and free of disease without recurrence or metastasis. One patient had lung metastases erradicated with mithramycin more than 6 years ago. Thus, at present, all 22 are alive and well.
The second series (22 patients) deals with patients who had involved nodes (four patients had incomplete lymphadenectomy). Eight patients received only chemotherapy after lymphadenectomy;
three are dead (these were treated in 1963, 1965, and 1971), of whom two had node recurrences and one lung metastases. These patients were treated with nitromin, cobalt, and mithramycin.

The remaining 5 patients in this group are free of disease. Fourteen patients have been irradiated with cobalt; three are dead two with node recurrences and one with lung metastases). These were patients treated years ago, with smaller doses of cobalt and chemotherapy. Ten patients manifest no evidence of disease; one had a lung metastasis that regressed with mithramycin + bleomycin and has now completely disappeared. Of 22 patients with involved nodes, 16 (73%) are alive and free of disease more than 3 years after surgery.
The third series consists of 13 patients who did not undergo lymphadenectomy. Nine patients received chemotherapy only, of whom eight are alive and well and one died of recurrence which appeared 1 year after the adjuvant treatment was discontinued. He had lung metastases and node recurrences. Of four patients who received cobalt as well as chemotherapy because their lymphangiogram showed involved nodes, three are alive and free of disease and one died of lung and liver metastases.

Toxicity

Chemotherapy, as given, was well tolerated by almost every patient (but three refused treatment because of vomiting). We have no treatment-related deaths, but this regimen is somewhat toxic for the bone marrow in patients previously treated with extensive irradiation. With regard to carcinogenesis, we can point out only one case of seminoma of the remaining testis 4 years after surgery and adjuvant chemotherapy for embryonal carcinoma without lymph node involvement (the patient received six courses of chemotherapy over 1 year). We have not carried out systematic studies of fertility in our patients, but we can say that after their treatment four patients begot children.

Results with Biologic Markers

α-Fetoprotein

All measurements were carried out between the 3rd and the 30th day after castration. Since 1974, quantity measurements have been carried out on 30 patients in the course of adjuvant chemotherapy. Thirteen (43%) had high levels over 20 ng/ml. In our series, ten patients had lymphadenectomy (seven and three N+) and three children had only castration. With the adjuvant treatment, all quantities measured became normal. Thereafter, all remained normal for 1 year or more.

HCG and LH

Measurements of HCG were carried out in 42 patients receiving adjuvant chemotherapy:
a) 28 had no trophoblastic elements in their testis; measurement was normal and remained so
b) 14 had trophoblastic elements, of whom three had predominant choriocarcinoma and high biologic levels of HCG before or just after castration – the measurement was normal in less than 1 month – and 11 had embryonal carcinoma with trophoblastic elements; five never had high levels of HCG but one had a high level of LH (all measurements were effected after castration); six had high levels of HCG during the course of their treatment.

Patient 1: 10 months after surgery, without any clinical signs, his HCG level was high; he therefore received mithramycin and had a normal level in 2 months. He has been well for 4 years.

Patient 2: had two abnormal measurements during adjuvant chemotherapy; as he had no clinical signs, we did not alter the treatment. He is alive and well 4 years later.

Patient 3: had one high level and received bleomycin; the next measurement was normal 1 month later. Then 4 months later he had gynecomastia. He then received vincristine and bleomycin; gynecomastia regressed in 2 months. He is alive and well 4 years later.

Patient 4: had gynecomastia and a high level of HCG just after lymphadenectomy. He received adjuvant chemotherapy, gynecomastia regressed, and HCG became normal; he is still normal 3 years later.

Patient 5: had high levels of HCG and LH during some months when chemotherapy was stopped because of surgery. We resumed the treatment and levels returned to normal and are still normal 2 years later.

Patient 6: had high levels of HCG less than 1 month after lymphadenectomy (he also had an elevated α-FP). He received adjuvant chemotherapy, and HCG became slowly normal 1 year later and is still normal 2 years later.

In the past, we have also carried out plasma-progesterone assays in some patients. Only four patients had a high level (more than 150 ng). These four patients had also a high level of HCG. But six other patients with a high level of HCG had a normal level of progesterone. We think that the level of HCG has a better diagnostic value than that of progesterone. The study of the level of α-FP and HCG is very important for follow-up. Variation in level may lead us to alter the type of chemotherapy used. In two cases, HCG became normal after a new drug (mithramycin in one case, vincristine + bleomycin in another case) was used. But our study does not allow us to draw significant conclusions as to the adjuvant chemotherapy to be preferred. Quantitative measurements prior to castration would be preferable.

Discussion

It is always difficult to draw significant conclusions from a nonrandomized trial. However, we can take into consideration that our cases are without exception consecutive. It is therefore possible to compare our series with those of others. At the congress in Florence in 1974, Lalanne [12] reported a retrospective study of ten French "Centre anticancéreux." The 3-year actuarial survival rate was 43% for embryonal carcinoma and 45% for teratocarcinoma. For Quivey [16] the 5-year actuarial survival rate was 56% for 75 patients with carcinoma. The rate varies according to the stage of the disease.

1. *For stage I:* 86% according to Staubitz and 73% according to Maier [13]. The overall 2-year disease-free survival in the series collected by Williams [24] was 87%. In our previous series without chemotherapy, there were four recurrences and three deaths of 11 patients with N^-.
2. *For stage II:* a 5-year survival rate of 40%–70% has been reported for patients with positive nodes. In the series collected by Williams [24] on patients treated with radiation and lymphadenectomy, the survival rate was 57%. The results of our series show:
   100% in stage I N^-
   73% in stage II N^+
   86% for the whole series.

This seems to show the advantage of adjuvant chemotherapy, but further controlled trials are needed.

We must try to improve our treatment protocol. The improvement must take into account the clinical objectives and currently available chemotherapy. The first objective is "cure with a minimum of sequelae." Some patients have perhaps been overtreated. The biologic follow-up with markers is now more accurate and more selective. With bleomycin, vinblastine, and cis-platinum, we have a more efficacious chemotherapy. However, toxicity is perhaps more considerable, i.e., treatment-related deaths, sequelae such as pulmonary fibrosis, renal failure, and deafness. For the discussion to be useful, treatment must be discussed stage by stage.

Stage I: N^0 and N^-

If α-FP and HCG are normal before and after surgery, adjuvant therapy may not be necessary, since the prognosis is very good. However, recurrence can occur with normal α-FP and in that case, biologic follow-up is impossible. A short adjuvant treatment over 6 months might be considered. If levels of α-FP or HCG are high, there is a risk of recurrence and adjuvant treatment with actinomycin D for 1 year would advisable.

Stage II: Inoperable Patients N^+

The discussion at present lies in the choice of the drugs that must be used for adjuvant chemotherapy. It seems possible to pursue the previously used treatment, i.e., association of actinomycin D, cytoxan, and methotrexate, if the first course is given very early, before lymphadenectomy, and the latter courses are given every month or 2 months over 1–2 years. Biologic follow-up must be frequent and accurate so as to allow a new combination of drugs if necessary, even before clinical recurrence. We can then use bleomycin, vinblastine, and cis-platinum and even mithramycin, as we did, because there is no crossresistance with actinomycin D. In patients with incomplete lymphadenectomy, one can use the most effective combination, i.e., vinblastine, bleomycin, actinomycin D, and cis-platinum, and possibly additional surgery and radiotherapy, followed by chemotherapy for 1–2 years.

References

1. Amiel, J. L., Curier, J., Vacant, J., Beurton, D., Lemaire, P., Rouesse, J., Droz, J. P.: Le traitement actuel des cancers du testicule. Nouv. Presse Med. *5,* 2928–2932 (1976)
2. Bourgeaux, C., Martel, N., Sizaret, P., Guerrin, J.: Prognostic value of alpha feto protein radio immuno assay in surgically treated patients with embryonal cell carcinoma of the testis. Cancer, *38,* 1658–1660 (1976)
3. Chigbuh, A., Pizzogaro, G.: The importance of gonadotrophin assays in the clinical follow-up of patients with germinal tumors of the testis. Tumori *62,* 7–18 (1976)
4. Comisarow, R. H., Grabstald, H.: Reexploration for retroperitoneal lymphnodes metastases from testis tumors. J. Urol. *115,* 569–571 (1976)
5. Einhorn, H. L., Furnas, B.: Improved chemotherapy in disseminated testicular cancer. J. Clin. Hematol. Oncol. *7,* 662–671 (1977)

6. Grigor, K. M., Detre, S. I., Kohn, J., Neville, A. M.: Serum alpha 1 fetoprotein levels in 153 male patients with germ cell tumors. Br. J. Cancer *35,* 52–58 (1977)
7. Hoffken, K., Schmidt, L. G.: Human chorionic gonadotropin (HCG) in monitoring the course of testicular tumors. Z. Krebsforsch. Klin. Onkol. *87,* 37–40 (1976)
8. Hussey, D. H., Luk, K. H., Johnson, D. E.: The role of radiation therapy in the treatment of germinal cell tumours of the testis other than pure seminoma. Radiology *123,* 175–180 (1977)
9. Johnson, S. A. N., Grudzinskas, J. G., Gordon, Y. B., Al Ani, A. T. M.: Pregnancy-specific beta 1 glyco protein in plasma and tissue extract in malignant teratoma of testis. Br. Med. J. *1977/I,* 951–952
10. Johnson, D. E., Bracken, R. B., Blight, E. M.: Prognosis for pathologic stage I non seminomatous germ cell tumours of testis managed by retroperitoneal lymphadenectomy. J. Urol. *116,* 63–65 (1976)
11. Kohn, J., Orr, A. H., McElwain, T. J., Bentail, M., Peckham, M. J.: Sera alpha fetoprotein in patients with testicular tumours. Lancet *1976/I* 433–436
12. Lalanne, C. M.: Radiotherapy of testicular cancer. XIth International Cancer Congress, Florence (1974)
13. Maier, J. G., Sulak, M. H.: Radiation therapy malignant testes tumors. Cancer *32,* 1217 (1973)
14. Lange, Ph., Mac Intire, K. R., Waldmann, T. A., Hakala, T. R., Fraley, F. F.: Serum alpha fetoprotein and human chorionic gonadotropin in the diagnosis and management of non seminomatous germcell testicular cancer. New Engl. J. Med. *295,* 1237–1240 (1976)
15. Newlands, E. S., Dent, J., Kardana, A., Searle, F., Bagshawe, Kd.: Serum alpha fetoprotein and HCG in patients with testicular tumours. Lancet *1976/II,* 744–745
16. Pommatau, E., Brunat, M., Chassard, J. L., Mayer, M.: The value of chemotherapy in the treatment of testicular dysembryoplastic tumors. J. Surg. Oncol. *8,* 211–215 (1976)
17. Pommatau, E., Brunat, M.: Cure of metastatic tumors by chemotherapy. Eur. J. Cancer *13,* 415–417 (1977)
18. Quivey, J. M., Fu, K. K., Herzog, K. A., Weiss, J. M., Phillips, T. L.: Malignant tumors of other testis. Analysis of treatment results and sites and causes of failure. Cancer *39,* 1247–1253 (1977)
19. Samuels, M. L., Lanzotti, U. J., Holoye, P. Y., Boyle, L. E., Smith, T. L., Johnson, D.: Combination chemotherapy in germinal cell tumors. Cancer Treat. Rev. *3,* 185–204 (1976)
20. Staubitz, W. J., Early, D. S., Magoss, I. V., Murphy G. P.: Surgical management of testis tumors. Journal Urologie *111,* 205 (1974)
21. Talerman, A., Haije, W. G., Baggerman, L.: Alpha 1 antitrypsin and alpha fetoprotein in sera of patients with germ cell neoplasm: value as tumour markers in patients with endodermal sinus tumour (yolk sactumour). Int. J. Cancer *19,* 741–746 (1977)
22. Talerman, A., Haije, W. G.: Alpha fetoprotein and germ cell tumours. A possible role of yolk sac tumor in production of alphafetoprotein. Cancer *34,* 1722–1726 (1974)
23. Wahren, B., Alpert, E., Esposti, P.: Multiple antigens as marker substances in germinal tumors of the testis. J. Natl. Cancer Inst. *58,* 489–498 (1977)
24. Williams, C.: Current dillemmas in the management of non seminomatous germ cell tumors of the testis. Cancer Treat. Rev. *4,* 275–297 (1977)

Adjuvant Chemotherapy of Testicular Carcinoma: Need for Evaluation of Curative Strategies

F. M. Muggia and E. M. Jacobs

Newer regimens including cis-diamminedichloroplatinum (DDP) have shown a striking therapeutic efficacy against advanced testicular cancer [22]. The impact of such chemotherapy on our overall approach to this disease will be described. Preceding the description of current trials, a review of staging concepts and the prognostic implications of histology and stage is essential to understanding the concepts underlying current strategies.

Staging of Testicular Cancer

Although widely accepted, the Walter Reed [17] and the Boden [3] systems of staging employ both clinical and pathologic criteria and, therefore, require modifications according to current concepts. In arriving at a more satisfactory staging system, an intergroup study sponsored by the National Cancer Institute has adopted the TNM systems of the UICC [29] or the American Joint Committee [1], which are identical, to classify the T and M compartments (Table 1). However, the definitions of the N compartment have been drastically altered according to suggestions by Whitmore and Golbey at the Memorial Sloan-Kettering Center. The TNM system offers unique advantages for surgicopathologic staging that is feasible after orchiectomy and retroperitoneal node dissection. However, clinical staging based on physical, radiographic, or laboratory findings is also desirable. A clinical staging system, which can be rendered equivalent to the surgicopathologic stage groupings from TNM findings, is presented in Table 2. Similar modifications have been recently proposed by other authors [15]. Subdivisions of clinical or pathologic stage II are primarily based on the very different prognoses of minimal versus more substantial involvement of retroperitoneal nodes [14, 28], also recognized by the Walter Reed system that distinguished between a microscopic retroperitoneal involvement (stage IB) and clinical or radiographic retroperitoneal involvement (stage II). It should also be noted that a persistently positive marker in a patient who has undergone resection of all disease areas in testis and retroperitoneum must be classified as clinical stage III, even though the surgicopathologic stage has been determined to be lower. As in malignant lymphomas, the designation of both clinical and surgicopathologic stages may be helpful in clinical trials since they reflect the extent of workup and histologic verification. Current staging proposals must be evaluated further in clinical trials to establish their prognostic validity.

Prognostic Implications of Histology and Stage

Trials apply to nonseminomatous germ cell tumors, since an entirely different strategy applies to the more radiosensitive pure seminomas. Because of the frequent compound nature of these tumors, various histologic classifications have been applied, the most prevalent being commonly referred to as the British system [7] or the American system (AFIP) introduced by

Table 1. TNM codes applied to testicular cancer

T – primary tumor		N – regional lymph nodes		M – distant metastases	
TX	Primary tumor assessment not carried out, or any category applicable	NX	Regional lymph assessment not carried out, or any category applicable	MX	Complete assessment of distal metastases not carried out, or any category applicable
T0	No evidence of primary tumor	N0	No evidence of involved nodes	M0	No evidence of distal metastases
T1	Tumor limited to body of testis	N1	Nodes not visibly enlarged at surgery but microscopic disease found on pathologic exam N1a 5 or fewer nodes + N1b > 5 nodes +	M1	Distal metastases present M1a Evidence of occult metastases based on biochemical markers and/or other tests M1b Single metastasis in single organ site M1c Multiple metastases in single organ site M1d Metastases in multiple organ sites
T2	Tumor extending beyond tunica albuginea	N2	Nodes enlarged and microscopically contain tumor but no extension beyond nodes into areolar tissue N2a Largest node < 2 cm and 5 or fewer nodes involved (both criteria) N2b Largest node > 2 cm and/or more than 5 nodes involved		
T3	Tumor including rete testis or epididymis	N3	Extension into adjacent areolar tissue (microscopic as well as gross). No gross residual tumor remaining after surgery		
T4a	Invasion of spermatic cords	N4	Tumor present in retroperitoneal nodes, retroperitoneal areolar tissue with gross residual tumor remaining		
T4b	Invasion of scrotal wall				

Table 2. Staging of testicular cancer[a, b]

Clinical staging		Surgicopathologic staging		
Stage	Findings	Findings	Stage	TNM class[c]
I	CXB (–), LAG (–), markers (–)[d]	RND (–): Negative nodes	I	T1–4 N0 M0
I	CXB (–), LAG (–), markers (–)	RND (+): Microscopic nodes	IIa	T1–4 N1 M0
II	CXB (–), LAG (–), markers (+)	RND (+): Microscopic nodes	IIa	T1–4 N1 M0
II	Abdominal mass (±), LAG (+), markers (±)	RND (+): Gross nodal disease definitely removed	IIb	T1–4 N2 M0
	Same	Possibly all removed	IIc	T1–4 N3 M0
	Same	Incompletely removed	IId	T1–4 N4 M0
IIIa	Mediastinal or supraclavicular mass (+), LAG (±), markers (±)	RND (+)	IIIa	TX NX M1
IIIb	Other metastases (+), LAG (±), markers (±)	RND (±)	IIIb	TX NX M1

[a] Adapted from Whitmore and Golbey by the NCI Testicular Intergroup Cooperative Study.
[b] CXB, clinical examination, X-ray, or biochemical findings other than markers; LAG, lymphangiogram; RND, retroperitoneal node dissection findings; ± refers to combination of negative or positive findings.
[c] See Table 1 for TNM code; T category as in UICC classification [29] but otherwise same as footnote a
[d] Markers: human chorionic gonadotropin, or its beta subunit, and α-fetoprotein constitute the basic biochemical markers in use. Note that if the marker is + with clinical stage I and negative RND, the surgicpathologic stage is actually III (M1a according to UICC: clinically occult metastases). This differs from the third category where + nodes are found at RND, although in this last instance additional occult metastases cannot be ruled out, particularly if marker continues to be abnormal after surgery.

DIXON and MOORE [10]. The World Health Organization (WHO) has proposed a modification of this classification to include additional types and subtypes, such as spermatocytic seminoma and yolk sac tumor, with the term teratoma reserved for mature or immature tumors that may contain areas of malignant degeneration of other than germ cell origin. The previously used term, teratocarcinoma, would now refer to embryonal and teratomatous mixtures and require definition of each element; as many as 40% of tumors may be in this latter category [21]. The prognostic implication of this new, more descriptive classification has not been fully established. At present, when developing therapeutic strategies, all the nonseminomatous germ cell tumors are considered together. The presence or absence of a biochemical marker and the surgicopathologic stage of disease are more important determinants of the strategy adopted. One exception is the presence of pure choriocarcinoma at orchiectomy; these patients are almost never in stage I and, therefore, retroperitoneal node dissection may even be unneeded.

An excellent outlook, always exceeding 80% cure rates, has been reported in patients with surgicopathologic stage I or in those with minimal retroperitoneal involvement found either at surgery [27] or converting to negative after preoperative radiotherapy (sandwich technique) [14, 16, 18]. However, when the retroperitoneal involvement was somewhat greater [> 2 cm masses according to 28], the prognosis, in spite of radiotherapy, was considerably worse (Table 3). Prior to use of the current chemotherapy regimens, patients with distant metastases or with unresectable retroperitoneal disease had a 5-year survival below 20% [4]. Several recent studies in patients with disseminated disease, in fact, have further indicated the importance of pretherapy tumor burden as a prognostic determinant of long-term response [11, 26]. Employing cytoreductive surgery to attain disease-free status after partial response from chemotherapy has been associated with some long-term survivors [6, 11, 20]. Thus, even in stage III, subclassification by bulk of disease may prove valuable.

Table 3. Results of stage II (retroperitoneal involvement) nonseminomatous testicular cancer[a]

Series (references)	All stage II			Comments
	Favorable	Unspecified	Unfavorable	
Staubitz et al. [27]		15/20 (3 yr survival)[b]		Surgery alone
Staubitz' review – 4 series (Walter Reed, Memorial, Skinner, Walsh) [27]		45/71 (2–5 yr survival)		RT, surgery embryonal only
Tyrrell and Peckham [28]	12/14 (3 yr NED)		5/15 (3 yr NED)	RT
Hussey et al. [14]	21/45 (3 yr NED)		3/17 (3 yr NED)	RT ± surgery
Maier and Mittemeyer [18]		26/32 (3 yr survival)		RT ± surgery ± RT
Lynch et al. [16]		10/14 (3 yr survival)		RT ± surgery RT

[a] NED, no evidence of disease; RT, radiotherapy.

[b] Excludes seven patients not fully resectable.

Chemotherapeutic Regimens

DDP has shown unprecedented effectiveness as a single agent in this disease (Table 4). Two combinations, VAB III [9] shown in Fig. 1 and PVB [11] in Table 5 stand out in therapeutic efficacy and number of patients treated. The addition of such treatment in patients at high risk of recurrence must therefore now be considered at the time of initial diagnosis.

Table 4. Single agent activity of DDP in testicular cancer

Reference	No. of patients	No. of remissions		Overall response rate (%)
		Complete	Partial	
[19]	10	6	3	90
[24]	22	1	14	68
[25]	22	1	8	40
[5, 8, 12, 23][a]	17	1	8	33
Total	86	16	36	60

[a] Series less than ten patients.

Table 5. PVB combination

(P) DDP	20 mg/m² as 15 min IV infusion on days 1–5, q 3 weeks for 3 courses
(V) Vinblastine	0.2 mg/kg IV days 1 and 2, q 3 weeks for 5 courses; then, 0.3 mg/kg IV q 4 weeks for 2 years (decreased 25% in cases of prior radiotherapy)
(B) Bleomycin	30 units IV weekly on days 2, 9, and 16 of each DDP course, and with DDP 6 h after vinblastine; then, weekly for 12 weeks (stopped at total dose of 360 units)

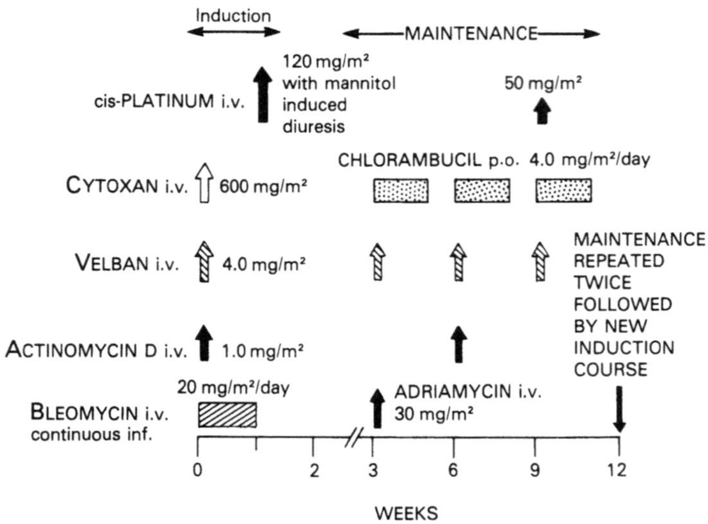

Fig. 1. VAB III. Germ cell tumors dosage schedule

Adjuvant Trials

Actinomycin D and chlorambucil have been used for years as "adjuvants" in an uncontrolled fashion. In 1974, under the sponsorship of the NCI, a protocol was launched to randomize patients with surgicopathologic stage II to receive postoperative radiotherapy or chemotherapy with actinomycin D and chlorambucil or both. The protocol never accrued more than a few patients because of knowledge of the successful sandwich technique [18] and the advent of more effective chemotherapy.

A modification of the VAB I treatment [31] was employed by Memorial Sloan-Kettering in 60 patients with surgicopathologic stage II [30]. Patients with five or fewer nodes positive and no larger than 2 cm in size, plus negative markers following dissection, were considered favorable; none of these patients has relapsed after a median follow-up of 17 months. In 35 patients with at least one unfavorable feature, relapse occurred in 11, with all but one of these occurring within 8 months. Subsequently, the VAB III protocol was employed in these unfavorable patients and only 1 of 11 has relapsed although the median follow-up is only 6 months.

Similarly, other studies have used varying regimens according to the risk of relapse. At the Sidney Farber Cancer Institute, patients with unfavorable surgicopathologic stage II receive PVB, whereas more favorable patients receive vinblastine and bleomycin, and still more favorable patients receive only actinomycin D. The Southwest Oncology Group has 44 stage II patients in a study comparing vinblastine and bleomycin preceding and following radiotherapy versus radiotherapy given as first treatment.

EINHORN has recently argued for delaying adjuvant chemotherapy in stage II patients until early relapse is observed [personal communication, May 1978]. This is based on the salvage of virtually all patients who relapse on no adjuvant treatment, who are then treated with PVB. Accordingly, an intergroup study has been established to begin testing immediate versus delayed chemotherapy with PVB or VAB III in patients with surgicopathologic stage II who have no residual disease clinically and no marker positivity following retroperitoneal dissection (Fig. 2). Finally, at the NCI, the value of cytoreductive surgery is being tested in more

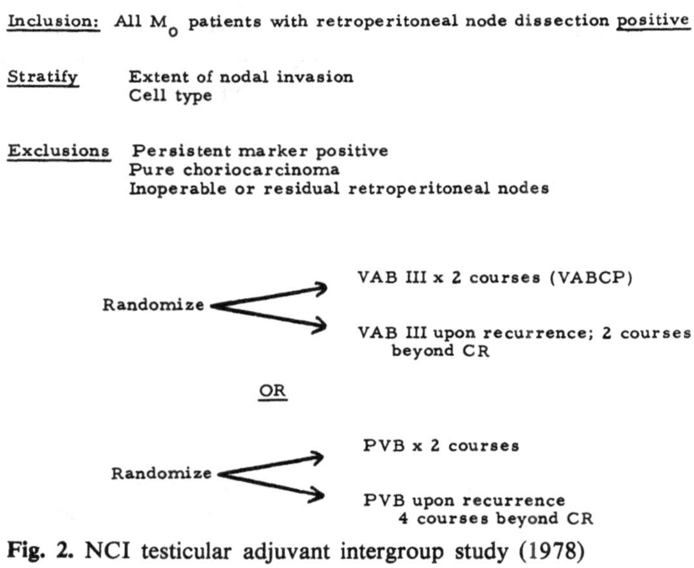

Fig. 2. NCI testicular adjuvant intergroup study (1978)

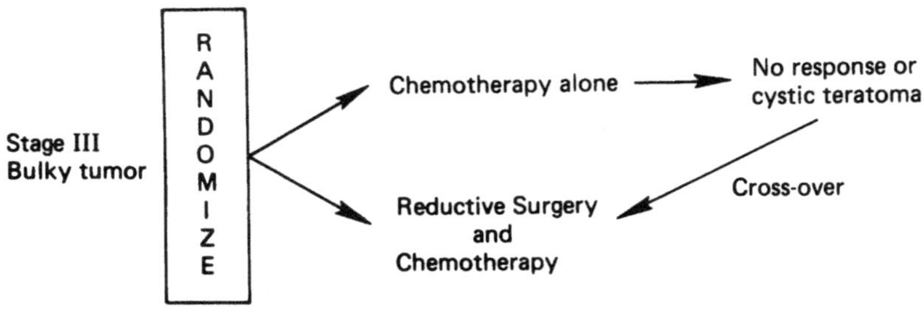

Fig. 3. NCI randomized clinical trial for bulky stage III non-seminomatous testicular tumor

advanced stages II and III (Fig. 3). This trial, which has already accrued more than 20 patients, will provide additional guidance on the value of gross disease removal in the durability of response resulting from currently available systemic therapies [2].

Conclusions

At present, radical orchiectomy, followed by clinical and laboratory staging, and then by surgicopathologic staging including bilateral retroperitoneal node dissection, represents the usual initial approach in patients with nonseminomatous germ cell tumors. In a sizeable percentage of patients beyond surgicopathologic stage I, relapse may be expected and these patients are obvious candidates for adjuvant chemotherapy. However, because of the great efficacy of new platinum-containing regimens and the expected rapidity of relapse in this disease, therapeutic strategies can reasonably test whether immediate chemotherapy versus chemotherapy on early relapse is preferred. Such studies are now underway, complemented by others evaluating the role of cytoreductive surgery in improving the results of chemotherapy. Results from such trials might point toward modifications in our initial approaches, including eventually foregoing retroperitoneal dissection. At this time, there appears to be little justification for using less than vigorous chemotherapeutic regimens; in addition, the role of radiotherapy and of surgery need to be reassessed particularly for the most favorable stages [16]. Close clinical and laboratory monitoring and early institution of aggressive treatments including chemotherapy upon relapse when it first becomes manifest may be an important alternate strategy to the use of adjuvant treatments in all patients. Evaluation of such strategies may only be obtained through carefully designed trials that include detailed staging procedures and classification. We urge that a classification, such as the one described here, be applied to trials in this disease.

References

1. American Joint Committee for Cancer Staging and End Results Reporting. 1977
2. Anderson, T., Walden, T., Javadpour, N., Anderson, T., Glatstein, E.: Recent advances in diagnosis and therapy of testicular germ cell neoplasms. Ann. Intern. Med. (in press) (1978)
3. Boden, G. L., Gibb, R.: Radiotherapy and testicular neoplasms. Lancet *1951 II,* 1195
4. Carter, S. K., Wasserman, T. H.: The chemotherapy of urologic cancer. Cancer *36,* 729–749 (1975)

5. Chary, K., Higby, D., Henderson, E., Swinerton, K.: Phase I study of high dose cis-diamminedichloroplatinum(II) with forced diuresis. Cancer Treat. Rep. *61,* 367–370 (1977)
6. Cheng, E., Cvitkovic, E., Wittes, R., Golbey, R.: Germ cel tumors (II): VAB II in metastatic testicular cancer. Cancer (in press) (1978)
7. Collins, D. H., Pugh, R. C. B.: Classification and frequency of testicular tumors. Br. J. Urol. *36,* [Suppl 1], 1, (1964)
8. Corder, M. P., Maguire, L. C., Witte, D. L., Panther, S. K., Lovett, J. M., Dietz, B. J.: Weekly outpatient cis-platinum(II) diamminedichloride (CPDD) and diuresis with dose-limiting myelosuppression. Proc. Am. Assoc. Cancer Res./Proc. Am. Soc. Clin. Oncol. *18,* 344 (1977)
9. Cvitkovic, E., Hayes, D., Golbey, R.: Primary combination chemotherapy (VAB III) for metastatic or unresectable germ cell tumors. Proc. Am. Assoc. Cancer Res. **17,** 296 (1976) (Abs.)
10. Dixon, F., Moore, R.: Tumors of the male sex organs. In: Atlas of tumor pathology. Section 8, Part 31b and 32, pp. 48–127. Washington D. C.: Armed Forces Institute of Pathology
11. Einhorn, L. H., Donohue, J. P.: Cis-diammine-dichloroplatinum, vinblastine, and bleomycin combination chemotherapy in dissemminated testicular cancer. Ann. Intern. Med. *87,* 293–298 (1977)
12. Hayes, D. M., Cvitkovic, E., Golbey, R. B., Scheiner, E., Helson, L., Krakoff, I. H.: High dose cis-platinum diammine dichloride. Amelioration of renal toxicity by mannitol diuresis. Cancer *39,* 1372–1381 (1977)
13. Higby, D. J., Wallace, H. J., Albert, D., Holland, J. F.: Diamminodichloroplatinum in the chemotherapy of testicular tumors. J. Urol. *112,* 100–104 (1974)
14. Hussey, D. H., Luk, K. H., Johnson, D. E.: The role of radiation therapy in the treatment of germinal cell tumors of the testis other than pure seminoma. Radiology *123,* 175–180 (1977)
15. Javadpour, N., Bergman, S.: Recent advances in testicular cancer. Curr. Probl. Surg. *25,* 1–64 (1978)
16. Lynch, D. F., McCord, L., Nicholson, T., Richie, J., Sargents, C.: Sandwich therapy in testis tumor: current experience. J. Urol. *119,* 612–613 (1977)
17. Maier, J. G., VanBuskirk, K. E.: Treatment of testicular germ cell malignancies. JAMA *213,* 97–98 (1970)
18. Maier, J. G., Mittemeyer, B. T.: Carcinoma of the testis. Cancer *39,* 981–986 (1977)
19. Merrin, C.: A new method to prevent toxicity with high doses of cisdiammine platinum (therapeutic efficacy in previously treated widespread and recurrent testicular tumors). Proc. Am. Assoc. Cancer Res./Proc. Am. Soc. Clin. Oncol. *17,* 243 (1976)
20. Merrin, C.: Multimodal treatment of advanced testicular tumor with cis-diammine dichloroplatinum (CPDD), bleomycin (BLEO), vinblastine (VLB), vincristine (VCR) and actinomycin D. Proc. Am. Assoc. Cancer Res. *18,* 298 (1977)
21. Mostofi, F.: Testicular tumors: epidemiologic, etiologic, and pathologic features. Cancer *32,* 1186–1201 (1973)
22. Muggia, F. M., Jacobs, E. M.: Chemotherapy of testicular cancer: Impact on curability. Princess Takamatsu Symposium (in press) (1978)
23. Nitschke, R., Starling, K., Land, V., Komp, D.: Cis-platinum (PDD) in childhood malignancies. Proc. Am. Assoc. Cancer Res. *17,* 310 (1976)
24. Osieka, R., Bruntsch, U., Gallmeier, W., Seeber, S., Schmidt, C.: Cis-diamminodichloro-platin in der Behandlung therapieresistenter maligner Hodenteratome. Dtsch. Med. Wochenschr. *101,* 191–195 (1976)
25. Rossof, A. H., Talley, R. W., Stephens, R. L.: Phase II evaluation of single high-dose cis-diamminedichloroplatinum in gynecologic and genitourinary neoplasia. Proc. Am. Assoc. Cancer Res. *18,* 97 (1977)
26. Samuels, M., Lancotti, V., Holoye, P., Howe, G.: Stage III testicular cancer: Complete response by substage to velban plus continuous bleomycin infusion (VB-3). Proc. Am. Assoc. Cancer Res. *18,* 146 (1977)

27. Staubitz, W. J., Early, R., Magoss, I., Murphy, G.: Surgical management of testis tumor. J. Urol. *111,* 205 (1974)
28. Tyrell, C., Peckham, M.: The response of lymph node metastases of testicular teratom to radiation therapy. Br. J. Urol. *48,* 363–370 (1976)
29. Union Internationale Contre le Cancer: TNM classification of malignant tumors, 2nd ed. Geneva, 1974
30. Vugrin, D., Cvitkovic, E., Whitmore, W., Golbey, R.: Prophylactic chemotherapy of testicular germ cell carcinomas (non-seminomas) Stage II following orchiectomy and retroperitoneal dissection. Proc. Am. Assoc. Cancer Res. *19,* 352 (1978)
31. Wittes, R. E., Yagoda, A., Silvay, O., Magill, G., Whitmore, W., Krakoff, I., Golbey, R.: Chemotherapy of germ cell tumors of the testis. I. Induction of remissions with vinblastine, actinomycin D, and bleomycin. Cancer *37,* 637–645 (1976)

Results of Cytostatic Therapy of Metastasizing Testicular Tumors

M. Hartmann and F. Körner

From 1 January 1974 to 1 April 1977 we treated 140 patients with malignant testicular tumors at the Urologic Department of the Federal Armed Forces Station Hospital Hamburg [6]. In 1977 alone we received 44 tumor patients, who, however, are not going to be considered in detail due to the short period of time they have undergone observation. Special attention is to be focused on the 60 patients who already had metastases when they came to our hospital or who developed metastases during the 1st year of treatment. All 60 patients were subjected to so-called controlled cytostatic therapy, which is theoretically based on cell kinetics.

Due to the efficacy of vincristine, bleomycin, and adriamycin on the different phases of the cycle of cell division (Fig. 1) [1, 4, 7, 16, 19, 21], these agents can be given in such a way that after a measurable time a partial synchronization of the tumor cells is achieved. The tumor cells, which pass through the cycle of cell division completely asynchronously, cumulate in the division phase, which is specifically blocked by the cytostatic agent [2, 5, 10, 11, 15, 18].

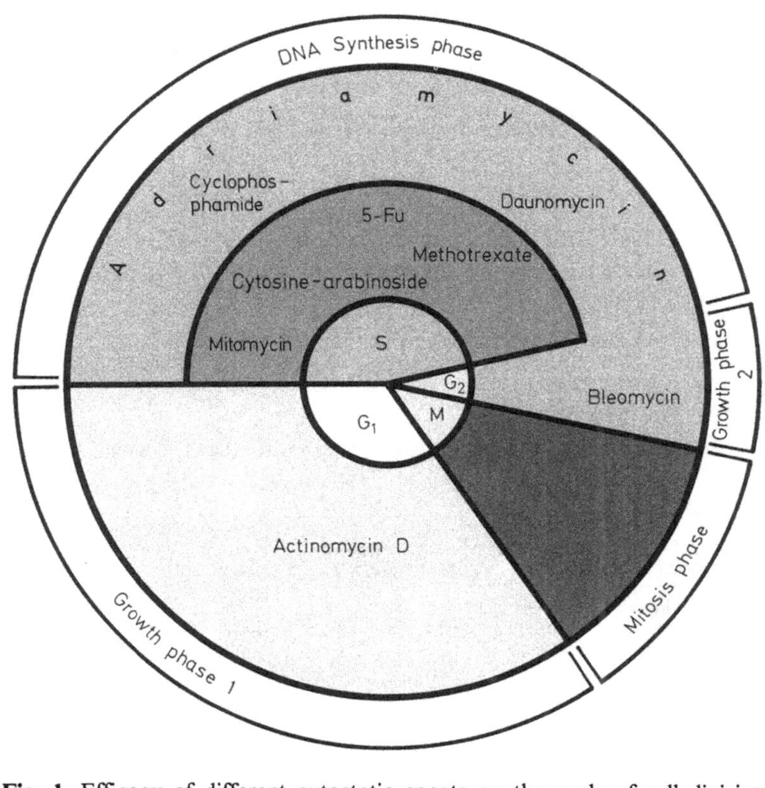

Fig. 1. Efficacy of different cytostatic agents on the cycle of cell division

When the DNA synthesis phase has been reached, a high dose of a cytostatic agent effective in this phase is applied. We use ifosfamid, an analog of cyclophosphamide [6, 9, 12–14]. The assessment of the cell-kinetic measuring data resulted in a time dosage scheme (Fig. 2) that has already been presented [13, 22, 23].

Since vincristine sulfate has proved to be the most effective agent and the one that is effective most frequently [22], it is used first until neurotoxic symptoms appear. The patients receive vincristine and ifosfamid twice a week. Then we change to bleomycin up to a maximum dose of 350 mg. This dose is given in 3-week cycles at intervals of 3 months over 1 year. If the metastases have not disappeared, either adriamycin is tried or a new vincristine series is started.

Figure 3 shows the therapeutic scheme we generally use if there is a seminoma or a malignant differentiated or an intermediate teratoma of type A [3, 20], in stage I. All other teratomas in stage I and all seminomas and teratomas in stage II with operable lymph node metastases are subjected to extended cytostatic therapy as described above (Fig. 4).

Vincristine ———— 8 h ———— Ifosfamid : 2 x/week
1.5 mg IV — 3 g in 500 ml levulose

Bleomycin ———— 24 h ———— Bleomycin ———— 15 h ———— Ifosfamid : 1x/week
15 mg IV — 15 mg IV — 3 g

Adriblastin ———— 24 h ———— Adriblastin ———— 24 h ———— Ifosfamid : 1x/week
50 mg/m² — 50 mg/m² — 3 g

Fig. 2. Therapy of metastasizing testicular tumors. Synchronization

I. Seminoma, MTD, MTIA in stage I:

Concurrent inguinal semitestectomy and lymphadenectomy;
during operation and on the postoperative day 3 g each of Isfosamid
Irradiation therapy (4000 rad), parailiacal and paraaortal
Permanent cytostasis treated orally with 250 mg Trophosfamid per day over 1 year
In case of absence of metastases termination of therapy after 15 months
Observation period of 5 years

Fig. 3. Therapy of malignant testicular tumors in stage I, scheme A

II. MTIB, MTA, MTT in stage I and all tumors in stage II
(lymphograph negative, retroperitoneal metastases not palpable)

Concurrent inguinal semitestectomy and lymphadenectomy;
during operation and on the postoperative day 3 g each Ifosamid
Partial cytostatic synchronization
Irradiation therapy: parailliacal, paraaortal, mediastinal, supraclavicular
Intermittent permanent cytostasis treated orally with 250 mg Trophosfamid per day
3 x cytostatic reinduction every 3 months over one year
In case of absence of metastases termination of therapy after 15 months
Observation period of 5 years

Fig. 4. Therapy of malignant testicular tumors in stages I and II, scheme B

III. Seminoma and all teratomas, with lymphographically positive inoperable retroperitoneal metastases, as well being in stages III/IV:

Inguinal semitestectomy;
duing operation and on the postoperative day 3 g each Holoxan
Partial cytostatic synchronization until operability
Retroperitoneal lymphadenectomy (neck dissection, thoracotomy, if necessary)
Partial cytostatic synchronization
Irradiation therapy: parailiacal, paraaortal, mediastinal, supraclavicular intermittent permanent cytostasis treated orally with 250 mg Trophosfamid per day
3 x cytostatic reinduction every 3 months over 1 year
In case of absence of metastases termination of therapy after 15 months
Observation period of 5 years

Fig. 5. Therapy of malignant testicular tumors in stages II, III, IV, scheme C

In cases in stages III and IV with inoperable metastases to lymph nodes in stage II the patients will first only be subjected to semitestectomy and then cytostatic treatment [20]. If regression of the metastases is achieved, retroperitoneal lymphadenectomy, irradiation therapy, and additional chemotherapy is then administered (Fig. 5).

The division of phases is based on the recommendations of Höffken and Schmidt [8], i.e.,

Stage I: tumor limited to testicle;

Stage II: metastases limited to retroperitoneum;

Stage III: metastases to the lymph nodes supraclavicular and/or inguinal and/or mediastinal;

Stage IV: Metastases to organs.

The breakdown of the 96 tumors treated (Table 1) indicates that only about one-third of the patients had no metastases. The relatively high proportion with teratoma is due to the young age of the patient group of conscripts [22].

Of the metastasizing tumors, 54 were teratomas, anaplastic teratomas occurring most frequently (Table 2). Nearly 50%, in fact 25 patients, were admitted to our department in stage IV, i.e., with metastases of organs (Table 3). Right from the beginning their prognosis was very unfavorable. There were some tumor patients in stage I at the start of therapy, five of whom entered stage IV within the observation period with a maximum period of latency of 15 months.

Table 1. Number of malignant testicular tumors from 1 January 1974 to 1 April 1977, as of 1 April 1978

Without metastases	
Seminoma	14
Teratoma	22
Total	36
With metastases	
Seminoma	5
Teratoma	54
Myoleiosarcoma	1
Total	60

Table 2. Histologic classification of metastasizing teratomas ($n = 54$), according to Collins and Pugh [3]

Malignant teratoma, differentiated	(MTD)	7
Malignant teratoma, intermediate, Type A	(MTIA)	10
Malignant teratoma, intermediate, Type B	(MTIB)	3
Malignant teratoma, intermediate, without Type	(MTI)	3
Malignant teratoma, anaplastic	(MTA)	20
Malignant teratoma, trophoblastic	(MTT)	7
Malignant primary teratoma, retroperitoneal	(prT)	4
Total		54

Table 3. Division of phases of metastasizing tumors at start of therapy (similar to Höffken and Schmidt [8])

	I	II	III	IV
Seminoma		4		1
MTD	2	2	1	2
MTIA	1	3		6
MTIB		1		2
MTI		1	1	1
MTA	1	11		8
MTT	1	3		3
prT		2		2
MYOLS	1			
Total	6	27	2	25

Table 4. Patients decreased up to 1 April 1978 (one patient with myoleiosarcoma not listed)

Tumor	n	%	Stage at start of therapy
MTD	6	86	1 × I, 2 × II, 1 × III, 2 × IV
MTIA	8	80	1 × I, 1 × II, 6 × IV
MTIB	2	67	2 × IV
MTI	2	67	II, III
MTA	13	65	1 × I, 5 × II, 7 × IV
MTT	5	71	1 × I, 2 × II, 2 × IV
prT	2	50	IV, IV
Seminoma	1	20	1 × II
Total	39		

At the end of a 51-months observation period (as of 1 April 1978), 40 of our patients with metastatic testicular tumors had died, i.e., 66.6% (Table 4). Of the deceased patients, 21 (54%) were already in stage IV at the start of therapy. Their survival time after our therapeutic program was initiated varied between 4 and 26 months (average 10 months). No substantial differences were revealed in the average survival time, which was 13 months in MTIA patients, 11 months in MTA patients, and 13 months in MTT patients.

We could not establish which of the teratomas was most aggressive according to the histologic classification. While the percentage fatality in the different classifications are essentially the same, additional data will be needed.

We have found out that the prognosis of survivors improves after therapy has been given for 15 months; the survival curves level off accordingly (Fig. 6). After this time we therefore stop our cytostatic therapy when patients are free of metastases. They are, however, subjected to monthly follow-up.

Of our 25 patients who were already in stage IV at the start of therapy, up to now 4 (16%) have survived and are in continuous complete remission according to the common definition. Of the stage II patients, 15 (55.5%) are alive and free of metastases. By way of comparison, 93% of the patients who came to us in stage I remained without metastases.

The 20 patients with metastasizing testicular tumors who survived continue in complete remission. We have had no case of partial remission. In three cases we were able to achieve a steady state of tumor growth over months. Therapy resistance to the applied cytostatic agents was noted in two cases.

In accordance with a recommendation of Scheef of a high-dosage single-drug [17], in 1977 we tried therapy with ifosfamid in our stage IV patients. According to our therapeutic scheme, these patients had not the slightest chance of achieving any tumor remission and some of them were also inoperable. For 5 consecutive days we administered 70–90 mg/kg body weight of this drug daily in infusions distributed over a short period of time. In the beginning we had to compensate for the toxic effects on the urinary tracts by daily infusions of 5–7 liters of liquid. For some time now, a highly effective antidote in the form of a drug called MESNA (in German: 2-mercaptoaethansulfonsaures natrium) has been available; at present this is being

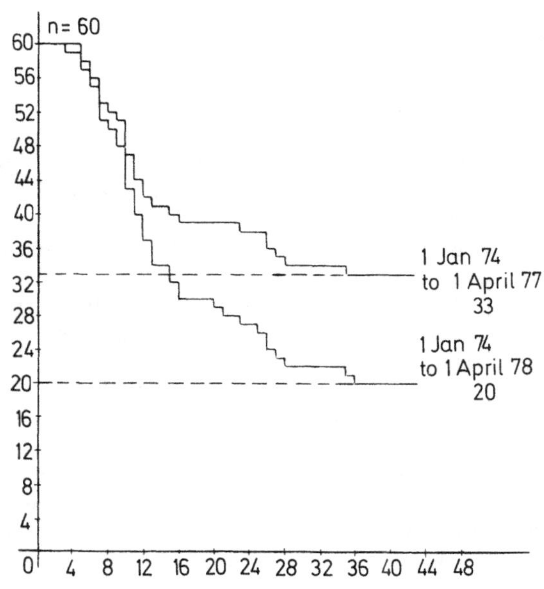

Fig. 6. Survival graph of 60 patients with metastasizing testicular tumors

clinically tested. We give it IV immediately at the end of the infusion and again after 4 and 8 h.

With antibiotic and antimycotic protection, in spite of leukocytic depression to 100–300, no serious complications arose although we conducted up to four cycles for each patient. Up to now we have treated ten patients in this way. We were able to achieve six partial remissions and two complete remissions, which are still fully effective. In two cases further tumor growth could not be prevented. This indicates that it may be possible to further prolong survival of young patients.

Summary

In many cases, metastases of malignant testicular tumors can be brought to remission by controlled cytostatic therapy. Metastases occurring after surgery do no force us to give up the patient, and even primarily inoperable patients should be subjected to an intensive cytostatic treatment, because at least a definite prolongation of live combined with an acceptable quality of life may be achieved.

Up to now, 33.3% of our patients with metastasizing testicular tumors have survived in complete remission (Table 5). The prognosis of the stage IV patients is still not favorable, although so far 16% have survived. They account for over half all cases of death.

Table 5. Summary of treatment results regarding 60 patients with metastasizing tumors (1 January 1974 to 1 April 1977; date of assessment: 1 April 1978)

Deaths	Complete remissions	Partial remissions	Steady state
40 = 66.6%	20 = 33.3%	–	–

References

1. Andreef, M.: Die Wirkung von Bleomycin auf die DNA-Reduplikation und Proliferationskinetik am Modell des Ehrlich-Tumor. Arzneim.-Forsch. *25,* 566–571 (1975)
2. Andreef, M.: Zellkinetik des Tumorwachstums. Stuttgart: Georg Thieme 1977
3. Collins, D. H., Pugh, R. C. B.: The pathology of testicular tumors. Br. J. Urol. *36* [Suppl. 2], 1 (1964)
4. Drings, P., Fritsch, H.: Erste Erfahrungen mit Bleomycin bei metastasierenden Tumoren. Therapiewoche *22,* 4569 (1972)
5. Göhde, W., Dietrich, W.: Impulsfluorometrie: ein neuartiges Durchflußverfahren zur ultraschnellen Mengenbestimmung von Zellinhaltsstoffen. A. Histochemistry [Suppl.] *10,* 429–437 (1971)
6. Hartmann, M.: Die sogenannte kontrollierte zytostatische Therapie maligner Hodentumoren. Tumor-Symposion of the Urological Department of the Federal Armed Forces Station Hospital. Hamburg, April 1978
7. Hartwich, G., Tschätsch, W., Lutz, H.: Zytostatische Kombinationsbehandlung mit Vincristinsulfat und Ifosfamid. Dtsch. Med. Wochenschr. *98,* 1203–1207 (1973)
8. Höffken, K., Schmidt, C. G.: Klassifikation und Stadieneinteilung der Hodentumoren. Dtsch. Med. Wochenschr. *102,* 143–150 (1977)

9. Jonas, U., Körner, Fr., Lund, S.: Therapie der metastasierenden Hodentumoren. Aktuelle Urologie *8,* 25–33 (1977)
10. Jonas, U., Altwein, J. E., Hohenfellner, R.: Hodentumoren: Klassifikation, Therapie, Prognose. Dtsch. Ärztebl. *18,* 1059–1068 (1978)
11. Klein, H. O., Lennartz, K. J., Groß, R.: In vivo- und in vitro-Untersuchungen zur Zellkinetik und Synchronisation menschlicher Tumorzellen. Dtsch. Med. Wochenschr. *97,* 1273 (1972)
12. Körner, Fr., Hartmann, M.: Die zytostatische Behandlung maligner Tumoren unter besonderer Berücksichtigung der sogenannten Teilsynchronisation. Verh. Dtsch. Ges. Urol. 26. Tagung, 167–169 (1975)
13. Körner, Fr.: Controlled chemotherapy Combinations in teratomas and seminomas. Pulsecytophotometry 2nd International Symposium, European Press Medicon, 326–334 (1976)
14. Lund, S., Körner, Fr.: Die Therapie metastasierender Hodentumoren. Hamburger Ärztebl. *7,* 184–185 (1975)
15. Nicolini, C.: The principles and methods of cell synchronisation in cancer chemotherapy. Biochim. Biophys. Acta *458,* 243–282 (1974)
16. Rathert, P., Terhorst, B., Lutzeyer, W.: Bleomycin bei malignen Genitaltumoren des Mannes. Urologe A *13,* 67 (1974)
17. Scheef, W., Hoefer-Janker, H.: Klinische Erfahrung mit Holoxan. International Holoxan-Symposion. Düsseldorf, March 1977
18. Schumann, J.: Impulscytophotometrie der DNS bei soliden Tumoren unter Cytostaticaanwendung in vivo und in vitro. Impulscytophotometrie-Symposion. Heidelberg, May 1973
19. Schumann, J., Göhde, W.: Die zellkinetische Wirkung von Bleomycin auf das Ehrlich-Karzinom der Maus in vivo. Strahlentherapie *147,* 298–307 (1974)
20. Skinner, D. G.: Advances in the management of non-seminomatous germinal tumours of the testis. Br. J. Urol. *49,* 553–560 (1977)
21. Umezawa, H., Ishijuka, K., Kimura, J., Iwanaga, J., Tatzeucki, T.: Biological studies on individual bleomycins. J. Antibiot. *21,* 592 (1968)
22. Weidner, J., Hartmann, M., Körner, Fr.: Holoxan in der kontrollierten zytostatischen Therapie metastasierender Hodentumoren. Holoxan-Symposion. Homburg (Saar), June 1977
23. Weidner, J., Körner, Fr.: Hodentumoren: bösartig – gutartig. Tempo Medical *7,* 43–55 (1978)

E. Digestive Tract Tumors

Treatment of Patients With Gastric Cancer by Surgery, Radiotherapy, and Chemotherapy: Preliminary Results of an EORTC Randomized Study

J. C. Goffin and D. Machin

Introduction

The 5-year survival rate of gastric cancer is between 8% and 9% and has not improved over the past 3 decades. In the American literature [1–3, 5, 6, 8, 9, 11], it is reported that the application of adjuvant chemotherapy after gastric resection has led to an improvement in the survival rate. Some studies in locally unresectable gastric cancer record an improved survival when 5-fluorouracil (5-FU) is combined with local radiotherapy [1, 10]. Reitemeier et al. [10] and Heidelberger et al. [4] pointed out that certain transplanted tumors showed a regression as well as prolonged survival when treated by irradiation therapy in addition to 5-FU. Working on this basis, Moertel et al. studied the effect of combined 5-FU and supervoltage radiotherapy and found that they gave significant objective asymptomatic palliation in some patients having gastrointestinal cancer [7]. It is thought that 5-FU acts as a radiosensitizor or at least as a synergistic adjuvant when given simultaneously with radiotherapy to the primary tumor. Moreover, 5-FU is given systematically and thus exerts its desirable effects on the floating cells in the circulation as well as on metastatic foci in distant organs.

Since 1972, the European Organization for Research on Treatment of Cancer (EORTC) Gastrointestinal Tract Cooperative Group has been conducting randomized study for patients with at least partially resectable gastric adenocarcinoma and no evidence of distant metastases after surgery. However, patients with a primary T1 tumor (UICC classification) falling in this category are excluded. The following centers have participated: Institut Médico-Chirurgical, Anderlecht, Belgium (M. Colard), Institut Jules Bordet and Hôpital Universitaire Saint Pierre, Bruxelles, Belgium (H. Bleiberg, A. Gerard, J. Sacre, and G. Storme), Centre Hospitalier Universitaire, Caen, France (M. Gignoux and P. Semama), Centre François Baclesse, Caen, France (A. Roussel), and Centre René Goffin, La Louvière, Belgium (J. C. Goffin and J. Michel).

Materials and Methods

The aim of this study is to compare four postoperative treatments: radiotherapy alone (treatment 1), radiotherapy associated with short-term chemotherapy (treatment 2), radiotherapy associated with long-term chemotherapy (treatment 3), and radiotherapy associated with short-term and long-term chemotherapy (treatment 4). Radiotherapy (XRT) is given on megavoltage machines via two parallel opposing fields, anterior and posterior. The fields cover the whole gastric region, including the small epiploon. The right and lower limits of the field are shown by metal clips placed at the level of the *Winslow hiatus* and at the level of the *genu inferior* of the duodenum.

Short-term chemotherapy (STC) is given in the form of 5-FU intravenously (IV). The daily dose is 375 mg/m^2 body surface area, given 4–6 h before the irradiation on the first 4 days only. Long-term chemotherapy (LTC) is given IV in the form of 5-FU. The biweekly dose is 750 mg/m^2 body surface, continued for 18 months or until obvious progression of disease is observed. This treatment starts 1 month after the end of radiotherapy.

Results

From July 1972 to May 1978, 104 patients from five institutions had been entered, 29 receiving treatment 1, 28 treatment 2, 22 treatment 3, and 25 treatment 4. Among these 104 patients, 59 are fully evaluable, 13 partially evaluable, 17 nonevaluable, and 15 not yet evaluable. Reasons for partial evaluability are: in two cases XRT was discontinued due to intolerance; in two others XRT was discontinued due to intolerance and no LTC received; in two cases there was local recurrence during XRT: two patients received no LTC; three were withdrawn early from LTC due to intolerance; and in four, LTC was stopped early. Reasons for nonevaluability are: no XRT given (1 case), XRT refusal by patient (1 case), death prior to start of XRT (4 cases), second-look surgery (1 case), surgical complications (2 cases), and data missing (8 cases).

The preliminary results are presented only for the 59 fully evaluable patients. The principal locations of primary tumors were 13 in the upper third of the stomach, 18 in the middle third, 25 in the lower third, and 3 linitis plastica. Regarding the UICC classification, 27 were tumors of deep invasion occupying not more than one-half of one region (T2), 24 were tumors with deep invasion occupying more than one-half but no more than one region (T3) and 8 tumors occupied more than one region or extended to the neighboring structures (T4).

The surgical procedures were: 29 distal subtotal gastrectomies according to Polya's technique, 8 subtotal gastrectomies according to Pean's technique, 3 proximal subtotal gastrectomies, 17 total gastrectomies, and 2 other nonspecified techniques. The primary tumor was totally resectable in 45 cases and partially resectable in 14 cases. No involvement of lymph nodes was observed in 14 cases; in 45 cases regional lymph nodes were involved including perigastric nodes only (Nx + a) and other nodes that are removable (Nx + b) or not removable (Nx + c).

Histologic evidence of residual tumor within the epigastric area was proven in 16 cases. Regarding the histologic grading, 34 were well-differentiated adenocarcinomas, 20 were poorly differentiated adenocarcinomas, and 5 were anaplastic carcinomas.

In the cases of penetration of the stomach wall, 3 were confined to mucosa including muscularis mucosae (P1), 9 involved submucosa and extended to or into but not through serosa (P2), 22 penetrated through serosa with or without invasion of contiguous structures (P3), and 25 diffusely involved the entire thickness of the stomach wall including linitis plastica.

As to toxicity, 2 of 66 patients (3%) died due to intolerance to XRT (infection and respiratory failure, stenosis of anastomosis) and 4 of 66 patients (4%) discontinued participation in the study due to intolerance to XRT. Toxicity to STC was almost absent. Of 23 patients, one (4%) died due to intolerance to LTC (nausea, vomiting, diarrhea) and 2 of 23 patients (9%) had LTC stopped due to intolerance (nausea, vomiting and diarrhea, leukopenia).

Table 1 shows the distribution of local recurrences. We noted 7 recurrences in treatment 1 (33%), 7 in treatment 2 (44%), 1 in treatment 3 (11%), and 2 in treatment 4 (17%). The overall significance was $P = 0.07$ (equal to overall probability associated with chi-squared test with three degress of freedom). There is some evidence that patients receiving treatment 2 have earlier local recurrences than those receiving the other treatments.

No significant difference was observed in the distribution of distant metastasis: 7 of 21 patients in treatment 1 (33%), 5 of 17 patients in treatment 2 (29%), 4 of 9 patients in treatment 3 (44%), and 4 of 12 patients in treatment 4 (33%). Table 2 suggests that treatment 4 is more successful in delaying the onset of distant metastases. A pairwise comparison of treatment 4 with treatments 1, 2, and 3 in turn gives successive probabilities of 0.11, 0.08, and 0.08.

Table 1. Number of local recurrences from start of radiotherapy by treatment group

Treatment group following surgery	No. of local recurrences	No. of patients
Radiotherapy alone	7 (33%)	21
Radiotherapy + short-term chemotherapy	7 (41%)	17
Radiotherapy + long-term chemotherapy	1 (11%)	9
Radiotherapy + short + long-term chemotherapy	2 (17%)	12
Total	17 (29%)	59

Table 2. Number of distant metastases from start of radiotherapy by treatment group

Treatment group following surgery	No. of distant metastases	No. of patients
Radiotherapy alone	7 (33%)	21
Radiotherapy + short-term chemotherapy	5 (29%)	17
Radiotherapy + long-term chemotherapy	4 (44%)	9
Radiotherapy + short + long-term chemotherapy	4 (33%)	12
Total	20 (34%)	59

Table 3. Number of deaths from start of radiotherapy by treatment group

Treatment group following surgery	No. of deaths	No. of patients
Radiotherapy alone	14 (67%)	21
Radiotherapy + short-term chemotherapy	10 (59%)	17
Radiotherapy + long-term chemotherapy	3 (33%)	9
Radiotherapy + short + long-term chemotherapy	4 (33%)	12
Total	31 (53%)	59

Table 3 show the distribution of deaths. We noted 4 deaths in treatment 1 (67%), 10 deaths in treatment 2 (59%), 3 deaths in treatment 3 (33%), and 4 deaths in treatment 4) (33%). Table 3 suggests that patients receiving treatments 3 and 4 have a better survival rate than those receiving either treatments 1 or 2.

Conclusions

The preliminary results of this controlled clinical study on resected gastric carcinomas comparing adjuvant therapy using radiation therapy and chemotherapy in the form of 5-FU in four different combinations show that:

In terms of local recurrence, distant metastasis, or survival, there seems to be no advantage to those patients receiving the STC; indeed, there is some evidence to suggest that patients receiving treatment 2 are receiving the worst treatment. The survival from start of treatment analysis suggests that treatments 3 and 4 are superior to treatments 1 and 2. However, for both time to local recurrence and to distant metastases, treatment 3 is more similar to treatments 1 and 2.

The average follow-up for the survival analysis is 55 weeks (76 for those patients still alive); a longer follow-up period will clarify the treatment comparisons.

References

1. Childs, D. S., Moertel, C. G., Holbrook, M. A., Reitemeier, R. J., Colby, M.: Treatment of unresectable adenocarcinomas of the stomach with a combination of 5-fluorouracil and radiation. Am. J. Roentgenol. *102,* 541–544 (1968)
2. Comis, R. L., Carter, S. K.: A review of chemotherapy in gastric cancer. Cancer *74,* 1576–1586 (1974)
3. Comis, R. L., Carter, S. K.: Integration of chemotherapy into combined modality treatment of solid tumors. III. Gastric cancer. Cancer Treat. Rev. *1,* 221–238 (1974)
4. Heidelberger, C., Griesbach, L., Montag, B. J., Mooren, D., Cruz, O., Schnitzerr, J., Grunberg, E.: Studies on fluorinated pyrimidines. II. Effect on transplanted tumors. Cancer Res. *18,* 305–317 (1958)
5. Hurley, J. D., Ellison, E. H., Carey, L. L.: Treatment of advanced cancer of the gastrointestinal tract with antitumor agents. Gastroenterology *41,* 557–562 (1961)
6. Jacobs, E. M., Reeves, W. J., Wood, D. A., Pugh, R., Braumwald, J., Bateman, J. R.: Treatment of cancer with weekly intravenous 5-fluorouracil. Cancer *27,* 1302–1305 (1971)
7. Moertel, C. G., Reitemeier, R. J.: Advanced gastrointestinal cancer. In: Clinical management and chemotherapy, p. 164. New York: Harper & Row 1969
8. Moore, G. E., Bross, I. D. J., Ausman, R., Nadler, S., Jones, R., Slack, N., Rimm, A. A.: Effects of 5-fluorouracil in 389 patients with cancer. Cancer Chemother. Rep. *52,* 641–653 (1968)
9. Nadler, S. H., Moore, G. E.: A clinical study of 5-fluorouracil. Surg. Gynecol. Obstet. *127,* 1210–1214 (1968)
10. Reitemeier, R. J., Moertel, C. G., Hahn, R. G.: Combination chemotherapy in gastrointestinal cancer. Cancer Res. *30,* 1425–1428 (1970)
11. Rochlin, D. B., Smart, C. R., Silva, A.: Chemotherapy of malignancies of the gastrointestinal tract. Am. J. Surg. *109,* 43–46 (1965)

Chemotherapy for Known Residual Disease After Resection of Gastric and Colorectal Cancer[1]

G. R. Giles and J. O. Lawton

Introduction

Palliative resections of colorectal and gastric carcinomata are normally justified on a clinical basis, in that removal of the primary tumour leads to symptomatic improvement or may prevent local complications. Clearly many of these patients still have a large tumour load after operation and under these circumstances, major surgery may not give other than a brief temporary extension in survival time.

Typical examples are local extensions of rectal cancers into the lateral pelvic wall or spread of a gastric cancer into the anterior surface of the pancreas. Equally common is an extensive lymph gland involvement found beyond the confines of normal surgical technique, for example, in the para-aortic regions. Another frustrating area of failure is the presence of small hepatic metastases in association with an otherwise operable primary tumour.

There is a need for additional therapy for these patients with residual malignant disease after surgery, which is in most instances too widespread to be encompassed by a radiotherapeutic approach. This report is concerned with a study of intermittent combination chemotherapy with a nitrosourea and an antimetabolite, given where possible for a period of 2 years after palliative resection of gastric or colorectal carcinoma.

Methods and Patients

Forty-eight patients underwent palliative resection of a colorectal adenocarcinoma and 25 patients had a palliative excision of a gastric carcinoma. At the time of resection of the primary malignancy, it was noted that the excision was not complete. The residual malignant disease was stratified as being due to: (a) local extension into neighbouring supportive structures, (b) lymph nodes not included in the en bloc specimen, or (c) distant disease, i.e. small liver metastases that appear to occupy less than 1% of the liver mass. After recovery from surgery, patients were randomised into two groups: the observation group were seen in the outpatient clinic where regular checks were made on full blood counts and liver function tests. Patients were examined every 8 weeks to determine the point of clinical recurrence. Chest X-rays were performed every 3 months. Liver scans were carried out if there was suspicion of liver metastases. Similar studies were carried out in the "treatment" group who received chemotherapy. Cytotoxic drugs were given to patients with gastric carcinoma in the form of 5-fluorouracil 325 mgm/m^2 IV daily × 5 every 6 weeks and BCNU (1-3-bis-(2-chloroethyl)-1-nitrosourea) 40 mgm/m^2 daily × 5 every 12 weeks. Patients with colorectal carcinoma received 5-fluorouracil 375 mgm/m^2 IV daily × 5 every 6 weeks plus MeCCNU

---

1 Work supported by Contract No. 1-CM-43727 from Division of Cancer Treatment, National Cancer Institute, National Institute of Health, Department of Health, Education and Welfare.

(1-(2-chlorethyl)-3-(4-methyl-cyclohexyl)-1-nitrosourea) 130 mgm/m^2 orally every 12 weeks. Patients receiving chemotherapy were followed in a similar manner to the observation group and underwent regular full blood counts to check for myelotoxicity. In most patients with colorectal cancer, plasma carcino-embryonic antigens were measured at intervals of 8 weeks. In the event of persistent reduction of the leucocyte and platelet counts, dosage reductions in drug therapy were made. Chemotherapy was given until the point of clinical recurrence or for a maximum of 2 years.

Results

Gastric Carcinoma

Thirteen patients were randomized to receive chemotherapy and 12 patients were maintained under observation. The two groups are well matched in terms of histological grading but differ in terms of gross morphology insomuch that three patients had carcinoma in the region of the cardia in the treatment group (none in the observation group) and three patients had lineitis plastica in the observation group (none in the treatment group). The extent and type of residual disease is detailed in Table 1 and shows the two groups to be comparable.

Unfortunately, there was one drug-related death in the treatment group. Of the remaining 12 patients in this group, only ten have been treated for 12 months or more, though all 12 patients in the observation group have been at risk for this period. During the 1st year of the treatment group four patients developed clinical recurrence (40%) and six have not. In the observation group, eight patients have developed recurrence (67%) and four have not. Similarly, the mortality in the treatment group was three patients (30%) and in the observation group six patients (50%).

Gastrointestinal drug toxicity was largely in the form of nausea and vomiting, which was seen in 92% of patients and in 49% of courses of treatment. Similarly, myelosuppression was found in 62% of patients mainly following nitrosourea treatment and in one patient this led to a fatal haematemesis 22 days following the first course of treatment, when the platelet count was 32×10^9/liter. As a result of toxicity, drug modifications were introduced in five patients (38%).

Colorectal Cancer

In all, 27 patients have received chemotherapy treatment and 21 patients have been randomized to observation. Whilst all patients receiving chemotherapy have been studied for 12 months or longer, only 16 of the observation group have been at risk for this period. Of the patients concerned in this report, the primary sites of tumour were: right colon 10, left colon

Table 1. Predominant residual disease (patients)

	Local	Nodal	Liver
Treatment group	5	7	1
Observation group	5	5	2

Table 2. Predominant residual disease

	Local	Nodal	Liver
Treatment group	14	8	5
Observation group	12	5	4

10, rectum 7 in the treatment group compared with right colon 3, left colon 7, rectum 6 in the observation group. Histological findings were similar in both groups. Table 2 details the site of the predominant residual disease in the two groups. As will be seen, the two groups are roughly comparable.

Of the 27 patients in the treatment group, 14 patients showed signs of clinical progression by 12 months (54%), which compares with 11 of the 16 patients in the observation group (69%). However, the mortality at 12 months was seven patients in the treatment group (27%) and 10 of 16 patients in the observation group (63%).

As in patients with gastric cancer, gastrointestinal drug toxicity was mainly nausea and vomiting and was found at some time in 25 patients though in only two patients was the symptom graded as severe. Only six patients had serious myelotoxicity in the form of severe depletion of platelets. However, in view of evidence of cumulative myelosuppression, adjustments in drug dosage were required in 12 patients. There was no evidence of hepatic toxicity.

Plasma CEA in Patients with Colorectal Cancer

The normal upper limit of CEA is taken to be 30 μg/ml in our survey and to accommodate the range of levels is best expressed by the log values. Table 3 summarises the results and demonstrates that as expected mean CEA levels are higher in patients with recurrent disease. There is, however, some evidence that chemotherapy results in a suppression of plasma CEA level in patients with and without recurrent malignancy during the 1st year. At this stage these differences are not statistically different. The observations may be of some assistance in judging the effect of adjuvant chemotherapy and in making a decision to continue therapy.

Table 3. Colorectal cancer: log CEA (normal limit 1.48)

	Patients	Mean log CEA at 6 months	12 months
Observation group			
No recurrence	7	1.13	1.75
Recurrent disease	6	2.60	–
Treatment group			
No recurrence	13	1.25	1.23
Recurrent disease	14	1.72	–

Discussion

At this time, the main hope for chemotherapy in gastrointestinal cancer would seem to be within the field of adjuvant therapy following radical surgery. The results of chemotherapy for patients with metastatic advanced disease do not suggest that gastric and colorectal carcinoma are particularly sensitive to cytotoxic agents either singly or in combination. However, such clinical trials are conducted in patients with large metastases, which may not be as sensitive as smaller tumour deposits. In this study we are reporting the effect of chemotherapy in patients whose clinical staging lies in an intermediate position between advanced disease and presumed microscopic metastases. The final results of this study will therefore be of some interest, not only to assess the effect of chemotherapy on the biological behaviour of the gastric and colorectal cancer but to determine whether it is worthwhile embarking on prolonged courses of combination chemotherapy in patients after palliative excision of gastric or colorectal cancer.

The reports of adjuvant chemotherapy trials in gastrointestinal cancer have been mainly concerned with the action of single agents, usually 5-fluorouracil (5-FU). Although it appears possible to improve the objective response rates in advanced disease by combining 5-FU with nitrosoureas and possibly vincristine, there is no indication as yet that these combinations will prove more effective in the adjuvant setting. Nevertheless, the combination of methyl CCNU and 5-FU would appear optimal for colorectal cancer. The choice of BCNU and 5-FU was based on the report of Kovach et al. [1] in which this particular nitrosourea seemed to have strong activity against gastric cancer.

The preliminary results of this study do not give much cause for hope that combination chemotherapy will have a marked effect on the point of clinical recurrence of either gastric or colorectal cancer. However, it may be that survival times will be prolonged in some patients, particularly in the case of colorectal cancer where the 1-year survival time in the treatment group was 73% compared to 41% in the observation group. Less impressive was a 12-month survival rate of 70% after chemotherapy for gastric cancer compared to 50% in the observation group. However, the groups are not yet completely studied and the time period is short. Statistical evaluation must await completion of the study.

A further controversial aspect of cytotoxic chemotherapy, given in an adjuvant setting, relates to the potential gains in delay of clinical recurrence and reduced mortality, which have to be balanced against the toxicity induced in the recipients. In this study the incidence of gastrointestinal disturbance following the use of nitrosoureas has been high but relatively shortlived and easily controlled by antiemetics. However, cumulative myelotoxicity has been a serious problem and necessitated reductions in drug doses in 17 of a total of 40 patients receiving treatment. Furthermore, it is necessary to record that one patient died of gastrointestinal haemorrhage at a time when the platelet count was suppressed and at its nadir following nitrosourea administration. This must be seen as a drug-related death. Despite this reservation, the study does seem to show that combinations of nitrosoureas and 5-FU can be given over prolonged periods of time without insurmountable problems. It seems justifiable to examine whether such treatments are effective in patients with tumour burdens that are less than those described in this study.

Acknowledgement

The group gratefully acknowledges the help of Dr. A. Malhotra in patient care and Professor Munro Neville, Chester Beatty Institute, London in CEA level estimation.

Reference

1. Kovach, J. S., Moertel, C. G., Schutt, A. J., Hahn, R. G., Reitemeier, R. J.: A controlled evaluation of 5-Fluorouracil and 1-3-bis-(2-chlorethyl)-1-nitrosourea used alone and in combination for therapy of advanced gastrointestinal cancer. Cancer 33, 563–567 (1974)

Adjuvant Treatment With Razoxane (ICRF 159) Following Resection of Cancer of the Stomach

J. M. Gilbert, P. Cassell, H. Ellis, Ch. Wastell, J. Hermon-Taylor, and K. Hellman

Introduction

Razoxane (ICRF 159) is an antimitotic drug that was developed at the laboratories of the Imperial Cancer Research Fund, London, England. The drug is related to the chelating agent EDTA and was found to be active in a wide range of experimental tumours (Fig. 1). It blocks cell cycle progression in the pre-mitotic or early mitotic phases of the cell cycle.
Razoxane has a profound antimetastatic effect in experimental tumours. "ICRF 159 completely inhibited metastasis formation in mice implanted with Lewis lung carcinoma and the dose had little influence on the rate of growth of the primary implant" [8]. Further studies showed that there was normalisation of the blood vessels at the periphery of the tumour, and it is thought that this may be related to the antimetastatic effect [6].
Razoxane is effective against a variety of human tumours [1] but this is the first report of its use in carcinoma of the stomach. The drug is active when taken orally and exceptionally well tolerated.

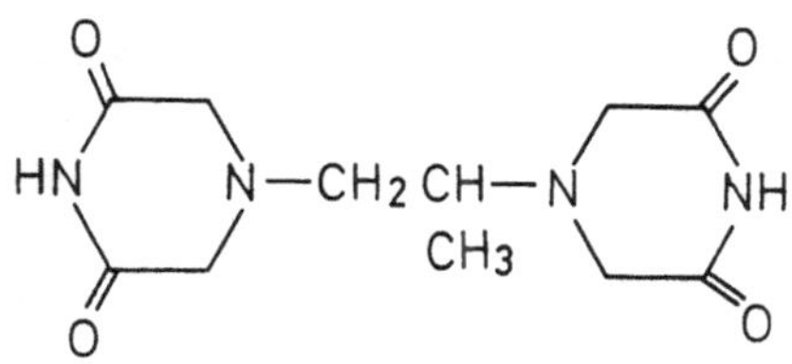

Fig. 1. ICRF 159

Patients and Methods

Sixteen patients with carcinoma of the stomach have received razoxane. The tumour was resected in all of these patients except one in whom it was by-passed. The first ten patients were treated with razoxane because the surgeon felt the resection was technically inadequate; three of these patients received other chemotherapeutic agents. The other six patients were allocated to razoxane treatment as part of the multicentre randomized controlled trial that has now been set up.
The patients who are part of the trial received razoxane in an oral dose of 125 mg twice daily Monday to Friday inclusive. The other patients received razoxane in a similar dosage but with a slightly different intermittent regime. The dose was reduced if the leucocyte count fell below 3000 cells/mm^3.

Results

The sixteen patients had a mean survival of 20.6 months and a median survival of 12.5 months. Those patients in whom the operative specimen showed evidence of extra-gastric spread histologically had a mean survival of 9.8 months with a median of 9.5 months (Table 1). If there was *no* evidence of extra-gastric spread in the operative specimen, the survival was a mean of 41.1 months with a median of 44 months (Table 2). The single patient who had a simple by-pass procedure survived for 27 months. Survival was not related to the degree of histological differentiation of the tumour cells. The survival curve is shown in Fig. 2.

Table 1. Carcinoma stomach (resected) + razoxane (ICRF 159): extra-gastric spread histologically in surgical specimen

Patient	Survival (months)	Differentiation
D. T.[a]	12	Well
H. B.	8	Poor
E. D.	5	Poor
T. F.	13	Poor
R. S.	8	Undifferentiated
J. D.	11	Well
D. McC.	18 +	Moderate
A. C.	17 +	Well
E. O.	3	Undifferentiated
E. B.	3	Poor
Mean	9.8	
Median	9.5	

[a] Plus other chemotherapy.

Table 2. Carcinoma stomach (resected) + razoxane (ICRF 159): no histological evidence of extra-gastric spread in surgical specimen

Patient	Survival (months)	Differentiation
K. J.[a]	62 +	Anaplastic
S. S.	54	Poor
G. C.	44	Well
G. R.	39 +	Anaplastic
W. C.	8 +	Well
Mean	41.1	
Median	44	

[a] Plus other chemotherapy.

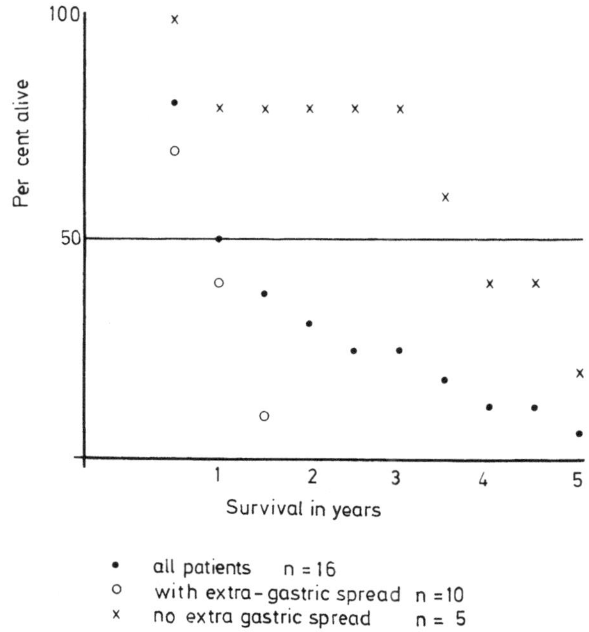

Fig. 2. Carcinoma of stomach and Razoxane (ICRF 159)

Discussion

The survival of patients in this series appears to be encouraging when compared to the figures published for carcinoma of the stomach from other centres in England. However, there is a marked difference between results published by specialist referral centres and general hospitals (Table 3). Twelve of the 16 patients in this series had their operation at Wexham Park Hospital, which is a district general hospital.

Costello et al. [4] reported a median survival of approximately 6 months if lymph nodes were involved and approximately 1 year if no nodes were involved (Fig. 3). The survival in this series is longer, especially in those patients without extra-gastric spread who had a median survival of 44 months.

The early experience with razoxane gave very good anecdotal evidence that the drug is active in carcinoma of the stomach. Five of the first ten patients survived more than 2 years following purely palliative gastric resections in which the surgeon felt that tumour had been

Table 3. Carcinoma of stomach crude 5-year survival (English series)

	Overall	Lymphatic spread	No lymphatic spread
Cassell 1976 [3] (St. Bartholomew's, London)	19.0%		
Brookes 1965 [2] (Birmingham)	5.0%		
Hawley 1970 [5] (St. Mark's, London)	19.4%	11%	40%
Costello 1977 [4] (Manchester)	8.5%	3%	21%

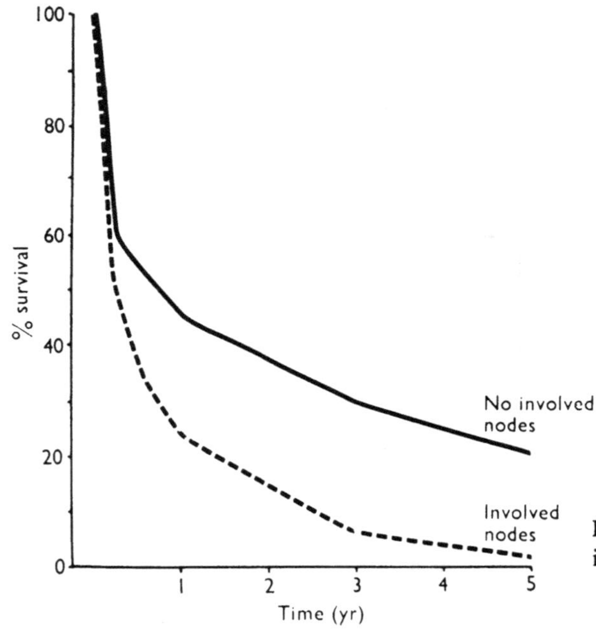

Fig. 3. Survival with and without involved lymph nodes. C. B. COSTELLO

left behind. One patient (G.C.) survived 44 months and developed signs of extensive metastases within 3 weeks of razoxane being inadvertently stopped. Another patient (J.U.) survived 27 months after a simple by-pass of his gastric carcinoma. Opacities on his chest X-ray disappeared soon after starting razoxane and at post mortem the tumour was still present in the stomach without any evidence of metastases. Ninety-six per cent of patients are dead within a year following a palliative by-pass operation for carcinoma of the stomach [7].

An autopsy has been performed on four patients, and there is some evidence that razoxane may have exerted an antimetastatic effect (Table 4). One patient (S.S.) is of special interest having survived 54 months despite disseminated disease as revealed at post mortem. WILLIS

Table 4. Carcinoma of stomach + razoxane (ICRF 159): pattern of metastases

Patient	Lungs		Liver		Lymph nodes		Survival (months)
	CXR	PM	Operations	PM	Operative specimen	PM	
S. S.	−	+	−	+	−	+	54
T. F.	−	−	−	−	+	+	13
J. U.[a]	+	−	−	−	?+	−	27
E. B.	−	−	−	−	+	−	3

[a] By-pass only.

[9] states that in a series of 85 post mortems performed on patients dying with carcinoma of the stomach, 22% had metastases in the lungs, 46% in the liver and 89% in lymph nodes. However, it is not stated in what proportion of these cases the primary tumour had been removed.

This series is part of a wider investigation of razoxane. A multicentre randomized controlled trial is now in progress to assess the effect of adjuvant razoxane compared to controls (no treatment or 5-fluorouracil). More than 100 patients with carcinoma of the stomach, pancreas, colon and rectum have so far entered this trial which began in January 1977, but it is too early tc assess the results at this stage.

Acknowledgement

We would like to thank Mr. R. Ramsay and Mr. E. J. Williams (Wexham Park Hospital) and Dr. O. K. Hjertaas (Prince Albert Community Clinic, Sakatchewan) for permission to report on their patients.

References

1. Bakowski, M. T.: ICRF 159, (±)1,2-di(3,5-dioxopiperazin-1-yl)propane NSC-129,943; Razoxane. Cancer Treat. Rev. *3,* 95–107 (1976)
2. Brookes, V. S., Waterhouse, J. A. H., Powell, D. J.: Carcinoma of the Stomach: a 10-year survey of results and of factors affecting prognosis. Br. Med. J. *1965/I,* 1577–1583
3. Cassell, P., Robinson, J. O.: Cancer of the Stomach: a review of 854 patients. Br. J. Surg. *63,* 603–607 (1976)
4. Costello, C. B., Taylor, T. V., Torrance, B.: Personal experience in the management of carcinoma of the stomach. Br. J. Surg. *64,* 47–51 (1977)
5. Hawley, P. R., Westerholm, P., Morson, B. C.: Pathology and prognosis of carcinoma of the stomach. Br. J. Surg. *57,* 877–883 (1970)
6. Le Serve, A. W., Hellmann, K.: Metastases and the normalization of tumour blood vessels by ICRF 159: A new type of drug action. Br. Med. J. *1,* 597–601 (1972)
7. Lundh, G., Burn, J. I., Kolig, G., Richard, C. A., Thomson, J. W. W., van Elk, P. J., Oszacki, J.: A co-operative international study of gastric cancer. Ann. R. Coll. Surg. Engl. *54,* 119–228 (1974)
8. Salsbury, A. J., Burrage, K., Hellmann, K.: Inhibition of metastic spread by ICRF 159: Selective deletion of a malignant characteristic. Br. Med. J. *4,* 344–346 (1970)
9. Willis, R. A.: The spread of tumours in the human body, 3rd Ed. p. 302. London: Butterworths 1973

Adjuvant Chemotherapy in Large-Bowel Cancer: Demonstration of Effectiveness of Single Agent Chemotherapy in a Prospectively Controlled, Randomized Trial[1]

T. B. Grage, G. J. Hill, G. N. Cornell, R. W. Frelick, and S. E. Moss

Introduction

Combining surgical resection and chemotherapy in the treatment of neoplasms has a sound biologic basis, and application of this principle has resulted in striking improvement in survival rates for a variety of malignancies, particularly in pediatric solid neoplasms.
Large-scale cooperative, prospectively controlled trials combining surgical treatment with adjuvant chemotherapy in the management of bowel cancer date back to 1967 and have been reviewed elsewhere [5, 8]. Most of these trials have not shown that the addition of chemotherapy has increased the disease-free interval and survival with the exception of the most recent Veterans Administration Surgical Adjuvant Group trial employing prolonged, intermittent treatment with 5-fluorouracil (5-FU) in which there is definite suggestion of treatment benefit in those patients receiving chemotherapy [2, 7–10, 15]. Evaluation of the treatment results in the Central Oncology Group trial (COG 7041) have been reported in the past and have consistently shown definite improvement in the duration of the disease-free interval and recurrence rate, particularly in certain unfavorable subgroups of patients with colorectal carcinoma [4–6]. This report is an update of the Central Oncology Group (COG) trial as of May 1978.

Description of Study

In 1971 the Central Oncology Group began a controlled clinical trial to determine the effect of long-term adjuvant chemotherapy with 5-FU upon survival and recurrence rates in patients with colorectal carcinoma who either underwent a curative or a palliative resection. The details of the trial have been presented elsewhere [5].
In summary, in the curative resection group only those patients were submitted to study who had an unfavorable prognosis as indicated by penetration of the tumor through the serosa or full thickness of the bowel wall, Dukes B, or invasion of the lymph nodes, Dukes C, or cancer in other organs removed as part of the primary resection. To the palliative group only those patients were entered in whom the primary tumor had been removed and there was histologic evidence of residual tumor. Criteria for exclusion of patients included "patients over 80 years, patients who were considered poor risk for chemotherapy because of inadequate nutrition, or patients with serious cardiopulmonary, hepatic, renal, or hematologic diseases believed to be unsuitable for adjuvant chemotherapy."
Allocation of patients to treatment group or control group was achieved by a centralized randomization procedure at the COG headquarters. To insure even distribution of unfavorable characteristics to treatment and control groups, patients were further stratified as to

1 This work was supported by Central Oncology Group Grants CA-12282 and CA-12271 and the Cancer Education Program Grant CA-19527 from the USPHS, National Cancer Institute.

primary site, whether in the colon or the rectum, absence or presence of lymph nodal involvement, and absence or presence of obstruction at the time of operation.

Those patients assigned to the chemotherapy group received 5-FU within 30 days after surgical resection, consisting of an initial intravenous loading course of 5-FU at a dose level of 12 mg/kg daily for 4 consecutive days, up to a maximum of 1.0 g of 5-FU, followed by 6 mg/kg/day on alternate days to the point of toxicity, or to a maximum of five doses. Weekly maintenance therapy was instituted as soon as toxicity from the loading course had subsided, at a dose level of 12 mg/kg, to a maximum of 1.0 g of 5-FU for a period of 1 year.

In the palliative group the primary purpose of the trial was to determine whether immediate administration of 5-FU increased the time-to-progression of disease and increased the survival. Those patients selected to receive 5-FU were started on chemotherapy within 30 days of resection and continued until there was clear-cut evidence of progression. Those patients randomized to surgical resection alone were followed at periodic intervals until there was evidence of progression and then started on 5-FU at the same dose and schedule. Progression of disease was defined as the appearance of new disease or an increase of 50% or more in the product of the diameters of measurable lesions. In other words, in the palliative group both groups of patients received 5-FU at one time during the course of their disease.

Patients whose disease recurred while on 5-FU or whose disease progressed were treated by a variety of chemotherapeutic agents, usually left to the discretion of the investigator. To insure a comparable end point, all patients were followed at periodic intervals and thoroughly reassessed every 3 months for evidence of recurrence or progression of their disease. The survival curves and duration of disease-free interval curves were calculated beginning with the day of definitive surgery, using the Kaplan-Meier life-table method, and the differences in the survival and disease-free interval curves were evaluated statistically using Gehans modification of the Wilcoxon test [3, 11].

Results

From August 1971 through November 1976 a total of 394 patients have been entered into the study. As of May 1978, 299 were acceptable for evaluation. Of the remaining 95 patients, 16 were ineligible because they did not meet study requirements, 38 were invalid due to improper drug administration, 31 were inadequate due to insufficient follow-up, and 10 were incomplete due to lack of reporting forms. Actually, the majority of the protocol violations were considered minor and these patients have been studied as a separate group. However, they will not be included in this report.

Of the 299 evaluated cases, 217 underwent a curative resection and 82 patients underwent a palliative resection. Follow-up in the curative group ranged 2—70 months, with a median of 28 months. In the palliative group minimum and maximum follow-up period was 2 and 56 months, respectively, with a median of 15 months.

Toxicity

Severe, life-threatening toxicity, primarily related to the intestinal tract, was of sufficient magnitude in seven patients to discontinue therapy entirely. The remaining patients tolerated the chemotherapy well with toxicity usually of mild to moderate degree. Some degree of leukopenia was seen in 60% of the patients, nausea and vomiting was seen in 46% of the patients, diarrhea in 53%, stomatitis in 20%, and thrombocytopenia in 36%. Less commonly seen were cerebellar toxicity, hyperpigmentation, and alopecia. There have been no drug-related deaths.

Curative Resection

Of 217 patients in the curative resection group, 98 received chemotherapy and 113 patients were treated by surgical resection alone (Table 1). In the chemotherapy group 58% of the patients are alive and free of disease, 12% have recurred, and 30% have died. Although the control group fared slightly worse, the differences are statistically not significant. Figures 1 and 2 show the overall disease-free interval and survival curves for the treated and the control groups. In neither case is the difference statistically significant, although it is nearly so in the case of disease-free interval ($P = 0.06$).

Table 1. Summary status of 211 patients undergoing curative resection for colorectal carcinoma

Treatment	Alive				Dead		Total	
	NED		Recurrence					
	#	%	#	%	#	%	#	%
Control	58	51	20	18	35	31	113	100
5 FU	57	58	12	12	29	30	98	100
Total	115	55	32	15	64	30	211	100

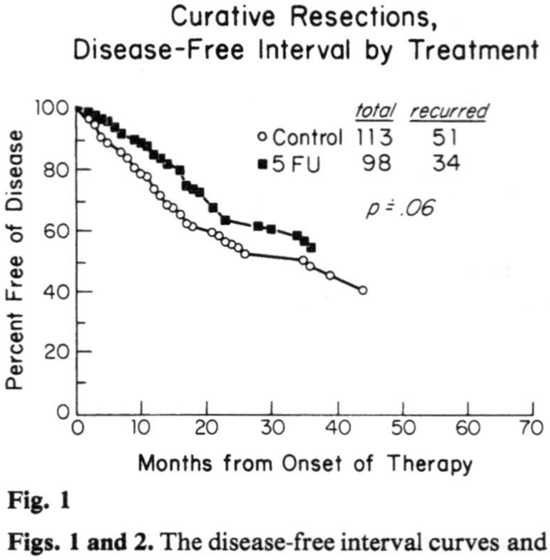

Fig. 1

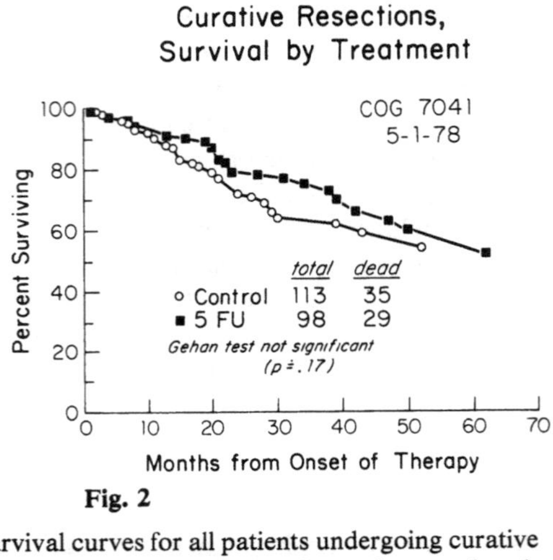

Fig. 2

Figs. 1 and 2. The disease-free interval curves and survival curves for all patients undergoing curative resection do favor the chemotherapy group, although only in the disease-free interval curve does it approach significance

Disregarding whether the patient received 5-FU or not and just comparing the stage of the disease, it is obvious that the prognosis for patients with Dukes C disease is significantly poorer than those with Dukes B both in terms of disease-free interval and survival (Figs. 3 and 4). In terms of the difference between the chemotherapy group and the surgical resection alone group, the Dukes C patients had a significantly longer disease-free interval, as reported in the past ($P = 0.003$), and are also favored in terms of survival ($P = 0.15$) (Figs. 5 and 6). As reported before, there is no difference between the treated and control group within Dukes B stage.

Regardless of whether the patient received 5-FU or not, patients whose primary tumor was located in the colon had a better prognosis than patients whose primary tumor was located in

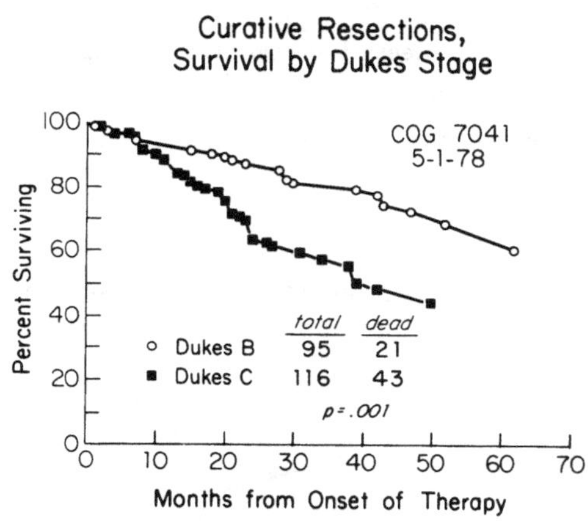

Fig. 3

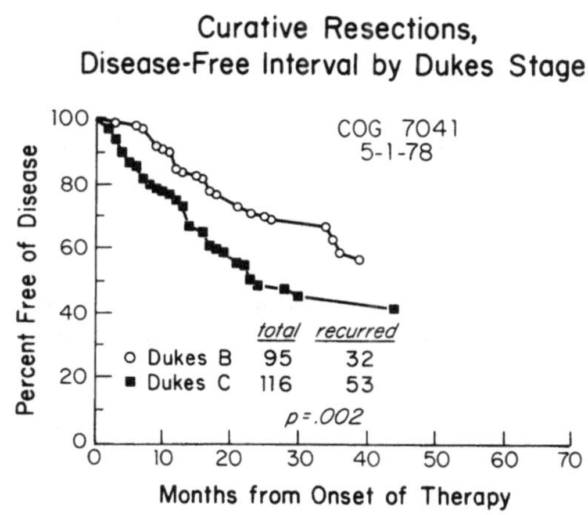

Fig. 4

Figs. 3 and 4. Involvement of lymph nodes by tumor confers a poorer prognosis than in patients with disease confined to the bowel wall

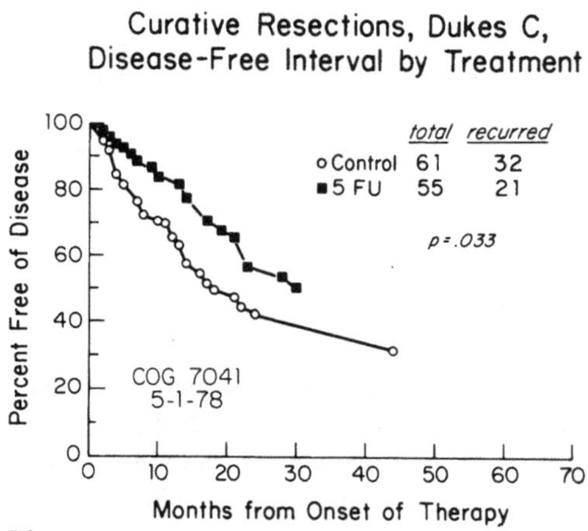

Fig. 5

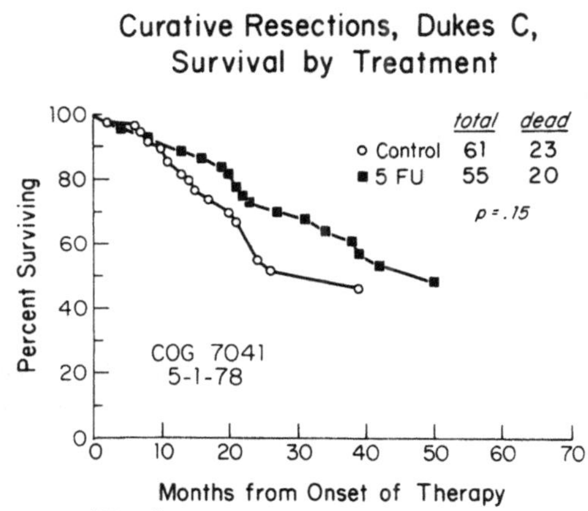

Fig. 6

Figs. 5 and 6. In patients with Dukes C lesions, the chemotherapy group has a significantly longer disease-free interval; survival is also better but not significantly

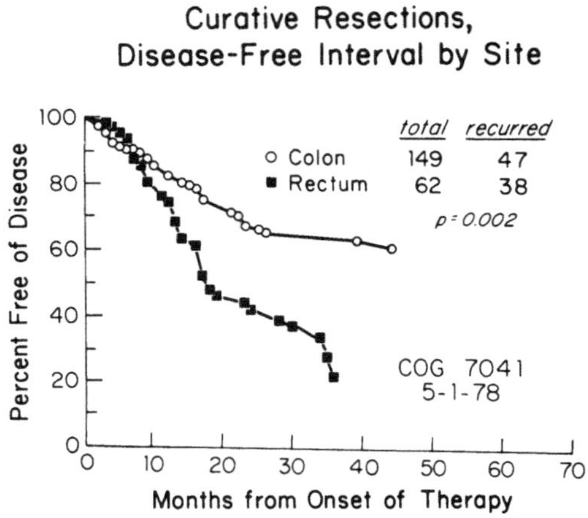

Fig. 7

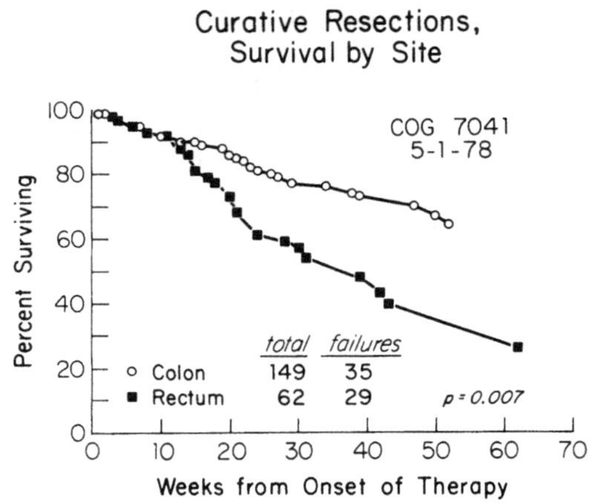

Fig. 8

Figs. 7 and 8. The curves by site clearly indicate the poorer prognosis in patients with rectal cancer as compared to patients with colonic cancer

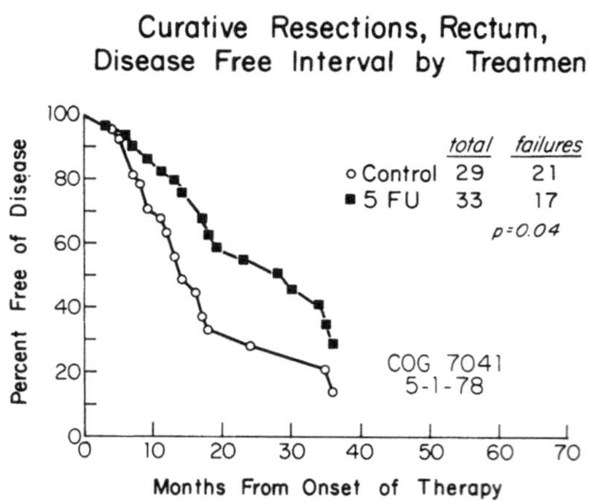

Fig. 9

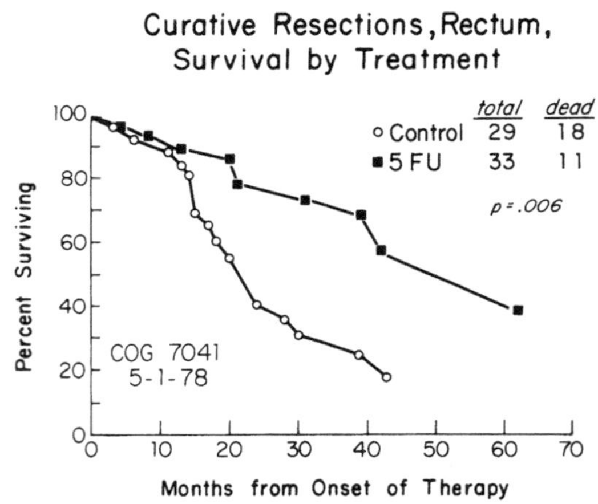

Fig. 10

Figs. 9 and 10. Both in terms of disease-free interval and survival, rectal cancer patients treated with 5-FU do significantly better than those treated by resection alone

the rectum, with respect to disease-free interval ($P = 0.002$) and survival ($P = 0.007$) (Figs. 7 and 8).

There was no difference in diesease-free interval and survival between the two treatment groups in patients with primary neoplasm located in the colon. In patients with the primary tumor located in the rectum, the chemotherapy group did significantly better than the control group in both disease-free interval ($P = 0.041$) and survival ($P = 0.006$) (Figs. 9 and 10).

When examining the treatment group only, in terms of disease-free interval and survival by toxicity, it is of interest that leukopenic patients (white count below 4000) have a significantly

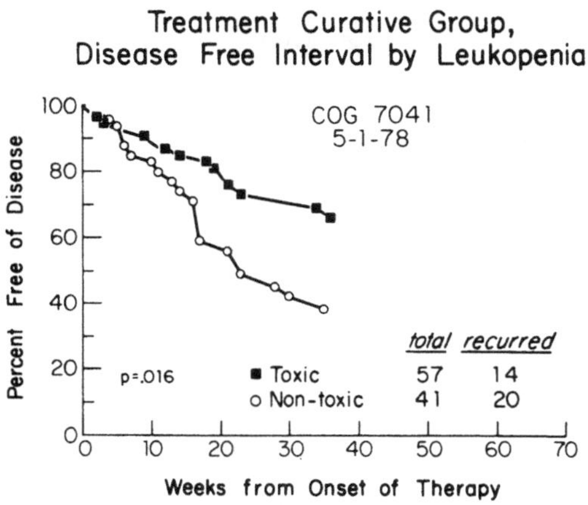

Fig. 11

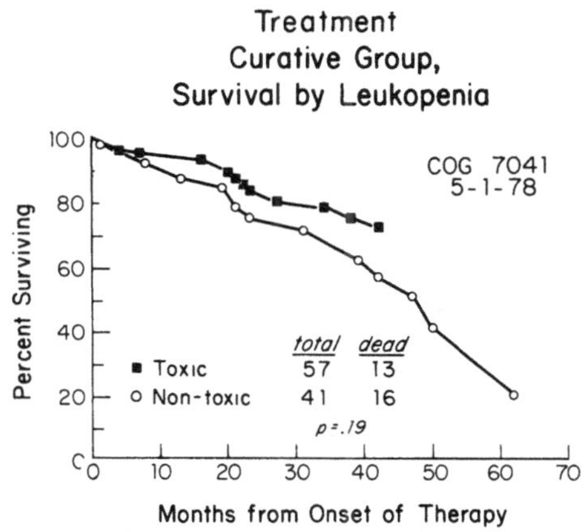

Fig. 12

Figs. 11 and 12. In the chemotherapy group, those patients treated to toxicity, in terms of leukopenia, have a significantly longer disease-free interval and appear to survive longer

longer disease-free interval than nonleukopenic patients ($P = 0.016$). However, this did not translate itself into prolongation of survival, although the leukopenic group is favored ($P = 0.19$) (Figs. 11 and 12). When examining disease-free intervals and survival by other toxicities such as nausea, vomiting, stomatitis, and thrombocytopenia and diarrhea, no significant differences were found.

Palliative Resection

Of 81 patients undergoing palliative resection, 83% have died in the control group versus 74% in the chemotherapy group; the difference is not significant (Table 2). When examining the asymptomatic interval curves and survival curves for the treatment and control groups, the treatment group is favored in both cases, but not significantly (Figs. 13 and 14).

Table 2. Summary results in 81 patients after palliative resection for colorectal carcinoma

Treatment	Alive				Dead		Total	
	Asymptomatic		Symptomatic					
	#	%	#	%	#	%	#	%
Control	2	5	5	12	35	83	42	100
5 FU	6	15	4	10	29	74	39	99
Total	8	9	9	11	64	79	81	99

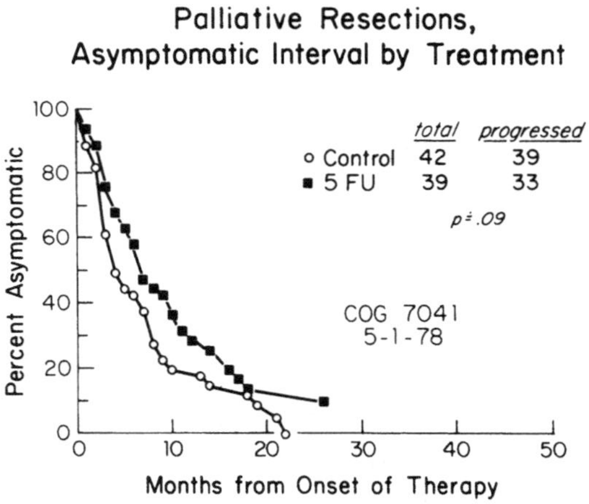

Fig. 13

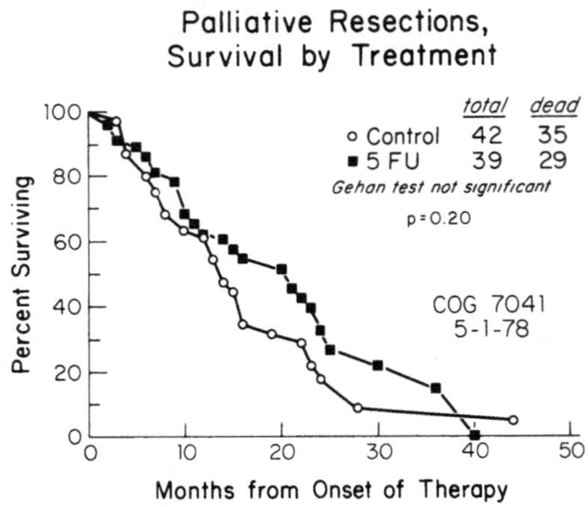

Fig. 14

Figs. 13 and 14. In the palliative group, chemotherapy with 5-FU shortly after resection appears to prolong the asymptomatic interval, but not significantly so, and there is no influence on survival

Discussion

Considering the large number of cases entered into the trial and the long period of follow-up, together with the prospectively randomized nature of the trial with stratification by prognostic indicators, it is becoming increasingly apparent that the addition of 5-FU to the treatment of patients with colorectal carcinoma confers a small, but significant benefit in terms of disease-free interval and survival in certain unfavorable subgroups of patients with this disease. Although the overall improvement is small, yet considering the relative ineffectiveness of a single agent such as 5-FU, this result is not surprising and in line with the results reported from the most recent study from the Veterans Administration Study Group [9].

One can only speculate why other trials, in which the same agent was used, did not show any improvement in their recurrence rates and disease-free interval. A clue may be provided by the observation that patients treated to toxicity have a better result than those in whom the drug did not result in leukopenia. In a previous phase III trial by the Central Oncology Group, a comparison of four dosage regimens of 5-FU, (1) an oral regime, (2) an intravenous regime without a loading course, (3) a nontoxic regime, and (4) an intravenous toxic regime with a loading course of 5-FU followed by weekly administration of 5-FU, reveals a clear superiority of the fourth dosage schedule over the other three schedules in the treatment of advanced colorectal cancer [1]. It appears that the dose and schedule of the chemotherapeutic agent do indeed matter and can significantly influence the outcome.

The demonstration that the addition of a single agent such as 5-FU confers some improvement to the surgical treatment of colorectal carcinoma provides grounds for increasing optimism. Since the addition of methyl-CCNU to 5-FU has been reported to result in a higher response rate in patients with advanced colorectal carcinoma, this may well translated itself into a more effective adjuvant chemotherapy program [14]. The Eastern Cooperative Oncology Group is conducting a colon cancer adjuvant trial comparing 5-FU alone in the form of 450 mg/m^2 intravenously, daily, for 5 days, every 5 weeks for 1 year to a combination regime consisting of 5-FU, 325 mg/m^2 intravenously, daily for 5 days, every 5 weeks, and methyl-CCNU 130 mg/m^2 orally, on day 1, every 10 weeks [13]. A total of 684 patients have been entered into this trial. Severe toxicity was seen in 33% with the combination chemotherapy versus 17% using 5-FU alone. The period of follow-up is simply too brief to be meaningful, and the codes as to the single agent group versus combination group have not been broken; however, the recurrence rates are 10% versus 13% and the death rate is 8% versus 7% in the two groups, a difference that is statistically not significant.

Summary and Conclusion

In a prospectively randomized study, the effect of adjuvant chemotherapy wity 5-FU on survival and recurrence rates was analyzed in 299 evaluable patients with colorectal carcinoma who either underwent a curative or a palliative resection. In the treatment group, chemotherapy consisted of the intravenous administration of 12 mg/kg daily of 5-FU for 4 consecutive days, then 6 mg/kg on alternate days, to the point of toxicity, or to a maximum of five doses, followed by 12 mg/kg weekly for 1 year. Some degree of drug toxicity was seen in the majority of patients, was rarely severe, and there have been no drug-related deaths. Analysis of the survival curves and disease-free interval curves reveal definite evidence of drug benefit in two unfavorable subgroups, namely patients with Dukes C tumors and in patients whose tumor was located in the rectum. In the chemotherapy groups, patients who were treated to toxicity (WBC less than 4000 mm^3), the disease-free interval was significantly longer than the nonleukopenic patients. We conclude that the addition of 5-FU to the surgical treatment of colorectal carcinoma provides a small, but significant benefit in patients with colorectal cancer in certain unfavorable subgroups, namely patients with Dukes C lesions and patients with rectal carcinoma.

Acknowledgement

We are most grateful for the dedicated help and assistance of our Data Manager, PHYLLIS MULTHAUF.

References

1. Ansfield, F., Klotz, J., Nealon, T. et al.: A phase III study comparing the clinical utility of four regimens of 5-Fluorouracil: A preliminary report. Cancer *39,* 34 (1977)
2. Dwight, R. W., Humphrey, E. W., Higgins, G. A., Keehn, R. J.: FUDR as an adjuvant to surgery in cancer of the large bowel. J. Surg. Oncol. *5,* 243 (1973)
3. Gehan, E. A.: A generalized Wilcoxon test for comparing arbitrarily singly-censored samples. Biometrika *52,* 203 (1965)
4. Grage, T., Cornell, G., Strawitz, J. et al.: Adjuvant therapy with 5-FU after surgical resection of colo-rectal cancer. ASCO Abs. 1149, p. 258 (May 1975)
5. Grage, T., Cornell, G., Strawitz, J. et al.: Adjuvant therapy with 5-FU after surgical resection of colo-rectal cancer. Am. J. Surg. *133,* 59 (1977)
6. Grage, T. B., Metter, G., Moss, S. E., Fletcher, W. S., Jonas, K., Meeker, W. R.: Adjuvant chemotherapy in large bowel cancer: A cautious reappraisal. Eur. J. Cancer (1978) (in press)

7. Grossi, C. E., Nealon, T. F., Rousselot, L. M.: Adjuvant chemotherapy in resectable cancer of the colon and rectum. Surg. Clin. North Am. *52,* 925 (1972)
8. Holden, W. D., Dixon, W. J., Kuzma, J. W.: The use of triethylenethiophosporamide as an adjuvant to the surgical treatment of colorectal carcinoma. Ann. Surg. *165,* 481 (1967)
9. Higgins, G. A., Humphrey, E. W., Juler, G. L. et al.: Adjuvant chemotherapy in the surgical treatment of large bowel cancer. Cancer *38,* 1461 (1976)
10. Higgins, G. A., Dwight, R. W., Smith, J. V. et al.: Fluorouracil as an adjuvant to surgery in carcinoma of the colon. Arch. Surg. *102,* 339 (1971)
11. Kaplan, E. L., Meier, P.: Non-parametric estimation from incomplete observations. J. Am. Stat. Assoc. *53,* 457 (1958)
12. Lawrence, W., Terz, J. J., Horsley, S. et al.: Chemotherapy as an adjuvant to surgery for colorectal cancer. Ann. Surg. *181,* 616 (1975)
13. Mansour, E. G.: Personal Communication. ECOG Protocol 2276: Surgical adjuvant study for resectable colon cancer.
14. Moertel, C. G., Schutt, A. J., Hahn, R. G. et al.: Brief communication: therapy of advanced colorectal cancer with a combination of 5-fluorouracil, methyl-1-3-cis (2-chloroethyl)-1-nitrosourea and vincristine. J. Natl. Cancer Inst. *54,* 69 (1975)
15. Rousselot, L. M., Cole, D. R., Grossi, C. E. et al.: A five year progress report on the effectiveness of intraluminal chemotherapy (5-fluorouracil) adjuvant to surgery for colo-rectal cancer. Am. J. Surg. *115,* 140 (1968)

Ongoing Trials in the Surgical Adjuvant Management of Colorectal Cancer

P. V. Woolley, G. A. Higgins, Ph. S. Schein

Even after complete surgical resection of apparent disease, adenocarcinoma of the colon has a significant mortality. When penetration into or through the muscularis (B1 and B2) has occurred, 5-year survival is no better than 50%–60%, while lymph node involvement (C) lowers the 5-year figure to about 25%. Current attempts to improve these survival figures involve the utilization of drugs that have activity in advanced disease, principally 5-fluorouracil (5-FU) and nitrosoureas, as well as immunotherapy and, in rectal cancer, radiation therapy. To date the margins of benefit that have been observed are small and clear interpretation of results requires carefully controlled trials that provide follow-up periods of several years. As a consequence, conclusions are derived slowly and many of the most important trials are still in progress. The present discussion reviews the status of ongoing trials, principally in the Veterans Administration Surgical Adjuvant Group (VASAG), and the Gastrointestinal Tumor Study Group (GITSG).

Although early trials by VASAG with thiotepa [1] and floxuridine (FUdR) [2] produced no improvement in survival at 5 years, the studies of current interest are those that used 5-FU in the postoperative period [3] and also the newest trial that uses 5-FU plus methyl-CCNU. In the first study of postoperative 5-FU, the patients were males with completely resected adenocarcinoma that had not been diagnosed preoperatively by sigmoidoscopic biopsy. These patients were stratified into three groups: (A) "curative resection" with no evidence of residual metastasis or tumor at a resection margin, (B) histologic proof that residual tumor was left behind either by biopsy or the finding of tumor at the resection margins, and (C) clinical evidence of tumor not proven histologically. These groups were randomized separately. Those patients randomized to 5-FU received 12 mg/kg body weight IV push on 5 successive days. Group A and group C patients received a second course about 7 weeks later, while group B continued to receive the drug courses at 6–8 week intervals until disease progression or patient death. A total of 496 patients were entered into this trial of whom 482 are included in the analysis (235 treated, 247 control). The survival rates of these patients are shown in Fig. 1. In 338 patients having "curative" resection, there is 58.2% 5-year survival in the 5-FU group as opposed to 48.0% in the control. In 84 group B patients, there is 35.7% survival at 18 months for those receiving the drug compared to 16.7% in controls. In 60 group C patients, there is 53.6% survival at 18 months in those receiving the drug and 31.3% in the control group.

In a second study, patients with large-bowel cancer at all sites, including rectum, were eligible for inclusion. Those actually included were patients who, upon resection, were found to have one or more unfavorable prognostic indicators: (1) presence of positive lymph nodes, (2) serosal involvement or invasion of perirectal fat, (3) blood vessel or lymphatic invasion, (4) involvement of an organ other than the colon. Patients were then divided into two groups, group A or curative resection and group B with proven residual disease or positive resection margin. The groups were randomized separately to receive or not receive 5-FU. The drug itself was given at a dose of 12 mg/kg/day for 5 successive days, and these courses were repeated at 6–8 week intervals. Patients in group A received the drug for 18 months and those

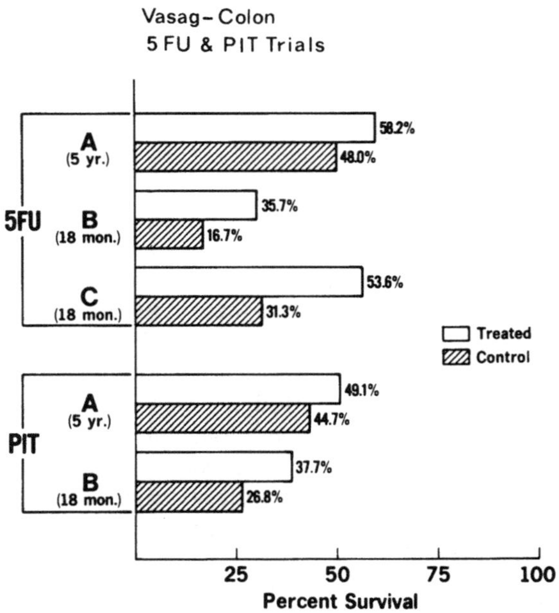

Fig. 1. Survival in the five components of the two trials, showing consistently better survival in patients receiving adjuvant 5-FU than in those treated by surgery alone

in group B until evidence of disease progression or death. There are 677 patients in this study who are eligible for analysis. In the 518 curative patients, survival at 5 years is 49.1% for patients receiving 5-FU and 44.7% for controls. For 159 patients in group B, survival is 37.7% at 18 months in the 5-FU group and 26.8% in controls (Fig. 1).

Further analysis of these groups of patients by the Mantel-Haenszel or log rank test of the difference between two survival curves has been done by comparing observed to expected deaths in each group, using uniform 30-day follow-up intervals (Fig. 2). The results show that survival in treated patients is consistently better than for controls for each operation group. In group A, B, and C the ratio of observed to expected deaths is 0.95, 0.85, and 0.77, respectively. None of the pairs of curves differ at the 5% level of significance; the P values for groups B and C are 0.13 and 0.09. When the three strata are pooled, to pose the question of whether two or more courses of 5-FU improve survival of the resection, mortality in treated patients averaged 81% of mortality in controls ($P = 0.05$). For the two operation groups of the PIT trial, observed/expected deaths were 0.92 in each case (Fig. 3). In the pooled group, mortality in treated patients averaged 85% of mortality in controls ($P = 0.08$).

Experience in the Central Oncology Group has also suggested a slight benefit for the use of adjuvant 5-FU after resection of carcinoma of the colon [3]. A study begun in 1971 has examined the effect of long-term adjuvant therapy with 5-FU upon survival and recurrence rates in patients who have undergone either palliative or curative resection. The trial is randomized and further stratified by site of disease. The drug schedule consists of an initial loading course of 5-FU at 12 mg/kg daily for 4 days, followed by 6 mg/kg/day on alternate days to the point of toxicity or to a maximum of five doses. Weekly maintenance is then carried out at 12 mg/kg/week for 1 year. Follow-up of this group has shown a general trent toward treatment benefit in the group undergoing curative resection, although survival

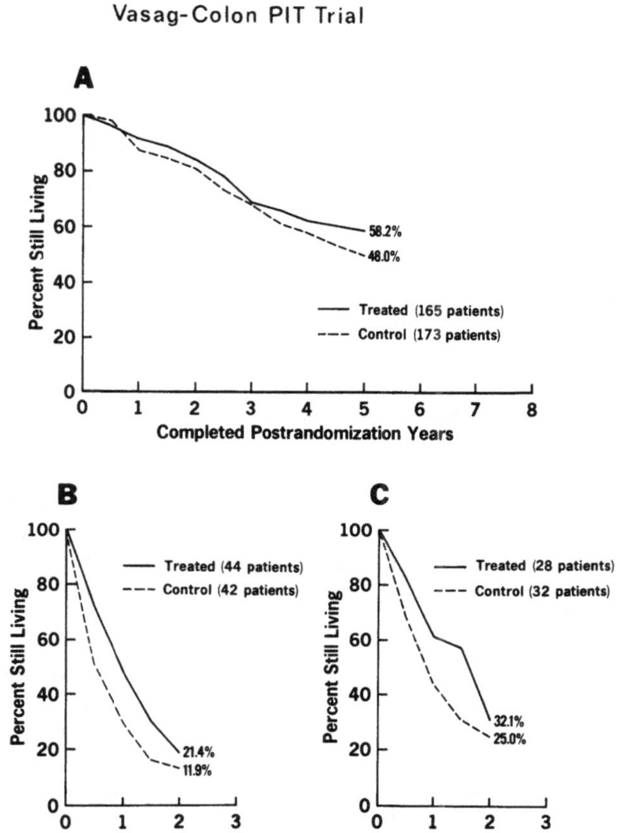

Fig. 2. Survival curves in the three components of the 5-FU trial showing improved survival in patients receiving adjuvant chemotherapy in (**A**) those having curative resection with no residual disease or tumor at a resection margin, (**B**) patients with microscopically proven residual disease, and (**C**) patients considered clinically palliative but without proven residual disease. Given for each curve are: N, the number of patients at the start of follow-up; O, the number of deaths observed during follow-up; E, the expected number of deaths with adjustment for numbers of men at risk during successive 30-day follow-up intervals. The probabilities that the difference between the paired curves are attributable to chance (MANTEL-HAENSZEL test) are (**A**) $P = 0.52$, (**B**) $P = 0.13$, (**C**) $P = 0.09$, pooled test $P = 0.05$

difference is not statistically significant ($P = 0.15$). In the patients with Dukes C disease, there is a prolongation of the disease-free interval in the treatment group ($P = 0.06$). There is also a survival benefit ($P = 0.18$). MAVLIGIT et al. [5] have presented evidence to suggest that adjuvant immunotherapy and chemotherapy are of benefit in resected Dukes C lesions. In 121 patients with such lesions treated either with BCG or BCG plus oral 5-FU, there was improved disease-free interval and survival as compared to a group of historical controls operated at M. D. Anderson between 1963 and 1973. There appeared to be no benefit of 5-FU/BCG as compared to BCG alone. While these data are provocative, the study is subject to objection on the basis of the use of oral 5-FU and of the use of historical controls.

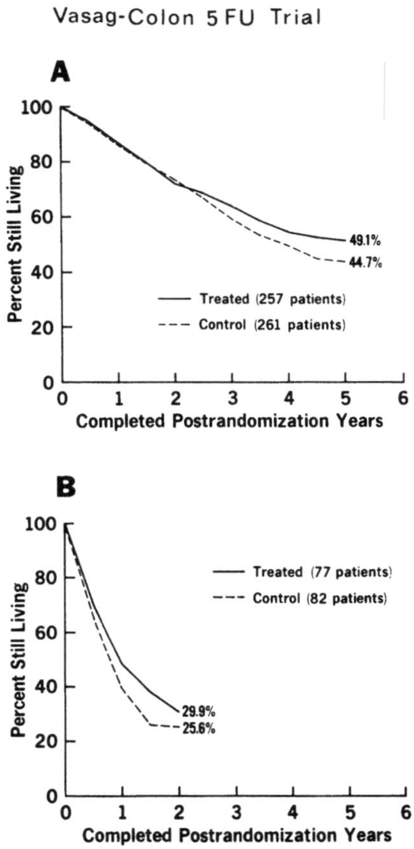

Fig. 3. Survival curves in the Prolonged Intermittent Therapy Trial showing improved survival in patients receiving adjuvant chemotherapy with 5-FU in both the (**A**) curative resection group and (**B**) patients with microscopically proven residual disease. Given for each curve are: N, the number of patients at the start of follow-up; O, the number of deaths observed during follow-up; E, the expected number of deaths with adjustment for numbers of men at risk during successive 30-day follow-up intervals. The probabilities that the differences are attributable to chance (MANTEL-HAENSZEL test) are (**A**) $P = 0.15$, (**B**) $P = 0.35$, pooled test $P = 0.08$

The Gastrointestinal Tumor Study Group has at the present time an ongoing trial for adjuvant therapy of adenocarcinoma of the colon following clinically curative resection. This consists of a four-armed study for which patient eligibility includes the complete surgical excision of a Dukes B2 (serosal penetration) or C (lymph node involvement) adenocarcinoma of the colon that was at least 12 cm from the anal verge. The study consists of a no treatment control group and treatment groups of 5-FU/methyl-CCNU, MER-BCG, and 5-FU/methyl CCNU + MER − BCG. At present, the study is still coded and accrual showed 75–80 patients in each group. Median follow-up is about 11 months. Additional studies within this group are directed at the adjuvant therapy of rectal cancer. A four-armed study is underway that compares no treatment to either radiation, chemotherapy with 5-FU and methyl-CCNU, or radiation plus chemotherapy. At present, accession into this protocol consists of about 30 patients in each group and the study is still coded. In summary, two of the most important studies of 5-FU to date, that of VASAG and that of COG, have shown suggestive evidence that adjuvant therapy of resected colon cancer produces at least a marginal benefit in terms of prolongation of disease-free remission and overall survival. Considering the fact that 5-FU produces objective responses in only 20% of cases of advanced colon cancer, these marginal effects may be as much as can be expected. The trials that are currently ongoing attempt to increase the yield by adding the active drug methyl-CCNU to the regimen, as well as immunotherapy in the form of MER. Since at least 2–3 years of follow-up are required before conclusions can be drawn from these trials, much of the available evidence is preliminary, and the next several years will teach us a great deal about this disease.

References

1. Dwight, R. W., Higgins, G. A. (Jr.), Keehn, R. J.: Factors influencing survival after resection in cancer of the colon and rectum. Am. J. Surg. *117,* 512–522 (1960)
2. Dwight, R. W., Humphrey, E. W., Higgins, G. A. et al: FUDR as adjuvant to surgery in cancer of the large bowel. J. Surg. Oncol. *5,* 243–249 (1973)
3. Grage, T. B., Metter, G. E., Cornell, G. N. et al: Adjuvant chemotherapy with 5-Fluorouracil after surgical resection of colorectal carcinoma (COG Protocol 7041): A preliminary report. Am. J. Surg. *133,* 59–66 (1977)
4. Higgins, G. A. (Jr.), Humphrey, E., Juler, G. L., LeVeen, H. H., McCaughan, J., Keehn, R. J.: Adjuvant chemotherapy in the surgical treatment of large bowel cancer. Cancer *38,* 1461–1467 (1976)
5. Mavligit, G. M., Gutterman, J. V., Malahy, M. A., Burgess, M. A., McBride, C. M., Juler, A., Hersh, E. M.: Adjuvant immunotherapy and chemotherapy in colorectal cancer (Dukes' Class C); prolongation of disease-free interval and survial. Cancer *40,* 2726–2730 (1977)

Clinical Studies on PSK: Combination Therapy of PSK With Surgery and Chemotherapy

T. Taguchi

Introduction

PSK is a polysaccharide preparation obtained from the mycelia of the CM-101 strain of Coriolus versicolor (Fr.) Quél in Basidiomycetes by hot-water extraction followed by sedimentation with ammonium sulfate saturation, dialysis, and drying. This preparation is a protein-bound polysaccharide containing about 38% protein, which consists of 18 kinds of amino acids such as aspartic acid, glutamic acid, etc.

PSK is a brown or brownish powder with a slightly characteristic odor without taste. When 1 g PSK is dissolved in water, the solution becomes brownish and slightly turbid, having a pH value of 6.6–7.2. When heated, this preparation gradually changes in color, to dark brown at about 120 °C, and finally decomposes. The average molecular weight of PSK measured by the ultracentrifugation technique is about 100,000, and it is stable against heat, light, and long storage.

As indicated in Table 1, the acute toxicity (LD_{50}) of PSK is low and there have been no abnormal findings due to oral administration of PSK in subacute and chronic toxicity tests (Table 2).

Clinical Studies

There are many reports on the effects of PSK combined with surgery and chemotherapy. Table 3 indicates the treatment schedule of stage IV stomach cancer, referred to as PLCC (postoperative long-term cancer chemotherapy) by Inoguchi et al. [2], in which the 3 year survival rate was 14.7% in the control group and 29.4% in the group treated with the PLCC schedule and PSK (Figs. 1 and 2).

Figure 3 indicates the results reported by Hattori et al. [1] on the treatment of stomach cancer. In this clinical study, based on the National Cancer Center system for the treatment of stomach cancer in Japan, 20 mg of mitomycin C on the day of operation and 10 mg on the following day were given, and PSK was administered orally from about 1 week after operation. Figure 4 indicates the results in 21 institutions [13] on the treatment of operable stage III stomach cancer with mitomycin C alone or mitomycin C plus PSK. After 2 years observation, a higher survival rate was found in the patients given mitomycin C and PSK. In this study, it was reported that the rate of appearance of leukopenia was low and the rate of completion of mitomycin C administration was higher in the patients given mitomycin C and PSK than those given mitomycin C alone. This result may suggest that PSK prevents side-effects of mitomycin C.

When PSK was combined with MF (mitomycin C plus 5-fluorouracil) for the treatment of recurrent stomach cancer, a 50% survival rate was reported at 6.4 months in the group treated with MF and at 12.0 months in the group given PSK plus MF (Fig. 5).

Table 1. Acute toxicity of PSK on mice, rats, dogs, and monkeys

Animal	Administration route	LD_{50} (mg/kg)	
		Female	Male
Mice	Intravenous	> 1,300	> 1,300
	Subcutaneous	> 5,000	> 5,000
	Intraperitoneal	> 5,000	> 5,000
	Oral	>20,000	>20,000
Rats	Intravenous	> 600	> 600
	Subcutaneous	> 5,000	> 5,000
	Intraperitoneal	> 5,000	> 5,000
	Oral	>20,000	>20,000
Dogs	Intravenous	> 320	> 320
	Oral	> 1,000	> 1,000
Monkeys	Intravenous	> 160	> 160
	Oral	> 5,000	> 5,000

Table 2. Subacute and chronic toxicity tests

Animals	Subacute toxicity (days)	Chronic toxicity (days)	Examination
Mice	30	180	Body weight Diet intake Hematological examination
Rats	30	180	Biochemical examination of serum
Dogs	30	180	
Monkeys	–	180	Urine test Findings upon autopsy Histopathological findings

Table 3. Regimens in postoperative long-term cancer chemotherapy

20 mg MMC during operation, upper half of body, I.V., one shot
20 mg MMC 4th week after operation, hospitalized, I.V., one shot
10 mg MMC 3 months after operation, as outpatient, I.V., one shot
10 mg MMC every 3 months for 2 years after operation as outpatient, I.V., one shot
800 mg/day of Futraful and 3 g/day of PSK from 7 days after operation, continued as long as possible

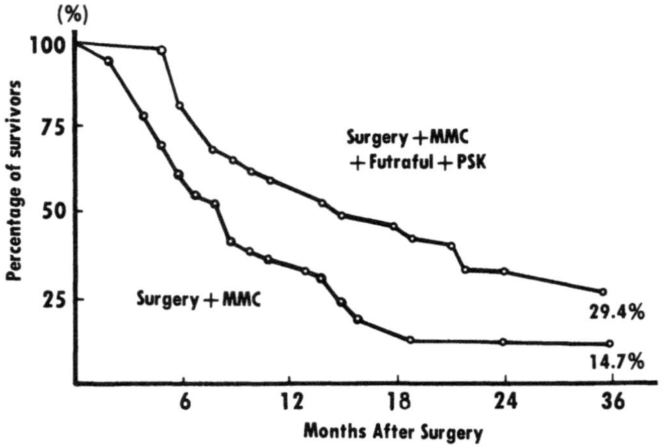

Fig. 1. Survival curve

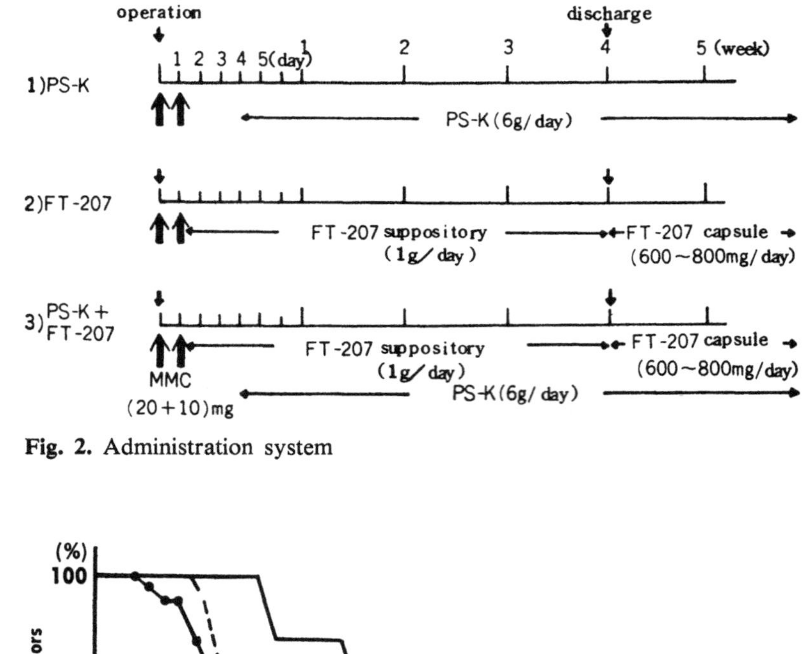

Fig. 2. Administration system

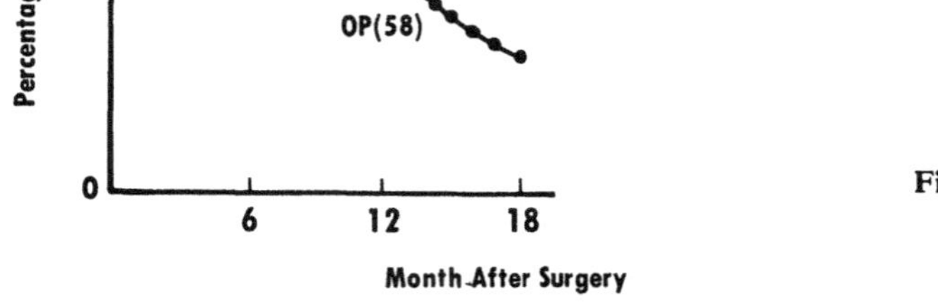

Fig. 3. Survival curve

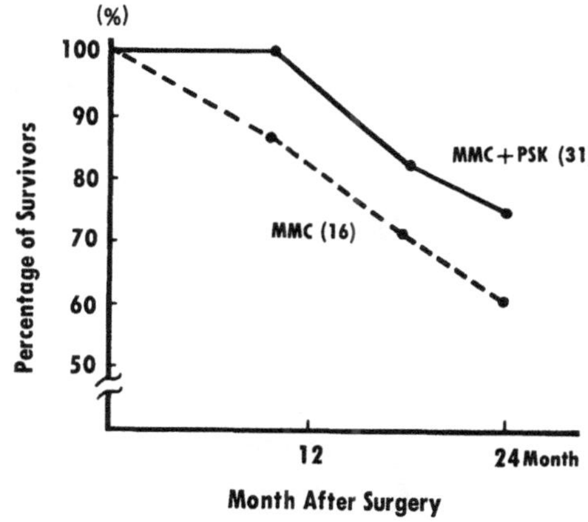

Fig. 4. Survival curve. Group I: Mitomycin C 4 mg/day, drip infusion 2 times/week, total 40 mg, Group II: Group I + PSK 6 g/day, orally, total more than 360 g

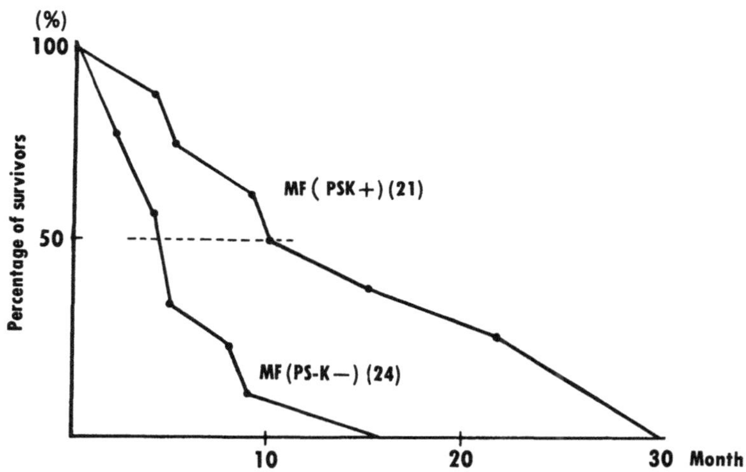

Fig. 5. Percentage of survivors of recurrent stomach cancer with MF therapy with or without administration of PSK

KOBAYASHI et al. [6], at the Laboratory of Pathology, Cancer Institute, Hokkaido University School of Medicine, similarly reported that various skin reactions such as PHA, PPD, CD, and SK-SD reactions were significantly positive in the cases of gastric cancer treated with surgery and PSK and/or chemotherapy compared with those not given PSK (Table 4). These results indicated that PSK possessed immunorestorative activity.

Conclusion

PSK possesses quite unique characteristics; it has (1) a different mode of action from conventional anticancer drugs, having a wide antitumor spectrum; (2) additive therapeutic effect by combination with other anticancer drugs; (3) apparent enhancement of antitumor effect and prolongation of survival time by combination of radiation and chemotherapy or

Table 4. Change of skin reactions after treatment with PSK in gastric cancer patients

Treatment	Antigen	Skin reaction[a]		
		Increase	No change	Decrease
Operation and PSK and/or chemotherapy	PHA	2/6	3/6	1/6
	PPD	1/6	3/6	2/6
	CD	2/6	3/6	1/6
	SK-SD	1/6	5/6	0/6
	Total	6/24 (25%)	14/24 (58%)	4/24 (17%)
Operation and/or chemotherapy	PHA	0/7	5/7	2/7
	PPD	0/7	7/7	0/7
	CD	0/7	4/7	3/7
	SK-SD	0/7	3/7	4/7
	Total	0/28 (0%)	19/28 (68%)	9/28 (32%)

[a] Evaluation of skin reaction changing was as follows: increase = more than 100% increase; decrease = more 50% decrease in diameter of reactions.

surgery and chemotherapy with PSK; (4) no special enhancement of hematopoietic toxicity of anticancer drugs, but rather restores it and improves total host conditions. From these observations, we can say that PSK will be one of the preparations valuable in combination modalities.

References

1. Hattori, T. et al.: Cancer Chemother. *4*, 587 (1977)
2. Kaibara, N. et al.: The 78th Congress of Japan Surgical Society. 1978
3. Kamitsuka, A. et al.: 31th Annual Meeting of the Japanese Society for Medical Mycology. 1977
4. Kimura, I. et al.: 36th Annual Meeting of the Japanese Cancer Association. 1977
5. Sobayashi, H. et al.: Cancer Res. *37*, 3042 (1977)
6. Kobayashi, H. et al.: 15th Congress of Japan Society for Cancer Therapy. 1977
7. Mizuno, D. et al.: GANN *67*, 685 (1977)
8. Nomoto, K. et al.: GANN *66*, 365 (1975)
9. Nomoto, K. et al.: GANN *66*, 649 (1975)
10. Nomoto, K. et al.: 35th Annual Meeting of the Japanese Cancer Association. 1976
11. Nomoto, K. et al.: 12th International Cancer Congress. 1978
12. Nomoto, K. et al.: 37th Annual Meeting of the Japanese Cancer Association. 1978
13. Shiba, S.: PSK Kenkyukai (1976)
14. Taguchi, T. et al.: Cancer Chemother. *2*, 13 (1975)
15. Taguchi, T. et al.: 12th International Cancer Congress. 1978
16. Yamada, K. et al.: GANN *67*, 97 (1976)

F. Bronchus Carcinoma

Role of Radiotherapy as an Adjuvant Therapy in Operable Bronchus Carcinoma

J. Stjernswärd

Based on a review of existing data on pre- and postoperative irradiation in operable non-small-cell lung cancer it is concluded that:
1. *Routine* postoperative irradiation in operable non-small-cell lung cancer is not prolonging survival.
2. Postoperative irradiation in operable lung cancers, even node positive should not be used routinely but only in controlled clinical trials, exploring its possible role alone or in combination with systemic therapies.
The biology of the disease, mostly with disseminated micrometastases outside the irradiated target volume, especially in a lymph node-positive patient, may be one of the explanations for why radiotherapy has thus far failed to change survival positively in operable non-small-cell lung cancer.
The role of radiotherapy in modern multi-modality adjuvant therapeutic approaches to non-small-cell lung cancer remains to be evaluated. It is suggested that local disease may be controlled, but due to the biology of the disease this will definitely not affect the survival. Consolidation radiation therapy ought to be valid if effect of systemic therapies will be achieved. Furthermore it can not be excluded that local radiotherapy may negatively effect the therapeutic outcome of other treatment modalities used for attacking systemic disseminated disease. The possible role of total- and half-body irradiation remains to be explored in well controlled clinical studies as well as the role of irradiation to special sites, e.g. privileged sites for chemo- and/or immunotherapy.

Influence of Postoperative Radiotherapy on Local Recurrence and Survival of Bronchial Epidermoid Carcinoma With Regard to Nodal Status: Preliminary Results of the EORTC Protocol 08741

L. Israel, A. Depierre, and R. Sylvester

Introduction

Protocol 08741 of the EORTC Lung Study group includes a first randomization following surgery between a control arm and radiotherapy (4500 rad in 4.5 weeks on the mediastinum) and a second randomization, in each of these two arms, intended to compare four groups, namely chemotherapy, immunotherapy, chemoimmunotherapy, and controls. The first part of this protocol, though not yet completed, can be analyzed since 372 patients have been entered from January 1974 to June 1977. A stratification by nodal status was made prior to randomization. This study was launched because of absence of data regarding the influence of nodal status on the radiotherapeutic results. Our preliminary data are represented in this report.

Statistical Considerations

A log rank test has been applied to the results to take into account both the numbers of failures and the time at which they are detected.

Local Recurrences

a) On the whole, there is no statistical significance between the local recurrence rate of N^+ and N^- cases (21.3% versus 21.5%) irrespective of their treatment.
b) Irrespective of the nodal status, radiation therapy is superior to controls in achieving local control (15% failures versus 26%; $P < 0.05$).
c) Among N_0 cases, which amount to 223, radiotherapy does not induce any significant reduction in local recurrence rates as compared to controls (19.4% versus 23.4%).
d) Among N^+ cases, which amount to 149, radiation therapy both decreases the recurrence rate (18.9% versus 31.5%) and delays the recurrence, the *P* value being at present at 0.07.

Distant Metastases

a) The distant metastases, irrespective of treatment, do not yet show a tendency to differ between N_0 and N^+ cases, either in numbers or in delay.
b) Irrespective of the nodal status, and taking into account the treatment only, there is no difference, in terms of disease-free interval, between radiation therapy and abstention.
c) This is also true among N_0 cases, where radiation therapy induces no difference.
d) Again this is true among N^+ cases, where no difference is seen between radiation therapy and abstention.

Comparing N^+ and N^- cases, less distant metastases appear in the N^- group in the absence of radiotherapy ($P = 0.08$). When radiotherapy is given, these differences disappear entirely, showing a slight tendency for radiotherapy to induce detrimental effects in N^- cases as far as disease-free interval from distant metastases is concerned.

Survival

Although it is still difficult to conclude due to the fact that patients with recurrences are still surviving, preliminary results not reaching the significant levels tend to show that survival is the same among N^+ patients, with or without radiation therapy, while in the N_0 group there is a tendency for patients not being irradiated to survive longer.

Conclusion

As one could have predicted, radiation therapy can only improve the local recurrence rate. This does not interfere with survival, because most of the patients are dying from distant metastases. There is even an unconfirmed indication that radiation therapy could be detrimental to N_0 patients. Thus, the field that remains for radiation therapy in the management of resected squamous cell carcinoma of the lung seems to be of very limited importance. To decide whether or not to keep including radiotherapy in our therapeutic strategies for N^+ patients one would have to know:

a) Whether chemotherapy can take care of local control as well as radiation therapy does – which does not seem to be the case in the present study.
b) Whether radiation therapy does not decrease the local and systemic effectiveness of chemotherapy. An answer will hopefully be provided when this study is completed.

Preliminary Trends of the EORTC Study Comparing Postoperative Chemotherapy, Immunotherapy, Chemoimmunotherapy or Abstention in Squamous Cell Bronchial Carcinoma

L. Israel, A. Depierre, and R. Sylvester

This is a very short interim report since, due to the stratification according to nodal status and the first random allocation to groups with and without radiotherapy, there are 16 subgroups among 310 patients available for analysis. For this reason, the EORTC expects no conclusive results before 2 additional years of follow-up. Nevertheless, some trends are beginning to appear that will be summarized below and should be considered as very preliminary.

Impact of Postoperative Medical Treatment Irrespective of Nodal Status and Radiotherapy

Chemotherapy given alone is worse than any other treatment method (abstention, immunotherapy, immunochemotherapy). This result may not be conceptually significant since no subgroups are considered, but it at least outlines the fact that, unlike immunochemotherapy, chemotherapy by itself may be detrimental in postoperative situations.

Impact of Postoperative Medical Treatment in N^- Cases

No significance has yet been reached. The only subgroup that seems to derive benefit from a medical treatment is the nonirradiated N^- subgroup receiving immunotherapy alone.

Impact of Postoperative Medical Treatment in N^+ Cases

No significance has yet been reached. The only subgroup that seems to derive benefit from a medical treatment, in terms of survival, is the nonirradiated N^+ subgroup receiving chemoimmunotherapy. It is too soon to evaluate a difference between this subgroup and the N^+ radiotherapy without medical treatment group.

Discussion

Although we would insist on the impossibility of drawing any firm conclusion as yet, it seems timely to consider the following points.

a) N^- cases should be considered good cases in terms of immune status [4, 5]. It thus seems that immunodepressing modalities such as radiation therapy or chemotherapy should be avoided, whereas nonspecific immune stimulation might be beneficial. It may well be that local stimulation such as the procedure advocated by Mc Kneally [6] will prove even better than distant stimulation for N^- cases.

b) N^+ cases have a far greater risk of devoping metastases. It has been shown in a previous paper that radiotherapy is useless in such cases in terms of survival. A systemic treatment must be tried instead. That it should consist of immunochemotherapy rather than of chemotherapy alone is not a surprise [1–3].

References

1. Israel, L.: Nonspecific immunostimulation in bronchogenic cancer. Scand. J. Resp. Dis. [Suppl.] *89,* 95–105 (1974)
2. Israel, L., Edelstein, R., Depierre, A., Dimitrov, N.: Daily intravenous infusions of Corynebacterium parvum in twenty patients with disseminated cancer: A preliminary report of clinical and biologic findings. J.N.C.I. *55,* 29–33 (1975)
3. Israel, L.: Nonspecific immune stimulation with corynebacteria in lung cancer. In: Lung cancer. Natural history, prognosis, and therapy. Israël, L., Chahinian, P. (eds.), Vol. I, pp. 273–280. New York-London: Academic Press 1976
4. Israel, L., Edelstein, R.: In vivo and in vitro studies on nonspecific blocking factors of host origin in cancer patients. Role of plasma exchange as an immunotherapeutic modality. Isr. J. Med. Sci. *14,* 105–130 (1978)
5. Israel, L.: An immunological look at the TNM classification therapeutic implications and strategies. Cancer Treat. Rep. (1978) (in press)
6. McKneally, M. F., Maver, C., Kansel, H. W.: Regional immunotherapy of lung cancer with intrapleural BCG. Lancet *1976/I,* 377–379

Adjuvant Chemotherapy of Post-Surgical Minimal Residual Bronchial Carcinomas

K. Karrer

Primary cancer of the lung was rare and always fatal before the early 1930s. It is now common and selectively curable [35]. Bronchogenic carcinomas today represent a great and growing problem. In 1914 the total number of deaths in the United States attributed to lung cancer was 317. In 1930 the figure was 2357, in 1940 it was 7121, in 1950 it was 18,313, and in 1960 deaths attributed to this cause numbered 36,420. In 1965 the total number of deaths from lung cancer was 53,000. It is estimated that more than 80,000 deaths per annum will occur by 1980 in the United States. Although female incidence of lung and bronchial cancer is considerably lower than male incidence, it has been increasing almost as rapidly as male incidence during the past 20 years [3]. Similarly, increasing figures are also reported from many other countries [7, 42, 43].

Although cancer of the lung has been a highly lethal disease, and even today many reports present the discouraging aspects, it is worthwhile to report that increasing experience warrants future optimism [34]. The first successful pneumonectomy for cancer of the lung was performed by Graham and Singer in 1933. Surgery has been established as the form of therapy in which cure might best be anticipated under circumstances where a preoperative assessment has accurately established the presence of limited primary disease. The therapeutic limitations of surgery are also now well recognized, and future progress in preventing or controlling this disease is contingent upon finding methods that will either supplant or enhance the therapeutic effectiveness of surgery [46]. The results of surgical resection of lung cancer are remarkably uniform throughout the world. The current mortality rate from surgical resection is 5%–10%.

Very importantly, there is general acceptance of the concept that lung cancer is a systemic disease at diagnosis in a majority of cases. It is agreed that therapies adjunctive to surgery must be actively investigated. Any material or truly meaningful improvement in survival will only be realized if effective adjuncts are employed. This excludes the unlikely possibility that some new therapy will be discovered that is, in itself, curative. That is to say that the contributions of surgery, with respect to their influence on survival, cannot be expected to change. The concept of biologic operability as opposed to technical resectability is preferable. Surgery has essentially reached its anatomic limit and it is felt that the future lies in chemotherapy, immunotherapy, and radiation therapy [33].

In spite of the efforts in early detection and aggressive therapy, the median survival of all patients from diagnosis to death remains less than 6 months and the 5-year survival rate remains less than 10%. Of the various modalities of treatment currently available, surgery has the best potential for long-term survivors. However, 50% of the patients have clearly inoperable tumors at the time of diagnosis, and 20% are found to be unresectable at the time of thoracotomy, leaving approximately 30% in whom resection is possible.

The results of surgical resection have been fairly accurately defined and correlated to stage by the TNM classification. An overall 5-year survival rate of approximately 25% has been reported in most series [28]. Among patients with the least tumor burden according to the TNM classification, i.e., $T_1 N_0 M_0$ (a tumor less than 3 cm in diameter without nodal or other metastases), representing approximately 7% of all lung cancer patients, the survival at 18 months is only 65%. In a series of 202 patients dying from whatever cause within 1 month after curative resection for bronchogenic carcinomas, local or distant metastatic disease was found at autopsy in 35% of patients, implying a much higher frequency of micrometastatic disease [37].

Observations that many grams of tumor cells could be destroyed by various methods using modern anticancer drugs led to the logical step of combining excision of all gross tumors with simultaneous chemotherapy. The idea was not new, being no different than the use of postoperative X-ray therapy, but there were several theoretical advantages. One was the use of adjuvant systemic therapy rather than two kinds of local therapy. However, if anticancer compounds can affect large tumor masses, it can be expected that small amounts of unrecognized tumor would be more susceptible to these agents when used in the immediate postoperative period.

Adjuvant chemotherapy has been successfully used in a number of experimental animal tumors. It was shown that surgery combined with chemotherapy was more effective than either of the modalities used alone. In addition, it has been observed that a combination of drugs was more effective than the single drugs, especially when there was obvious residual tumor after surgery.

The reproducibility of these experiments has been quite encouraging in advancing the principles of adjuvant chemotherapy. The beneficial effects of chemotherapy in the situation are presumably due to control of residual cancer cells, often in the form of micrometastases that exist at the time of resection of the primary tumor. Micrometastases, by virtue of a higher growth fraction, are more responsive to chemotherapy than the advanced tumor. Early treatment by-passes the problem of the more resistant nonproliferative or resting cells that predominate in advanced metastatic disease [8, 11, 12, 14–20, 22, 31, 41].

Based on the animal data, the concept of adjuvant chemotherapy has been extended to the treatment of many human cancers. Adjuvant chemotherapy, which is increasingly employed in the clinic, is defined as the improvement of the cure rate of cancer by the addition of chemotherapy to ostensibly curative surgery. Because of the large number of complex factors involved in the adjuvant chemotherapy of solid tumors, extensive clinical trials are necessary before any rational modification of the drug or dose schedule is justified. Systemic cytostatic therapy is considered best for such general therapy, but at present there is no drug available that has a completely specific action against tumor cells, and chemotherapeutic effectiveness still depends on the adjustment of the relative toxic effects of known drugs on both tumor and host cells. Today, no other available methods are as effective as chemotherapy in producing tumor inhibition [23].

For this reason, adjuvant chemotherapy studies have been carried out in Vienna since 1954 in patients with bronchial carcinomas [8]. Also in the United States the Veterans Administration Surgical Adjuvant Cooperative Study Group was organized in 1957. Survival curves of almost 3000 patients who had surgical resection of lung cancer and 4-day treatment with 30 mg nitrogen mustard showed no beneficial effect from this drug therapy. An almost identical study of university hospitals in the United States confirmed these results [13, 45].

These trials of chemotherapy in the surgical adjuvant setting have largely been focussed on two hypotheses that are now discredited: (1) that short-term exposure to drugs at the time of surgery might delay or prevent recurrence by killing tumor cells that were "seeded" by the operation and (2) that alkylating agents are likely to be effective in killing micrometastatic lesions [29].

As administration of the drug in a short immediate postoperative period produced no general change of survival [6, 48], long-term chemotherapy was therefore introduced [49]. Several reports indicated partially positive results [1, 21, 24, 26, 36, 38, 39].

But also from similar studies a failure of effectiveness has been seen [5, 32, 40] and additionally negative results have been reported by the Swiss Group [4]. But the different dose schedules and different drugs used make comparisons difficult.

The efficacy of the chemotherapy seems to be dependent on the dose schedule and the stage and nature of the disease. Of particular importance seems also the consideration of different subgroups: as for instance, as also reported by the Veterans Administration Group in the United States, a cooperative trial using 740 mg cytoxan in two courses within 5 postoperative weeks, demonstrating in the whole group of 845 curative and 163 palliative resected patients no beneficial effect of cytoxan; but in the subgroup of oat cell carcinoma, the survival was substantially better than in the controls [13].

From the consideration of these results as well as of experimental studies on appropriate animal model systems, the Viennese Working Group has introduced the concept of a high-dosed intermittent long-term combined polychemotherapy, including intervals without treatment for recovery, as the optimal balance possible at present between the desired tumor inhibitory effect and undesirable and unfavorable immunosuppression [21].

Besides this trial with a four-drug polychemotherapy of the Viennese Working Group, the Veterans Administration Surgical Adjuvant Group carried out a trial using cyclophosphamide and methotrexate in an alternating sequence at 5-week intervals for a period of 18 months and compared it with an untreated control group. The results of this study were disappointing, showing no difference in the 5-year survival between the two groups. The toxicity was minimal, with 50% of the treated patients showing no leukopenia. However, only 50% of the prescribed dose of chemotherapy was actually administered [44].

In Japan, a trial employing a two-drug combination of chromomycin-A_3 and mitomycin-C, given intermittently in courses over a 3-year period was initiated. The authors report a 5-year survival rate of 50% in the treated group as compared to 22% in a retrospective control group [26].

There are currently also five other ongoing trials with adjuvant chemotherapy: the Veterans Administration Surgical Adjuvant Group is investigating a combination of hydroxyurea and CCNU with a no-treatment control group (protocol 26). Lung cancer patients of all cell types with no microscopic evidence of residual disease are entered in this trial. The chemotherapy is to continue for 1 year in the treatment group. The results of this trial should soon be available.

The Working Party for Therapy of Lung Cancer is evaluating the role of CCNU in stages I and II nonsmall cell carcinoma with a control group of no chemotherapy (WPL-protocol 7351). Chemotherapy is continued for a period of 2 years. Protocol 7551 has been designed recently to include resectable stage III large cell carcinoma and adenocarcinoma as well in the CCNU trial. A similar study is being done in the U.S.S.R. as part of the U.S.-U.S.S.R. Agreement for Health Cooperation.

The lung group of the European Organization for Research on Treatment of Cancer (EORTC) is investigating the role of combined chemotherapy and immunotherapy in nonsmall cell carcinoma. The chemotherapy consists of a combination of cyclophosphamide, methotrexate, and CCNU, and BCG is the immunotherapeutic agent [28]. As mentioned above, a randomized clinical trial was initiated in 1969 to determine whether a high-dosed intermittent long-term polychemotherapy can increase the survival rate and/or survival time of patients who have undergone radical surgery for bronchial carcinomas at the I. Surgical

Department of the Hospital of Vienna-Lainz (Prof. Dr. H. Denck) in cooperation with the Ludwig Boltzmann Institute for Clinical Oncology (Prof. Dr. H. Denck, Doz. Dr. G. Alth, OMR Dr. R. Titscher and Doz. Dr. H. Sighart). For constructive collaboration we are thankful to the colleagues of these institutions, in particular to OA Dr. N. Pridun and OA Dr. E. Zwintz.

In order to attain a maximal destruction of small tumor foci in the whole body, the highest possible dose, limited according to the resulting side-effects, should be administered. All patients were randomized after surgery. The stratification of the patients was performed thereafter according to the TNM classification based on the histologic examination of the operation specimens, Feinstein's classification, and the histologic main types [2, 9, 27]. Thus, four groups of patients are categorized: squamous cell, adenocarcinoma, small cell, and all other types of carcinoma, termed "diverse;" no unknown histologic type is included in this study.

Radical surgery is defined as the removal of the whole primary tumor together with the surrounding involved tissue. This is performed by lobectomy, bilobectomy, or pneumonectomy, according to the localization and size of the primary tumor. The regional lymph nodes are also removed by this procedure. Additional lymph nodes are also removed if macroscopically involved. The operation specimen is examined by the same pathologist. The cutting board and the extent of the primary tumor as well as the labeled, removed lymph nodes are evaluated in anatomic relationship. This provides the evidence for the subsequent postoperative TNM staging. No X-ray treatment was used at this stage. Both groups of patients received the same general medical care at equal intervals.

Chemotherapy was carried out as follows: 1–2 weeks after surgery, the first intravenous infusion of 500 ml of 5% levulose containing 12 mg/kg cyclophosphamide, 12 mg/kg 5-FU, 0.5 mg/kg methotrexate, and 0.1 mg/kg vinblastine was administered. This infusion was repeated a second and a third time at intervals of 7 days. The protocol requires the administration of 13 such series of three infusions within 3 years after surgery. The first series of three infusions is given within the usual time required for hospitalization for this type of operation. Subsequent infusions are given in the outpatient clinic. The hematogram is determined before chemotherapy is started. The minimum hematologic level must be 4 million erythrocytes, 4000 leukocytes, and 100,000 platelets per mm^3. During therapy a leukocyte count is required twice weekly; if the leukocyte and platelet counts fall below 4000 or 100,000 per mm^3, respectively, the intervals without treatment are prolonged. The chemotherapy protocol was followed as closely as possible; no reduction of schedule of chemotherapy was used. However, the interval of treatment was prolonged as made necessary by low white blood counts. The chemotherapy is given in the outpatient clinic of the hospital where the blood counts are also performed. Patients from outside of Vienna are also treated (i.e., chemotherapy administration) and examined in the outpatient clinic mentioned above. Close cooperation with the referring family physician is important. Therefore, the general practitioner is informed by an explanatory letter and asked to provide psychologic support, advice, and care of the patient. The private physician is only requested to treat the general physical condition of the patient, but no cytostacic chemotherapy is administered by him.

As indicated in Fig. 1, many of these patients (predominantly from outside Vienna) are not willing to undergo regular chemotherapy. This is often because the patient does not understand his diagnosis and prognosis, which one is usually not told in Austria. Therefore, treatment is unfortunately not administered to all patients as would be required according to the protocol. Because they are convinced neither of the necessity for the long-term therapy nor of the rationale of the adjuvant chemotherapy, not only the patients themselves but also

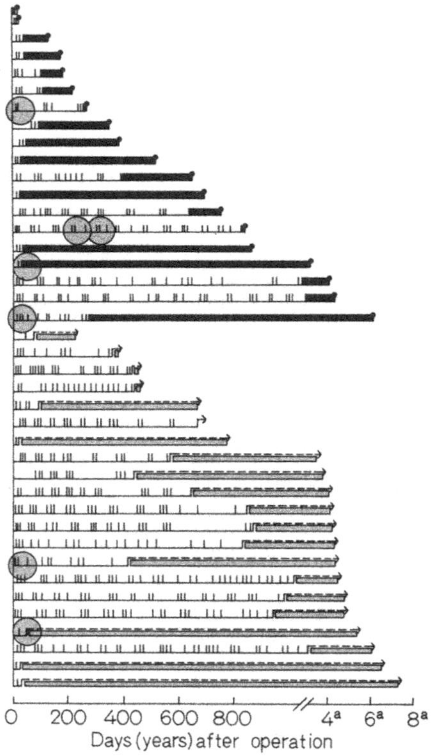

Fig. 1. Observation or survival time with number of infusions administered and length of intervals without treatment for each patient operated on for bronchial squamous cell carcinoma in stage $T_2N_aM_0$. ⊥⊥⊥, infusions; ——● deaths; – – – –→ observation period after chemotherapy; ● leukopenia below 2000 leukocytes/mm³

some of the private physicians involved do not cooperate in supporting the maintenance of the protocol schedule.

The preliminary evaluation of this study on 1 January 1978 is based on 588 patients. The parameter used for the evaluation of the chemotherapy administered is the survival time from the point of surgical tumor removal up to the patient's demise. Of the 588 patients, 339 received only surgical treatment (randomized controls). To define different prognostic groups of bronchogenic carcinomas and their reactions to the uniform therapy, detailed stratifications were used. This was accomplished by a definite description and classification of the tumor at the time of resection, using the TNM system [2], the Feinstein categories [9] and histologic major types [27]. Calculation of the life table survival curves is based on all randomized patients, including the postoperative mortality without exception even in the case of protocol violation or deviation [10, 47]. The establishment of criteria for defining whether or not treatment is adequate appears premature at the present stage of the investigation. The following TNM staging is used:

Stage I	Stage II	Stage III	Stage IV
T1NaM0 T2NaM0	T1NbM0 T2NbM0	T1NcM0 T2NcM0 T3Na,bM0	T3NcM0 T4Na,b,cM0 TxNxM1
A	**B**	**C**	
T1NaM0 T2NaM0 T3NaM0	T1NbM0 T2NbM0 T3NbM0	T1,2,3NcM0 T4Na,b,cM0 TxNxM1	

Table 1. Number of bronchial carcinoma patients treated with radical surgery and adjuvant chemotherapy

TNM stages																	
Histo	I				II				III				IV				Total
	S	A	O	D	S	A	O	D	S	A	O	D	S	A	O	D	
Feinstein 1	13	7	1	5	3	6	—	—	4	1	1	3	—	3	—	1	48
2	6	3	2	1	5	1	—	3	5	—	2	—	2	—	1	1	32
3	26	5	2	6	13	8	3	1	9	4	1	1	13	5	6	2	105
4	1	—	—	—	1	—	—	—	3	1	—	1	3	1	—	—	11
5	10	2	1	2	7	2	1	1	6	2	1	—	8	2	1	—	46
U	1	1	—	—	1	—	—	—	1	—	1	—	1	—	—	1	7
Total	57	18	6	14	30	17	4	5	28	8	6	5	27	11	8	5	
Grand total	95				56				47				51				249

S squamous; *A* adenocarcinoma; *O* oat cell; *D* diverse carcinoma; *U* Feinstein category unknown.

Table 1 shows the number of patients treated both surgically and with chemotherapy, grouped according to TNM stages, Feinstein categories, and the three major cell types (squamous cell, adenocarcinoma, oat cell, and all others, i.e., "diverse" tumor types). Diverse histology means all histologic types other than the three main cell types already mentioned, and no "unknown" histologic type is included in this group. In accordance with the Viennese School of Surgery, the oat cell carcinoma is also included for surgery.

The age distribution shows a significant peak between the ages of 60 and 65 in both sex groups. Only a few patients older than 70 years of age were operated on. The male : female ratio was 5 : 1.

The percentage of asymptomatic patients (Feinstein category 1 shown in Table 1) is quite similar to that of the original distribution recorded by Feinstein, indicating that no particular measures of early diagnosis were effective. Table 2 summarizes the infusions given to only 239 patients of the 249 randomized patients, as ten randomized patients died postoperatively before chemotherapy.

Table 2. Bronchial carcinomas treated by radical surgery: with or without leukopenia after chemotherapy

TNM stages	I			II			III			IV			Total	Grand total
Leucocytes not below	No. of pat.	Admin. infusions	No. of inf.	No. of pat.	Admin. infusions	No. of inf.	No. of pat.	Admin. infusions	No. of inf.	No. of pat.	Admin. infusions	No. of inf.	Patients	Infusions
2000	83	1–45	1072	49	1–42	551	44	1–40	405	38	1–35	352	214	2380
1500	3	2–13	17	5	3–33	79	–	–	–	5	1–26	41	13	137
1000	5	3–32	57	–	–	–	2	14–38	52	2	2–30	32	9	141
700	1	11	11	–	–	–	–	–	–	2	4– 6	10	3	21
Total	92	1–45	1157	54	1–42	630	46	1–40	457	47	1–35	435	239	2679

Detailed information is provided in Fig. 1, where the occurrence of leukopenias is also documented for one group of patients ($T_2N_0M_0$) for example. Alopecia, cystitis, and infections have been rare so that they have been omitted from this preliminary evaluation. No second primary neoplasm has yet been observed.

The treatment was well tolerated, causing only minor side-effects, such as vomiting and nausea for 1–2 days. Loss of hair and diarrhea were also rare. No patient required hospitalization due to side-effects. Most of the patients stayed away from work only for the day of infusion. It seems particularly important that the rate of leukopenia appears lower than a comparably high-dosed single-drug therapy would cause. Table 2 also demonstrates the important finding that only 25 of 239 patients developed leukopenia below the leukocyte level of 2000/mm^3. Spontaneous recovery from leukopenia was seen in most cases and only in some cases was the administration of cortisone and/or blood transfusion necessary. Only a few patients received antibiotics and γ-globulin prophylactically. It seems important that the occurrence of leukopenia during one treatment period is often followed by normal acceptance of the same treatment given later (Fig. 1). Chemotherapy was always begun and administered according to the protocol in hospital after operation. Continuation of this intermittent chemotherapy was followed much more rigorously by those patients living in the city of Vienna than those living outside Vienna, as already mentioned above. The crude survival rate of the patients is calculated according to the life table method. The number of patients at the time of operation, 36 and 60 months thereafter, represents the number of the patients at risk at this given time. The survival rates of patients with combined treatment and those of the control patients are subdivided into TNM stages A, B, and C (Fig. 2). The steepness of the curves in Fig. 2 demonstrates that the prognosis worsens with advancing TNM stage. These findings permit no significant statistical difference but do support a passing tendency of improvement in some of these patients.

Figure 3 shows the survival curves of the groups of the same patients, subdivided into Feinstein categories. On the left side the patients with Feinstein 2 or 4 (i.e., that of patients with slow growing tumors) are depicted; the therapy administered seems to decrease the survival rate of the treated group. On the right side the group of patients with Feinstein 3 or 5

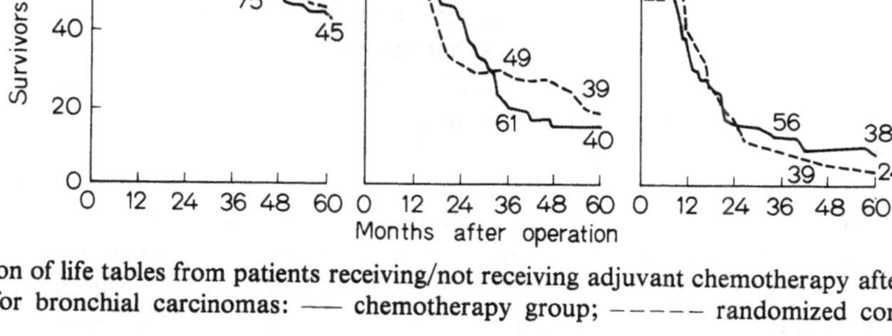

Fig. 2. Comparison of life tables from patients receiving/not receiving adjuvant chemotherapy after radical surgery for bronchial carcinomas: —— chemotherapy group; ----- randomized controls

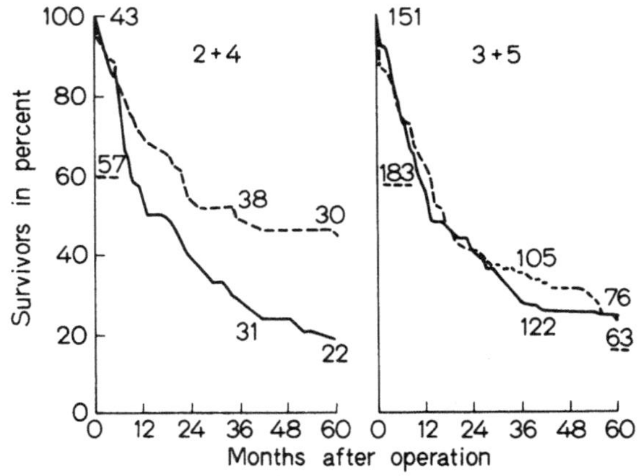

Fig. 3. Comparison of life tables from patients receiving/not receiving adjuvant chemotherapy after radical surgery for bronchial carcinomas. Feinstein classification 2 + 4 and 3 + 5: —— chemotherapy group; ---- randomized controls

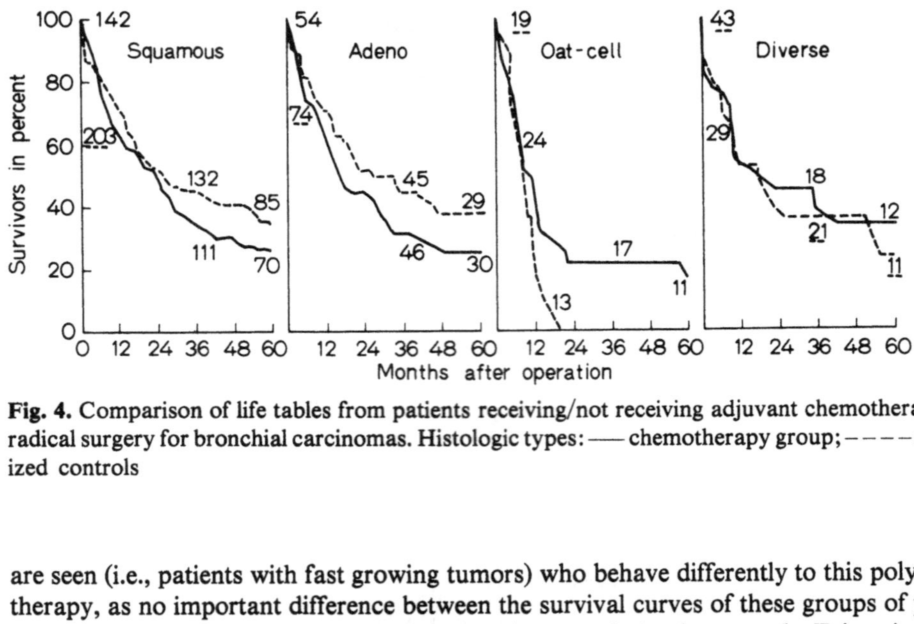

Fig. 4. Comparison of life tables from patients receiving/not receiving adjuvant chemotherapy after radical surgery for bronchial carcinomas. Histologic types: —— chemotherapy group; ---- randomized controls

are seen (i.e., patients with fast growing tumors) who behave differently to this polychemotherapy, as no important difference between the survival curves of these groups of patients can be observed. This demonstrates that there is a correlation between the Feinstein categories and differences in prognosis and in sensitivity to the chemotherapy given. The slower growing tumors have a better prognosis than the faster growing tumors. However, the sensitivity to the chemotherapy used shows the opposite.

Figure 4 demonstrates the different effectiveness of this adjuvant chemotherapy on the patients of histologically different groups without regard to TNM staging or Feinstein categories. Figure 5 depicts the life table curves of the selected patients in Feinstein categories 3 and 5, subdivided into TNM stages I, II, and III + IV. Within the subgroups demonstrated in Fig. 5, a tendency for the treatment to be beneficial can be seen in stages I and II.

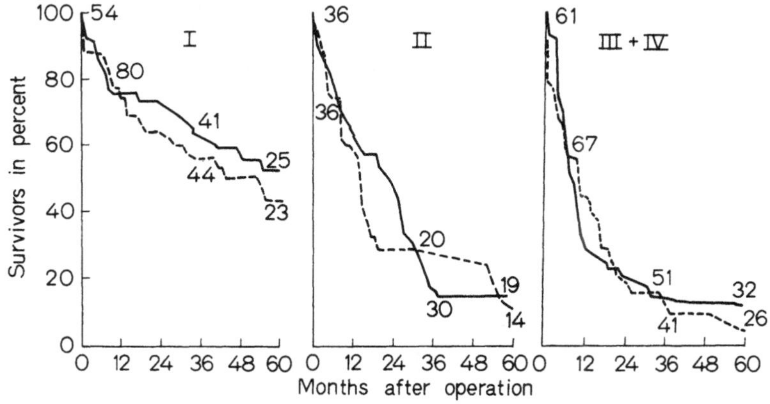

Fig. 5. Comparison of life tables from patients receiving/not receiving adjuvant chemotherapy after radical surgery for bronchial carcinomas. Feinstein categories 3 + 5, subdivided into TNM stages: —— chemotherapy group; – – – – – randomized controls

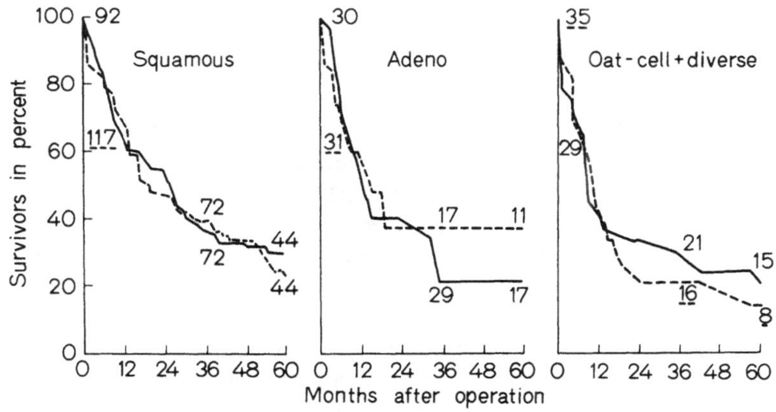

Fig. 6. Comparison of life tables from patients receiving/not receiving adjuvant chemotherapy after radical surgery for bronchial carcinomas. Feinstein categories 3 + 5, subdivided into histologic types: —— chemotherapy group; – – – – – randomized controls

Figure 6 shows the same patients as in Fig. 5, but subdivided into the three histologic main groups.

It is of interest that there seems to be a positive tendency, even in the groups with squamous cell carcinoma. The subdivision of the squamous cell carcinoma by degree of histologic differentiation expressed by the presence or absence of keratinization results in an apparent difference between these two groups. The group with keratinization shows a more favorable prognosis, whereas it shows a lower sensitivity to the chemotherapy used. The recent evaluation of this adjuvant chemotherapy as of 1 January, 1978 confirms the results of the preliminary evaluation as of 1 January, 1977 [25], which led us (DENCK, PRIDUN) to the decision to change the protocol used since autumn 1969 and to divide the patients after radical operation before the adjuvant therapy according to the histologic classification.

Table 3. Bronchogenic carcinomas "radically" operated for cure

Histologic		
Squam, adeno, or large cell		Small or div. cell
TNM		
I, II	III, IV	I–IV
Randomized		
At Lausanne for Ludwig Trial using coryneb. parv i. pleur.	At Vienna for pilot studies with diff. immunother.	At Vienna for polychemoth. + local X-ray treat.

The patients with bronchogenic squamous, adenocarcinoma, or large cell tumors with TNM stages I or II are going to be treated within the framework of the international Ludwig Lung Cancer Study Group [30] intrapleurally with a preparation of corynebacterium parvum for nonspecific immunostimulation. Since the start in July 1977, about 300 of these selected patients have already been randomized in this study. Four hundred can be expected by fall of 1978, so that with 1 more year of observation time, at the end of 1979, the first results about changes in the duration of the disease-free interval would be available. Patients with tumors of equal histologic types but with TNM stages III or IV are going to be treated within pilot studies of different types of immunotherapies.

For patients with small-cell-type tumors – who are also receiving surgery according to the Viennese School of Surgery – and with all other different histologic types of bronchogenic carcinomas, we are using polychemotherapies and local X-ray treatment.

This decision was based on the observed differences of the treatment efficacy in patients with various biologically different tumor types, as seen in the evaluations of the high-dosed intermittent four-drug- polychemotherapy. This preliminary evaluation of combined modality treatment certainly encourages the continuation of these kinds of studies. Considering the variety of prognostic factors and types of tumors involved, including differences in the sensitivity to a given drug combination and/or dose, it might become necessary and/or advantageous to select various other therapeutic agents that act as specifically as possible on the different kinds of tumors. The results shown seem to support the hypothesis that the dose schedule used was not adequate for slow growing tumors and for squamous cell and adenocarcinoma.

Therefore, it seems advantageous to change the dose schedule or the combination of drugs used for the adjuvant treatment for this group of tumors. This does not necessarily mean that the dose used is optimal for faster growing tumors.

With the improvements in early diagnosis, the resectability rate is likely to be increased and the proportion of patients requiring effective adjuvant treatment will be greater. Seventy-five percent of patients with surgically resectable tumors still die of recurrent disease. It is precisely in this potentially curable group that adjunctive chemotherapy would be expected to be most effective. The reviewed previous studies should be used as a guide for further activity that would be expected to be beneficial, when available chemotherapeutic agents are used optimally in the adjuvant situation.

Notwithstanding reservations on the degree of effectiveness of chemotherapeutic agents in advanced lung cancers, further study of single agents alone or combined with immunotherapy appears urgent. At present the evidence of benefit from combination chemotherapy in advanced lung cancers is not impressive in terms of survival gain. In evolving strategy for adjuvant studies, it would appear most reasonable for now to evaluate the effectiveness of additional single agents. In addition, every effort should be made to evaluate new combinations of chemotherapeutic agents to find better activity in advanced disease and then move these combinations into adjuvant treatment. However, all therapeutic modalities, including single agent or combination chemotherapy and immunotherapy must be introduced in well-designed, controlled clinical studies. To overcome difficulties already observed, adequately large international cooperative studies are preferable. Such studies could provide the information needed to substantially improve the treatment of lung cancers.

References

1. Adelberger, L., Wörn, H.: Erfahrungen und Aussichten der kombinierten chirurgisch-zytostatischen Behandlung des Bronchialkarzinoms. Mitteilungsdienst der Ges. z. Bekämpf. d. Krebskrankh. *2,* 521 (1962)
2. Arnal, M. L., Dold, U., Ehlers, C. Th., Gögler, E., Hamperl, H., Karrer, K., Oberhofer, G., Ott, G., Pascher, W., Proppe, A., Scheibe, O., Schmolling, E., Spiessl, B., Thurmayer, R., Wildner, E. P.: Zur Klassifizierung der Geschwulstkrankheiten. Der „gesicherte" TNM-Schlüssel (Erweiterungsvorschlag zu den „General Rules" der UICC). Methods Inf. Med. **6,** 70 (1967)
3. Axtell, L. M., Asire, A. J., Myers, M. H.: Cancer patient survival *5.* DHEW Publication no. (NIH) 77-992. Washington, D. C.: U.S. Government Printing Office 1976
4. Brunner, K. W., Marthaler, Th., Müller, W.: Unfavourable effects of long-term adjuvant chemotherapy with Endoxan in radically operated bronchogenic carcinoma. Eur. J. Cancer *7,* 285 (1971)
5. Buyze, E. A. C., Nelemans, F. A.: A study of postoperative cytostatic medication in patients with operable carcinoma of the lung. Arzneim. Forsch. *23,* 860 (1973)
6. Crosbie, W. A., Candar, H. H., Belcher, J. R.: A control trial of vinblastine sulfate in the treatment of carcinoma of the lung. Br. J. Dis. Chest *60,* 28–35 (1966)
7. Cutler, S. J., Young, J. L.: Third National Cancer Survey: Indicence Data. Washington, D. C.: U.S. Government Printing Office 1975
8. Denk, W., Karrer, K.: Modellversuch einer Rezidivprophylaxe des Karzinoms. Wiener Klin. Wochenschr. *67,* 986 (1955)
9. Feinstein, A. R.: Symptomatic patterns, biologic behavior and prognosis in cancer of the lung. Ann. Intern. Med. *61,* 27 (1964)
10. Fisher, R. A.: Fishers exakter Vierfeldertest. In: Statistische Auswertungsmethoden. Sachs, L. (ed.), p. 365. Berlin, Heidelberg, New York: Springer 1969
11. Friedl, H. P., Karrer, K., Kühböck, J.: The relation of tumour size to the results of chemotherapy in malignant tumours. Eur. J. Clin. Biol. Res. *16,* 268–272 (1971)
12. Friedl, H. P., Karrer, K.: Adjuvant Chemotherapy on Metastasizing Experimental Tumors. Proc. VIIth Int. Congr. Chemotherapy, Prague: Advances in Antimicrobial and Antineoplastic Chemotherapy. Hejzlar, M. (ed.), pp. 285–286. München, Berlin, Wien: Urban & Schwarzenberg 1972

13. Higgins, G. A. (Jr.): Use of Chemotherapy as an Adjuvant to Surgery for Bronchogenic Carcinoma. Cancer *30,* 1383–1387 (1972)
14. Humphreys, S. R., DeWys, W. D., Karrer, K.: A model System for the Selection of Drugs for Chemotherapy of Metastasis. Proc. 5th Int. Congr. Chemotherapy, Vienna, June 26–July 1, B 9/17 1967
15. Humphreys, S. R., Karrer, K.: Relationship of dose schedules to the effectiveness of adjuvant chemotherapy. Cancer Chemother. Rep. *54,* 379–392 (1970)
16. Karrer, K., Humphreys, S. R., Goldin, A.: Relationship of drug toxicity to chemotherapeutic effektiveness. Antimicrob. Agents Chemother. 539–543 (1965)
17. Karrer, K.: Experimentelle Studien zum Problem der Tumormetastasierung I bis III. Klin. Med. *20,* 313 (1965)
18. Karrer, K., Humphreys, S. R., Goldin, A.: Ein neues experimentelles Modell zum Studium der Beeinflußbarkeit der Metastasierung maligner Tumoren. Krebsforsch. Krebsbek. *6,* 166–169 (1967)
19. Karrer, K., Humphreys, S. R., Goldin, A.: An experimental model for studying factors which influence metastases of malignant tumours. Int. J. Cancer *2,* 213–223 (1967)
20. Karrer, K., Humphreys, S. R.: Continuous and limited Courses of Cyclophosphamide (NSC-26271) in Mice with pulmonary Metastasis after Surgery. Cancer Treat. Rep. *51,* 439–449 (1967)
21. Karrer, K., Denck, H.: Weitere Vorschläge zur chemotherapeutischen Rezidivprophylaxe des Bronchuskarzinoms. Wiener Med. Wochenschr. *121,* 112–120 (1971)
22. Karrer, K.: Relations of dose schedules of adjuvant chemotherapy in experimental systems and in clinical trials. Poc. VIIth Int. Congr. Chemotherapy, Prague: Advances in Antimicrobial and Antineoplastic Chemotherapy. Hejzlar, M. (ed.), pp. 765–768. München, Berlin, Wien: Urban & Schwarzenberg 1972
23. Karrer, K.: Surgical adjuvant therapy. Proceedings of the XIth International Cancer Congress, Florence 1974. Excerpta Medica Int. Congr. Series No. 353, *5,* 68–73 (1974)
24. Karrer, K., Pridun, N., Denck, H., Sighart, H.: Polychemotherapie bei Patienten nach radikaler Operation wegen Bronchus-Karzinom. Österr. Z. Onkologie *3,* 127–141 (1976)
25. Karrer, K., Pridun, N., Denck, H.: Chemotherapy as an adjuvant to surgery in lung cancer. Cancer Chemother. Pharmacol. (in press) (1978)
26. Katsuki, H., Shimada, K. et al.: Long-term intermittent adjuvant chemotherapy for primary, resected lung cancer. J. Thorac. and Cardiovasc. Surg. *70,* 590 (1975)
27. Kreyberg, L., Libow, A. A., Uehlinger, E. A. W.: International histological classification of tumors. 1. Histological typing of lung tumors. Geneva: WHO 1967
28. Legha, S. S., Muggia, F. M., Carter, S. K.: Adjuvant chemotherapy in lung cancer. Cancer *39,* 1415–1424 (1977)
29. Livingston, R. B.: Combined modality approaches in lung cancer. In: Adjuvant therapy of cancer. Salmon, S. E. (ed.), pp. 191–205. Amsterdam, Oxford, New York: North-Holland 1977
30. Ludwig Lung Cancer Study Group: Search for the possible Role of "Immunotherapy" in operable Bronchial non-small Cell Carcinoma (Stage I and II): A Phase I Study with Corynebacterium parvum Intrapleurally. Cancer Immunol. Immunother. (in press) (1978)
31. Mayo, J. A., Laster, W. R. (Jr.), Andrews, C. M., Schabel, F. M. (Jr.): Success and failure in the treatment of solid tumors – III "Cure" of metastatic Lewis lung carcinoma with methyl-CCNU and surgery-chemotherapy. Cancer Treat. Rep. *56,* 183–195 (1972)
32. Miller, A. B.: (A medical Research Council Working Party) Study of cytotoxic chemotherapy as an adjuvant to surgery in carcinoma of the bronchus. Br. Med. J. *1972/II,* 421–428
33. Mountain, C. F.: The surgeon's viewpoint on collaborative research on lung cancer. Cancer Treat. Rep. *4,* 307–309 (1973)
34. Overholt, R. H., Oliynyk, Cady, B.: The current status of primary cancer of the lung.
35. Overholt, R. H., Neptune, W. B., Ashraf, M. M.: Primary cancer of the lung. Ann. Thorac. Surg. *20,* 511–519 (1975)

36. Pavlov, A., Pirogov, A., Trachtenberg, A., Volkova, M., Maximov, T., Matveeva, T.: Results of combination treatment of lung cancer patients: surgery plus radiotherapy and surgery plus chemotherapy. Cancer Treat. Rep. *4,* 133 (1973)
37. Perloff, M., Holland, J. F.: Surgical adjuvant chemotherapy. Ann. Rev. Med. *28,* 475–488 (1977)
38. Pfeiffer, K. M., Middendorp, U. G., Marthaler, Th.: Cytostatische Rezidivprophylaxe operierter maligner Tumoren. Schweiz. Med. Wochenschr. *96,* 903 (1966)
39. Poulsen, O.: Prae- und postoperative cytostatische Behandlung von Lungencarcinomen mit Cyclophosphamid. Arzneim. Forsch. *11,* 238 (1961)
40. Scadding, J. G.: Study of cytotoxic chemotherapy as an adjuvant to surgery in carcinoma of the bronchus. Br. Med. J. *1971/II,* 421
41. Schabel, F. M., (Jr.): Experimental basis for adjuvant chemotherapy. In: Adjuvant therapy of cancer. Salmon, S. E. (ed.), pp. 3–14. Amsterdam, Oxford, New York: North-Holland 1977
42. Schottenfeld, D., Houde, R. W.: The changing pattern of cancer morbidity and mortality and its implications. Med. Clin. North Am. *50,* 613 (1966)
43. Segi, M., Kurihara, M.: Cancer mortality for selected sites in 24 countries. No. 6 (1966/67), Jpn. Cancer Soc. 110 (1972)
44. Shields, T. W., Robinette, C. D., Keehn, R. J.: Bronchial carcinoma treated by adjuvant cancer chemotherapy. Arch. Surg. *109,* 329–333 (1974)
45. Slack, N. H.: Bronchogenic carcinoma: nitrogen mustard as a surgical adjuvant and factors influencing survival. Cancer *25,* 987 (1970)
46. Vincent, R. G., Takita, H., Lane, W. W., Gutierrez, A. C., Pickren, J. W.: Surgical therapy of lung cancer. J. Thorac. Cardiovasc. Surg. *71,* 581–591 (1976)
47. Wilcoxon, F., Mann, H. B., Whitney, D. R.: U-Test. In: Statistische Auswertungsmethoden. Sachs, L. (ed.), p. 293. Berlin, Heidelberg, New York: Springer 1969
48. Wingfield, H. V.: Combined surgery and chemotherapy for carcinoma of the bronchus. Lancet *1970/I,* 470–471
49. Wurnig, P., Scheuba, G., Karrer, K.: Vorläufige Ergebnisse der chemotherapeutischen Rezidivprophylaxe mit Mitomen beim operierten Bronchuscarcinom. Acta Union Internationale Contre le Cancer, XVI, 935–936, 1960

Attempt at Immunotherapy With Living BCG in Patients With Bronchus Carcinoma

P. Pouillart, T. Palangie, P. Huguenin, P. Morin, H. Gautier, A. Baron, and G. Mathé

Introduction

Squamous cell carcinoma of the bronchus still appears to be one of the most lethal of all malignancies. Under actual therapeutic conditions cure can be anticipated only when complete surgical resection is possible. Bronchogenic carcinoma responds poorly to chemotherapy [2, 5, 10] and in some trials no beneficial effect of systematic application of a "preventive" chemotherapy protocol after surgery was found [1]. Radiotherapy appears generally ineffective [3, 9], but recent results have demonstrated that it can increase the median survival when applied after surgery in patients with lymph node involvement.
In 1973, we drew attention to the prognostic significance of responses of skin tests to recall antigens in patients with resected non-oat-cell bronchus carcinomas [4]. In patients with more advanced disease, similar prognostic significance of immunologic status was found [7]. Another trial demonstrated that applications of BCG three times a week for 3 weeks could induce a conversion of skin test reactivity to recall antigens. A significant correlation was observed between conversion of skin reactivity and prognosis [8]. The aim of the present trial was to study the therapeutic effect of immunotherapy with living BCG applied after surgical resection of squamous cell carcinoma of the lung.

Patients and Methods

The trial began in June 1973; 55 patients entered this trial after surgical resection of a squamous cell carcinoma of the bronchus. Patients were selected at random for the group to be submitted to BCG applications (28 patients) and no further treatment after surgery (27 patients). The distribution according to age and sex is shown in Fig. 1. We classed 12 patients in the BCG group and 13 in the control group as stage I and 16 patients in the BCG group and 14 in the control group as stage II (Table 1). The 28 patients submitted to immunotherapy received weekly applications of Pasteur Institute living BCG (75 mg) on a scarified area of 20 cm^2 on the proximal portion of one of the limbs. This immunotherapy was given for 18 months.

Survey of the Patients

The condition of the patients was monitored in three ways: clinically, radiologically, and immunologically. Clinical examination of the patients was systematically repeated monthly and routine radiologic survey of the lungs was also obtained. A fibroscopic examination was repeated every 4 months. Radioisotopic scanning of the bones, of the brain, and of the liver

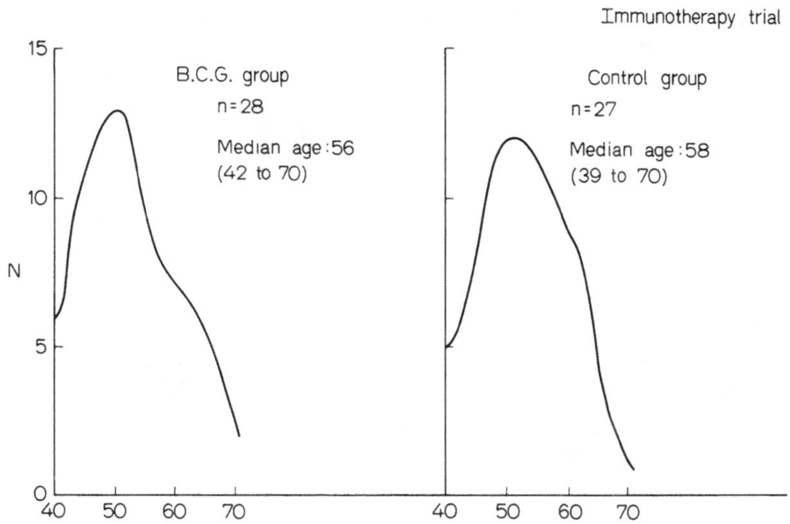

Fig. 1. Distribution of patients according to age. Only one woman entered this trial and was randomly allocated to BCG group

Table 1. Distribution of patients according to anatomic staging

	BCG	Control
Stage I	12	13
Stage II	16	14
Total	28	27

were repeated every 6 months or whenever any suspicious symptoms developed. During evolution, the delayed skin hypersensitivity to recall antigens was checked every 2 months for 6 months and then every 4 months for 2 years. Finally, the average survival time of both groups of patients was studied and presented actuarially.

Results

The application of BCG was well tolerated. Some patients manifested fever for 12 h after applications of BCG. No other complications were observed in this group of patients. In the group of patients treated with BCG 11 patients of 28 (39.2%) died of their tumor and 15 of 28 (53.5%) relapsed. In the control group, 15 of 27 died (55.5%) and 19 of 27 relapsed (70.3%) (Table 2).

Comparison of the actuarial survival curves (Fig. 2) shows a significant difference between the two groups at 24 and 30 months, but this difference disappears at 42 months. If we consider only the shapes of the actuarial curves of remission, there is no difference at any time between the groups of treatment (Fig. 3).

Table 2. Situation of the total population of patients entered in the immunotherapy trial

	Patients receiving BCG	Controls
Number of patients	28	27
Median time since entering trial	40 months	44 months
Number of patients in relapse	15/28 (53.5%)	19/27 (70.3%)
Number of patients who died of tumor	11/28 (39.2%)	15/27 (55.5%)
Number of patients who died of other disease	1	2

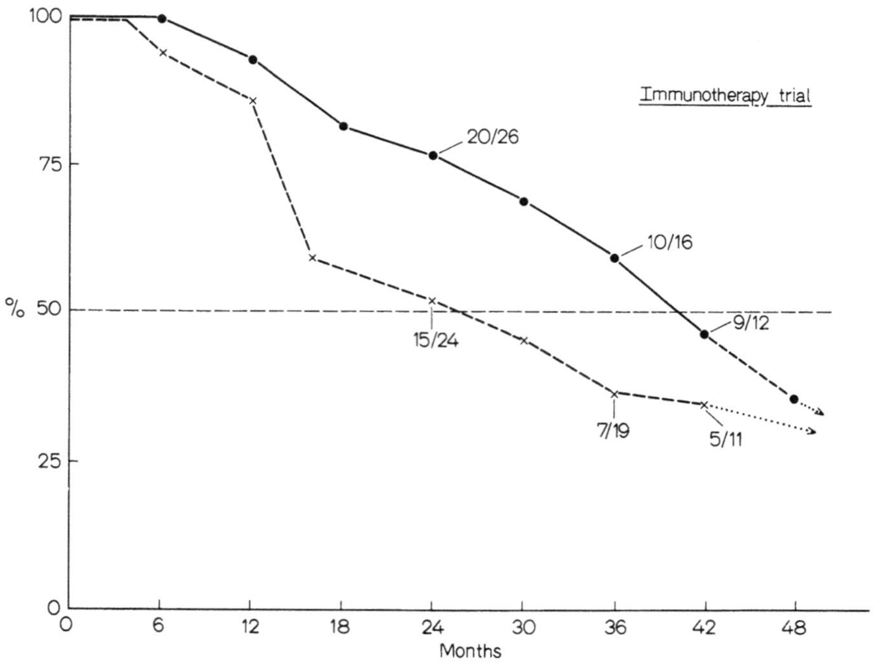

Fig. 2. Actuarial survival curves of two groups of patients. ●——●: BCG group; ×- - - -×: control group

The chance of surviving for 30 months is 68% in the immunotherapy group, and only 45% in the non-treated group. However, in the BCG group, 49% of the patients are alive and free of disease against 38% at the same time in the control group. The actuarial remission curves and actuarial survival curves appear more nearly parallel in the control group than in the BCG

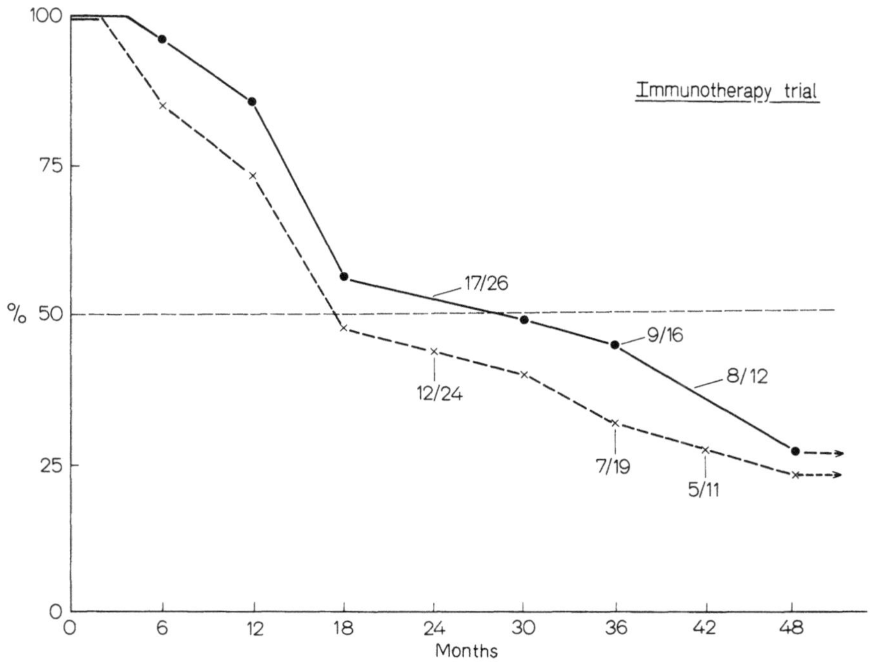

Fig. 3. Actuarial remission curves of two groups of patients. ●——●: BCG group ($n = 28$); ×- - - -×: control group ($n = 27$)

Table 3. Mean interval between relapse and death

	BCG group	Control group
Number of patients	28	27
Number of patients in relapse	15	19[a]
Mean interval between first manifestation of relapse and death[b]	6.6 months	4.5 months

[a] One patient appears free of disease more than 36 months after ralapse.
[b] After relapse, the patients were started on a chemoimmunotherapy protocol of treatment.

group (Figs. 4 and 5). A possible explanation is provided by the different intervals of time observed between relapse and death in the different treatment groups (Table 3).
The distribution of patients according to stage I or II shows that the survival rate is significantly higher for stage I patients under immunotherapy than for control patients. But we have observed no difference in survival between the two groups in stage II patients (Figs. 6 and 7).

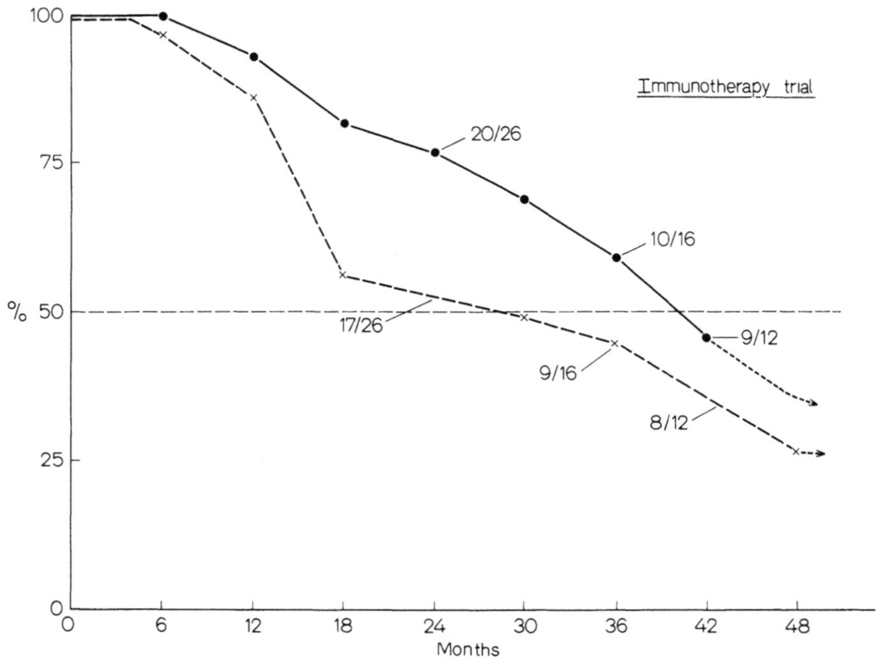

Fig. 4. Actuarial survival curve and actuarial remission curve of BCG group. ●——●: suvival curve; x- - - -x: remission curve

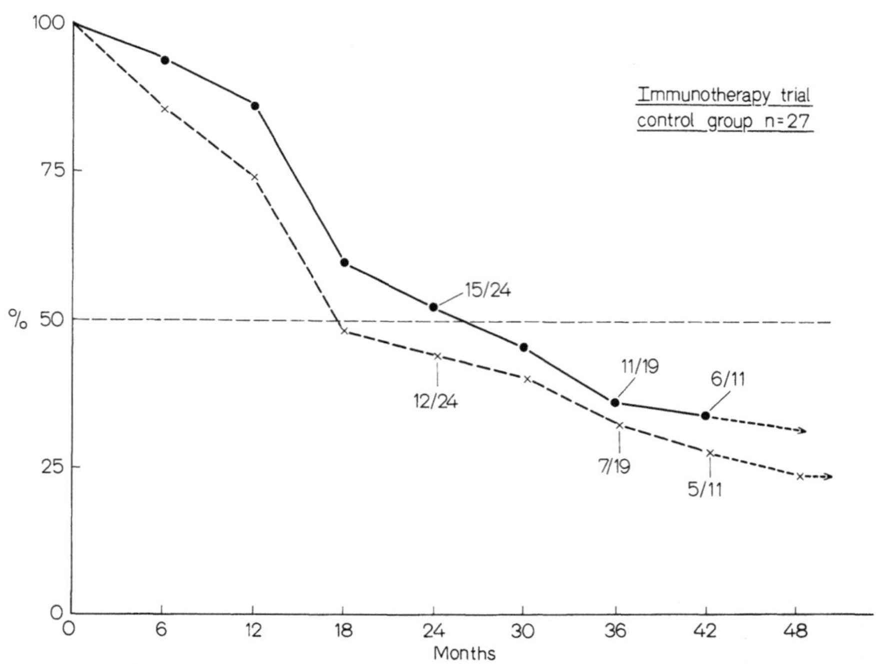

Fig. 5. Actuarial survival curve and actuarial remission curve of control group. ●——●: survival curve; x- - - -x: remission curve

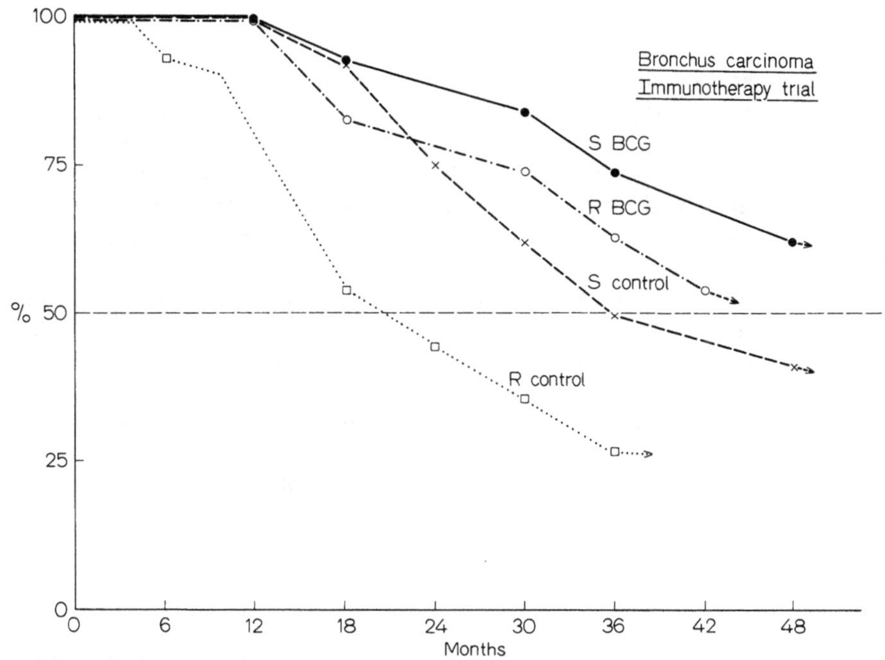

Fig. 6. Actuarial survival curve and actuarial remission curve of stage I patients. ●——●: survival, BCG group; ×- - - -×: survival, control group; ○–·–·–○: remission, BCG group; ○– – – –○: remission, control group

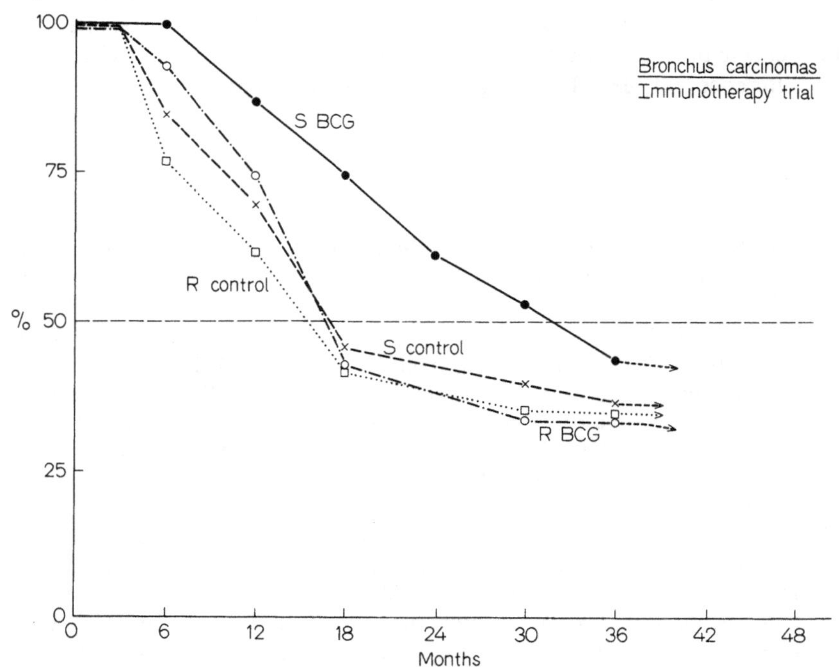

Fig. 7. Actuarial survival curve and actuarial remission curve of stage II patients. ●——●: survival, BCG group; ×- - - -×: survival, control group; ○–·–·–○: remission, BCG group; ○– – – –○: remission, control group

Discussion

Radical surgery remains the only effective means of treatment for patients with squamous cell carcinoma of the bronchus. However, the small percentage of patients apparently cured 5 years after satisfactory surgery encourages one to investigate complementary therapeutic means liable to improve results already obtained. In this trial we have studied in two randomized groups of patients the role of BCG applied systematically and regularly after surgery. The chance of survival is significantly higher at 30 months for the treated group than for the control group, but this difference disappears at 42 months.

Comparison of stage I and stage II patients shows a significant difference in survival at 42 months for patients treated with BCG, but no difference is observed at any time for stage II patients. These results confirm once again the efficacy of BCG in cases where the tumor mass has been reduced as much as possible [6].

The immunotherapy study is continuing along different lines and the aim now is to compare BCG with other systematic adjuvant immunotherapy. With improved results, immunotherapy would rapidly be made part of the prescribed routine for the treatment of patients suffering from epidermal bronchial cancers.

Conclusion

After surgery, 55 patients with resectable squamous cell carcinoma of the bronchus were randomized to two treatment groups: 28 patients received weekly applications of BCG, 27 patients were considered as the control group and received no further treatment. The comparison of the survival curves obtained showed that BCG appears effective only for stage I patients and the difference from the control group is significant at 42 months. We observed no difference between the two groups for stage II patients.

References

1. Brunner, K. W., Marthaler, T. H., Muller, W.: Unfavorable effects of long terme adjuvant chemotherapy with endoxan in radically operated bronchogenic carcinoma. Eur. J. Cancer *7*, 285 (1971)
2. Edmonson, E. J., Lagalos, St., Stolbach, L., Perlia, Ch. P., Bennett, J. M., Mansour, E. G., Horton, J., Regelson, W., Commings, F. J., Israel, L., Brodsky, I., Smider, B. T., Creech, R., Carbone, P. P.: Mechlorethamine (NSC 762) plus CCNU (NSC 79037) in the treatment of inoperable squamous and large cell carcinoma of the lung. Cancer Treat. Rep. *60*, 625–627 (1976)
3. Hansen, H. H., Muggia, F. M., Andrews, R., Selawry, O. S.: Intensive combined chemotherapy and radiotherapy in patients with non resectable bronchogenic carcinoma. Cancer *30*, 315–324 (1972)
4. Israel, L., Mugica, J., Chahinian, P.: Prognosis of early bronchogenic carcinoma. Survival curves of 451 patients after resection of lung cancer in relation to the results of pre-operative tuberculin skin tests. Biomedicine *19*, 68–72 (1973)
5. Linvingston, R. B., Fee, W. H., Einhorn, L. H., Burgess, M. A., Freireich, E. J., Gottlieb, J. A., Farber, M. O.: B.A.C.O.N. (bleomycin, adriamycin, CCNU, oncovin and nitrogen-mustard) in squamous lung cancer. Experience in fifty patients. Cancer *37*, 1237–1242 (1976)
6. Mathé, G., Pouillart, P., Lapeyraque, F.: Active immunotherapy of L1210 leukemia applied after the graft of tumor cell. Br. J. Cancer *23*, 814 (1969)

7. Pouillart, P., Botto, G., Gautier, H., Huguenin, P., Baron, A., Laparre, C., Hoang Thi, H. T., Parrot, R., Mathé, L. G.: Relation entre l'état immunitaire et la réponse à la chimiothérapie. Résultats chez 64 malades avec cancers bronchiques épidermoïdes inopérables. Nouv. Presse Méd. *5,* 1037 (1976)
8. Pouillart, P., Palangie, T., Huguenin, P., Morin, P., Gautier, H., Baron, A., Mathé, G., Lededente, A., Botto, G.: Cancers épidermoïdes bronchiques inopérables. Etude de la signification pronostique de l'état immunitaire et résultats d'un essai d'immunorestauration par le B.C.G. Nouv. Presse Méd. *7,* 265–269 (1978)
9. Roswitt, B., Patno, M. E., Rapp, R., Veinberg, A., Feder, B., Stuhlbarg, J., Reid, C. B.: The survival of patients with inoperable lung cancer: large scale randomized study of radiation therapy versus placebo. Radiology *90,* 668–671 (1968)
10. Vincent, R. G., Pickren, J. W., Fergen, T. B., Takita, H.: Evaluation of methotrexate in the treatment of bronchogenic carcinoma. Cancer *36,* 873–880 (1975)

Adjuvant Therapy With Levamisole in Resectable Lung Cancer

W. K. Amery, J. Cosemans, H. C. Gooszen, E. Lopes Cardozo, A. Louwagie, J. Stam, J. Swierenga, R. G. Vanderschueren, and R. W. Veldhuizen

Introduction

Several controlled studies in lung cancer have evaluated the adjuvant use of cytostatic chemotherapy. The results of these investigations, and particularly of the carefully randomized ones, have been disappointing as they range from a significant difference, to the disadvantage of chemotherapy [4], to some suggestion of benefit only [5]. In view of these data, two different attitudes can be taken in making further efforts to develop an effective adjuvant treatment modality for resectable lung cancer patients who are known to be seriously at risk of relapsing within the first few years after their operation. One research path is to continue using cytostatic chemotherapy but to more carefully select the drug(s) to be used, e.g., by relying on the known effects of these drugs in advanced cancer, and to scrutinize the intensity of the chemotherapeutic regimen to be given [7]. It seems obvious that this is a very delicate task as judged from the limited effectiveness of the wide range of available chemotherapeutic agents in advanced lung cancer, and, also, from the lack of well-established guidelines to choose a therapeutic scheme to be followed in the adjuvant setting. Moreover, if some amount of unexpected, divine intervention fails to occur, we will continuously have to deal with the sometimes very unpleasant side-effects of these drugs, even if such adverse effects may at first glance appear acceptable from the treating oncologist's point of view: he is accustomed indeed to see more severe side-effects from more intensive treatment with the same drugs in patients with advanced malignancies.

Another approach to find effective types of adjuvant treatment in lung cancer is to look for other treatment modalities that are not cytotoxic. Theoretically, immunotherapy is probably the most appealing one. Thousands of articles have been published on the possibilities of clinical immunotherapy in cancer. Sometimes one has the awkward feeling of dealing with two opposing camps in this respect, i.e., the one that considers it too early or meaningless to initiate clinical evaluations of immunotherapy and the other that feels that the time has come to thoroughly evaluate this new therapeutic modality. If such two camps really exist, the authors of this article will in all probability be considered as belonging to the "pro" group, since they have actually become involved in a clinical study of this matter. However, there appears to be very little reason for having two camps if one gives serious consideration to the counterarguments that are presented. One such argument is that we do not yet know exactly how immunotherapy works and that we first ought to know before we give such a treatment to the patients. This looks very much like a perfectionist's attitude. It might well be sound if we were sure that we knew everything about the intricate machinery of the host defense mechanisms; obviously, we are still far from having achieved that goal. Also, such an attitude fails to appreciate the lessons from the history of medicine that show that a lot is still to be learnt empirically, as the mechanism of action of most well-established medicines was found only after they were used in the clinic for a long time. Only one more counterargument will be dealt with here: it is sometimes argued that only very slight effects can be expected from immunotherapy. This point can only be clearly proved or invalidated by carefully conducted

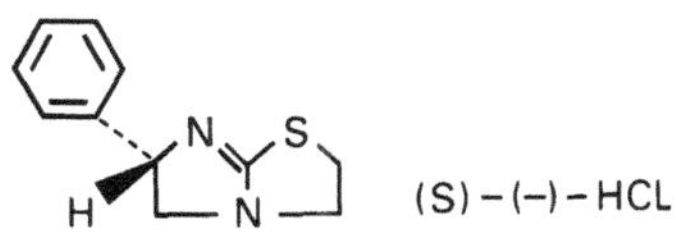

(S)-(-)-2,3,5,6-tetrahydro-6-phenylimidazo [2,1-b] thiazole hydrochloride

Fig. 1. Structural formula of levamisole

clinical trials. Moreover, even if the results of such studies confirmed that prediction, a slight effect obtained in a devastating disease like lung cancer, where adjuvant therapy efforts have failed so far, would be progress (certainly if this effect is not obtained at the cost of substantial toxicity).

For the study reported here, levamisole (Fig. 1) was selected as the immunotherapeutic agent to be used as an adjunct to surgery. This drug is known to behave as an antianergic chemotherapeutic agent that both restores the functions of the cellular compartments of the immune system if these are deficient and has thymomimetic properties [11]. The rationale for using levamisole in this setting has been discussed at more length elsewhere [1, 10] and will, therefore, not be repeated here.

Material and Methods

This study was started during the first half of 1972 and all 211 patients were in the study for at least 2 years, as required by the protocol, by the end of 1977. Ninety-six patients received levamisole and the other 115 a placebo. As reported elsewhere [3], the two medication groups were well comparable as regards sex (96% of the patients were males), age (median = 63 years), weight (median = 72 kg), erythrocyte sedimentation rate (median = 22 mm), skin test reactivity to PPD and to DNCB at the start, daily use of cigarettes, tumor location, type of surgery, largest tumor diameter, regional extent of the cancer, and duration of anesthesia. There was no difference regarding the number of patients with the different histologic types of cancer (63.5% had squamous cell carcinoma), except for adenocarcinoma that was somewhat more frequently found in the control group (15% of the levamisole patients against 26% of the controls: $P = 0.06$, two-tailed chisquare test). When the protocol of this study was prepared, no established TNM classification system of lung cancer was available yet. The preoperative tumor load was assessed by two measures. Firstly, the largest diameter of the tumor (range: 1–15 cm; median 4 cm) was measured after its removal and its fixation by the pathologist. Secondly, a category grouping system, slightly adapted from Slack [9], was used to describe the regional extent of the tumor; within this system, category 1a is the only category where there is no evidence that the tumor could have left or had already left the primary site. Further details about these two assessments are to be found in earlier reports on this study [1, 10]. Randomization, stratified by the three cooperating centers, has been used to assign the patients to double-blind treatment with either levamisole or the placebo. The medication consisted of tablets, containing 50 mg or a placebo, and was separately coded for each participating patient. The treatment was started 3 days before the operation and such 3-days courses were repeated every 2 weeks for 2 years or until relapse was established. A fixed dose, i.e., one tablet t.i.d., was given on the treatment days. Any use of cytostatics, corticosteroids, or irradiation treatment was prohibited as long as no evidence of relapse was found, but appropriate anticancer treatment was obviously permitted in the case of proven recurrence.

Recurrence and carcinomatous or other death rates were calculated by means of the actuarial method using a commonly available computer program [6].

Results

Outcome

If all types of mortality are considered, a significant reduction is found 18 and 21 months after surgery in the patients of the levamisole group. A separate analysis of the cancer death and of the non-tumor deaths shows that this reduction is due to a diminished cancer mortality with levamisole since the other causes of death occurred to a similar extent in the two medication groups (Fig. 2). Similarly, a reduction in the number of tumor recurrences is found in the levamisole patients (not shown).

Since in all previous interim analyses of this study, a substantial group of patients had been found to have been underdosed; recurrence and death rates were reanalyzed with respect to

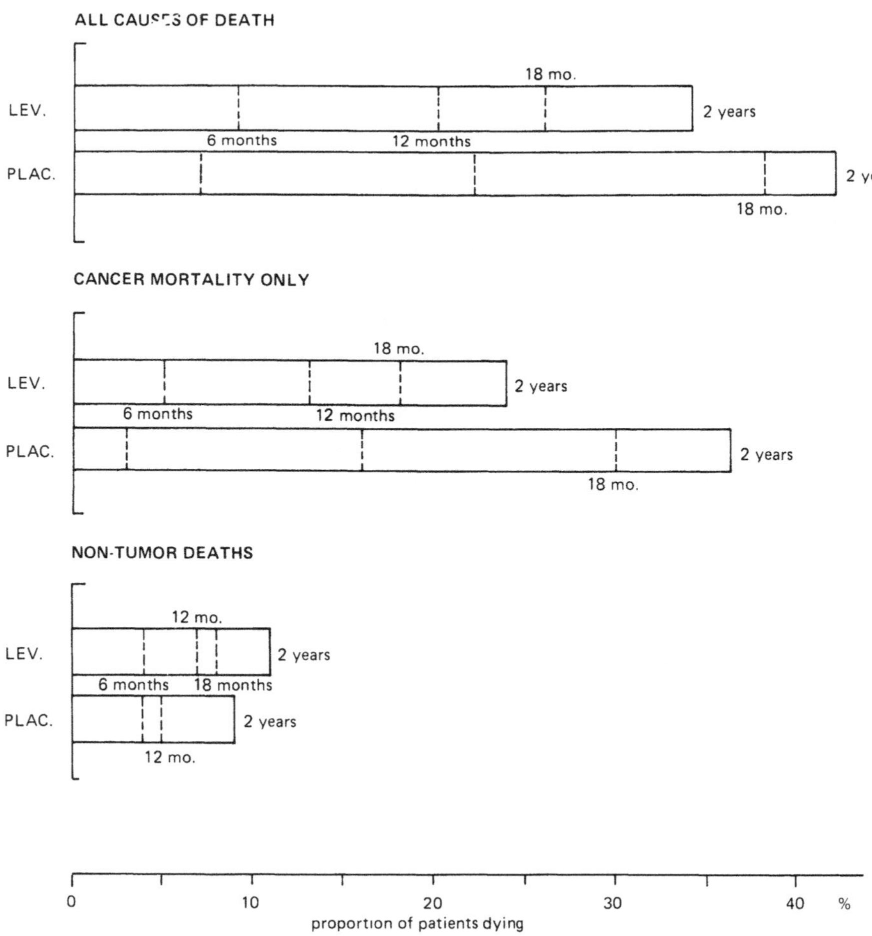

Fig. 2. Death rates (actuarial estimates)

the relative dose (expressed as mg/kg per day) each patient has taken. The details of this analysis are given elsewhere [3]. In each of the treating centers and in the first as well as the second half of the study, those patients whose daily dose was 2.1 mg/kg or less (i.e., those weighing more than 70 kg) did not benefit from the levamisole treatment, whereas a very significant superiority of levamisole to the placebo was evident in the patients who had received the higher daily doses (median: 2.3 mg/kg). This is illustrated in Fig. 3. The

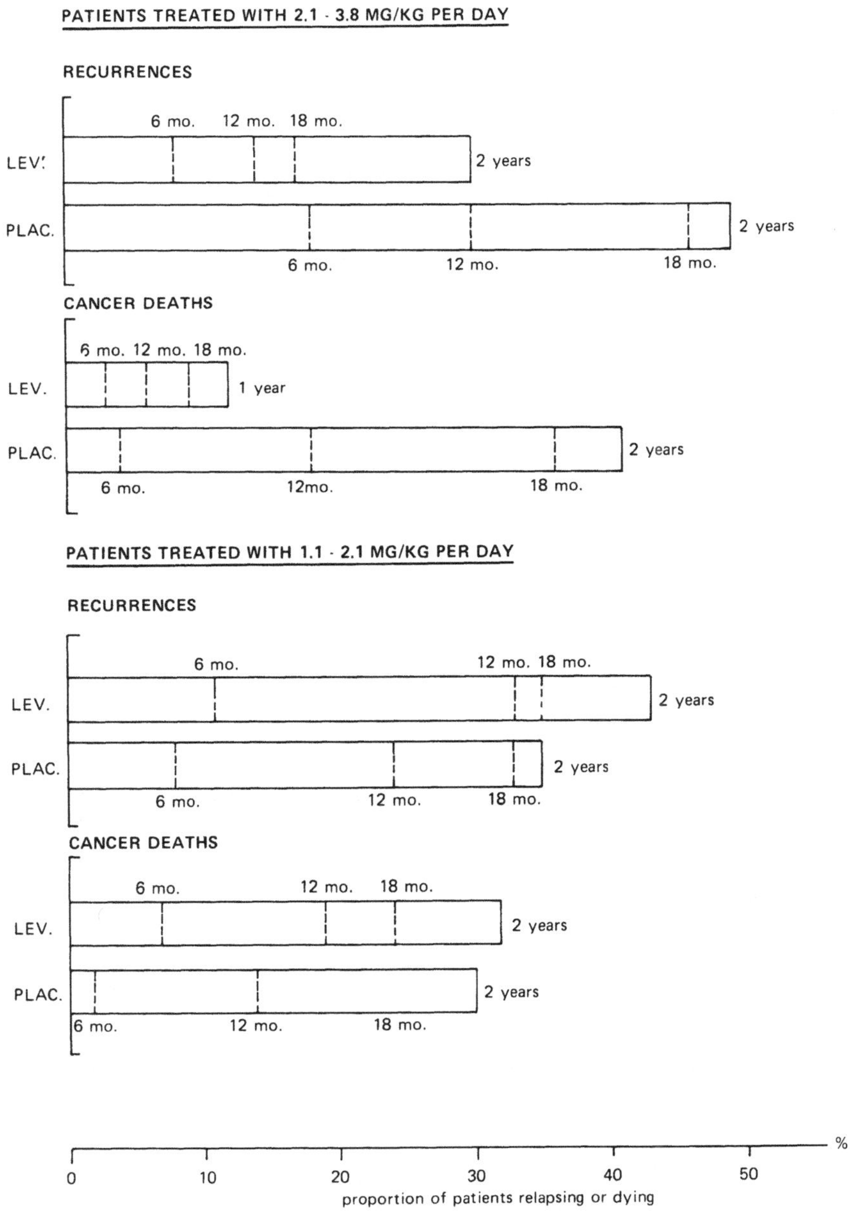

Fig. 3. Recurrence and death rates as related to dose

remainder of the analysis was, therefore, restricted to the latter group, i.e., the group of adequately dosed patients.

It was of interest to see whether the results obtained with levamisole could be predicted from the skin tests obtained at the start of the study. Only the tests with 10 IU of PPD and with 50 μg of DNCB will be discussed here as tests with higher doses of DNCB had only been obtained in a much smaller number of patients. The two tests considered here appear to have some predictive value (DNCB more for early recurrences and PPD more for later recurrences) regarding the risk of recurrence in the control group, but they are not helpful in

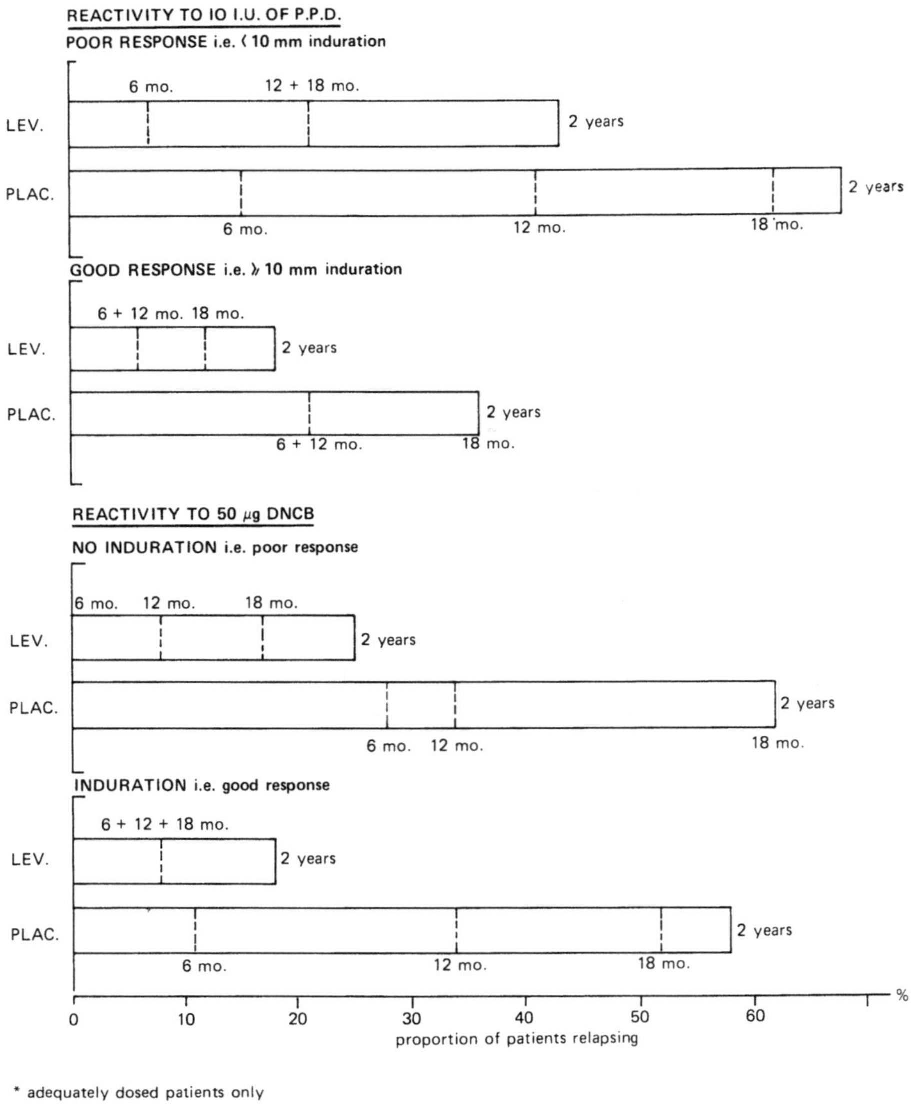

Fig. 4. Recurrence rates (adequately dosed patients only) as related to skin test reactivity at start

predicting an effect of levamisole as fewer recurrences are seen with levamisole both in the well and the poorly responding patients (Fig. 4).
The tumor load seemed to be a somewhat more reliable variable. As expected, more recurrences in the control group were found among those patients who had more advanced disease at the time of surgery. However, levamisole was only slightly superior to the placebo in preventing recurrences in those patients who had small tumors (i.e., 3 cm largest diameter) and almost no difference was found between the two treatments in patients who belonged to the regional grouping category 1a, the prognostically most favorable group. On the other

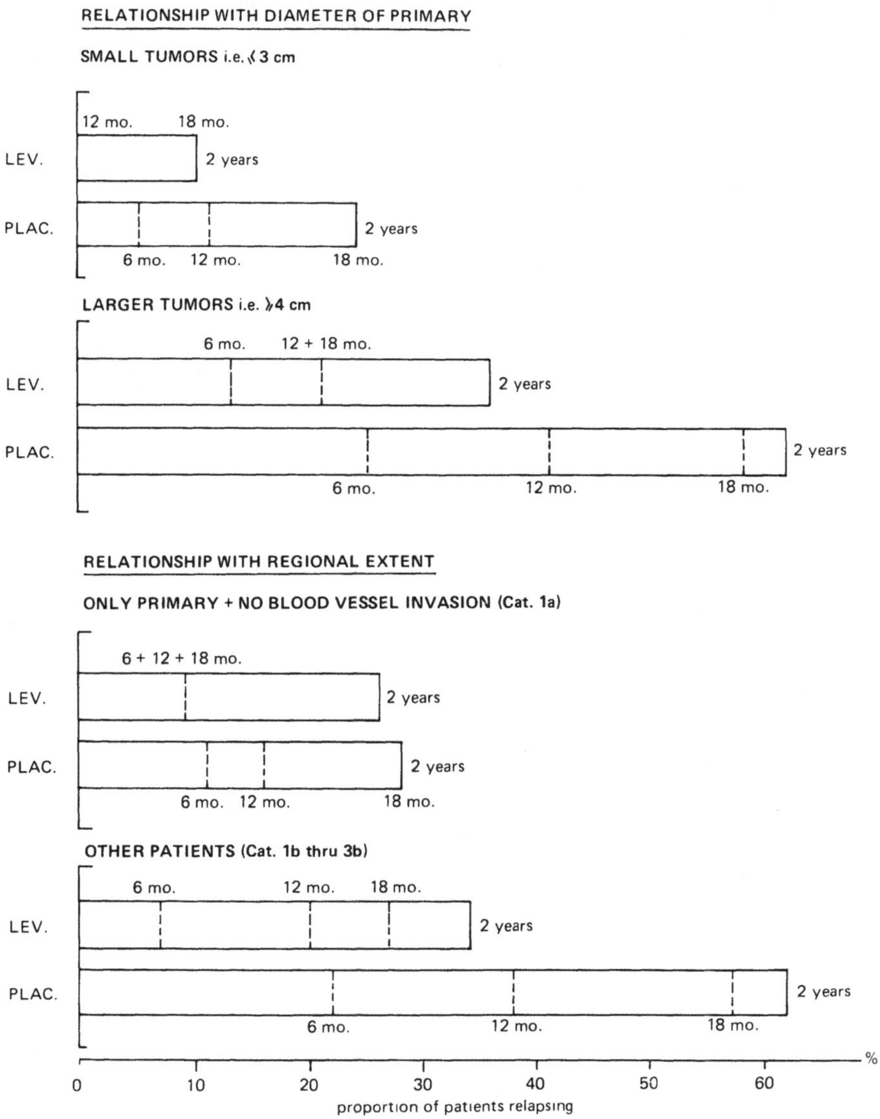

* adequately dosed patients only.

Fig. 5. Recurrence rates (adequately dosed patients only) as related to tumor extent

hand, the beneficial effect observed with levamisole appeared to be primarily due to an ameliorated prognosis in the patients who had more advanced and/or more extended tumors before the operation (Fig. 5).

The recurrence rate observed within the first 2 years in the control group varied from 36% (adenocarcinoma) over 52% (squamous cell carcinoma) to 56% (other + mixed types) of the patients. Levamisole appeared to be significantly superior to the placebo in each of the three histologic subgroups. This is illustrated in Fig. 6; it may be worth noting that the absence of recurrences in the adenocarcinoma patients treated with levamisole should not be taken at face value as the number of such patients was very limited (only five). The more important conclusion from this analysis seems to be that levamisole appears to be helpful whatever the histologic type of the bronchial cancer is and that the relative excess of adenocarcinoma cases in the control group cannot account for the results that have been observed.

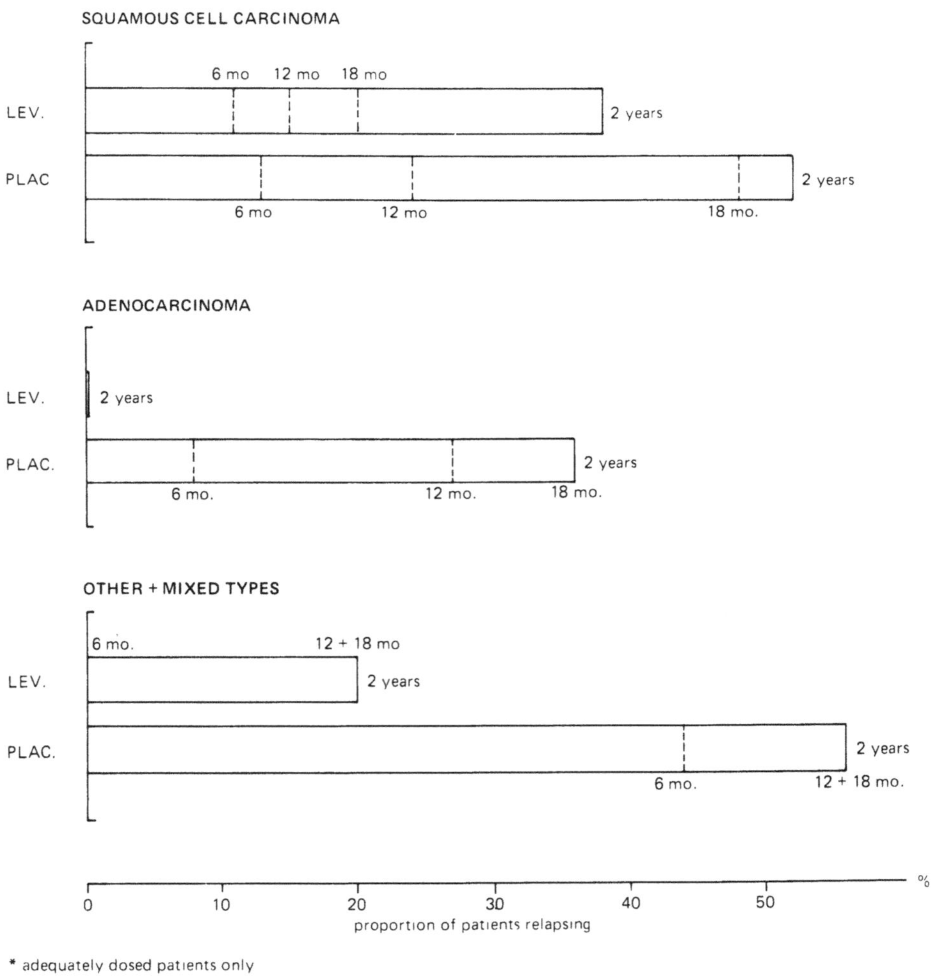

Fig. 6. Recurrence rates (adequately dosed patients only) as related to tumor histology

Table 1. Site of first recurrence[a]

Site of 1st recurrence	No. of patients			
	Levamisole		Placebo	
Intrathoracic				
Same lung	2	5/40 (12.5%)	2	9/52 (17.3%)
Other lung	2		3	
Mediastinum	0		4	
Mediastinal nodes	1		0	
Distant				
Bone	2	5/40 (12.5%)	6	17/52 (32.7%)
Brain	1		6	
Liver	1		4	
Esophagus	1		0	
Kidney	0		1	

[a] Adequately treated patients only (levamisole: No. = 40; placebo: No. = 52).
[b] May also be stem bronchus close to carina after pneumonectomy.

The site of the first recurrence was a final point of interest in this analysis, since there is some indication that levamisole could preferentially inhibit metastasis formation [2]. Again, this aspect was evaluated in the subgroup of adequately dosed patients. The results are given in Table 1. Levamisole may be marginally superior to the placebo in preventing intrathoracic recurrences (which account for only one-third of the relapses in the control group), but significantly less remote recurrences are found in the levamisole group than in the controls.

Safety

As mentioned above, the incidence of non-tumor deaths was not changed by levamisole treatment. Therefore, there seems to be no indication that levamisole could be dangerous if it is used as an adjuvant treatment modality in cancer surgery.

Also regarding side-effects, the incidence in the two groups was not markedly different. Somewhat more patients had gastrointestinal complaints with levamisole (24%) than with the placebo (22%), and these complaints were usually mild in the two groups. Nervousness and/or sleep disorders were somewhat more frequent with levamisole (5% against 2% with the placebo) and the same accounts for allergic side-effects, particularly drug fever and symptoms suggestive of the beginning of influenza; these were reported in 7% of the levamisole patients and only 5% of the placebo controls (the drug was stopped for this reason in 2% of the levamisole patients and 1% of the controls), but no cases of allergic agranulocytosis [8] occurred in this study.

Discussion and Conclusions

Lung cancer is a very difficult disease to treat and, despite carefully planned therapy, most patients die from this malignancy. Only a minority of lung cancer patients are still operable when first diagnosed, and surgery alone is known to fail in a large proportion of them. The slightly ameliorated prognosis after surgery observed during the last decade in such patients is not sufficient reason for much hope either, as it merely reflects the use of more stringent criteria to label a patient as operable. A more efficient treatment for lung cancer is badly needed. As long as no entirely new treatment approaches are detected, our main hope is based on a more efficient use of the available treatment modalities, including immunotherapy. Cure is the ultimate goal of treatment, but if this cannot be obtained, ensuring the prolongation of the patient's life and keeping that life comfortable are worth pursuing. As discussed in the introduction, we have decided to evaluate the potential usefulness of levamisole as an adjunct to surgery in resectable lung cancer patients. It is our conviction that our findings prove that the prognosis of such patients can be ameliorated and that levamisole is an agent that is very well suited for that purpose since it combines efficacy, at least if it is adequately dosed, with a minimum of inconvenience for the patient.

Summary

In view of the discouraging results that have been obtained so far with the use of cytotoxic chemotherapy as an adjunct to surgery, a double-blind placebo-controlled evaluation of the adjuvant use of levamisole was conducted in 211 resectable lung cancer patients, following these patients for 2 years after their operation. Levamisole (or the placebo) was given for 3 days every 2 weeks and the dose level ranged 1.1–3.8 mg/kg per day (a fixed dose of 3 × 50 mg was given to all patients). It appeared that recurrences and carcinomatous deaths had occurred significantly less often in patients who had received a high dose (i.e., 2.1–3.8 mg/kg: patients weighing 70 kg or less) but not in the patients who received a lower dose. Patients who had more advanced cancers at the time of surgery seemed to have profited more from the treatment, but the results did not seem to depend upon the histologic type of the tumor or on the immune status of the patients as estimated from the skin test reactivity at the start. There was also suggestive evidence that levamisole may be more effective in preventing hematogenous dissemination than in inhibiting recurrences in the lung or the mediastinal tissues. Levamisole, if dosed adequately, appears to be a very suitable adjuvant treatment in resectable lung cancer patients as judged from its efficacy and its lack of troublesome side-effects.

Acknowledgement

We wish to thank all the other members of our study group who contributed to the success of this trial: Mr. E. Denissen for his coordination efforts, Dr. W. Tanghe for reviewing all pathology material, and Mr. G. De Ceuster, Dr. L. Desplenter, Mr. J. Dony, Prof. A. Drochmans, and Dr. P. A. J. Jansen for their valuable role as consultants. Thanks is also due to Mrs. N. Smets-Raeymaekers for her substantial help in the computer processing.

References

1. Amery, W. K.: Double-blind levamisole trial in resectable lung cancer. Ann. N.Y. Acad. Sci. *277*, 260–268 (1976)
2. Amery, W. K., Spreafico, F., Rojas, A. F., Denissen, E., Chirigos, M. A.: Adjuvant treatment with levamisole in cancer. A review of experimental and clinical data. Cancer Treat. Rev. *4*, 167–194 (1977)
3. Amery, W. K.: Final results of a multicenter placebocontrolled levamisole study of resectable lung cancer. Cancer Treat. Rep. (in press) (1978)
4. Brunner, K. W., Marthaler, T., Muller, W.: Unfavourable effects of long-term adjuvant chemotherapy with Endoxan in radically operated bronchogenic carcinoma. Eur. J. Cancer *7*, 285–294 (1971)
5. Crosbie, W. A., Kamdar, H. H., Belcher, J. R.: A controlled trial of vinblastine sulphate in the treatment of cancer of the lung. Br. J. Dis. Chest *60*, 28–35 (1966)
6. Dixon, W. J. (ed.): B.M.D., Biomedical Computer Programs. Berkeley: University California Press 1973
7. Legha, S. S., Muggia, F. M., Carter, S. K.: Adjuvant chemotherapy in lung cancer. Cancer *39*, 1415–1424 (1977)
8. Rosenthal, M., Breysse, Y., Dixon, A. St. J., Franchimont, P., Huskisson, E. C., Schmidt, K. L., Schuermans, Y., Veys, E., Vischer, T. L., Jannsen, P. A. J., Amery, W. K., Brugmans, J., De Cree, J., Symoens, J., MacNair, A. L.: Levamisole and agranulocytosis. Lancet *1977 I*, 904–905
9. Slack, N. H.: Bronchogenic carcinoma: nitrogen mustard as a surgical adjuvant and factors influencing survival. Cancer *25*, 987–1002 (1970)
10. Study Group for Bronchogenic Carcinoma: Immunopotentiation with levamisole in resectable bronchogenic carcinoma: a double-blind controlled trial. Br. Med. J. *1975/I*, 461–464
11. Symoens, J., Rosenthal, M.: Levamisole in the modulation of the immune response: the current experimental and clinical state. J. Reticuloendothel. Soc. *21*, 175–221 (1977)

Specific Active Immunochemotherapy in Lung Cancer: A Survival Study

T. H. M. Stewart, A. C. Hollinshead, J. E. Harris, S. Raman, R. Belanger, A. Crepeau, A. F. Crook, W. E. Hirte, D. Hooper, D. J. Klaasen, E. F. Rapp, and H. J. Sachs

In this report we give the survival data on 52 patients with stage I cancer of the lung who have been treated in Ottawa. A year has passed since the last figures for survival were published [15, 16]. We also indicate survival data for the small numbers of patients who were included in this study and who had either stage II or stage III disease. The rationale and design of this study has been reported in detail [14] as has the preparation and characterization of antigens used for immunisation [6]. The usefulness of such antigens in monitoring patients progress following curative surgery has also been reported [16].

Method and Materials

Patients were drawn from those having surgical removal of their tumour at the Ottawa Civic Hospital, the National Defence Medical Centre, Ottawa and the Ottawa General Hospital. Careful staging for TNM [10] was assured by preoperative radiography, scans, mediastinoscopy and postoperative consideration of the notes of the surgeon and pathologist. From August 1972 to May 1978 we evaluated 52 patients with stage I disease. Of these, 16 patients acted as a control group; they were operated upon by the same surgeons and would have been included in the treatment groups but for a delay of more than 30 days following surgery when they were unavailable for randomization. The remaining 36 patients were randomized into one of three treatment groups. Group I consisted of eight patients who received methotrexate (MTX) followed by citrovorum rescue once a month, for 3 months. Group II comprised 15 patients who received soluble allogeneic antigen (matched for histology) homogenized with Freund's complete adjuvant (FCA) once a month for 3 months. Group III comprised 13 patients who were immunized 7–9 days after administration of MTX with citrovorum rescue once a month for 3 months. In Table 1 we have summarized all the relevant characteristics of the patients with stage I disease.

The preparation of soluble allogeneic lung cancer antigens has already been described in detail [4, 14] as have their characterization with recognition of oncofoetal antigens, tumor-associated antigens and a herpes simples virus tumor-associated antigen [6]. The mean total quantity of antigen given to patients in the immunotherapy group was 1495 μg, with a range of 1125–2200 μg. The mean total quantity of antigen given to the immunochemotherapy group was 1610 μg (range 900–3000 μg). An average of 500 μg of antigen in 0.5 ml was homogenized with an equal volume of FCA (Difco Laboratories, Detroit, Michigan), which contains 10 mg of killed mycobacterium hominis per 10 ml, made up of 8.5 ml Bagol-F (mineral oil) and 1.5 ml Arlacil (mannide manolliate). The homogenate was given intradermally into the deltoid region of the arm, the thigh and again the arm at monthly intervals. The details of the care of the ensuing ulcer have been described already [14]. Methotrexate (Lederle Laboratories) was given by rapid intravenous infusion, 300 mg and then 700 mg was infused over a period of 6 hours. A normal creatinine clearance is mandatory and the urine is alkalinized by giving sodium bicarbonate 1.2 gm every 6 h per os starting 24 h before the

Table 1. Data on the three groups of patients: stage I chemotherapy and concomitant controls, immunotherapy and immunochemotherapy

		MTX & controls	Immunotherapy	Immuno-chemotherapy
Total patients		24	15	13
Male		19	11	9
Median age		57	55	57
Age range		39–74 years	46–71 years	45–66 years
Performance status at surgery	0	3	5	3
	1	21	10	10
Total pneumonectomy		6	2	5
Right sided		14	7	5
Hilar node involvement		3	1	2
Mean follow-up period		35 months	36 months	40 months
Cell type				
Epidermoid well-differentiated		9	7	5
Epidermoid poorly-differentiated		3	1	4
Adenocarcinoma		10	4	4
Anaplastic large cell		1	2	0
Anaplastic small cell		1	0	1

0 asymptomatic; *1* symptomatic ambulant.

infusion and continuing during the folinic acid rescue period of 60 h. The urine pH is monitored every 6 h to ensure that the pH remains above 6. Delayed hypersensitivity reactions (DHR) to allogeneic and occasionally autologous soluble cancer antigen were tested on subsequent visits of the patients following the initial 3-months course of treatment. The skin test dose has been 100 μg of antigen, unless dilution, dose responses were measured [14]. Induration at 48 h, measured by the technique of Sokal [12], was recorded over the two greatest diameters. Results are expressed as the surface area of an elipse. Readings less than 5 mm in diameter were scored as negative. Biopsies of the test sites have been done for histologic confirmation of a delayed hypersensitivity reaction.

Results

We divided our patients into two groups, those who were not immunized, some of whom received methotrexate, and those who were immunized, some of whom received methotrexate. For a comparison of survival statistics, we compared only those patients who had stage I cancer. We do not have enough patients in stage II and stage III to allow a meaningful comparison. Our nonimmunized group consisted of 24 patients, stage I; of these, 16 were control patients followed for a mean of 37 months and eight patients who received methotrexate followed for a mean of 34 months. Six control patients have died and one developed a metastasis proven at craniotomy at 24 months. Of the eight patients who received methotrexate, four have died. Our immunized group was made up of 28 patients, all stage I. Fifteen of these received the allogeneic antigen in FCA, followed for a mean of 36 months, and 13 had a

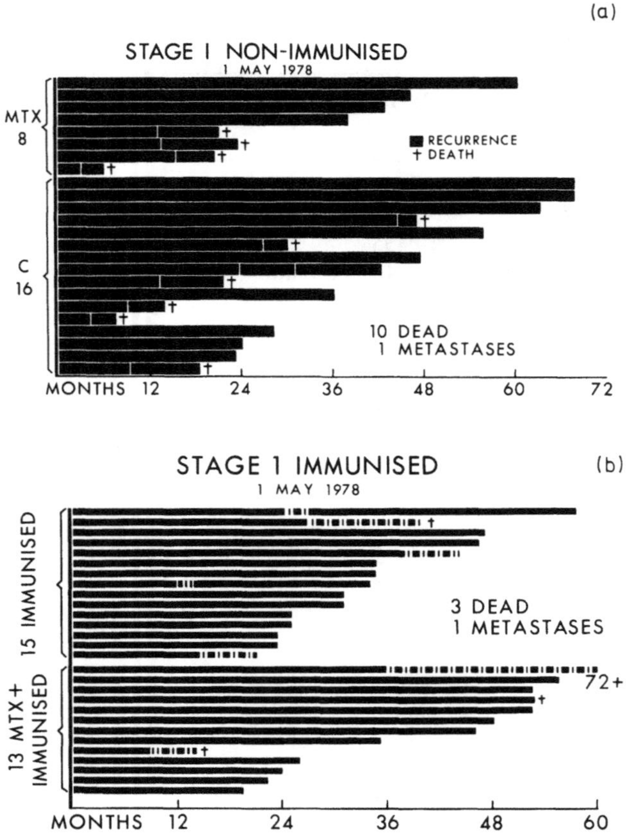

Fig. 1. Status of patients with stage I cancer. **a** The status of patients who were not immunized and who had a stage I cancer of the lung removed surgically. Eight of these patients received methotrexate and citrovorum rescue postoperatively. Of the 24 patients, ten have died and one had an intrecerebral metastasis removed at 24 monts. **b** The status of patients who have been immunized. In the 15 patients immunized, one died at 40 months, two had local recurrence and one has cerebral metastases. Of the 13 patients who received immunochemotherapy, two have died of their disease

combination of methotrexate and immunization with antigen plus FCA, followed for a mean of 40 months. Of those who were immunized only, one had a stump recurrence at 21 months, received radiotherapy and is at present alive and free of disease 58 months after surgery. A second patient in this group developed a stump recurrence at 26 months, received irradiation and chemotherapy and died at 40 months after surgery. A third patient with two primaries in the right lung had a recurrence around the sleeve resection of his right upper lobe lesion at 12 months and is well and free of disease at 36 months after the first surgery. Two other patients have failure, one with cerebral metastases at 15 months, alive at 24 months, the other local mediastinal recurrence at 41 months, alive at 48 months. Of those that received immunochemotherapy, one died at 14 months of a cerebral metastasis. He had a 9-cm poorly differentiated epidermoid carcinoma that was contiguous with the visceral pleura. One patient developed a stump recurrence at 36 months and eventually died at 72 months. He was our first and only patient in whom crude membranes were used, plus methotrexate [14]. One woman

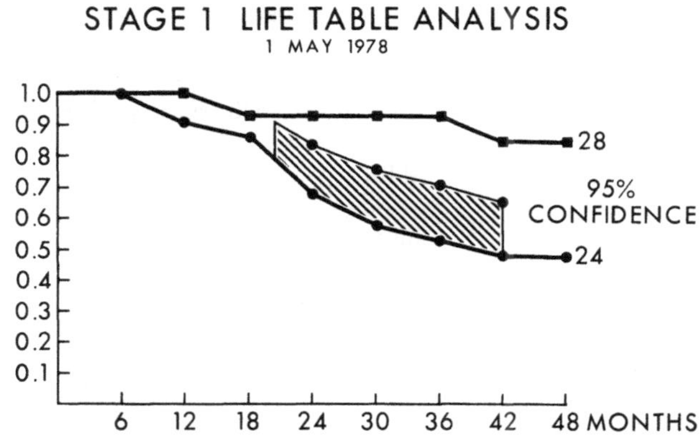

Fig. 2. Life table analysis of the survival difference between the two stage I groups of patients in control, with or without MTX (24, lower line) and immunized, with or without MTX (28, top line). The 95% confidence band becomes significant after 18 monts

died at 51 months of staphylococcal pneumonia without evidence of recurrence. No other patients in this group has had a recurrence or metastases.

In Fig. 1 we have compared the survival data of our two groups in stage I. The classic life table analysis (Fig. 2) of survival for stage I patients using the method of Cutler and Ederer [1] shows a significant separation between the groups after 18 months, extending to 42 months. The 2-year survival of our 24 nonimmunised patients is 68% and in a further 4 months this will be real survival, not based on life table methods. It compares with the 65% survival of 155 controls in the Canadian Study of oral BCG in the adjuvant therapy of lung cancer [8]. Thus, our controls are no worse or better than the concurrent Canadian experience. The number of patients with stage II are seven in all; three randomized to receive immunotherapy, two to immunochemotherapy and two to MTX. Both patients in the immunochemotherapy group are free of disease at 22 and 30 months. Two patients have died in the immunised group, at 6 and 18 months, and one is free of disease at 32 months. One patient given MTX died at 8 months, the other has had metastases since 25 months, alive at 36 months. All ten patients with stage III disease have died, and no difference in longevity is seen with immunisation or immunochemotherapy.

Skin Testing

We have previously reported stronger delayed hypersensitivy reactions (DHR) to skin testing with cancer antigens in these patients who received immunochemotherapy. In Table 2 we show two such patients that illustrate the induction of a very strong DHR to cancer antigen when immunised following MTX. The first patient had an oat cell carcinoma removed. She was immunised with epidermoid antigen as we had no supply of allogeneic oat antigen at the time and we had previously shown that a patient with epidermoid lung cancer gave a strong reaction to oat cell antigen [13], suggesting shared antigens between oat cell carcinoma and epidermoid carcinoma. Within 4 months this woman had a 6-cm DHR to epidermoid antigen and a 5.7-cm reaction to anaplastic large cell antigen. A month later she gave a 4-cm DHR at

Table 2. Serial skin testing in two patients with cancer and recall antigens. Both patients received immunochemotherapy. A strong reaction is seen within 3 months to cancer antigen

Patient J. F., oat cell carcinoma T1N1M0 (surgery 23 May 1974)

Antigen	MTX			1975 Sept	1975 Nov	1978 April
	June	July	August			
Randomised to immunochemotherapy						
Epidermoid 100 μg	3	4	40	60		47
Autologous	ND	ND	ND	ND	40	30
Anaplastic large	ND	ND	ND	57		
D	–	–	–	–		–
P	–	15	20	26		26
V	20	30	20	46		75
M	–	–	–	6		ND

Patient F. P., Squamous cell carcinoma T1N0M0 (surgery 8 May 1975)

Antigen	MTX				1975 Oct	1978 April
	May	July	August	September		
Randomised to immunochemotherapy						
Epidermoid 100 μg	–	15	25	77	10	45
D	5	10	11	26	21	–
P	15	20	17	33	35	42
V	–	12	18	24	55	102
M	8	–	–	21	ND	ND

ND not done.

48 h with a response to as little as 500 ng [14]. This autologous reactivity was retained 4 years later, with 3 cm of induration toward her own soluble oat cell antigen.
The second patient showed 7.7 cm of reaction by the 4th month following immunochemotherapy. A month later this was reduced to 1 cm. Three years later, free of disease, he showed a 4.5-cm reaction. In Table 3 we show skin reactions of six patients from this phase II trial tested with 100 μg of pooled soluble cancer antigen derived from allogeneic epidermoid and adenocarcinoma of the lung. The asterisk indicates the pooled antigen. It can be seen that strong reactions are seen to both lots. These pooled antigens will be used in a large multicenter trial in Canada that will test the findings of this trial.

Discussion

We believe that this phase II study is the first attempt at specific immunotherapy of cancer in man using soluble antigens. Thus, it has been a source of great satisfaction that in recent years others have identified tumour-associated antigens in lung cancer in man. Sega et al. [11] in

Table 3. In order to test for biologic activity of pooled allogeneic antigen (*) to be used in a multicenter trial, six patients were skin tested. Note reactivity to stored autologous antigen in J. F. (4 years storage) and A. L. (3 years storage)

Antigen, patient J. F., 47 months after surgery for oat cell carcinoma	
	48 h induration
Epidermoid* 100 μg	35 × 47
Autologous oat 100 μg	30 × 30
Dermatophytin	Negative
PPD	26 × 20
Varidase	75 × 50
Antigen, patient E. C., 56 months after surgery for epidermoid adenocarcinoma	
	48 h induration
Adenocarcinoma*	27 × 22
Epidermoid*	37 × 32
Dermatophytin	Negative
PPD	40 × 41
Varidase	25 × 32
Antigen, patient F. P., 36 months after surgery for epidermoid carcinoma	
	48 h induration
Epidermoid*	45 × 31
Dermatophytin	Negative
PPD	42 × 35
Varidase	102 × 67
Antigen, patient A. L., 36 months after surgery for epidermoid carcinoma	
	48 h induration
Epidermoid*	47 × 54
Autologous oat 20 μg	43 × 36
Dermatophytin	10 × 10
PPD	20 × 14
Varidase	40 × 32
Antigen, patient A. T., 20 months after surgery for epidermoid adenocarcinoma	
	48 h induration
Epidermoid*	20 × 19
Adenocarcinoma*	21 × 22
Dermatophytin	10 × 10
PPD	25 × 25
Varidase	27 × 27
Antigen, patient A. L., 26 months after surgery for adenocarcinoma	
	48 h induration
Adenocarcinoma*	15 × 12
Dermatophytin	23 × 26
PPD	32 × 33
Varidase	27 × 32

1974 reported on tumour antigens in squamous cell carcinoma of lung, comparable to those used in our study [5]. MOHR et al. [9] described an alveolar cell carcinoma-like antigen, FROST et al. [2] described a bronchogenic carcinoma antigen unlikely to be related to histocompatibility between individuals. VIZA et al. [17] described at least one tumour-associated antigen was present in some lung tumours. WATSON et al. [18] identified tumour-associated antigens in squamous cell carcinoma of the lung and in some other histological types of lung cancer, adenocarcinoma alveolar and anaplastic carcinoma. More recently attempts are being made to develop a radioimmunoassay for a tumour-associated antigen in lung cancer by GAFFAR et al. [3]. This programme of immunochemotherapy extends the disease-free interval in patients with stage I cancer of the lung. Skin rections are sometime very strong following immunochemotherapy, but as soon as the effect of MTX is removed, the reaction reverts to a weak one, to slowly strengthen over the subsequent months in patient F.P.

If the effect of MTX is to delete suppressor cells [7], it is a transient effect, but late testing at 18 months after surgery shows maintenance of the early strong response. Thus, chemotherapy may favourably influence the strength of a DHR to cancer antigen, and this can be seen early and in late testing. We have already discussed the importance of such skin reactivity [15]. The multicenter trial in Canada will have three groups in a total of 300 patients with stage I and II lung cancer following curative surgery; 100 will serve as controls, 100 will receive FCA once a month and 100 will receive FCA homogenised with appropriate allogeneic pooled cancer antigen. The results of such a trial may settle the question as to whether soluble antigens homogenised with FCA will improve upon any favourable effect given by nonspecific stimulation with FCA used alone.

References

1. Cutler, S. J., Ederer, F.: Maximum utilization of the Life Table Method in analyzing survival. J. Chronic Dis. *8*, 699–712 (1958)
2. Frost, M. J., Rogers, G. T., Bagshawe, K. D.: Extraction and preliminary characterization of a human bronchogenic carcinoma antigen. Br. J. Cancer *31*, 379–386 (1975)
3. Gaffar, S. A., Braatz, J. A., Kortright, K. H., Princler, G. L., Herberman, R. B., McIntire, K. R.: Isolation and characterisation of a human lung tumour associated antigen and developement of a radio immunoassay. A.A.C.R. Abs. *424*, 106 (1978) 69th Annual Meeting
4. Hollinshead, A. C., Stewart, T. H. M., Herberman, R. B.: Delayed hypersensitivity reactions to soluble membrane antigens of human malignant lung cells. J. Natl. Cancer Inst. *52*, 327–338 (1974)
5. Hollinshead, A. C., Sega, E., Stewart, T. H. M.: A comparison of lung cancer antigens. Tumori *6*, 125–8 (1975)
6. Hollinshead, A. C., Stewart, T. H. M.: Lung tumour antigens. In: Proc. 3rd Int. Symp. Cancer Detection Prevention. Nieburg, H. E. (ed.). Basel: E. Karger (in press) (1977)
7. Kourounakis, L., Kapusta, M. A.: Restoration of diminished T-cell function in adjuvant induced disease by methotrexate. J. Rheumatol. *3*, 346–354 (1976)
8. Miller, A. B.: Personal communication. (1978)
9. Mohr, J. A., Nordquist, R. E., Rhoades, E. R., Coalson, R. E., Coalson, J. J.: Alveolar cell carcinoma-like antigen and antibodies in patients with Alveolar cell carcinoma and other cancers. Cancer Res. *34*, 1904–1907 (1974)
10. Mountain, C. F., Carr, D. T., Anderson, W. A. D.: A system for the clinical staging of lung cancer. Am. J. Roentgenol. *120*, 130–138 (1974)

11. Sega, E., Natali, P. G., Ricci, C., Mineo, C. T., Citro, G.: Lung cancer tumour associated antigens. Isolation by gel filtration and characterisation by immunodiffusion. IRCS *2,* 1278 (1974)
12. Sokal, J. E.: Measurements of delayed skin test response. New Engl. J. Med. *293,* 501–502 (1975)
13. Stewart, T. H. M., Hollinshead, A. C., Herberman, R. B.: Soluble membrane antigens of human malignant lung cells. Cancer detection and prevention. Maltoni, C. (ed.), p. 638. Amsterdam: Excerpta Medica 1973
14. Stewart, T. H. M., Hollinshead, A. C., Harris, J. E.: Immunochemotherapy of lung cancer. Ann. N.Y. Acad. Sci. *277,* 436–466 (1976)
15. Stewart, T. H. M., Hollinshead, A. C., Harris, J., Raman, S., Belanger, R., Crepeau, A., Crook, A., Hirte, W., Hooper, D., Klaassen, D., Rapp, E., Sachs, H. J.: Specific Active Immunochemotherapy in lung cancer: A survival study. Can. J. Surg. *20,* 370–377 (1977)
16. Stewart, T. H. M., Hollinshead, A. C., Harris, J., Raman, S., Belanger, R., Crepeau, A., Crook, A., Hirte, W., Hooper, D., Klaassen, D., Rapp, E., Sachs, H. J.: A survival study of Specific Active Immunochemotherapy in lung cancer. Neoplasm Immunity: Solid tumour therapy. Cripsen, R. G. (ed.), pp. 37–48. Chicago: Franklin Institute 1977
17. Viza, D., Louvier, M., Phillips, J., Boucheix, C., Guerin, R. A.: Solubilization of an antigen associated with certain bronchial tumours. Eur. J. Cancer *11,* 765–770 (1975)
18. Watson, R. D., Smith, A. G., Levy, J. G.: The detection by immunodiffusion of tumour associated antigenic components in extracts of human bronchogenic carcinoma. Br. J. Cancer *32,* 300–309 (1975)

Patterns of Recurrence After Regional BCG Immunotherapy of Bronchial Cancer

M. F. McKneally, C. Maver, S. Kellar, L. Lininger

Background

The specificity of the immune response and its biologic compatibility with the normal tissues of the host are responsible for its great appeal to clinical scientists as a therapeutic intervention in patients with early or minimal residual cancer. Because carcinoma of the bronchus appears to be a carcinogen-induced cancer and because carcinogen-induced cancers are frequently, at least minimally immunogenic, this tumor seems a reasonably logical target for immunotherapeutic attack.

The first reported experiences with regional immunotherapy of carcinoma of the bronchus were inadvertent experiments. TAKITA [10] and RUCKDESCHEL [9] reported a beneficial effect of postoperative infection in the pleural space following putatively curative surgical resection for lung cancer. In an attempt to reproduce this natural experiment in immunotherapy, 116 patients were entered into a randomized prospective trial of intrapleural BCG immunotherapy following surgical resection during the interval from April 1973 to November 1977. The methods of preoperative screening, surgical treatment, and postoperative follow-up have been previously reported [6, 7]. Staging followed the criteria of the Joint Committee on Lung Cancer Staging [8]. The essential element of the trial was the administration of 10^7 colony-forming units of Tice BCG into the pleural space in the early postoperative period. Patients so treated, and their randomized concurrent control counterparts, were subsequently treated with isoniazid 300 mg/day starting on the 14th post-injection day and continuing for 12 weeks. All patients were seen at regular intervals at 1, 3, 6, 12, 18, 24, 30, 36, 42, 48, 54, and 60 months after treatment. Chest X-rays, physical examinations, skin tests, and blood chemical profiles were performed at each follow-up visit. No patient was lost to follow-up, and appropriate scans and local X-ray studies were performed when symptoms of recurrence were detected.

Prior permission for postmortem examination was not required for entry into the study, and patients were often hospitalized for the terminal phase of their illness in community hospitals, for the convenience and comfort of the family and the patient. Consequently, the pattern of recurrence is documented on clinical grounds in 39 of the 50 patients with recurrent disease. With this limitation, we have compared the pattern of recurrence in the treatment and control arms in the hope of increasing our understanding of the mechanism of regional immunotherapy in patients with minimal residual disease following surgical resection.

Results

Our experience with minimal residual disease following surgical excision of carcinoma of the bronchus was somewhat less favorable than the experience reported from some other centers [4] but generally followed the pattern of early recurrence and death that has been the hallmark of this highly malignant tumor [8]. Recurrent lung cancer developed in 17 of 36 stage I control

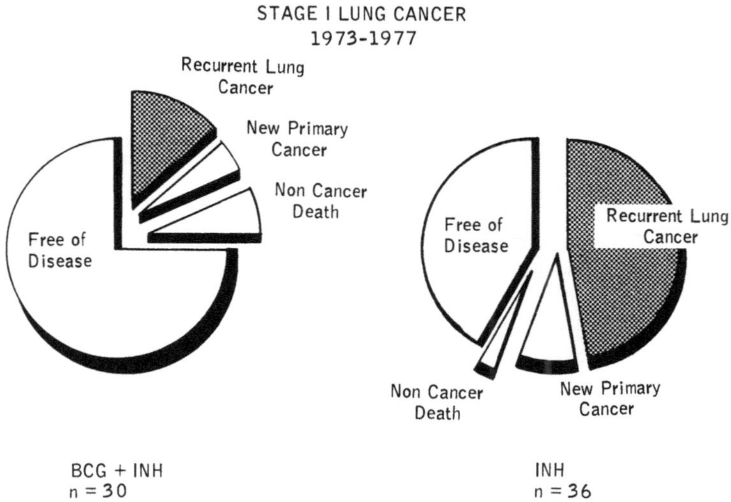

Fig. 1. Regional immunotherapy with intrapleural BCG reduced the number of recurrences following surgical excision of lung cancer ($P < 0.0009$)

patients. Among 30 patients treated with intrapleural BCG after surgery, recurrent lung cancer developed in four patients. Analysis of the censored survival data using GEHAN's statistic [1] rejects the hypothesis that intrapleural BCG is no better than the control ($P < 0.0009$). These results are illustrated in Fig. 1.

Among 36 stage I control lung cancer patients, three have developed new primary cancers in other organs without evidence of recurrence of lung cancer. Two of these were laryngeal cancers and the third a prostatic cancer. A fourth patient developed a new cancer in the contralateral lung, composed of cells of a different type from those in the original lesion. This new stage I tumor has been resected and the patient is free of disease.

Seventeen control patients developed evidence of recurrent lung cancer. Seven patients developed clear-cut local recurrences of cancer in the chest, evident on follow-up chest X-rays or at postmortem examination. One additional patient developed a nodule in the lung associated with disseminated metastases, which suggested that the lung lesion was a blood-borne metastasis, and another developed regional recurrence in the scalene lymph nodes.

These observations suggest that local failure was a fairly frequent finding in control patients with putatively complete surgical excision of stage I lung cancers. Seven of 17 (41%) of the failures were associated with local recurrence in this group of patients. Six patients, 17% of the total, failed because of disseminated metastases to the brain, spine, small intestine, liver, or bone, without evidence of local recurrence. Four of the patients with local recurrence had disseminated metastases as well.

The patients in the stage I BCG immunotherapy group had a lower overall incidence of recurrent lung cancer ($P < 0.0009$). One patient developed a new primary colon cancer without evidence of recurrent lung cancer. No stage I BCG patient had evidence of a local recurrence at the site of excision or in regional lymph nodes. One patient developed a single ipsilateral nodule in another lobe 4½ years after the original resection. This nodule when excised was of the same histologic type as the original primary tumor. A second patient developed a similar ipsilateral single nodule 18 months after the original excision, composed of cells of the same cell type as the original tumor. Both of these lesions could be interpreted as blood-borne metastases or as new primary carcinomas.

The data suggest that regional immunotherapy with a single dose of intrapleural living BCG reduced the number of local recurrences. The treatment may also have influenced distant

Table 1. Patterns of recurrence in stage I lung cancer

	INH	BCG + INH
Local recurrence	7/17 (41%)	0/4 (0%)
Metastatic or new primary tumor in lung	2/17 (12%)	2/4 (50%)
Distant metastases	7/17 (41%)	2/4 (50%)
Indeterminate	1/17 (6%)	0/4 (0%)

Table 2. Patterns of recurrence in stage II and III lung cancer

	INH	BCG + INH
Local recurrence	3/11 (27%)	5/18 (28%)
Metastatic or new primary tumor in lung	0/11 (0%)	1/18 (6%)
Distant metastases	8/11 (73%)	11/18 (61%)
Indeterminate	0/11 (0%)	1/18 (6%)

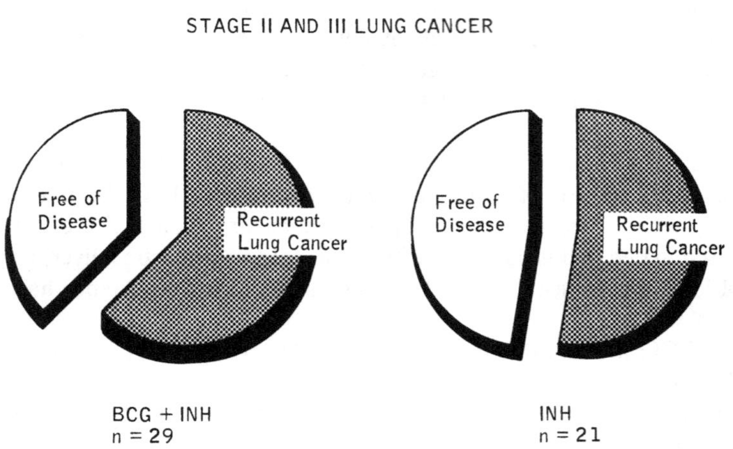

Fig. 2. Recurrence of stage II and III lung cancer was not reduced by regional immunotherapy with intrapleural BCG

metastases. The number of recurrences in the BCG-treated group is low, so that inferences about the pattern of recurrence cannot be made with confidence. These results are summarized in Table 1.

Recurrence of locally advanced, but resectable lung cancer in stage II and III was not reduced by intrapleural BCG treatment (Fig. 2). Eighteen of 29 (62%) patients treated with BCG and INH and 11 of 21 (52%) patients treated with INH alone developed recurrent cancer. The apparent local effect of regional administration of BCG in the pleural space was not evident in the pattern of recurrence observed in these patients (Table 2).

Discussion

The pattern of failure after surgical treatment of lung cancer depends upon the distribution of minimal residual disease microscopically or grossly present within the patient immediately following surgical resection. This distribution has been carefully documented by MATTHEWS, who found residual local and systemic cancer foci in 33% of 254 patients autopsied within 30 days of putatively curative surgical resection [5].

Our patients conformed to the patterns of recurrence described by MATTHEWS, with the exception that patients who could be expected to have the smallest amount of residual tumor (stage I) showed an apparent reduction in local recurrence of cancer after regional BCG administration. The cause for this reduction could be maldistribution of cases at risk, as the number of patients in this subset is small. If the mechanism is immunologic, two hypotheses might be tested for conformity to the patterns of recurrence. Elimination of residual tumor cells may have resulted from the generation of nonspecific cellular and extracellular factors in the field of local infection. This hypothesis fits the observation that local recurrence was reduced in BCG-treated stage I patients. It could be invoked to explain a reduction in distant metastases, but would conform less well to such an observation, because the size and doubling time of the distant metastases identified in early postoperative autopsies [5] suggest that they are present from before the time of surgery and do not disseminate subsequently, e.g., from local residual tumor.

The alternate immunologic hypothesis postulates the development of specific immunity by reason of bacterial stimulation of the immune response at a time when subtle or minimally immunogenic tumor antigens might be coresident in the lymphoid apparatus. Specific immunity developed against these tumor antigens might then result in immunologic injury to systemically disseminated metastases outside the infected region. Such an effect has been demonstrated in line 10 hepatomas treated regionally with BCG in strain 2 guinea pigs. HANNA and PETERS [2] have shown that such local treatment results in regional control of the tumor but also causes systemic immunity that can protect against rechallenge with the same tumor at distant sites. We suspect that the difference in the incidence of recurrences recorded in our stage I lung cancer patients is related to development of systemic specific immunity to tumor-associated antigens [3] generated during the period of regional immunologic stimulation of BCG organisms, but we cannot validate this inference from the distribution of sites of recurrence documented in this review.

The distribution of recurrences in stage II and III patients conforms to the hypothesis of specific immunity, although the basis for this inference is less secure. If nonspecific destruction of residual tumor cells were the only mechanism activated by BCG, this effect might still be detectable locally even in patients with these more advanced stages of disease, whose risk of residual occult distant metastases is high after surgery [5]. The fact that the reduction in local recurrences observed in stage I patients was not seen in stage II and III patients might be interpreted to mean that the observation in stage I patients is unreliable or that a nonspecific local effect seen in stage I patients was overwhelmed in stage II and III by reason of larger amounts of residual tumor persisting locally. The interpretation that specific immunologic competition prevented the local effect is supported by the studies of HANNA and PETERS [2]. These investigators found that regionally administered BCG caused regression of local lesions and arrested the growth of regional lymph node metastases. When the stage of disease was artificially advanced by the administration of tumor cells intravenously, the local skin tumor and regional lymph node metastases escaped from BCG-mediated regression. We postulate that a similar mechanism might be operative in our patients.

The paradigm that specific immunity is responsible for the apparent beneficial effect of postoperative intrapleural BCG is encouraging though unproven. It implies the possibility of selective toxicity against tumor cells, the sine qua non of successful systemic cancer therapy. If the surface characteristics of tumor cells are sufficiently antigenic to allow their identification by specifically immunized cells, further augmentation of specific immunity should be beneficial to these patients. The hypotheses suggested by the data from this preliminary trial can be tested more reliably when the patterns of recurrence become clear in larger cooperative trials of regional BCG immunotherapy currently in progress.

Acknowledgement

Supported by National Cancer Institute contract NO-1-CB-53940, grant #RO1-CA-17346, U.S. Public Health Service General Clinical Research Center Grant #2-Mo-1-RR-00749, and the New York State Kidney Disease Institute, Division of Laboratories and Research, an agency of the New York State Department of Health. The authors wish to acknowledge the significant contributions made by RALPH D. ALLEY, HARVEY W. KAUSEL, THOMAS M. OLDER, ERIC D. FOSTER, JOSEPH B. MCILDUFF, BERNARD POLLARA, BARBARA RICHARDSON, MARTIN FILARDI, ROSALIE JENNINGS, MAUREEN JUSSEN, MANCIA PROPP, and the patients, residents, and referring physicians participating in this study.

References

1. Gehan, E.: A generalized two-sample Wilcoxon test for doubly censored data. Biometrika *52,* 650–653 (1965)
2. Hanna, M. G., Peters, L. C.: Efficacy of intralesional BCG therapy in guinea pigs with disseminated tumor. Cancer *36,* 1298–1304 (1975)
3. Hollinshead, A. C., Stewart, T. H. M.: Lung tumour antigens. Procedures 3rd International Symposium Ca. Nieburg, H. E. (ed.). Basel: E. Karger (in press) (1978)
4. Martini, N., Beattie, E. J.: Results of surgical treatment in stage I lung cancer. J. Thorac. Cardiovasc. Surg. *74,* 499–505 (1977)
5. Matthews, M. J., Pickren, J., Kanhouwa, S.: Who has occult metastases? In: Perspectives in lung cancer. Williams, T. E. et al. (eds.), pp. 9–17. Frederick E. Jones Memorial Symposium in Thoracic Surgery. Columbus (Ohio), 1976. Basel: Karger 1977
6. McKneally, M. F., Maver, C., Kausel, H. W.: Regional immunotherapy of lung cancer with intrapleural BCG. Lancet *1976 I,* 377–379

7. McKneally, M. F., Maver, C., Kausel, H. W., Alley, R. D.: Regional immunotherapy with intrapleural BCG for lung cancer. J. Thorac. Cardiovasc. Surg. *72,* 333–338 (1976)
8. Mountain, C. F.: Assessment of the role of surgery for control of lung cancer. Ann. Thorac. Surg. *24,* 365–373 (1977)
9. Ruckdeschel, J. C., Codish, S. D., Stranahan, A., McKneally, M. F.: Postoperative empyema improves survival in lung cancer: Documentation and analysis of a natural experiment. N. Engl. J. Med. *287,* 1013–1017 (1972)
10. Takita, H.: Effect of postoperative empyema on survival of patients with bronchogenic carcinoma. J. Thorac. Cardiovasc. Surg. *59,* 642–644 (1970)

Intrapleural BCG in Operable Lung Cancer

P. B. Iles, D. F. Shore, M. J. S. Langman, and R. W. Baldwin

Introduction

Bacille Calmette-Guérin (BCG) has been administered to patients with a wide range of malignant disease, including malignant melanoma [4, 5], leukaemia [7, 17], colorectal cancer [8], and lung cancer [3, 18] in the hope of improving the patients' survival by enhancing the patients' nonspecific immunity or macrophage responses. It has also been used in conjunction with tumour-derived substances to try and enhance tumour-specific immune responses [7, 12].

McKneally et al. [9–11] have reported that intrapleural BCG (Tice strain) given after resection of lung cancer prolongs the survival of patients who had localised disease. This finding is in keeping with data from animal studies indicating that the greatest benefit from BCG is obtained when administered to the tumour site and when the tumour bulk is at a minimum [1, 6].

Following the reports of McKneally et al. [9] we sought to confirm the value of this mode of adjuvant immunotherapy using Glaxo BCG, since this strain is readily available in the United Kingdom and has been shown to retard the intrapleural and intrapulmonary growth of injected tumour cells in experimental animals [14–16]. We began a controlled, randomised prospective study of intrapleural Glaxo BCG at the City Hospital, Nottingham in May 1976 and extended the study to the Sheffield Royal Infirmary and the Northern General Hospital, Sheffield in November 1976.

Patients and Methods

All patients having resections for lung cancer in the Nottingham and Sheffield hospitals were eligible for the study. Preoperative investigations included measurement of pulmonary function, routine haematology and biochemistry and skin test with tuberculin (Heaf test). Other investigations (isotope scanning, etc.) were performed if indicated. Patients were considered for entry into the study on the 3rd to 5th postoperative day, before their intercostal drainage tubes were removed. We excluded patients with cardiovascular instability or with a swinging fever.

Patients who agreed to take part in the trial, which had the prior approval of the hospital ethical committee, were randomly allocated to control or BCG-treated groups using previously prepared randomised individual envelopes. BCG-treated patients were given a single intrapleural injection of 1×10^7 [18] viable units of Glaxo intradermal vaccine (one ampoule). The injection was given via the intercostal tube and flushed in with saline just before the tube's removal in those patients undergoing lobectomy. The BCG was given by thoracentesis in patients undergoing pneumonectomy. All patients received BCG from the same batch. Those patients who developed a febrile reaction considered to be due to BCG were given soluble aspirin. The patients were discharged on the 10th or 11th postoperative day, according to the

Table 1. Staging

Stage I	Tumour < 3.0 cm in diameter; hilar nodes may or may not contain tumour or Tumour > 3.0 cm; without involvement of adjacent structures or hilar lymph nodes
Stage II	Tumour > 3.0 cm; hilar nodes contain metastatic tumour
Stage III	Tumour invading mediastinal structures or chest wall, or mediastinal nodes contain tumour, or invasion into blood vessels

practice of that surgical team. Fourteen days after the BCG, 300 mg/day isoniazid was started and continued for 8 weeks. Control patients were given an 8-week supply of placebo (lactose) tablets, similar in appearance to isoniazid and did not receive any intrapleural injection.

Patients were followed up to determine their survival and were reviewed regularly as outpatients by their surgical team, with the exception of a few patients living at a distance who returned to the supervision of the referring chest physician. The progress of these patients was determined by communication with the chest physician and general practitioner.

The preoperative investigations were repeated at intervals during the follow-up. Tumour recurrences or metastases were treated with chemotherapy, radiotherapy or conservative measures as appropriate. Resected tumours were staged and histologically typed without knowledge of the treatment category of the patient. The staging used was essentially that of McKneally et al. [9, 10], but with the inclusion in stage III of any patient with histological evidence of invasion of pulmonary vessels by tumour (Table 1).

The overall survival of the two groups of patients was plotted graphically by the life table analysis method [2] to obtain the maximum information from the data: difference in death rates were analysed by the log rank test [13] and two-tailed P values derived. The significance of differing survival rates within subgroups of patients was tested using the "χ^2 test for trends" and also the log rank test in the manner described by Peto et al. [13].

Results

Survival Data

Ninety-two patients with lung cancer entered the study in its first 20 months. The two treatment groups are well matched, with the exception of the distribution of anaplastic (including small cell) cancer (Table 2). The excess of such tumours in the patients allocated BCG treatment has occurred by chance. There is an equal distribution of these tumours in the two treatment groups in the stage II and III cancer patients but there are six in the stage I BCG-treated patients compared with only one in the stage I controls.

The survival of the 52 stage I patients is shown graphically in Fig. 1, and the patients with anaplastic cancer are indicated. There is a trend of benefit in the BCG-treated patients, with 5

Table 2. Patient distribution

Tumour histology	Control		BCG	
Squamous	30	(68%)	29	(60%)
Adenocarcinoma	8	(18%)	7	(15%)
Alveolar cell	1	(2%)	2	(4%)
Anaplastic	5	(11%)	10	(21%)
(oat cell)	(2)		(3)	
Total	44	(100%)	48	(100%)

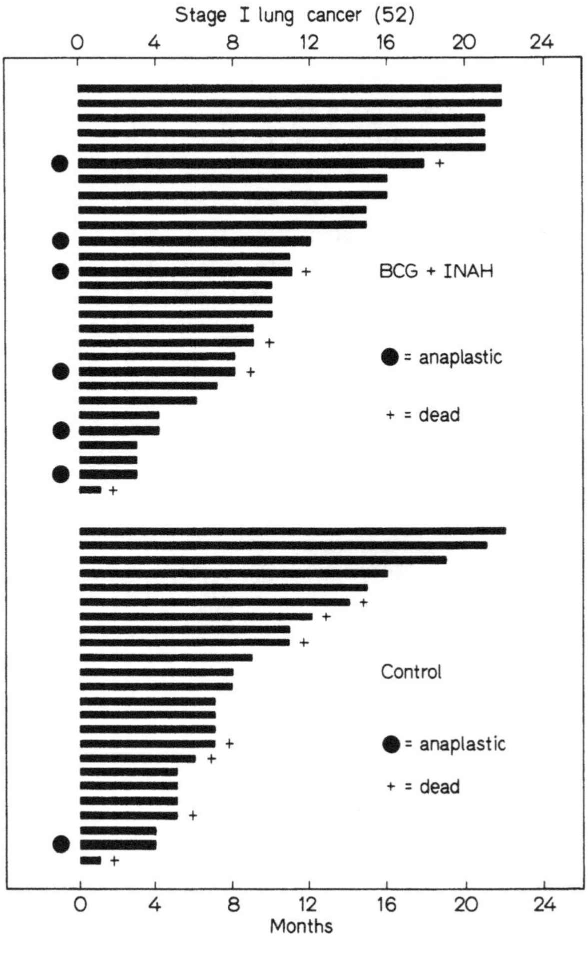

Fig. 1. Survival of stage I patients

deaths in 28 compared with 7 in 24 control patients. When the results of treatment in stage I patients with non-anaplastic carcinoma are considered alone, there is a more pronounced trend, with only 2 deaths in 22 BCG-treated patients compared with 7 in 23 control patients (Fig. 2).

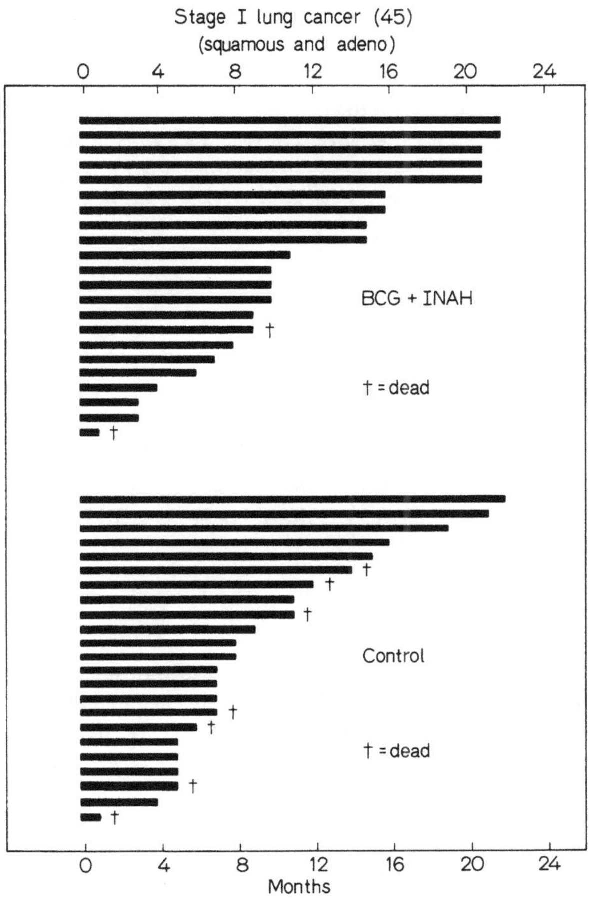

Fig. 2. Survival of stage I patients with non-anaplastic carcinoma

Discussion

Our data, although indicating some benefit from Glaxo BCG, do not show the same marked effect as that reported by McKneally et al. using Tice BCG [9–11]. There are three points in which our studies differ. Firstly, by including into stage III all patients with evidence of tumour within pulmonary vessels, our study has relatively more stage III and relatively fewer stage I and II patients and may lead to a slightly enhanced prognosis of the stage I patients. The second point of difference is in our treatment of control patients with lactose-containing tablets rather than isoniazid. We have no reason to suppose that lactose enhances patients' survival. The third, and probably most crucial difference between our studied lies in our use of Glaxo strain BCG, whereas McKneally's group used Tice strain.

There have certainly been differences in the clinical effects observed following BCG treatment. Only half of our patients had any febrile response at all, and this was usually brief and mild. Only in four instances was discharge from hospital delayed because of fever, and then by only 2–3 days. In contrast, McKneally et al. have indicated that febrile responses occurred in almost every case after Tice BCG and that discharge from hospital was delayed by an average of 5 days [9].

The two strains of BCG differ in other respects such as viability, with Glaxo strain having the higher proportion of viable units. We used the same number of viable units as McKneally's group (1×10^7 units), but this would be accompanied by fewer non-viable organisms. There is no way of knowing if the number of these non-viable units should also be taken into account, or if some other more subtle difference between BCG strains is important. Similarly, there is no good evidence regarding the relationship between post-BCG fever and survival. Too few of our patients have died to draw any firm conclusions, but 5 of the 11 BCG-treated patients to die had a fever following BCG.

Acknowledgements

We are most grateful to Mr. R. C. Barclay, Mr. A. G. Norman, Mr. F. D. Salama, Mr. G. H. Smith and Mr. D. G. Taylor for permission to include their patients in this study, and also to the Chest Physicians and General Practitioners for their co-operation and assistance. We wish to thank Mrs. B. Mullinger of Glaxo Laboratories Ltd. for supplies of BCG. The study was supported by the Cancer Research Campaign.

References

1. Bast, R. D., Zbar, B., Borsos, T., Rapp, H. J.: N. Engl. J. Med. *290,* 1413 (1974)
2. Cutler, S. J., Ederer, F.: J. Chron. Dis. *8,* 699 (1958)
3. Edwards, F. R., Whitwell, F.: Thorax *29,* 654 (1974)
4. Eilber, F. R., Morton, D. L., Holmes, E. C., Sparks, F. C., Ramming, K. P.: N. Engl. J. Med. *294,* 237 (1976)
5. Gutterman, J. U., McBride, C., Freireich, E. J., Mavligit, G., Frei, E. (III), Hersh, E. M.: Lancet *1973/I,* 1208
6. Laucius, J. F., Bodurtha, A. J., Mastrelangelo, M. J., Creech, R. M.: J. Reticuloendothel. Soc. *16,* 347 (1974)
7. Mathé, G., Amiel, J. L., Schwarzenberg, L., Schneider, M., Cattan, A., Schlumberger, J. R., Hayat, M., de Vassal, F.: Lancet *1969/II,* 697
8. Mavligit, G. M., Burgess, M. A., Seibert, G. B., Jubert, A. V. et al.: Lancet *1976/I,* 871
9. McKneally, M. F., Maver, C., Kausel, H. W.: Lancet *1976/I,* 377
10. McKneally, M. F., Maver, C., Kausel, H. W., Alby, R. D.: J. Thorac. Cardiovasc. Surg. *72,* 333 (1976)
11. McKneally, M. F., Maver, C., Kausel, H. W.: Lancet *1977/I,* 1003
12. McIllmurray, M. B., Embleton, M. J., Reeves, W. G., Langman, M. J. S., Deane, M.: Br. Med. J. *1976/I,* 540
13. Peto, R. et al.: Br. J. Cancer *35,* 1 (1977)
14. Pimm, M. V., Baldwin, R. W.: Int. J. Cancer *15,* 260 (1975)
15. Pimm, M. V., Hopper, D. G., Baldwin, R. W.: Br. J. Cancer *34,* 368 (1976)
16. Pimm, M. V.: Lancet *1976/II,* 95
17. Powles, R. L. et al.: Br. J. Cancer *28,* 365 (1973)
18. Roscoe, P., Pearce, S., Ludgate, S., Horne, N. W.: Cancer Immunol. Immunother. *3,* 115 (1977)

G. Head and Neck Tumors

Adjuvant Chemoimmunotherapy of Head and Neck Cancer

S. G. Taylor, G. A. Sisson, and D. E. Bytell

Introduction

Adjuvant systemic therapy in head and neck cancer has not been actively studied because regional recurrences have focused attention on the need for improved regional therapy and because additive toxicity with radiation therapy has discouraged use of effective regimens of chemotherapy. Randomized multi-institution studies have shown no differences in disease-free survival after 2 years [15, 28]. However, improved disease-free survival for the first 8–12 months was observed in a few studies [14, 21]. Such a duration of effect from methotrexate in the treatment of gross residual disease would be unusual and suggested that a more aggressive approach to adjuvant treatment might yield more long-lasting beneficial results. With improved local control from more effective surgery and radiation therapy, systemic metastases have caused an increased percentage of treatment failures accentuating the need to re-examine systemic adjuvant therapy [13]. Response rates to chemotherapy have also improved with the use of methotrexate and leucovorin in a weekly schedule [20] and use of combination drug therapy [3] although duration of response remains short. These developments are background to our current approach to adjuvant therapy trials.

Adjuvant Chemotherapy

We have reported a pilot study of 17 patients with advanced head and neck cancer treated with three cycles of moderate dose methotrexate with leucovorin given over 2 weeks prior to surgery or radiation therapy [27]. Methotrexate was begun at a dosage of 240 mg/M^2 given as intermittent IM injections of 60 mg/M^2 every 6 h for four doses and followed, 6 h after the last injection, by leucovorin orally, first 40 mg and then 10 mg every 6 h for 7 doses. After a 24-h rest, the cycle was repeated with a 50% dose escalation of the methotrexate if no mucositis or hematologic toxicity (WBC $\leq$ 4000 and platelets $\leq$ 125,000) was evident. A third cycle was delivered after another 24-h rest with a further 50% escalation in dosage if no toxicity was present. The occurrence of mild mucositis or a depressed white count between 4000 and 2500 or a platelet count between 125,000 and 75,000 resulted in no dose escalation. If oral ulceration or more severe blood count depression was apparent, the dosage was held until recovery and only two cycles were given.

The study included seven stage III patients and ten stage IV patients. Currently all patients have been followed for 3–5 years and eight (47%) remain disease-free. Three of the patients considered failures had second primaries as the cause of failure (one colon and two head and neck lesions), and one patient died of a myocardial infarction 4 years after treatment, still disease-free. Two of the patients who failed remain alive, one salvaged and one with persistent disease. We would have expected less than 20% of patients disease free with such advanced lesions. While these results were not definitive, they did suggest long-term benefit from the adjuvant treatment. We attributed part of the beneficial effect to escalation of methotrexate dosage. Clifford also has achieved encouraging long-term results with aggressive (more toxic) combination therapy (see report of this meeting). We have subsequently used this methotrexate regimen in a randomized study examining the benefit of adjuvant chemoimmunotherapy compared to adjuvant chemotherapy.

Adjuvant Chemoimmunotherapy Study

Study Design

Design of a randomized study in head and neck cancer posed certain unique problems. Although some corrections for imbalance in patient sampling can be made post facto [18], an

Table 1. Prognostic categories for head and neck cancer study

Site	Stage	Estimated % 3-Year NED			
		0–10%	11–30%	31–50%	51–70%
Buccal mucosa	II				×
Fl. mouth	III			×	
Ant. tongue	IV	×			
Palate	II			×	
Naso, oro	III		×		
Hypopharynx	IV	×			
Alveolar ridge	II			×	
	III			×	
	IV	×			
Sinus	II				×
	III		×		
	IV	×			
Supraglottic	III			×	
Glottic	III				×
Subglottic	III		×		
All larynx	IV	×			
Peristomal recurrence	Above		×		
	lat. or below	×			
Cervical esophagus	II		×		
	III	×			
	IV	×			

Table 2. Stratification variables for adjuvant chemoimmunotherapy study in head and neck cancer

Prognostic category
51%–70% expected 3-yr NED survival
31%–50% expected 3-yr NED survival
11%–30% expected 3-yr NED survival
0 –10% expected 3-yr NED survival
Histologic grade
Well or moderately well differentiated
Poorly differentiated or anaplastic
Skin test reactivity
One test > 10 mm or two tests > 5 mm each
Nonreactivity
Standard therapy
Surgery
Radiation therapy
Both

equal distribution of prognostic variables between the two treatments is desirable for a comparative study. The large number of site-stage combinations in head and neck cancer precluded an even distribution of patients using the usual methods of stratification and randomization. Our technique for balancing the two treatment groups as to site of origin and stage was to define the risk of treatment failure at 3 years for each specific site and stage. We divided patients into prognostic categories based on their relative risk of failure as determined by the 3-year disease-free survival results published by the American Joint Committee [1] and, for laryngeal stomal recurrence, on the experience of Sisson [24]. Table 1 displays the four possible prognostic categories for each site and stage using the staging system of the American Joint Committee for Staging [5]. Other stratification variables were the histologic grade of the tumor, skin test reactivity to four common recall antigens including candida, mumps, PPD, and varidase, and the planned standard therapy (Table 2). Treatment of the initial patient in any stratum was randomly assigned using a table of random numbers. Each subsequent patient entered into the same stratum was given the alternative treatment using the method of systematic sampling.

Treatment

The chemotherapy was unmodified from the pilot study except that repeat 2-week courses were also given following surgery and radiation therapy every 3 months for 1 year. Because of the rapid development of resistance by this tumor, repeated intensive courses were thought to be possibly more effective than more frequently repeated but less vigorous treatments. If radiation therapy was given, the second course of chemotherapy was delayed for at least 6 weeks after completion of radiation therapy. The initial dose of methotrexate for each course was always 60 mg/M^2 × 4 independent of dose escalation of previous courses. We have also used sodium bicarbonate to alkalinize the urine during methotrexate treatment [19].

Immunotherapy began 2 weeks after completion of surgery and radiation therapy. Patients randomized to receive immunotherapy received 10^6 Tice strain BCG organisms intradermally on alternate sides of the neck. Those patients randomized to immunotherapy whose tumor was available for vaccine preparation were also given 1×10^6 neuraminidase-treated cells mixed with BCG using a modification of Simmons technique [23]. A single cell suspension was obtained, washed two times, and treated with vibrio cholera neuraminidase (Behring Diagnostics) 25 U per 10^6 cells for 1 h at 37° C. Cell viability varied between 20% and 80% by trypan blue exclusion, being negatively influenced by more than one passage through the mesh screen during preparation of the single cell suspension. Cells were then radiated to 10,000 rad, washed in phosphate buffered saline, and stored quick-frozen at −70° in 0.1 cc quantities (1×10^6 cells) until use. BCG, with the cell vaccine if available, was given every 2 weeks for six treatments and then monthly for 1 year.

Evaluation of Response

Assessment of tumor eradication following surgery and/or radiotherapy was made by complete ENT evaluation including direct laryngoscopyand biopsy of any suspicious areas at monthly intervals. To qualify as being grossly disease free (NED), patients had to have all gross tumor resected at surgery or have complete shrinkage of tumor with radiation. However, positive histologic margins or residual induration did not exclude a patient from being NED. Patients not rendered NED were removed from study and were followed for survival. These patients should not be included in the randomized study results because they were treated palliatively with other therapy and no immunotherapy was given.

Results

Patient Characteristics

Fifty patients have been entered between December 1974 and December 1977. There were 40 males and ten females with an age range of 37–71. Twenty-eight patients were assigned to adjuvant chemotherapy and 22 to adjuvant chemoimmunotherapy. The characteristics of the two patient groups are described in Tables 1 and 2. All the evaluated characteristics were evenly distributed except for histology. The division of patients into prognostic categories appeared successful in maintaining an even balance of patients by site and stage (Table 3). The predominance of moderately well differentiated tumors in the chemoimmunotherapy group and of well and poorly differentiated tumors in the chemotherapy group is evident, but not statistically significant (Table 4). Analysis of the data has shown that this imbalance did not affect the results.

Treatment Results

Thirty-nine of the 50 patients (78%) became grossly disease free with the combination of preoperative chemotherapy and standard therapy and were eligible for follow-up. Eight patients (four in each group) had gross unresectable disease or refused surgery. These were all

Table 3. Patient characteristics divided by treatment group

Characteristic	Treatment group	
	Chemotherapy (No. = 28)	Chemoimmunotherapy (No. = 22)
Sex: M/F	22/6	18/4
Age range (mean)	38–71 (57)	37–70 (59)
Prior therapy		
None	18	14
Surgery	3	1
Radiation	3	4
Both	4	3
Stage		
II	3	2
III	7	7
IV	18	13
Tumor Site		
Oral cavity	7	7
Paranasal sinuses	1	0
Oropharynx	1	4
Nasopharynx	1	0
Hypopharynx	2	4
Larynx	9	6
Cervical esophagus	1	1

stage IV patients who had received prior therapy. In addition, there were three treatment deaths, one from chemotherapy and two from surgery (all stage IV patients).

The recurrence rate for the chemotherapy group was 50% and for the chemoimmunotherapy group was 35%. This difference is not statistically significant. We have further examined those patients who received neuraminidase-treated tumor cells in comparison to those who did not. Four patients randomized to immunotherapy received a vaccine prepared from their own tumor plus BCG.

Table 5 includes an analysis of the immunotherapy group by whether or not tumor cells were given. Three of the four patients who received cells plus BCG have recurred versus 3 of 13 who received BCG without cells. Two of the four patients who received cells had stage III disease and two had stage IV disease. There were two stage II, five stage III, and six stage IV patients in the BCG subgroup, demonstrating no imbalance in disease stage between the group that received cells versus the group that did not. The small number of patients precludes any statistical conclusions as to the effectiveness of the tumor cell vaccine. However, immunotherapy with BCG plus cells is not likely to be more effective than BCG alone. With the difficulty in obtaining an autochthonous tumor preparation and the possibility of tumor enhancement or abrogation of BCG effectiveness with our method of preparation, we have discontinued the vaccine and are continuing the study using BCG only as the immunotherapy.

Table 4. Patient stratification variables divided by treatment groups

	Treatment group	
	Chemotherapy (No. = 28)	Chemoimmunotherapy (No. = 22)
Stratification variable		
Prognostic category		
51%–70%	0	0
31%–50%	7	5
11%–30%	3	4
0 –10%	18	13
Skin tests	20	17
Reactive		
Nonreactive	7	4
Not done	1	1
Histology		
Well	7	2
Moderately well	13	18
Poorly diff.	8	2
Standard therapy		
Surgery	12	12
Radiation	7	4
Both	9	6

Table 5. Results of adjuvant chemoimmunotherapy in head and neck cancer

Treatment	No. of patients				
	Total	Continue NED	Recur	Not NED	Died Rx.
Chemotherapy	28	11	11	4	2
Chemoimmunotherapy					
Total	22	11	6	4	1
Without cells	13	10	3		
With cells	4	1	3		

An analysis by histologic type is displayed in Table 6. The expected trend favoring a well-differentiated histology has not occurred. While it is possible that the chemotherapy has been more effective against the more poorly differentiated histologies negating histology as a risk factor, a larger series of patients is required to evaluate the prognostic effect of tumor differentiation with chemotherapy.

Table 6. Recurrence in disease-free patients (NED) by adjuvant treatment and histologic type

Histology	No. of patients by treatment		
	Chemotherapy	Chemoimmunotherapy	Total
Well			
NED	1	2	3
Recur	5	0	5
Moderately well			
NED	6	9	15
Recur	4	4	8
Poorly diff.			
NED	4	0	4
Recur	2	2	4

Toxicity

Dose-limiting toxicity from the chemotherapy was usually oral stomatitis both from the initial and subsequent courses of therapy. Only four patients (8%) developed thrombocytopenia and/or severe leukopenia requiring a delay in surgery. One drug-related death occurred. This patient developed severe pancytopenia and stomatitis concomitant with transient renal failure and jaundice. He expired from bronchopneumonia with a white count less than 500. No sodium bicarbonate had been given during methotrexate therapy. Since the routine administration of sodium bicarbonate, such renal failure has not occurred in 24 patients so treated. He represents the only drug-related death in 85 patients treated in our combined series. Stomatitis has been a much more severe problem during the course given following surgery and especially radiation therapy, requiring a substantial reduction in methotrexate dosage. Eighty-seven percent of patients had oral ulcerations following radiation therapy but only 40% had similar reactions with the initial course. Moreover, after radiation therapy the stomatitis occurred earlier, often preventing dose escalation and limiting the number of cycles of methotrexate to two (Table 7). Such compromise in dosage supports the use of methotrexate prior to standard therapy and questions the value of its use within the first 6 months following radiation therapy. Two postoperative deaths occurred. One patient had a carotid blowout following an unsuccessful attempt to remove extensive neck disease. The second patient developed meningitis from a fistula following a craniofacial resection of extensive ethmoid sinus cancer. Neither death was drug-related.

Nonspecific Immunologic Monitoring

As a possible marker of the response to immunotherapy, we have longitudinally followed various nonspecific tests of immune function and compared them to the pretreatment values. These tests included delayed hypersensitivity reactions to candida, mumps, PPD and varidase, lymphocyte thymidine uptake as a measure of blastogenic response to a media control

Table 7. Number of patients receiving dose escalation and experiencing mucositis from adjuvant methotrexate with leucovorin. A comparison of the initial course with that given following surgery or radiation therapy

	Course 1	Course 2	
		No radiotherapy	S/P radiotherapy
Dose escalation			
0	11	7	10
1	19 } (77%)	5 } (50%)	4 (29%)
2	17 }	2 }	
Severity of mucositis			
None	11	2	
Mild	17	2	2
Ulceration	19 (40%)	9 (69%)	12 (87%)

and to phytohemagglutinin (PHA), the percentage of T cells as the total T cells using neuraminidase-treated sheep RBCs (SRBC), and immediate, "active", E rosettes as described by WYBRAN [31] and quantitative immunoglobulins including IgM, IgG, and IgA. These tests were performed prior to therapy and then every 3 months following therapy.

As a means of examining the influence of various disease and treatment factors on these tests and in order to assess the pattern of change in these tests with time, we have used the technique of multiple regression analysis. Each value has been made a function of potential influencing variables attempting to establish a linear relationship between changes in the test values and the defined disease and treatment-related characteristics. With this technique the significance of any relationship can be calculated and the contribution of selected variables to the observed variance of the lab value estimated.

The results in the first 40 patients have been tested for significant relationships. The variables we have included are (1) the randomized treatment groups, to assess the influence of immunotherapy on follow-up test values, (2) the disease status divided into continuously disease-free, recurring following a disease-free status, or never disease-free, (3) random variation due to individual patient characteristics other than disease status and treatment as indicated by the study number, (4) changes with increasing time from the point of initial treatment, and (5) whether or not radiation therapy was included in the standard therapy plan. We have indicated the total contribution of these variables taken together as overall variance, "r^2". The test's value is indicated by the significance p. Table 8 displays the results of this analysis. Several conclusions are possible from these results. The major factor influencing PPD reactivity was whether or not BCG was given, but there was less effect from BCG on the other skin tests. Lymphocyte blastogenesis did not have any monitoring value being so strongly influenced by random variability but was depressed to a greater degree following radiation therapy than following other treatment. We and others have demonstrated a decreased percentage of T cells in patients with head and neck cancer prior to treatment [4, 26]. The current analysis supported the inability to normalize this depressed T cell population with any of the treatments given or with time from initiation of treatment. Finally, the immunoglobulins may be affected more than previously appreciated by giving BCG immunotherapy and with increasing time from treatment. There was a decrease in IgM and IgA in

Table 8. Multiple regression analysis of changes in the immunologic parameters monitored in the follow-up period in comparison to the pretherapy value and to each other

Parameter	Treatment group	Disease status	Study No.	Time	± RT	r^2	*P*
Skin test							
PPD	.009	NS	NS	.002	NS	.36	.001
Total	.03	.08	NS	NS	NS	.21	.023
Lymphocyte blastogenesis							
Control	.06	.06	NS	NS	NS	.12	.09
Stimulated	NS	NS	.009	NS	NS	.11	NS
Index	NS	NS	.007	.05	.003	.22	.002
% T cells							
Total	NS	NS	NS	.08	NS	.13	NS
Active	.06	NS	NS	NS	.001	.27	.01
Immunoglobulin							
IgM	.04	.03	NS	.03	NS	.56	.02
IgG	NS	NS	NS	NS	NS	.25	NS
IgA	NS	.04	NS	.009	NS	.50	.04

NS, not significant with $P \geq 0.1$.

those patients not successfully rendered disease free accounting for the significant variance seen with disease status. An increase in the same immunoglobulins (IgM and IgA) was demonstrated in NED patients during the longitudinal follow-up from the time of therapy. None of these tests appear to be useful markers for disease status. The immunoglobulins demonstrated a definite pattern but this was in "not NED" patients whose status was already known. BCG immunotherapy had limited effect on the nonspecific immunologic tests monitored.

Discussion

Immunotherapy of head and neck cancer has had limited study. One report has observed an improved survival when BCG was combined with multiagent chemotherapy over chemotherapy alone in advanced cancer [22]. Remission rate (40% versus 50% for the chemotherapy only group) was, however, not affected. Disease stage, a known prognostic factor in head and neck cancer treated with chemotherapy [16] was not mentioned in that study so one cannot adequately evaluate the significance of the results. Donaldson has published positive results with a combination of methotrexate, isoniazid, and BCG in head and neck cancer [2]. However, his results have become less impressive in subsequent reports as more advanced patients have been entered under controlled conditions [8]. Two subsequent randomized studies, one using methotrexate, BCG, and INH [30], and one using methotrexate and MER [9], have failed to demonstrate any value of immunotherapy in palliative therapy of head and neck squamous cancer. It may be concluded from these studies that current nonspecific immunotherapy has had a limited role in controlling gross metastatic disease.

There is more sound experimental basis for using immunotherapy as an adjuvant to radiation or surgery in head and neck cancer after all gross disease has been removed. Such an approach has been successful in early lung cancer, including squamous cell histology, whereas in late disease categories the same immunotherapy has been valueless [16]. Unfortunately, few randomized studies of adjuvant immunotherapy in head and neck cancer exist. An encouraging preliminary report using levamisole is suggesting benefit from that agent in a randomized study [29]. While it is premature to make any conclusions as to the efficacy of adjuvant immunotherapy in head and neck cancer, the current trends would hopefully stimulate other comparative trials.

The failure to achieve improved results using an autochthonous tumor cell vaccine may possibly be related to the method of preparation or the dose given. We have utilized the method of Simmons, which he found highly tumor specific and effective in animal models [23]. Others have questioned treatment with neuraminidase prior to freezing the cells and the method of quick freezing [2]. The dosage of the cell vaccine is more likely to be a critical factor. Using neuraminidase-treated cells or tumor antigen extract, different doses have been found to increase or decrease tumor growth [12, 17, 25]. These observations appear timely in view of the current interest in specific immunotherapy. It should be equally emphasized, however, that failure to find benefit from a particular dosage of tumor cells or antigen preparation does not exclude effectiveness from other dose levels or preparation methods.

This study has included very advanced disease patients, reflecting the aggressiveness of our surgeons in managing this disease. With 38% of patients having received prior treatment and 62% having stage IV disease, 78% were successfully made disease free and 44% of the total series (56% of NED patients) remain so after a median follow-up of 18 months. Over the last 1 year, we have included stage II primaries other than larynx. Chemotherapy regressions tend to be more dramatic in these earlier stage patients as described by others [6, 20]. One patient had no microscopic evidence of tumor at resection of an originally 4 × 3 cm alveolar ridge primary (biopsy confirmed) following preoperative chemotherapy. A randomized study is currently in progress to further define the value of this chemotherapy.

We have demonstrated the usefulness of a division of patients with head and neck cancer into prognostic categories rather than a division based on stage and site of origin. Such a division based on risk may more accurately reflect expected disease course avoiding an imbalance of prognostic factors if patients had been stratified by anatomic regions. The variable disease course seen in head and neck cancer would appear to make such an approach a worthwhile consideration for future studies.

References

1. American Joint Committee for Cancer Staging and End Results Reporting. Chicago (Ill.) 1965, 1972, 1976
2. Bekesi, J. G., Holland, J. F., Roboz, J. P.: Specific immunotherapy with neuraminidase-modified leukemia cells. Med. Clin. North Am. *61*, 1083–1100 (1977)
3. Caradonna, R., Paladine, W., Goldstein, J. et al.: Combination chemotherapy with high dose cis-diammine-dichloroplatinum (II), methotrexate, and bleomycin for epidermoid carcinoma of the head and neck. Proc. Am. Soc. Clin. Oncol. *C 378*, 401 (1978)
4. Catalona, W. J., Sample, W. F., Chretien, P. B.: Lymphocyte reactivity in cancer patients: correlation with tumor histology and clinical stage. Cancer *31*, 65–70 (1973)

5. Chandler, J. R., Guillamondegui, O. M., Sisson, G. A. et al.: Clinical staging of cancer of the head and neck: A new "new" system. Am. J. Surg. *132,* 525–528 (1976)
6. DeConti, R. C.: Phase III comparison of methotrexate with leucovorin vs. methotrexate alone vs. a combination of methotrexate plus leucovorin, cyclophosphamide and cytosine arabinoside in head and neck cancer. Proc. Am. Soc. Clin. Oncol. *C 46,* 248 (1976)
7. Donaldson, R. C.: Methotrexate plus bacillus Calmette-Guerin (BCG) and isoniazid in the treatment of cancer of the head and neck. Am. J. Surg. *124,* 527–534 (1972)
8. Donaldson, R. C.: Chemoimmunotherapy for cancer of the head and neck. Am. J. Surg. *126,* 507–512 (1973)
9. Donaldson, R., Banda, F., Keehn, R.: Methotrexate plus MER for head and neck cancer. Immunity: Solid tumor therapy. Crispen, R. G. (ed.), pp. 243–248. Franklin Inst. 1977
10. Eilber, F. R., Morton, D. L.: Adjuvant chemoimmunotherapy in advanced lesions of the head and neck. Am. J. Roentgenol. Rad. Ther. Nucl. Med. *126,* 1082–1087 (1976)
11. Feinstein, A. R.: Clinical Biostatistics. pp. 385–413. St. Louis: C. V. Mosby 1977
12. Froese, G., Berczi, I., Sehon, A. H.: Neuraminidase-induced enhancement of tumor growth in mice. J. Natl. Cancer Inst. *52,* 1905–1908 (1974)
13. Jesse, R. H., Lindberg, R. D.: The efficacy of combining radiation therapy with a surgical procedure in patients with cervical metastatis from squamous cancer of the oropharynx and hypopharynx. Cancer *35,* 1163–1166 (1975)
14. Knowlton, A. H., Percarpio, B., Bobrow, S. et al.: Methotrexate and radiation therapy in the treatment of advanced head and neck tumors. Radiology *116,* 709–712 (1975)
15. Kramer, S.: Methotrexate and radiation therapy in the treatment of advanced squamous cell carcinoma of the oral cavity, oropharynx, supraglottic larynx, and hypopharynx. Can. J. Otolaryngol. *4,* 213–218 (1975)
16. McKneally, M. F., Maver, C.: Regional immunotherapy using intrapleural BCG and isoniazid for resectable lung cancer: Results in the first 100 cases. In: Adjuvant therapy of cancer. Salmon, S. E., Jones, S. E. (eds.), pp. 207–216. Amsterdam: Elsevier/North Holland 1977
17. Pellis, N. R., Kahan, B. D.: Specific tumor immunity induced with soluble materials: Restricted range of antigen dose and of c challenge tumor load for immunoprotection. J. Immunol. *115,* 1717–1722 (1975)
18. Peto, R., Pike, M. C., Armitage, P. et al.: Design and analysis of randomized clinical trials requiring prolonged observation of each patient. Br. J. Cancer *34,* 585–612 (1976)
19. Pitman, S., Landwehr, D., Jaffe, N., Frei, E., III: Methotrexate citrovorum: Effect of alkalinization on nephrotoxicity and of weekly schedule on response. Proc. Amer. Assoc. Cancer Res. *17,* 129 (1976)
20. Pitman, S. W., Miller, D., Weichselbaum, R., Frei, E., III: Weekly high dose methotrexate with leucovorin rescue as initial adjuvant therapy in advanced squamous cell carcinoma of the head and neck: A pilot study. In: Adjuvant therapy of Cancer. Salmon, S. E., Jones, S. E. (eds.). Amsterdam: North Holland 1977
21. Richard, J. M., Sancho, H., Lepintre, Y. et al.: Intra-arterial methotrexate chemotherapy and telecobalt therapy in cancer of the oral cavity and oropharynx. Cancer *34,* 491–496 (1974)
22. Richman, S. P., Livingston, R. B., Gutterman, J. U. et al.: Chemotherapy versus chemoimmunotherapy of head and neck cancer: Report of a randomized study. Cancer Treat. Rep. *60,* 535–539 (1976)
23. Rios, A., Simmons, R. L.: Experimental cancer immunotherapy using a neuraminidase-treated non-viable frozen tumor vaccine. Surgery *75,* 503–507 (1974)
24. Sisson, G. A., Bytell, D. E., Becker, S. P.: Mediastinal – 1976: Indications and new techniques. Laryngoscope *87,* 751–759 (1977)
25. Sparks, F. C., Breeding, J. H.: Tumor regression and enhancement resulting from immunotherapy with *Bacillus Calmette-Guerin* and neuraminidase. Cancer Res. *34,* 3262–3269 (1974)

26. Taylor, S., Bytell, D., Sisson, G. A. et al.: Chemoimmunotherapy as adjuvant to surgery and radiotherapy in stage III–IV head and neck squamous cancer patients. Neoplasm immunity: solid tumor therapy. Crispen, R. G. (ed.), pp. 249–266. Chicago: Franklin Inst. 1977
27. Taylor, S. G., IV, Bytell, D. E., DeWys, W. D.: Adjuvant methotrexate and leucovorin in head and neck squamous cancer. Arch. Otolaryngology (1978) (to be published)
28. von Essen, C. F., Joseph, L., Simon, G. et al.: Sequential chemotherapy and radiation therapy of buccal mucosa carcinoma in So. India. Am. J. Roentgenol. Radium Ther. Nucl. Med. *102,* 530–540 (1968)
29. Wanebo, H. J., Hilal, E. Y., Strong, E. W.: Randomized trial of levamisole in patients with squamous cancer of head and neck. Am. Soc. Clin. Oncology C 189 (1978)
30. Woods, J. E., DeSanto, L. W., Ritts, R. E. (Jr.): A controlled study of combined methotrexate, BCG, and INH therapy for squamous cell carcinoma of the head and neck. Surg. Clin. North Am. *57,* 769–778 (1977)
31. Wybran, J., Fudenberg, H. H.: Thymus-derived rosette-forming cells in various human disease states: Cancer, lymphoma, bacterial and viral infection and other diseases. J. Clin. Invest. *52,* 1026–1032 (1973)

Adjuvant Treatment of Tongue and Floor of the Mouth Cancers

H. Szpirglas, Cl. Chastang, and J. Ch. Bertrand

Introduction

Chemotherapy of head and neck cancers gives objective responses in about 30% of the cases, sometimes spectacular but never durable enough to significantly after prognosis. One of its limitations seems to be related to the tumor mass. It is, therefore, important to test chemotherapy on the residual cells, which are not visible, but are responsible for local, regional, or distant relapses after apparently satisfactory local treatment. These residual cells are also the proposed target for adjuvant *immunotherapy*.

Materials and Methods

Since January 1974 we have treated 136 patients, with squamous cell (epidermoid) carcinoma of the oral cavity. Of the patients, 95 had cancer of the anterior tongue or the floor of the mouth, which will only be considered in this study.
The staging was either stage A corresponding to T1–T2 N0 tumors treated only by electrosurgery or stage B corresponding to T3 N0 and T1-T2-T3 N^+ tumors of which there were two groups: one treated by surgery alone, the other by surgery followed by radiotherapy when invasion of lymph nodes was found histologically after neck dissection. Patients with extremely large tumors and those associated with fixed nodes are associated with only transient complete remissions were not considered in this trial.

Randomization

Patients in remission after initial treatment were randomized into three groups:
1. No treatment;
2. Chemotherapy;
3. Immunotherapy.

Chemotherapy

The protocol we chose was the one we used frequently in 1973 and combined methotrexate (400 mg per month given by intravenous infusion) followed by intramuscular injection of 100 mg of citrovorum factor and bleomycin in two 15-mg doses intramuscularly per week. The total dose of bleomycin never exceeded 450 mg in 15 weeks of treatment because of the cumulative toxicity of this product. Methotrexate was administered for 2 years.

Immunotherapy

Immunotherapy consisted of subcutaneous or intramuscular injection of 2 ml of Corynebacterium parvum every week for 2 years. The Corynebacterium parvum vaccine was furnished by Merieux Laboratories with new lots delivered every 2 months. Some minor modifications in preparation could therefore have affected the vaccine.

Routine Observation

An evaluation was made at least every 2 months and included a locoregional examination and a general examination to detect local recurrence, evolution or recurrence in lymph nodes, and metastatic spread. A clinical assessment, in addition to its usefulness in the detection of metastases, permitted the evaluation of tolerance to adjuvant treatments.

Results

This trial initiated in January 1974 used a computer program prepared by the INSERM Unit 88. The file was brought up to date on 15 June 1978. We used the classic methods of statistical analysis and *the log rank test* to compare the recurrence and survival curves.

Distribution

The distribution of the 95 patients is shown in Table 1.

Table 1. Distribution of 95 patients with floor of mouth and tongue cancers entered on the randomized adjuvant trial

			No. treat.	Chemo.	Immuno.
Stage A:	Surgery	45 pts	16	16	13
Stage B:	Surgery	27 pts	10	8	9
	Surgery + Radiotherapy	23 pts	7	8	8

Recurrences

Overall analysis: the rate of recurrence reached 50% for all patients by 2 years. After 2 years, of the 37 patients still at risk there was only one recurrence at 27 months. Figure 1 shows the remission curves for the different adjuvant treatments for all patients. A significant difference is not evident according to the log rank test ($P = 0.60$). However, we observed a delay in the onset of recurrences in the groups receiving chemotherapy or immunotherapy. The difference

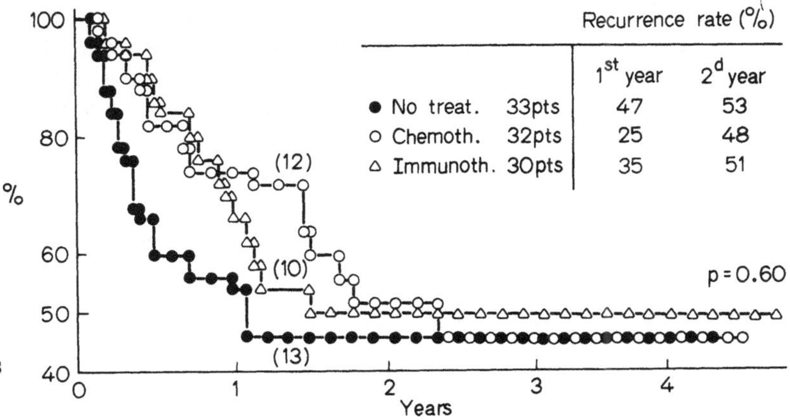

Fig. 1. Remission curves for different adjuvant treatments

in recurrence rate diminished with time. At 1 year, 25% of the patients under chemotherapy, 35% of those under immunotherapy, and 47% of those under simple observation had recurrences. At 2 years, we observed 48% recurrences under chemotherapy, 51% under immunotherapy, and 53% of nontreated patients.

Analysis by Patient Group

For stage A (T1-T2 N0, surgery only: 45 patients), the overall recurrence rate reached 45% at 2 years. Of the remaining 17 patients still at risk, there were no recurrences (Fig. 2). There was no significant difference shown by the log rank test, but with adjuvant therapy a delay in the time to recurrence was observed:

1. Recurrence at 1 year: no treatment 44%, chemotherapy 19% and immunotherapy 33%. However, this favorable effect seems to diminish in time without disappearing entirely.
2. Recurrence at 2 years: no treatment 50%, chemotherapy 46%, and immunotherapy 41%.

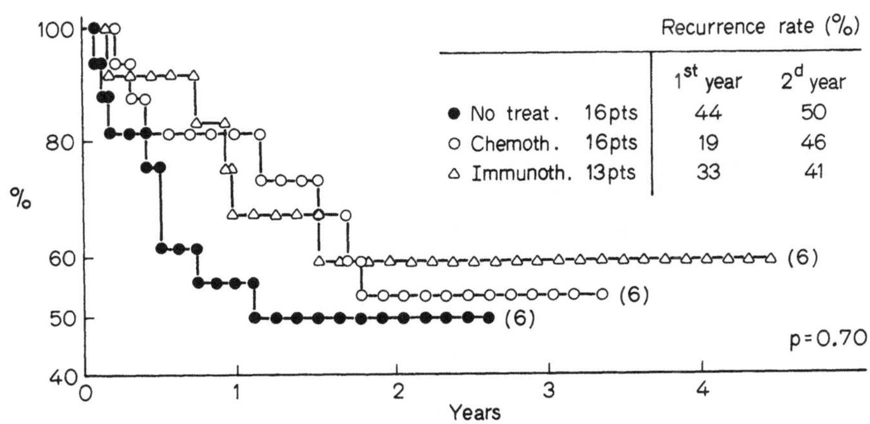

Fig. 2. Disease-free interval and recurrence rate for stage A (T1-T2 N0) patients

For stage B (surgery only: 27 patients), the overall recurrence rate reached 61% at 2 years. Seven patients had no recurrence beyond 2 years (Fig. 3). The log rank test was not significant ($P = 0.43$). A delay in the onset of the recurrences was always noted with adjuvant treatment. The favorable, but diminished effect remained for the group undergoing chemotherapy:

1. Recurrence at 1 year: no treatment 67%, chemotherapy 25%, and immunotherapy 38%.
2. Recurrence at 2 years: no treatment 67%, chemotherapy 55%, and immunotherapy 69%.

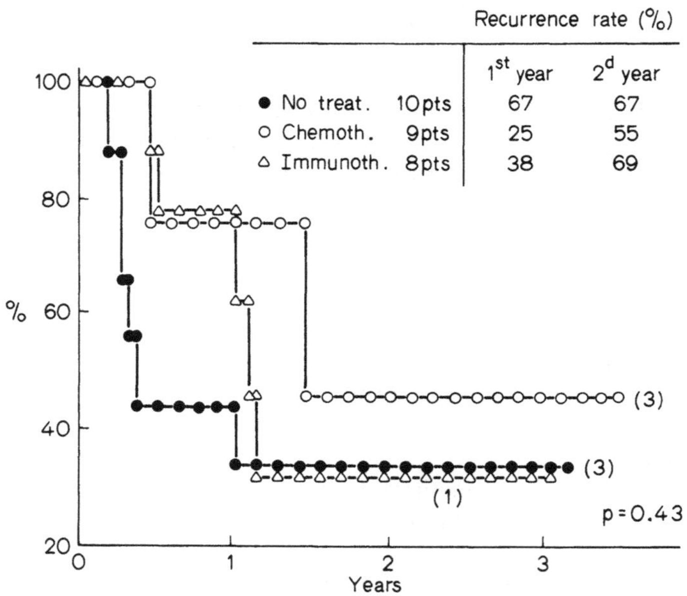

Fig. 3. Disease-free interval and recurrence rate for stage B (surgery only) patients

For stage B (surgery + radiotherapy: 23 patients), we observed 46% recurrences at 2 years, and one patient of ten remaining after 2 years relapsed (Fig. 4). The log rank test was not significant ($P = 0.92$). Contrary to groups 1 and 2, the three curves run parallel. There was no delay in recurrence under treatment, and at 3 years patients without adjuvant treatment had fewer recurrences.

1. Recurrence at 1 year: no treatment 29%, chemotherapy 42%, and immunotherapy 38%.
2. Recurrence at 2 years: no treatment 43%, chemotherapy 42%, and immunotherapy 53%.

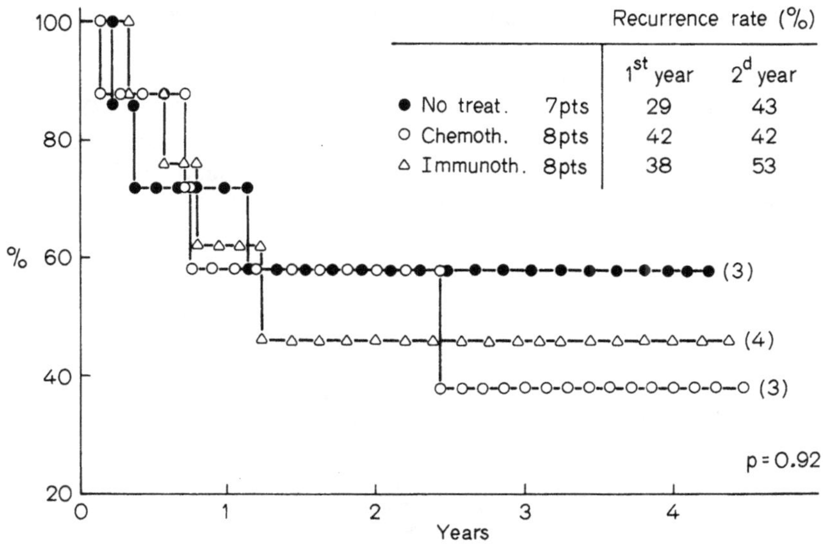

Fig. 4. Disease-free interval and recurrence rate for stage B (surgery + radiotherapy) patients

Nature of Recurrences

The study of the nature of the recurrences showed a significant difference depending on whether or not the patient had adjuvant treatment, regardless which type ($P = 0.05$) (Fig. 5). While the total number of recurrences was comparable in each group, the patients treated with chemotherapy or immunotherapy developed 2 lymph node evolutions and 25 local recurrences, while nontreated patients presented 6 lymph node evolutions and 11 local relapses. We did not observe spread to lymph nodes in patients receiving chemotherapy; however, we observed two metastatic evolutions during chemotherapy in the surgery + radiotherapy group. One of these occurred 2 months after randomization and after methotrexate alone and can hardly be attributed to treatment. The other, however, occurred after 26 months, even though the locoregional area was free of relapse.

Recurrences
15.06.78 - 46 Cases

	No treat. 17	Chemoth. 15	Immuno. 14
Local recur.	11	13	12
Node evol.	6	—	2
Metast.	—	2	—

	Stage A surgery			Stage B surgery			Stage B surgery + radioth.		
	No treat.	Chemoth.	Immuno.	No treat.	Chemoth.	Immuno.	No treat.	Chemoth.	Immuno.
Local recurrence	5	7	4	3	4	4	3	2	4
Node evolution	3	—	1	3	—	1	—	—	—
Metastic evol.	—	—	—	—	—	—	—	2	—

Fig. 5. Nature of recurrences according to adjuvant treatment

Overall Survival According to Adjuvant Treatment

For all 95 patients, Fig. 6 shows that the evolution was rigorously the same, whatever the adjuvant treatment (the log rank test was not significant, $P = 0.93$). The study of the overall survival in relation to staging (Fig. 7) shows a short-term prognostic improvement that does not prove to be significant ($P = 0.14$). At 2 years, the survival of the stage A patients is 90%, compared to 80% for stage B surgery alone and 63% for stage B surgery + radiotherapy.

		Survival rate (%)			
	years	1	2	3	4
● No treat.	33pts	88	81	58	58
○ Chemoth.	32pts	87	84	58	58
△ Immunoth.	30pts	86	79	70	58

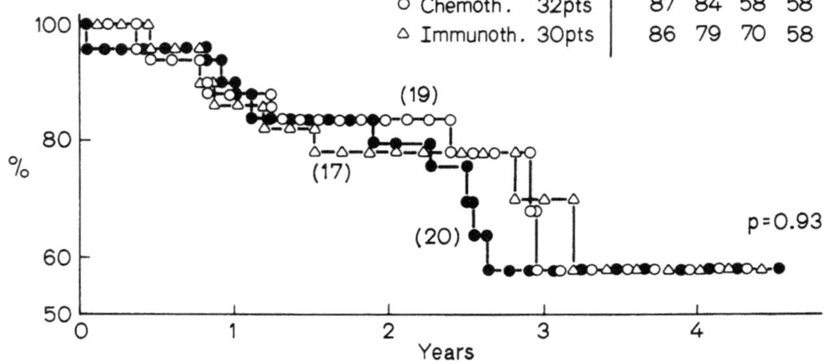

Fig. 6. Overall survival according to adjuvant treatment

		Survival rate (%)			
		1st year	2d year	3d year	4th year
● Stage A: surg.	45pts	95	90	59	59
○ Stage B: surg.	27pts	84	80	66	66
△ Stage B: surg.+ rad.	23pts	73	63	52	45

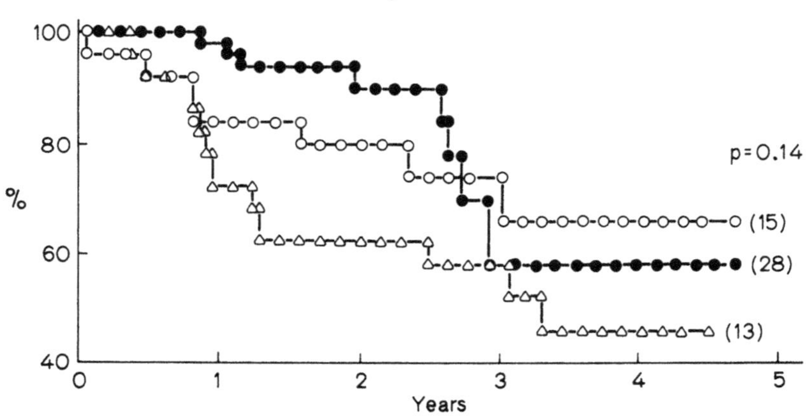

Fig. 7. Overall survival according to staging

However, in the 3rd year, four deaths were recorded among the 15 patients having reached 2 years in the first group, and the survival rates after that are completely comparable. This may be considered when dealing with high risk or low risk patients.

Survival in Each Group

For stage A (T1-T2 N0), *a significant difference* appears depending on the adjuvant treatment ($P = 0.01$). Of the four deaths between 2 and 3 years in this group, three were nontreated patients (Fig. 8). Of the 16 nontreated patients six died, while the egality hypothesis predicted two deaths. In contrast, one death was recorded among 16 patients receiving chemotherapy compared to 3.2 expected, and one death was recorded among 13 patients receiving immunotherapy compared to 2.7 expected. Except for one patient for whom the cause of death was unknown, all the deaths were observed after recurrence and were due to progressive cancer.

For stage B (surgery only), analysis of survival does not show a significant difference ($P = 0.67$) (Fig. 9). The curves were superimposable. One of the two deaths recorded in the nontreated group was of a patient without recurrence.

For stage B (surgery + radiotherapy), up to 1 year, the three curves were also superimposable (Fig. 10). After 1 year, no additional deaths were observed among the nontreated patients,

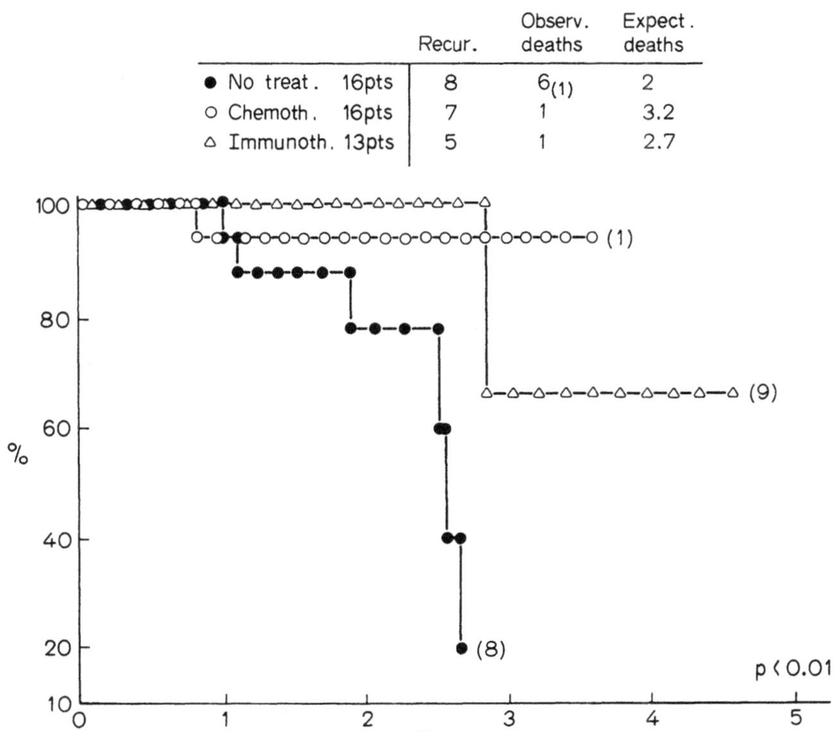

Fig. 8. Survival according to adjuvant treatment for stage A (T1-T2 N0) patients

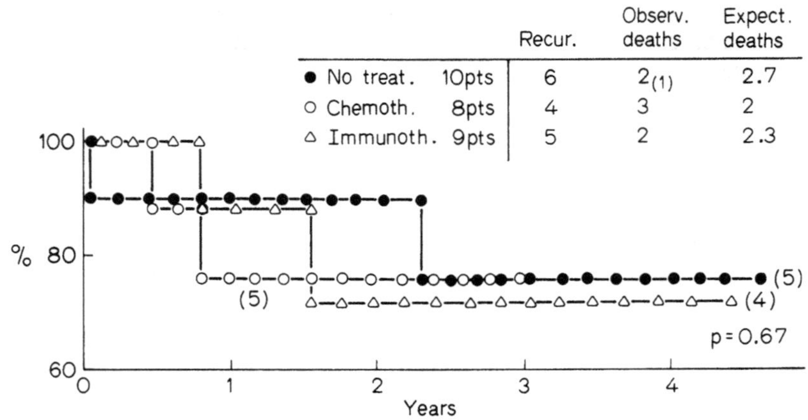

Fig. 9. Survival according to adjuvant treatment for stage B (surgery only) patients

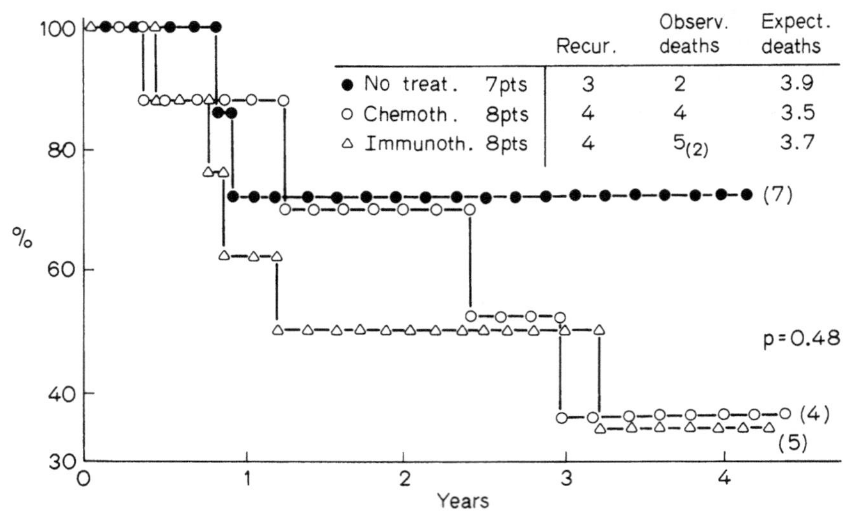

Fig. 10. Survival according to adjuvant treatment for stage B (surgery + radiotherapy) patients

while three deaths were recorded among the patients undergoing adjuvant therapy. The log rank test was not significant ($P = 0.48$). It is noteworthy that two of the deaths recorded in the immunotherapy group were not due to cancer.

Survival After Recurrence

Figure 11 shows that the group of patients undergoing chemotherapy had the least favorable course after recurrence, which is logical because previously untreated patients could receive palliative chemotherapy after recurrence.

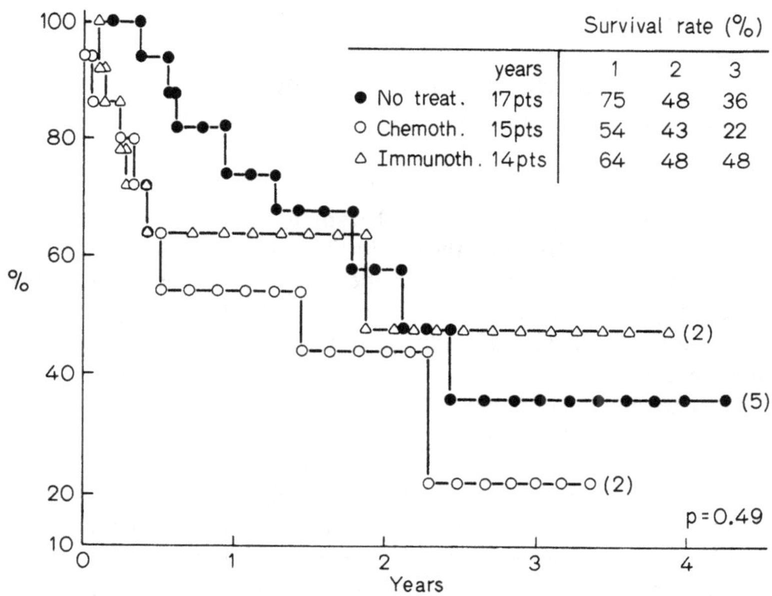

Fig. 11. Survival after recurrence according to adjuvant treatment

Conclusion

The results presented here were disappointing, considering the encouraging results we found after the first analysis 2 years ago. This may depend on the choice of therapies, and other programs of adjuvant chemotherapy and immunotherapy are presently employed. We can see, however, that adjuvant treatment can delay the recurrences but does not decrease the recurrence rate and adds nothing when patients have previously received radiotherapy. While it may seem paradoxical that patients with small tumors would benefit more from adjuvant treatment, this result could be anticipated if treatment is of limited potency.

Summary

Since January 1974, 95 patients with anterior tongue and floor of the mouth cancers were included in a randomized trial. After stratification according to staging and initial treatment, one-third of the patients received chemotherapy for 2 years (methotrexate 400 mg followed by citrovorum factor 100 mg + bleomycin 30 mg/week, during the first 15 weeks), one-third of the patients received immunotherapy with weekly C. parvum injections during 2 years, while the remaining third did not receive any treatment. If adjuvant treatment seems to delay recurrence it did not significantly decrease the recurrence rate. Survival is also not significantly modified by adjuvant treatment and was better for patients with small tumors. Patients who previously received radiotherapy did not benefit from adjuvant therapy.

First Results of a Randomized Trial on Immunotherapy of Head and Neck Tumors

J. L. Amiel, H. Sancho-Garnier, C. Vandenbrouck, F. Eschwege, J. P. Droz, G. Schwaab, P. Wibault, M. Stromboni, and A. Rey

Trials of active nonspecific immunotherapy as adjuvant therapy for tumors have increased dramatically in number since the results that have been published on acute leukemia [6] and melanoma [3, 5, 7–9]. In spite of considerable work [4], the justification of immunotherapy in cancerology has made hardly any progress, and the results remain controversial [10]. In numerous cases, the actual conditions of the trials undertaken do not seem satisfactory. An example is the application of immunotherapy to patients still carrying massive tumoral growths, despite the fact that this contravenes experimental data [1] and also discredits the interpretation because of many other intervening factors; furthermore, the influence of the symptomatic treatments necessarily associated confuses the observed results.

Sometimes the methodology of the trial allows right conclusions. A trial where the association of chemotherapy and immunotherapy is compared with immunotherapy alone can hardly demonstrate as evidence the proper efficacy of immunotherapy. Besides, numerous trials dealing with historical comparisons, if they sometimes have a real interest, are never totally convincing, however sophisticated they are. Finally, in some cases, the behavior of immunotherapy-treated and untreated groups may differ by such a small percentage rate that it is doubtful that the effect can be shown with a reasonable number of patients in a suitable time period. Consequently, it appears to us that an immunotherapy trial on solid tumors can really give results only if certain conditions are met:

1. The trial must be randomized;
2. Immunotherapy must be used by itself and compared to the absence of adjuvant therapy;
3. The group of patients participating in the trial must be homogenous with regard to the clinical state, i.e., to be without detectable tumor growth;
4. The criteria needed to assess the result has to be an objective one, i.e., disease-free interval, survival rate;
5. The response of the group studied must be bad enough to evidence a difference between treated and untreated patients if any.

Furthermore, these conditions assume that the patients are in complete remission after locoregional treatment and that they cannot benefit from any other kind of treatment such as chemotherapy.

All these stipulations are apparently met in cases of larynx and hypopharynx tumors that have been locally treated in a radical way by surgery and radiotherapy [2]. Although patients could be considered to be in complete remission, they have a high percentage of recurrences that lead to low survival rates. Systematic chemotherapy has given poor results and is very difficult to apply regularly to such patients who are often alcoholic and in a generally poor condition.

In 1973 we decided to begin a randomized clinical trial within the head and neck department of the Gustave Roussy Center. Patients with epithelioma of the larynx or hypopharynx capable of total surgery, either with or without radiotherapy, were eligible. All the diagnoses have been histologically confirmed by biopsy. The pathologic examination of the surgical specimen permits us to ascertain the completeness of the resection. Metastasis, second primary tumor, (except skin epithelioma), contraindications to BCG therapy, previous chemotherapy or radiotherapy, and incomplete macroscopic resection were the criteria for ineligibility. The delay between the end of the first therapeutic sequence (surgery with or without radiotherapy) must be less than or equal to 1 month.

The first treatment for each patient is surgical. The type of the intervention depends upon the sites and the extension of the tumor, i.e., in laryngeal tumor immediate total laryngectomy or partial laryngectomy for patients not previously treated, secondary total laryngectomy for patients having recurrence after first partial laryngectomy, and laryngopharyngectomy for hypopharynx tumor. Except for secondary total laryngectomy, surgery is followed with radiotherapy on the tumoral bed and on the area of the cervical nodes. The dose is 5000–6000 rad according to the target volume.

At the end of this sequence and if the patient is still eligible for the trial, he is given at random a BCG treatment or nothing (control group). Three vials of live Pasteur BCG are applied once a week on scarifications (areas: 5 cm × 5 cm) on the limbs. After having verified the patients reactions, the BCG can be followed up usually by the family doctor for a period of 1 year. However, the patients should be examined every 2 months at the hospital.

The determined criteria for assessment are, on the one hand, the survival curve and, on the other hand, the development of carcinologic events, i.e., local or regional recurrences, metastasis, and second primary tumor. Between January 1974 and May 1977, 129 patients were randomized into the two groups. One case from each group was erroneously included (contraindications to the BCG treatment), and they have been excluded from the present analysis, which is made up of 62 cases in the BCG group and 65 in the control group. Table 1 gives the distribution according to the type of surgery that was the stratification criterion. Tables 2, 3, and 4 describe the distribution according to the main prognostic factors, i.e., tumor sites, TN (from UICC classification), and histologic node involvement. No statistical differences between the two groups have been observed.

Figure 1 shows the histogram of the duration of the BCG treatment for the patients who have already finished it. Twenty cases did not receive the 1 year of BCG. In eight cases, treatment was stopped due to a development of recurrences or metastasis or second primary; in 11 other cases the patients refused the follow-up, and in one case the BCG was terminated after 1 month because of the negativity of the tuberculin skin test.

In the two groups, 50% of the patients have had at least a 2-year follow-up; one-third have been followed for at least 3 years. No patients have been lost to follow up and all the causes of

Table 1. Distribution of patients stratified by type of surgery

	Without BCG	With BCG	Excluded
Total pharyngolaryngectomy or total laryngectomy (salvage)	42	39	1 (Without BCG)
Primary total laryngectomy	23	23	1 (With BCG)
Total	65	62	2

Table 2. Distribution of patients according to tumor site

	Hypopharynx		Supraglottis		Glottis		Subglottis		Marginal zone	
Without BCG	42%	(27)	18%	(12)	5%	(3)	17%	(11)	18%	(12)
With BCG	32%	(20)	24%	(15)	10%	(6)	16%	(10)	18%	(11)

Table 3. Distribution of patients according to TN classification (UICC)

	T1		T2		T3		T4		N0+N1a+N2a		N1b+N2b		N3	
Without BCG	5%	(3)	16%	(9)	79%	(46)	–		49%	(28)	17%	(10)	34%	(20)
With BCG	4%	(2)	–		91%	(50)	5%	(3)	45%	(25)	20%	(11)	35%	(19)

Table 4. Distribution of patients according to histologic node involvement

	N–		N+R–		N+R+	
Without BCG	32%	(18)	19%	(11)	49%	(28)
With BCG	25%	(14)	28%	(16)	47%	(27)

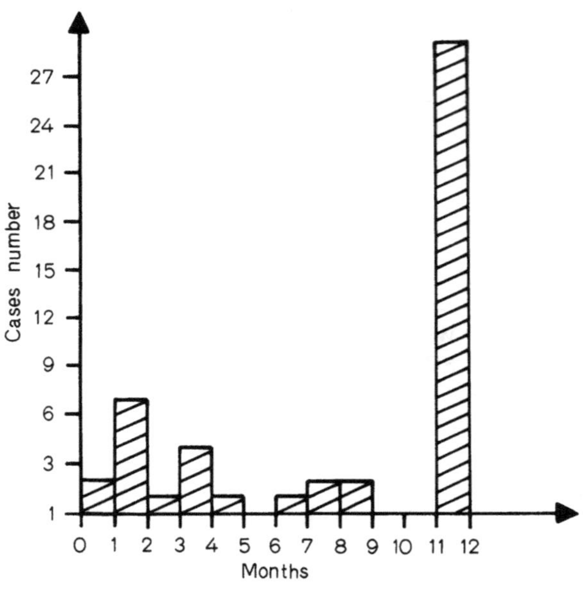

Fig. 1. Distribution of duration of BCG therapy (patients still on treatment are excluded)

Table 5. Patient status

	Alive	Dead	Causes of death		Carcinologic evolution Alive + dead
			Cancers	Others	
Without BCG	41 (4 with recurrences)	24	21	3	25
With BCG	48 (2 with recurrences)	14	11	3	13

Table 6. Detailed causes of death

	Cancers	Others
Without BCG	8 Local recurrences 3 Local recurrences + metastasis 1 Local recurrence + second primary 5 Metastases 3 Second primary tumor	1 Car crash 1 Arteritis 1 Gastric ulcus
With BCG	5 Local recurrences 1 Local recurrences +metastasis 4 Metastases 1 Second primary tumor	1 Postsurgical hemorrhage 2 Ruptures of carotid artery

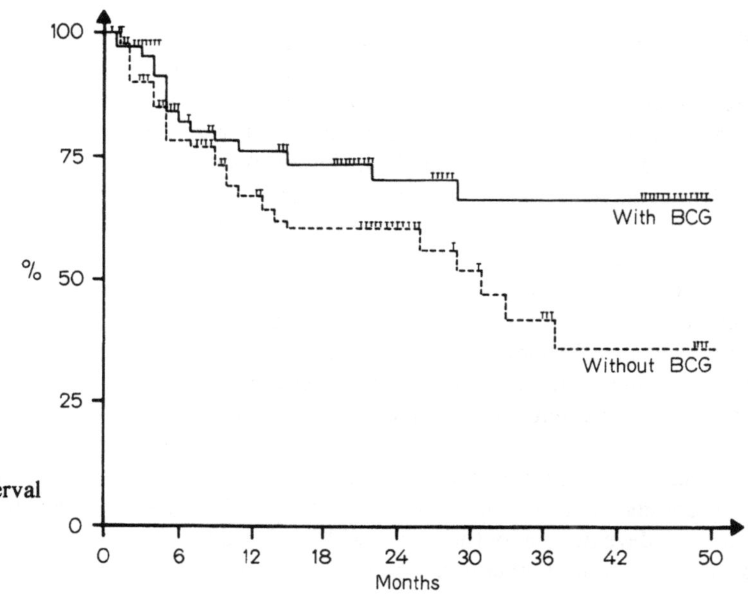

Fig. 2. Disease-free interval (June 1978)

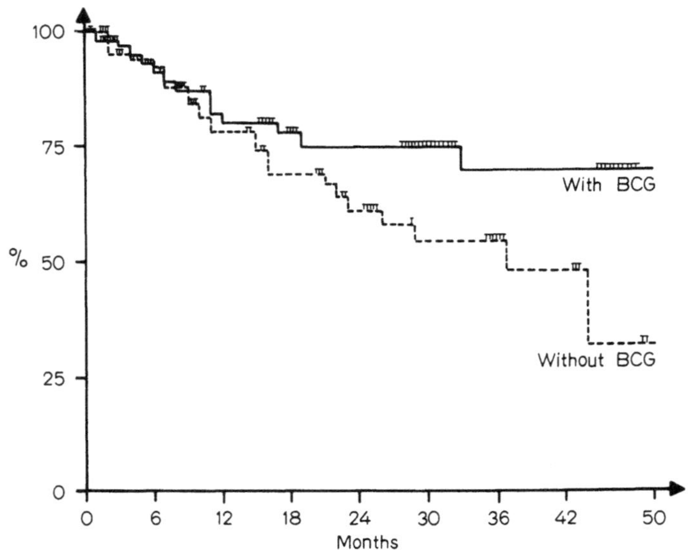

Fig. 3. Survival curves (Kaplan and Meier) (June 1978)

death are known. The first results were analyzed generally (Tables 5 and 6) and then (Figs. 2 and 3) in more depth, taking into account the time element. In both methods the group of patients treated by BCG seems to differ from the control group in a lower number of deaths and by an even lower number of carcinologic events. The differences are not, however, statistically significant when one compares the curves by the log rank test.

Discussion

The results of this trial have already brought out a difference (nonsignificant) between the group treated by BCG and the control group. The difference was noticed in spite of interfering factors such as deaths due to other than cancer-related causes and premature termination of immunotherapy because of lack of discipline. The group of randomized patients with BCG who refused it is, however, numerically low (18%) considering the usual lack of compliance of such patients who are often alcoholic and unstable. In this subgroup of 11 patients, there are four carcinologic events that do not vary from the other 25 of 65 observed in the group without BCG.

It is interesting to note that the difference between the two groups becomes more evident with time, which is logical for immunotherapy. In fact, we know by animal experimentation that active and specific immunotherapy can only act on a very small number of malignant residual cells. It is thus logical that the difference between the two groups is especially evident for later cancer-related events. The frequent initial recurrences that are due to larger residuals of neoplasic cells have less chance to be influenced by immunotherapy. It remains to be seen whether or not the two curves will converge later on; if they do, it would mean that we would have obtained only a prolongation of the disease-free interval instead of a definitive cure. Any expected development of the curves will furnish indications on how to adjust techniques and duration of immunotherapy, which were empirically fixed previously.

We have already found these results interesting: immunotherapy by BCG is better supported than was supposed and better accepted than we had hoped at the beginning of the trial. Immunotherapy seems to have efficacy after complete locoregional treatment in laryngeal and hypopharyngeal tumors. We hope that the results of this trial will in the long run and in the initial analysis of our trial will be substantiated with more cases and longer followup.

References

1. Amiel, J. L., Berardet, M.: Factor time for active immunotherapy after cytoreductive chemotherapy. Eur. J. Cancer. *10,* 89 (1974)
2. Amiel, J. L., Sancho, H., Vandenbrouck, C.: Note préliminaire sur un essai d'immunotherapie active par le BCG pour des tumeurs ORL. Bull. Cancer. *63,* 287–288 (1976)
3. Eibler, F. R., Morton, D. L., Holmes, E. D., Sparks, F. C., Ramming, K. P.: Adjuvant immunotherapy with BCG in treatment of regional-lymphnode metastasis from malignant melanoma. N. Engl. J. Med. *294,* 237–240 (1976)
4. International Registry of Tumor Immunotherapy: Compendium of Tumor Immunotherapy Protocols. N° 5. September 1977
5. Jewell, W. R., Thomas, J. H., Sterchi, J. M., Morse, P. A., Humphrey, L. J.: Critical Analysis of Treatment of Stage II en Stage III Melanoma Patients with immunotherapy. Ann. Surg. *183,* 543–549 (1976)
6. Mathe, G., Amiel, J. L., Schwarzenberg, L., Schneider, M., Cattan, A., Schlumberger, J. R., Hryat, M. de Vassal, F.: First results of active immunotherapy in the treatment of acute lymphoblastic leukaemia in man. Lancet *1969/1,* 697
7. McCulloch, P. B., Dent, P. B., Blajchman, M., Muirhead, W. M., Price, R. A.: Recurrent malignant melanoma: effect of adjuvant immunotherapy on survival. CMA J. *117* (1977)
8. Morton, D. L., Eilber, F. R., Holmes, E. C., Sparks, F. C., Ramming, K. P.: Present status of BCG immunotherapy of malignant melanoma. Cancer Immunol. Immunother. *1,* 93–98 (1976)
9. Newlands, E. S., Oon, C. J., Roberts, J. T., Elliott, P., Mould, R. F., Topham, C., Madden, F. J. F., Newton, K. A., Westbury, G.: Clinical trial of combination chemotherapy and specific active immunotherapy in disseminated melanoma. Br. J. Cancer. *34,* 174 (1976)
10. UICC: Controlled Therapeutic Trials in Cancer. Technical Report Series *14,* Geneva 1974

Adjuvant Trial of Levamisole in Patients With Squamous Cancer of the Head and Neck: A Preliminary Report[1]

H. J. Wanebo[2, 3], E. Y. Hilal[2], E. W. Strong[2], C. M. Pinsky[2], V. Mike[2], and H. F. Oettgen[2]

The goal of this study was to evaluate whether adjuvant therapy with the immune modulator levamisole could reduce the recurrence rate and possibly increase the survival rate in patients with squamous cancer of the head and neck. A secondary goal was to evaluate whether this type of immunotherapy could affect the known immunosuppression of these patients.
A double-blind study was initiated in which patients were randomized after surgery to receive levamisole or a placebo. Levamisole was given as tablets, 150 mg three times weekly on alternate weeks for a planned 2-year period. Prior to randomization, all patients were stratified according to *type of disease*, primary or recurrent; *site of disease*, oral cavity, pharynx or larynx; and *stage* I–IV. All patients had careful clinical follow-up at 2-month intervals and in addition received immunologic tests at 2–4 month periods.

Background

In squamous cancer of the head and neck, recurrence at the primary site or in the neck is the most common cause of death. The rate of recurrence varies with the type of disease, primary or secondary, the site, and the stage. In the study by Farr et al. of 1405 patients with squamous cancer of the mouth and pharynx (MSKCC) the recurrence rate ranged from 30% for cancer of anterior tongue to 73% for base of tongue [5]. The 5-year cure rate ranged from 42% for primary cases to 20% for secondary cases. The cure rate also related to stage with 5-year survival figures of 89% for stage I, 59% for stage II, 33% for stage III, and 8% for stage IV.

A second major feature of head and neck squamous cancer is the accompanying immunosuppression [3, 6, 8, 15, 16]. Approximately 30–50% of these patients have depressed immune function studies as demonstrated by skin tests and in vitro lymphocyte function studies prior to treatment [6, 16]. There is a significant correlation of the patient's recurrence rates with the DNCB response in patients with stage I and II cancer [6]. There is no correlation of any of the in vitro tests with prognosis.

Levamisole is a phenylimidazothiazole that had been initially developed as an antihelminthic agent. It was first demonstrated to have immunorestorative effects by Renoux and Renoux, who found that it increased the protective effect of antibrucella vaccination in mice [10, 11]. Since then a rapidly expanding literature has documented the immunopotentiating effects of this compound (recently reviewed by Symoens, 1977) [14].

---

1 This work was supported by Contract No. NO1-CB-53875 Division of Cancer, Biology and Diagnosis, from the National Cancer Institute, National Institute of Health, Department of Health, Education and Welfare, and generous funds from the Cancer Research Institute (New York). Dr. Wanebo was a recipient of the American Cancer Society Junior Clinical Faculty Fellowship.

2 Memorial Sloan Kettering Cancer Center, New York, NY 10021.

3 Present address: Department of Surgery, University of Virginia Medical Center, Charlottesville, VA 22901.

Controlled clinical trials have provided evidence of antitumor effects of this agent in man [1, 2]. ROJAS et al. have reported significant beneficial effects of levamisole on recurrence rates and survival in a double-blind study comparing levamisole to placebo as adjuvants to radiotherapy of stage III and IV breast cancer [12]. AMERY et al. have also shown clinical benefit of levamisole in a double-blind placebo-controlled clinical trial of levamisole in resectable bronchogenic carcinoma [1–2]. Here, levamisole when given in a proper dose (2.5 mg/kg/day) significantly reduced distant metastases during the first 2 years and was preferentially of benefit to patients with large or more extensive primary tumors [1–2].

Materials and Methods

Patient Accession and Randomization

Between July 1975 and July 30, 1978, 80 patients were entered into the study, of whom 65 were evaluable [17]. All patients had squamous cancer of the oral cavity, pharynx, or larynx and had been stratified according to type of disease (primary or recurrent), site of primary, and stage of disease, prior to being randomized to receive levamisole or placebo. There were 31 evalable patients in the levamisole group and 34 in the placebo group. The patients were comparable in prognostic factors including type of disease, site and stage of the primary cancer, DNCB reactivity, lymphocyte count, and lymphocyte response to phytohemagglutinin. The distribution of the two treatment arms is shown in Table 1.

Treatment Plan

After randomization, treatment with 150 mg levamisole or placebo three times weekly on alternate weeks was scheduled for 2 years unless recurrence or excessive toxicity occurred.

Table 1. Clinical characteristics

Characteristic	Treatment group	
	Levamisole (31 patients)	Placebo (34 patients)
Type of disease		
Primary	24	29
Recurrent	7	5
Site of primary		
Oral cavity	23	22
Pharynx	1	5
Larynx	6	6
Unknown	1	1
Stage of disease		
I	7	7
II	6	8
III	17	18
IV	1	1

Immunologic Methods

All patients were skin tested and had lymphocyte counts and lymphocyte function studies performed prior to initiation of the study. Patients were tested for pre-existing delayed hypersensitivity to Dermatophyton-O (1 : 100, Hollister Stier Laboratories, Yeadon, PA.), mumps skin test antigen (Eli Lilly and Co., Indianapolis, Ind.), intermediate strength tuberculin (Parke-Davis Co., Detroit, Mich.) and streptokinase/streptodornase (Lederle Laboratories, Pearl River, N.Y.). The antigens were injected intradermally in volumes of 0.1 ml. The tests were read at 48 h and considered positive when the diameter of induration was 5 mm or more.

Sensitization and challenge with 2,4-dinitrochlorobenzene (DNCB) was carried out according to the method of Eilber and Morton [4]. DNCB 2000 μg dissolved in 0.1 ml of acetone was applied to the inner aspect of the upper arm, within the confines of a plastic ring measuring 2 cm in diameter, and allowed to evaporate. It is rare for patients or controls to show de novo sensitivity to this dose at 48 h. Prior hypersensitivity to DNCB was excluded by control tesing with 100, 50, and 25 μg DNCB in 0.1 ml accetone applied simultaneously to the ipsilateral forearm and read at 48 h. All testing sites were covered for 48 h and kept dry. All sites were examined for erythema and induration after 2 weeks. If there was no reaction at the 100 and 25 μg sites, the patients were rechallenged on the ipsilateral extremity with the 100, 50, and 25 μg DNCB. The reaction was considered positive if there was induration of 5 mm or greater at 48 h at the challenge sites.

In Vitro Tests

Stimulation of Lymphocytes by Mitogens and Antigens

Lymphocyte transformation in vitro was performed using a micro method [16]. Lymphocytes were obtained from heparinized blood on Ficoll-Hypaque ("Lymphoprep") density gradients and resuspended in RPMI 1640 with Hepes buffer, glutamine (0.25 ng/ml), penicillin 10 units/ml, streptomycin 10 units/ml, heparin 10 IU/ml, and 15% pooled normal human serum. Lymphocyte culture was performed in flat bottom microtiter plates (Falcon 3040) by adding 100,000 lymphocytes in 200 λ of medium. Transformation of lymphocytes was measured in terms of incorporation of C^{14} thymidine, which was added after 72 h (for mitogens) or 120 h (for antigens) and then incubated 24 h. Cultures were performed in triplicate. Dilutions of mitogens or antigens that had been prepared in advance and stored at −20° C were freshly thawed and added to the cultures in 25 μl volumes. The concentrations of phytohemagglutinin (PHA-P) used were 500, 250, 50, 10, and 5 μg/ml, conconavallin A (Con A, Difco) at 125, 42, 15, and 5 μg/ml, pokeweed mitogen (PWM, Gibco) at 2000, 400, and 80 μg/ml. The following antigen preparations were used in four tenfold dilutions: *Candida albicans* (Hollister Stier Laboratories) 1 : 10 dilution, streptokinase/streptodornase (Lederle) 24,000 units in 2 ml, *Staphylococcus aureus* 1×10^9 organisms/ml (heat inactivated), *Escherichia coli* 1×10^9 organisms/ml (heat inactivated), mixed bacterial vaccine prepared from *Streptococcus marcescens* and *Streptococcus hemolyticus* (MBV) 1 : 10 dilution, and mumps antigen (Lilly mumps skin test antigen) 1 : 10 dilution.

Statistical Methods

Curves for time to recurrence were calculated by the Kaplan Meier product limit procedure [7]. For the comparison of the distributions of times to recurrence for two or more groups, the log rank test was applied [9]. This test can detect differences in the distributions of the two groups while controlling for other factors thought to be associated with prognosis. All reported P values refer to two-sided tests.

Results

Pretreatment Immunologic Characteristics

Most patients had immunologic tests performed prior to enrollment into the study (Table 2). Fourteen of 57 patients tested (25%) were DNCB negative. The lymphocyte count was $< 1200/mm^3$ in 16 of 41 patients (39%). The response of isolated lymphocytes to PHA was < 15,000 cpm in 26 of 43 patients (60%); the response to Con A was < 10,000 cpm in 27 of 43 patients (63%) and to PWM was less than 5000 cpm in 25 of 39 patients (64%). These cutoff points were chosen somewhat arbitrarily at the tenth percentile of expected responses in lymphocyte cultures from normal controls. There was no significant difference between the levamisole and placebo group with respect to these pretreatment immunologic characteristics. Preliminary analysis of serial immunologic studies has not shown meaningful change on therapy. The DNCB data is shown in Table 3. Neither the lymphocyte levels nor mitogen responses have yet shown a consistent trend.

Table 2. Pretreatment Immunologic characteristics

Characteristic	Treatment group	
	Levamisole	Placebo
DNCB	6/27[a]	8/30
Absolute lymphocyte count	8/21	8/20
Lymphocyte response to PHA	15/22	11/21
Lymphocyte response to Con A	16/22	11/21
Lymphocyte response to PWM	12/21	13/18

[a] Number abnormal/number tested.

Table 3. DNCB response

	Levamisole		Placebo	
	Positive total	%	Positive total	%
Pre Rx	20/26	77	19/26	73
Month 3	16/20	80	17/20	85
Month 7	12/16	75	14/15	93

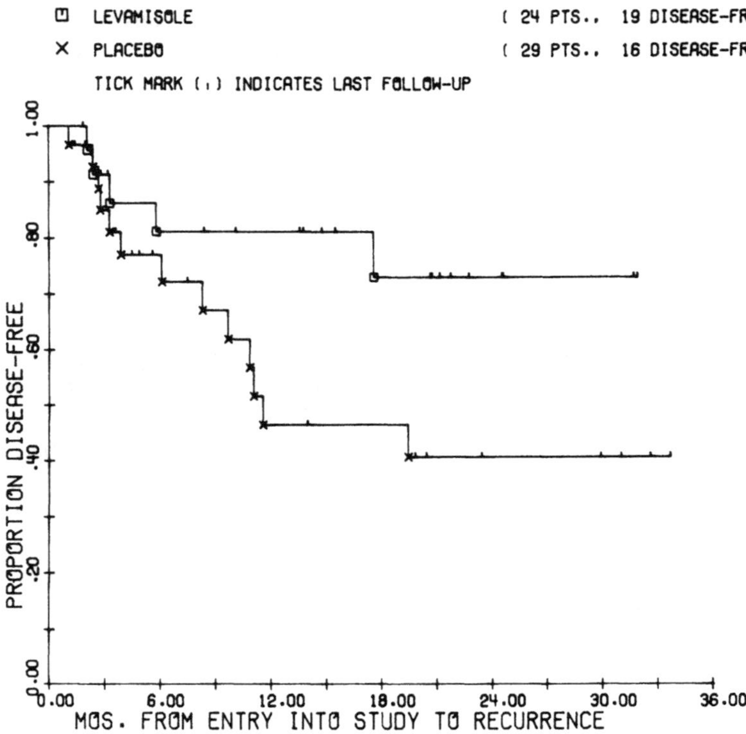

Fig. 1. Recurrence distributions of patients with no prior definitive surgery. The advantage for the levamisole-treated patients has borderline statistical significance ($P < 0.06$)

Recurrence

Statistical analysis was carried out on the recurrence experience of 65 evaluable patients, all of whom had at least 1 month of follow-up; 53 of these patients had no definitive surgery prior to entry into the study. The levamisole and placebo groups were compared as a whole, but a more extensive analysis focused on the 53 primary operable patients. The data were considered in terms of stage, site, and pretreatment DNCB status.

The curves for time to recurrence are shown in Fig. 1 for the two groups of primary patients. The observed difference in distribution of recurrence times has borderline statistical significance ($P < 0.06$); the corresponding analysis for the entire group of 65 patients yielded $P > 0.1$.

Comparison of the levamisole and placebo groups by site revealed a statistically significant difference in favor of levamisole for patients with cancer of the oral cavity ($P < 0.01$); the corresponding curves are shown in Fig. 2. There was no significant difference with respect to cancer of the pharynx or larynx; the overall difference, after adjustment for site of disease, was similarly not significant.

For the primary operable patients, there were no recurrences in stage I and IV (ten and two patients, respectively). The curves for stages II and III are shown in Fig. 3. In stage II patients, there was a statistically significant difference, again in favor of levamisole ($P < 0.02$). The observed difference for stage III patients was not significant, and the overall significance level, after adjustment for stage, was borderline.

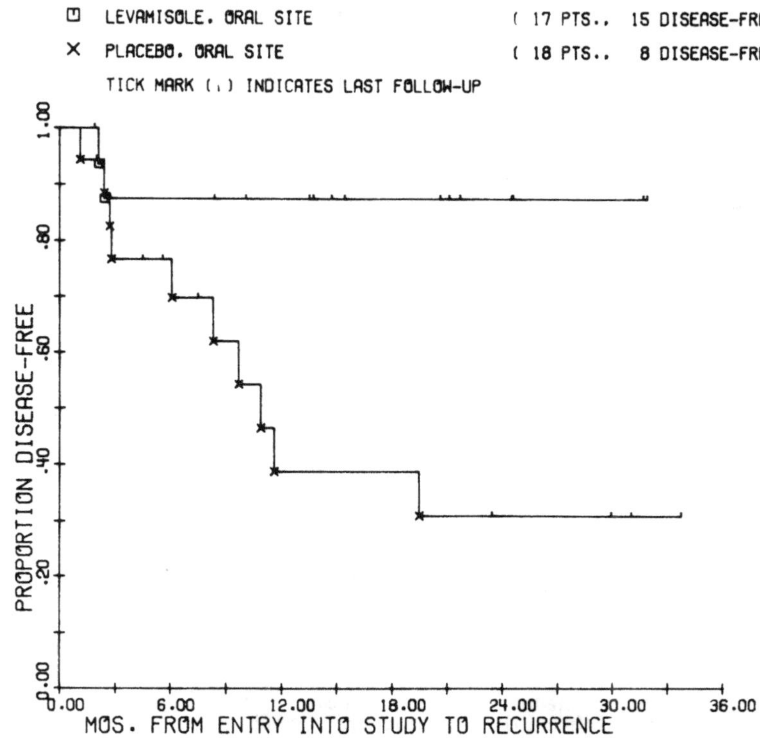

Fig. 2. Recurrence distributions of patients with oral cavity cancer who had no prior definitive surgery. The time to recurrence is significantly longer in the patients who received levamisole ($P < 0.01$)

It is important to note that among stage II patients, four of five of the levamisole group and five of six of the placebo group had cancer that originated from the oral cavity. When the data were further broken down according to site *and* stage, only one significant difference emerged, and this was for the "oral site, stage II" subgroup.

Figure 4 shows the curves for time to recurrence for patients grouped according to pretreatment DNCB status. These groups are not significantly different. Controlling for other covariates and comparison of the levamisole and placebo groups with adjustment for DNCB again yielded no significant differences.

Toxicity

There was considerable minor toxicity associated with this protocol. Of 65 evaluable patients, 40 (62%) experienced some subjective toxicity and most patients had more than one side-effect. The major side-effects were in the gastrointestinal and central nervous systems. Treatment was stopped in five patients (four from the levamisole and one from the placebo group). Diarrhea in three of these patients and hives in one patient were primary reasons for discontinuance of therapy. Marked granulocytopenia, which reversed after stopping levamisole, was seen in one patient. Side-effects were frequent in the placebo-treated patients; 17 of 34 had at least one side-effect, compared with 23 of 31 in the levamisole group.

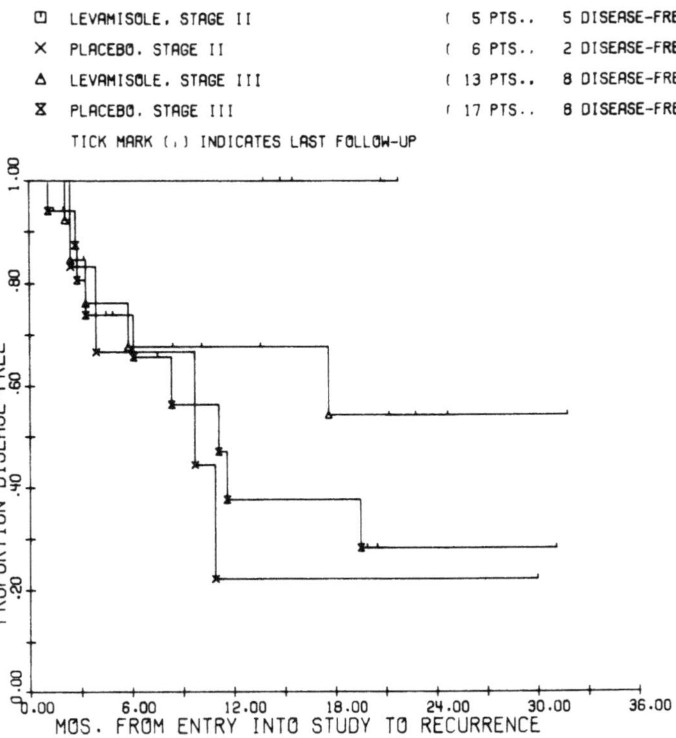

Fig. 3. Recurrence distributions of patients with stage II or stage III disease. For stage II patients, the time to recurrence is significantly longer in those who received levamisole ($P < 0.02$); the difference in patients with stage III disease is not statistically significant

Radiation

Although patients were not specifically stratified according to radiotherapy, approximately the same proportion had received either preoperative or postoperative radiation. There were 12 patients who had received radiation in the placebo group (ten preoperative and two postoperative). In the levamisole group, there were 14 patients who had been treated with radiation (ten preoperative and four postoperative).

Discussion

This is a preliminary report of a randomized double-blind study comparing levamisole with placebo as surgical adjuvant treatment for head and neck cancer patients. The study groups were comparable with respect to selected prognostic factors: type, site and stage of disease, and pretreatment immune function (DNCB, lymphocyte count, and mitogen response). The difference in the distribution of times to recurrence of the entire group of levamisole and placebo patients was not significant; the comparison for primary disease patients yielded borderline significance. Analysis of the data for the primary patients by site and stage revealed some suggestive differences within these subgroups. In particular, there was a significant

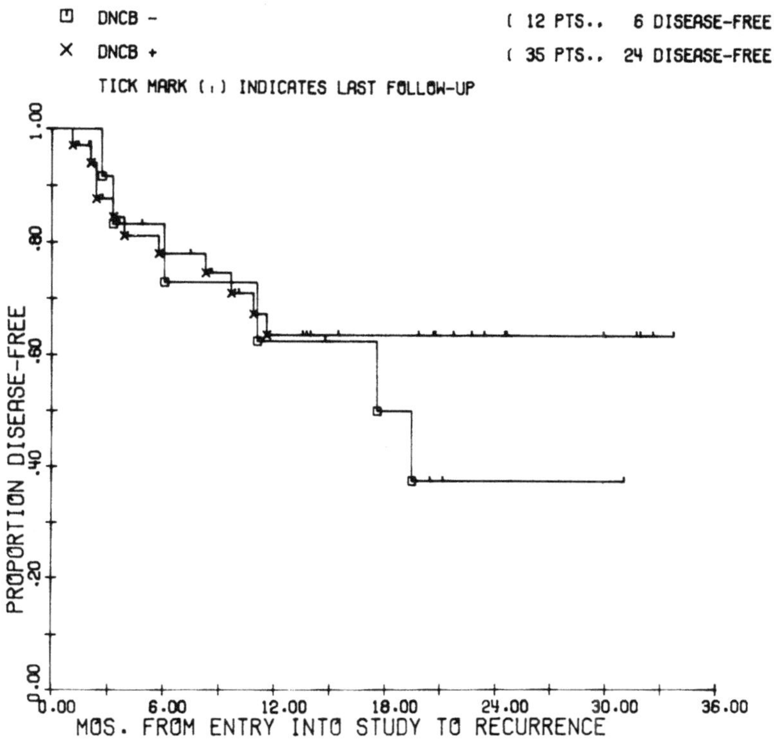

Fig. 4. Recurrence distributions according to pretreatment DNCB skin test reactivity. No difference is seen

difference in recurrence rates in favor of levamisole for patients with cancer of the oral cavity and for stage II patients. Considering site and stage simultaneously resulted in one significant difference, for stage II patients with oral cancer. No differences were found related to pretreatment DNCB status.

Due to the relatively small sample sizes involved in the various subgroups and the fact that many significant tests were carried out in the course of this analysis, the results reported must be interpreted with caution, in the context of exploratory data analysis.

It is remarkable that most of the patient experienced minor side-effects. In particular, the development of side-effects in half of the placebo-treated patients should be noted. On the other hand, only five patients had toxicity severe enough to discontinue treatment (and one of these was receiving placebo).

It has been reported that patients with operable squamous cell carcinoma are frequently immunodeficient [3, 6, 8, 15, 16]. The results of this study once again confirm that observation. The lack of correlation between DNCB skin test results and recurrence is at variance with our previous experience [6]. This discrepancy is not as suprising as it seems since the correlation was only seen in stage I and II patients in our previous studies [6], and few recurrences have occurred in such patients to date in the present study.

Preliminary analysis of immunologic studies has not shown significant changes in DNCB skin tests, lymphocyte levels, nor mitogen responses between the levamisole and placebo-treated patients. This may reflect the insensitivity of these tests to reflect subtle immune changes exerted by levamisole, or perhaps levamisole exerts its effects on other cell systems not measured by the assays used. Additional immunologic tests might include measurements specific for monocyte-macrophage function and the use of mixed lymphocyte culture techniques [3].

Summary

A preliminary report is made of a randomized double-blind study comparing levamisole with placebo as surgical adjuvant treatment of patients with squamous cancer of the head and neck. The study groups were comparable according to the prognostic factors of *type* (primary or recurrent), *site* (oral cavity, pharynx, larynx), and *stage* of disease and were also similar in pretreatment immune function and in radiation exposure. Of 65 evaluable patients, 31 were treated with levamisole and 34 received placebo. Although there was no difference in the distribution of the time to recurrence of the overall treatment group, there was a difference of borderline significance in favor of levamisole in the primary disease patients ($P < 0.06$). Further analysis of subgroups in the primary disease category showed decreased recurrence rates in patients receiving levamisole who had cancer of the oral cavity $P < 0.01$ or who had stage II disease, $P < 0.02$. Considering site and stage simultaneously, the only significant difference was in stage II patients with oral cancer. The above results, though encouraging, must be viewed with caution due to small sample sizes and relatively short follow-up of most patients.

References

1. Amery, W. K.: Double blind placebo controlled clinical trials of Levamisole in resectable bronchogenic carcinoma. Control of Neoplasia by Modulation of the Immune System. Chirigos, M. (ed.), pp. 197–203. New York: Raven Press 1977
2. Amery, W. K.: Immunopotentiation with Levamisole in resectable bronchogenic carcinoma: A double blind controlled trial. Br. Med. J. *3*, 461–464 (1975)
3. Berlinger, N. T., Hilal, E. Y., Oettgen, H. F., Good, R. A.: Deficient cell-mediated immunity in head and neck cancer patients secondary to autologous suppressive immune cells. Laryngoscope. (1978) (in press)
4. Eilber, F. R., Morton, D. L.: Impaired immunological reactivity and recurrence following cancer surgery. Cancer *25*, 362–367 (1970)
5. Farr, H. W., Arthur, K.: Epidermoid carcinoma of mouth and pharynx. J. Laryngol. Otol. *86*, 243–253 (1972)
6. Hilal, E. Y., Wanebo, H. J., Pinsky, C. M., Middleman, P., Strong, E. W., Oettgen, H. F.: Immunologic evaluation and prognosis in patients with head and neck cancer. Am. J. Surg. *134*, 469–473 (1977)
7. Kaplan, I. I., Meier, P.: Nonparametric estimation from incomplete observations. J. Am. Statis. Assoc. *53*, 457–481 (1958)
8. Lundy, J., Wanebo, H. J., Pinsky, C. M., Strong, E., Oettgen, H. F.: Delayed hypersensitivity reaction in patients with squamous cell cancer of the head and neck. Am. J. Surg. *128*, 530 (1974)
9. Peto, R., Pike, M. C.: Conservation of the approximation $\Sigma(O\text{-}E)^2/E$ in the logrank test for survival data or tumor incidence data. Biometrics *29*, 579–584 (1973)
10. Renoux, G., Renoux, M.: Effet immunostimuland d'un imidothiazole dans l'immunisation des souris contre l'infection par Bruella Abortas. C.R. Acad. Sci. *272*, 349–350 (1971)

11. Renoux, G., Renoux, M.: Stimulation of anti-brucella vaccination in mice by tetramisole, a phenyl-imidothiazole salt. Infect. Immun. *8*, 544–548 (1973)
12. Rojas, A. F., Mickiewicz, E., Feierstein, J. N., Glact, H., Olivari, A. J.: Levamisole in advanced human breast cancer. Lancet *1*, 211–215 (1976)
13. Rojas, A. F., Feierstein, J. N., Glact, H. M., Varela, O. A., Pradier, R., Olivari, A.: Clinical action of Levamisole and effects of radiotherapy on immune response. Control of Neoplasia by Modulation of the Immune System. Chirigos, M. (ed.), pp. 159–174. New York: Raven Press 1977
14. Symoens, J.: Levamisole, an antianergic chemotherapeutic agent: An overview. Control of Neoplasia by Modulation of the Immune System. Chirigos, M. (ed.), pp. 1–25. New York: Raven Press 1977
15. Tarpley, J. L., Potvin, C., Chretien, P. B.: Prolonged depression of cellular immunity on cured laryngopharyngeal cancer patients treated with radiation therapy. Cancer *35*, 638–644 (1975)
16. Wanebo, H. J., Jun, M. Y., Strong, E. W., Oettgen, H. F.: T cell deficiency in patients with squamous cell cancer of the head and neck. Am. J. Surg. *130*, 445–451 (1975)
17. Wanebo, H. J., Hilal, E. U., Pinsky, C. M., Strong, E. W., Mike, V., Hirshaut, Y., Oettgen, H. F.: Randomized trial of Levamisole in patients with squamous cancer of the head and neck: A preliminary report. Cancer Treat. Rep. (in Press) (1978)

H. Urological Tumors

Adjuvant Chemotherapy Following Radical Radiotherapy in T3 Bladder Carcinoma

B. Richards, A. Akdas, P. Corbett, R. W. Glashan, M. R. G. Robinson, and P. A. Smith

Introduction

The results of treatment of deeply infiltrating bladder cancers (T3 in the UICC classification or B2 and C in the American classification) are dismal, whatever the method of treatment of the local disease. No matter whether the primary treatment is radiotherapy [12, 14], surgery [13] or a combination [14], 40% of patients die within 12 months, about 50% in 2 years, and about 70% within 5 years (Fig. 1).

Rider and Evans, reviewing 281 cases of bladder cancer treated with radical radiotherapy found that 195 (69.4%) died within 3 years [12]. Of these, 96 (34.2%) died of distant metastases that were not evident at the time of local treatment. Less than half this number (39%–14%) died of failure of local treatment within this period. There might be a substantial increase in survival if the micrometastases present at the time of primary treatment could be destroyed by adjunctive therapy, a form of treatment that has been advocated by Prout [11] and by DeKernion [3]. It is unfortunate that relatively few of the available cytostatic drugs have been properly evaluated in bladder cancer. A recent search found adequate information in only eight (Table 1).

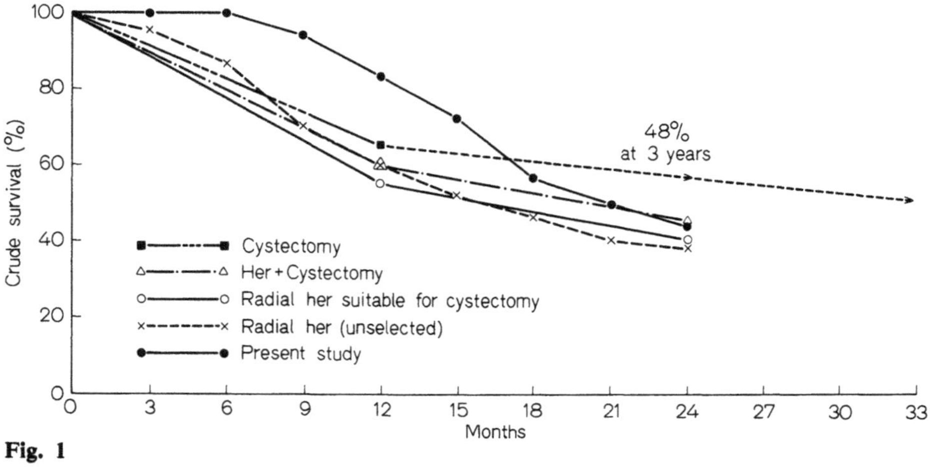

Fig. 1

Table 1. Cytostatic agents evaluated against bladder cancer

Drug	Remission rate (authors definition)	
	Alone	In combination
Adriamycin	40/168	40/111
Bleomycin	5/36	5/5
Cis platinum	8/23	11/18
Cyclophosphamide	18/47	14/39
5-FU	39/90	23/49
Methotrexate	29/77	–
Mitomycin-C	13/51	–
VM-26	5/30	5/27

The studies from which this information was drawn deal mainly with patients with advanced disease and give a conservative assessment of the results that could be obtained if the agents were used at an earlier stage. There have been few reports of adjuvant chemotherapy in the primary treatment of T3 bladder cancer. 5-Fluorouracil has been used in combination with radiotherapy [4, 7, 10, 15], and EDLAND, WEAR, and ANSFIELD reported a lower incidence of distant metastases when radiotherapy was combined with chemotherapy than when it was used alone [4] though this has not been confirmed [10]. More recently, MERRIN and BECKLEY have reported the preliminary results of adjuvant chemotherapy with adriamycin and cyclophosphamide in six patients with B and C cancers treated with radical cystectomy [9].

We have been impressed with the effect of adriamycin and 5-fluorouracil given in combination to patients with advanced bladder cancer [2] and wished to set up a prospective randomised study to test the effect of adjuvant chemotherapy with these agents following radical radiotherapy for T3 bladder lesions.

Since radiotherapy and chemotherapy may be toxic in combination, we carried out a pilot investigation on 18 unselected patients with T3 bladder cancers to see whether the combination was safe and tolerable to the patient. The toxicity proved to be acceptable [5]. The 2-year follow-up of this small group is now available. The survival of these patients is better than expected and forms the basis of this report.

Patients

Eighteen patients with T3 bladder cancers, aged 44–76 years (mean = 65 years) were entered into the study. There were 14 males and 4 females. The histological grade of the tumours is shown in Table 2.

Table 2. T3 bladder cancer – histological grading

Well differentiated	2
Moderately differentiated	9
Poorly differentiated	7
Total	18

The criteria for entry to this study were T3, Nx, M0 or Mx. No patients had symptomatic evidence of metastases, though they were not specifically excluded in every case. None of the patients had additional primary tumours, serious intercurrent disease, renal failure, liver disease, impaired bone marrow or peptic ulceration.

Methods

All patients received a radical course of radiotherapy to the bladder and lateral pelvic wall, followed after at least 4 weeks by adriamycin, 50 mg/m^2, and 5-fluorouracil, 500 mg/m^2, intravenously at 3-week intervals to a maximum dose of 550 mg/m^2 of adriamycin. Chemotherapy was given as an out-patient with appropriate modification for bone marrow toxicity. Treatment was discontinued if toxic symptoms demanded it. Prophylactic digoxin was not given.

Toxicity

The cardiac toxicity of adriamycin was the most serious problem. Cardiac failure developed in five patients and contributed to the death of three. These patients had received 10, 10, 9, 8 and 6 cycles of chemotherapy respectively. This high incidence of cardiac toxicity was surprising as it is rare if less than 550 mg/m^2 of adriamycin has been given [1, 8]. It might have been less if the patients had been given prophylactic digoxin, as suggested by Guthrie and Gibson [6]. Haematological toxicity was mild. The haemoglobin tended to fall by 1–2 g/100 ml over four cycles, but only one patient required transfusion. The total white count often fell below 4000/mn^3 at the nadir but failed to regain this level at 3 weeks on only two occasions. Four patients declined further chemotherapy after 4, 4, 5 and 8 cycles because of nausea and vomiting.

Results

Of the 18 patients, 15 (83%) survived 1 year, 10 (56%) survived 18 months, and 8 (44%) 2 years. It is relevant to note that seven of the eight survivors are free of disease as judged by cystoscopy and EUA biochemical tests and bone scan. In one patient there has been a superficial recurrence of carcinoma that has been easily treated with fulguration.

Discussion

Recent series of patients with category T3 carcinomas of the bladder report 1-year survivals of 55%–65% whether the treatment was surgery [13], radiotherapy [12, 14] or a combination of the two [14]. The survival rate of 83% at 1 year in this study was unexpected. The numbers are small and the difference does not persist at 2 years (Fig. 1), but these results suggest that adjuvant chemotherapy in T3 bladder cancer is unlikely to reduce survival and that it would be appropriate to initiate a randomised controlled prospective study to assess whether it is beneficial. Such a study has been set up by the Yorkshire Urology Cancer Research Group. It has been running for 1 year and now contains 46 patients.

References

1. Cortes, E. P., Lutman, G., Wanka, J., Wang, J. J., Pilkren, J., Wallace, J., Holland, J. F.: Adriamycin cardiotoxicity: a clinicopathological correlation. Cancer Chemother. Rep. *6,* 215 (1975)
2. Cross, R. J., Glashan, R. W., Humphrey, C. S., Robinson, M. R. G., Smith, P. H., Williams, R. E.: Treatment of advanced bladder cancer with Adriamycin and 5-Fluorouracil. Br. J. Urol. *48,* 609–615 (1976)
3. De Kernion, J. B.: The chemotherapy of advanced bladder carcinoma. Cancer Res. *37,* 2771–2774 (1977)
4. Edland, R. W., Wear, J. B., Ansfield, F. J.: Advanced cancer of the urinary bladder. An analysis of results of radiotherapy alone versus radiotherapy and concomitant 5-Fluorouracil; a prospective randomized study of 36 cases. Am. J. Roentgenol. *108,* 124–129 (1970)
5. Glashan, R. W., Houghton, A. L., Robinson, M. R. G.: A toxicity study of the treatment of T3 bladder tumors with a combination of radiotherapy and chemotherapy. Br. J. Urol. *49,* 669–672 (1977)
6. Guthrie, D., Gibson, A. L.: Doxorubicin cardiotoxicity: possible role of digoxin in its prevention. B.M.J. *2,* 1447–1449 (1977)
7. Kaufman, J. J., Langdon, E. A., Stein, J. J., Burt, F. B.: Cancer of the bladder. Combined 5-Fluorouracil and cobalt 60 teletherapy. Calif. Med. *101,* 334–340 (1964)
8. Lefrak, E. A., Pitha, J., Rosenheim, S., Gottlieb, J. A.: A clinicopathological analysis of Adriamycin cardiotoxicity. Cancer *33,* 302–314 (1973)
9. Merrin, C., Beckley, S.: Adjuvant chemotherapy for bladder cancer with Doxorubicin hydrochloride and cyclophosphamide: preliminary report. J. Urol. *119,* 62–63 (1978)
10. Prout, G. R., Slack, N. H., Bross, I. D. J.: Irradiation and 5-Fluorouracil as adjuvants in the management of invasive bladder carcinoma. A c-operative Group report after 4 years. J. Urol. *104,* 116–129
11. Prout, G. R.: The role of surgery in the potentially curative treatment of bladder carcinoma. Cancer Res. *37,* 2764–2770 (1977)
12. Rider, W. D., Evans, D. H.: Radiotherapy in the treatment of recurrent bladder cancer. Br. J. Urol. *48,* 595–601 (1976)
13. Wajsman, C., Merrin, C., Moore, R., Murphy, G. P.: Current results from treatment of bladder tumours with total cystectomy at Roswell Park Memorial Institute. J. Urol. *113,* 806–810 (1975)
14. Wallace, D. M., Bloom, H. J. G.: Management of deeply infiltrating (T3) bladder carcinoma: controlled trial of radical radiotherapy versus pre-operative radiotherapy and radical cystectomy. Br. J. Urol. *48,* 587–594 (1976)
15. Woodruff, M. W., Murphy, W. T., Hodson, J. M.: Further observations on the use of combination 5-Fluorouracil and supervoltage irradiation therapy in the treatment of advanced carcinoma of the bladder. J. Urol. *90,* 747 (1963)

Adjuvant Therapy of T1 Bladder Carcinoma: Preliminary Results of an EORTC Randomized Study[1]

C. Schulman, R. Sylvester, M. Robinson, P. Smith, A. Lachand, L. Denis, M. Pavone-Macaluso, M. De Pauw, and M. Staquet

Introduction

Superficial bladder tumors (T1, P1 of the TNM Classification [19] or Jewett Stage O and A) are usually treated by transurethral resection (TUR). However, recurrence of the tumor after complete resection occurs in about 60% of the patients [9, 10] with a significant percentage of these recurrences showing a higher degree of malignancy [10]. In 10% of the cases the tumor progresses to invasive carcinoma [7] and the 5-year survival rate following TUR is about 62% [12].

Several adjuvant treatments to TUR have been advocated in an attempt to increase the survival rate, the duration of the disease-free interval, and to reduce the recurrence rate. Thiotepa, adriamycin, epodyl, bleomycin, BCG, pyridoxine, and VM-26 have all been suggested as intravesical agents of possible benefit [1, 2, 3, 4, 5, 6, 8, 11, 13, 14, 21, 22]. Periodic instillation of thiotepa, a cytotoxic alkylating agent, has been used for more than 15 years both for prophylaxis and for the treatment of recurrent T1 bladder tumors, but its true effectiveness remains to be demonstrated [8, 20, 21]. Staquet [18] has recently reviewed nine nonrandomized studies with intravesical thiotepa and found a success rate ranging 24%–100%.

Objectives of the Study

This randomized clinical trial was designed by the EORTC Genito-Urinary Tract Cancer Cooperative Group to compare:

1. The disease-free interval;
2. The recurrence rate;
3. The number of patients with an increase in the T or G classification,

in category T1 carcinoma of the bladder after TUR alone or TUR followed by bladder instillations of thiotepa or VM-26 for 1 year [17].

Selection of Patients

Criteria for Admission

All patients with a biopsy proven primary or recurrent T1 papillary carcinoma of the bladder that was resectable transurethrally were considered eligible for the trial. T1 lesions are defined

---

1 EORTC Genito-Urinary Tract Cooperative Group Protocol 30751.
This investigation was supported by grant 5R10 CA11488-09, awarded by the National Cancer Institute, DHEW, Bethesda, Md., United States.

according to the 1974 TNM classification and represent tumors with no microscopic infiltration beyond the lamina propria. All visible lesions were completely resected. In addition, neither induration nor a mass could be palpated on bimanual examination under anesthesia after TUR. In the case of urinary infection, the start of the trial was delayed until control of the infection.

Criteria for Exclusion

1. Presence of another cancer or previous local or systemic cancer chemotherapy;
2. Bladder lesions other than papillary lesions;
3. General condition such that an expected survival for the duration of the study was unlikely;
4. Expected difficulties of follow-up related to overt psychosis, marked senility, or too large distance between patient's home and investigator's center;
5. White blood cell count (WBC) below 4500/mm^3 and/or platelet count below 150,000/mm^3
6. Bladder papillomatosis not resectable by TUR.

Design of the Trial

Three weeks after TUR, the following treatments were randomly allocated to eligible patients after stratification for primary or recurrent cases: treatment group 1, intravesical thiotepa; treatment group 2, intravesical VM-26; and treatment group 3, no treatment. Thiotepa and VM-26 are administered for 1 year starting 1 month after TUR. All patients entering the trial are followed for 5 years or until death, whichever comes first.

Therapeutic regimen

The drugs, 30 mg of thiotepa in 30 ml sterile water or 50 mg of VM-26 in 30 ml normal saline, were instilled into the bladder and retained for 1 h. The drug instillation was started 1 month after TUR, given every week for 4 weeks, and then once every 4 weeks for 11 months (total: 15 instillations) unless a recurrence occurred. If a recurrence was observed during the instillation treatment, a new complete schedule with the same regimen was repeated after TUR. Thus, 1 month after TUR, the drug instillation was started again every week for four instillations and then once every 4 weeks. The total duration of treatment was limited to 12 months beginning after the first TUR. Nitrofurantoin (Furadantine) was given after each instillation at 3×100 mg/day for 3 days.

WBC and platelet counts were obtained before each chemotherapy administration. In the case of hematologic toxicity, drug administration was delayed until WBC $\geqslant$ 4000/mm^3 and platelets $\geqslant$ 150,000/mm^3. Chemotherapy was also delayed whenever cystitis was present at the time of instillation. If severe drug-induced cystitis occurred, the drug was given in a total solution volume of 60 ml for the following administrations. If severe drug-induced cystitis occurred again, no further instillations were given. Urinalysis was also performed before each drug instillation. Treatment was temporarily interrupted in the case of urinary infection until control of the infection was achieved.

Evaluation of Therapy

Cystoscopy was repeated every 12 weeks during the 1st year, every 16 weeks during the 2nd year, and then every 26 weeks during the following 3 years. All visible lesions seen on cystoscopy were biopsied with recurrence being established *only* by histologic examination of the biopsy material. The free interval was defined as the time interval between TUR and the date of the first positive biopsy.

Results

From 20 participating institutions in six different countries, 340 patients have been admitted to this protocol from November 1975 to April 1978. While the analysis that is presented here is based on the 215 patients for whom follow-up is available, a similar analysis yielding essentially the same results was made eliminating 16 ineligible or nonevaluable patients from the calculations. Kaplan-Meier curves are used to estimate the time until the first recurrence and differences between the curves are tested using the Logrank and Gehan generalized Wilcoxon test procedures [15]. Two-tailed significance levels are reported in the text. A comparison of the recurrence rates (number of recurrences per patient months of observation) is performed using a chi square test statistic [16]. The primary aim of the study was to discover if thiotepa or VM-26 when compared to no treatment significantly increased the duration of the disease-free interval. Hence, Kaplan-Meier curves giving the time until first recurrence have been calculated for each treatment group. Figure 1 gives a comparison of the time until first recurrence between primary and recurrent patients, and the difference is

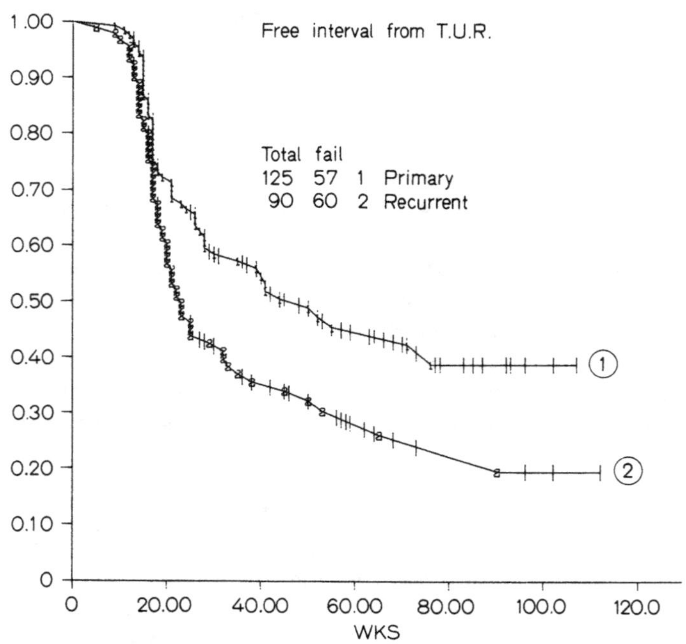

Fig. 1. Kaplan-Meier curves for the time until first recurrence, a comparison of primary and recurrent patients

significant at $P = 0.01$. The median time to first recurrence is approximately 45 weeks for primary patients and 23 weeks for recurrent patients. If we compare the three treatment groups with respect to the time until first recurrence (Fig. 2), we find that overall there is no significant difference between thiotepa, VM-26, and no treatment. The same conclusion is valid among primary patients (Fig. 3) and among recurrent patients (Fig. 4).

The number of patients in each treatment group with follow-up is indicated in the second line of Table 1 and the number of patients with recurrences per treatment group is given in line 3. For the purposes of this paper the word "recurrence" will refer to a visit at which one or more tumors have reappeared in the bladder (with histologic confirmation) after having been removed previously by TUR. From Table 1 we see that the percentage of patients with at least one recurrence is 49.3 for thiotepa, 62.0 for VM-26, and 52.2 for no treatment. Ignoring the time at which the first recurrence occurred, the difference between these percentages is not

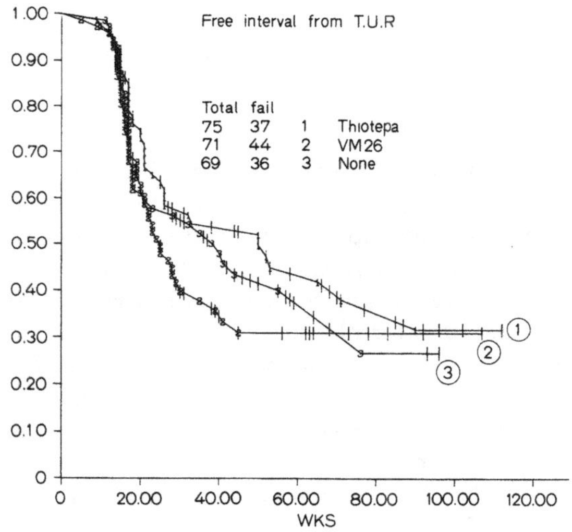

Fig. 2. Kaplan-Meier curves for the time until first recurrence, a comparison of thiotepa, VM-26, and no treatment in all patients

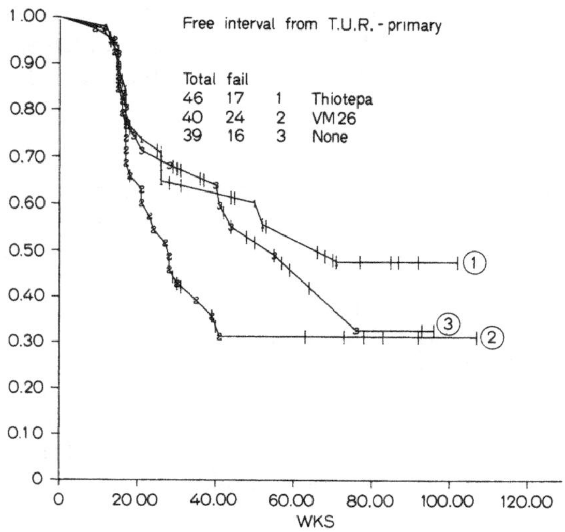

Fig. 3. Kaplan-Meier curves for the time until first recurrence, a comparison of thiotepa. VM-26, and no treatment in primary patients

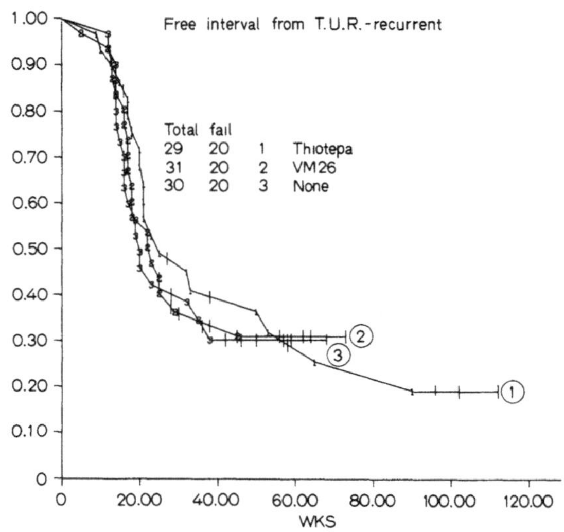

Fig. 4. Kaplan-Meier curves for the time until first recurrence, a comparison of thiotepa, VM-26, and no treatment in recurrent patients

significant. In the lower part of Table 1 recurrence rates are determined for each treatment by dividing the total number of visits at which recurrences were present by the total patient months of follow-up for all patients in a treatment group. The average duration of follow-up for all patients is approximately 10 months; however, some patients have been followed for as long as 2 years. The recurrence rates per 100 patient months of follow-up are 6.93 for thiotepa, 10.12 for VM-26, and 9.97 for no treatment. Comparisons reveal that the recurrence rate for thiotepa is significantly lower than that for either VM-26 ($P = 0.03$) or no treatment ($P = 0.04$), but there is no significant difference between VM-26 and no treatment. Tables 2 and 3 repeat these analyses for primary patients and recurrent patients separately. In each case the recurrence rate for thiotepa is lower than that for no treatment or for VM-26, but overall the differences are not statistically significant ($P = 0.11$ for primary patients and $P = 0.17$ for recurrent patients).

Table 4 presents the number of patients with recurrences showing a higher degree of malignancy (increase in G classification) while Table 5 presents the number of patients with recurrences for which there has been an increase in the T classification. The number of patients showing an increase in both the G and T classifications is given in Table 6. Overall

Table 1. Recurrences by treatment (all patients)

	Thiotepa	VM 26	No treatment	Total
No. of patients randomized	115	116	109	340
No. of patients with follow-up	75	71	69	215
No. of patients with recurrences	37	44	36	117
Percent with recurrences	49.3	62.0	52.2	54.4
Total No. of recurrences	58	69	68	195
Total months of follow-up	837	682	682	2201
Recurrence rate/100 patient months	6.93	10.12	9.97	8.86

there are no significant differences between the three treatment groups with respect to changes in the G and/or the T classifications; however, among primary patients there has been a higher incidence of increases in the T classification in patients treated with VM-26 (P = 0.01).

Table 2. Recurrences by treatment (primary patients)

	Thiotepa	VM 26	No treatment	Total
No. of patients randomized	71	70	69	210
No. of patients with follow-up	46	40	39	125
No. of patients with recurrences	17	24	16	57
Percent with recurrences	37.0	60.0	41.0	45.6
Total No. of recurrences	23	36	26	85
Total months of follow-up	462	417	386	1265
Recurrence rate/100 patient months	4.98	8.63	6.74	6.72

Table 3. Recurrences by treatment (recurrent patients)

	Thiotepa	VM 26	No treatment	Total
No. of patients randomized	44	46	40	130
No. of patients with follow-up	29	31	30	90
No. of patients with recurrences	20	20	20	60
Percent with recurrences	69.0	64.5	66.7	66.7
Total No. of recurrences	35	33	42	110
Total months of follow-up	375	265	296	935
Recurrence rate/100 patient months	9.33	12.45	14.19	11.75

Table 4. Patients with recurrences showing a higher degree of malignancy

	Thiotepa	VM 26	No treatment	Total
Primary patients	2/46	4/40	0/39	6/125
Recurrent patients	3/29	2/31	5/30	10/ 90
Total	5/75	6/71	5/69	16/215

Table 5. Patients with recurrences showing an increase in the T category

	Thiotepa	VM 26	No treatment	Total
Primary patients	0/46	4/40	0/39	4/125
Recurrent patients	3/29	3/31	4/30	10/ 90
Total	3/75	7/71	4/69	14/215

Table 6. Patients with recurrences showing a higher degree of malignancy and an increase in the T category

	Thiotepa	VM 26	No treatment	Total
Primary patients	0/46	4/40	0/39	4/125
Recurrent patients	2/29	2/31	2/30	6/ 90
Total	2/75	6/71	2/69	10/215

Discussion

The preliminary results from this study indicate that while neither thiotepa nor VM-26 significantly increase the duration of the disease-free interval as compared to no treatment, thiotepa does appear to decrease the overall recurrence rate. This result agrees with the results of previous studies [2] that advocate the prophylactic use of intravesical thiotepa. Since thiotepa has failed to decrease the number of patients who had recurrences and does not delay the time until the first recurrence, its activity can only be considered to be minimal. Thus, the EORTC Genito-Urinary Tract Group is in the process of implementing other protocols for the testing of new intravesical or oral agents in the treatment of T1 bladder carcinoma.

Summary

This paper reports the preliminary results of an ongoing clinical trial in patients with category T1 bladder cancer who are randomized after transurethral resection to receive either thiotepa, VM-26, or no treatment. While there are no significant differences between the three treatment groups with respect to the time until first recurrence, thiotepa has significantly reduced the recurrence rate as compared to either VM-26 ($P = 0.03$) or no treatment ($P = 0.04$) among the 215 patients for whom follow-up information is currently available.

References

1. Abbassian, A., Wallace, D. M.: Intracavitary chemotherapy of diffuse noninfiltrating papillary carcinoma of the bladder. J. Urol. *96,* 461 (1966)
2. Byar, D., Blackard, C.: Comparisons of placebo, pyridoxine, and topical thiotepa in preventing recurrence of stage T1 bladder cancer. Urol. *10,* 556 (1977)
3. Drew, J., Marshall, C.: Effect of topical tiotepa on recurrence rate of superficial bladder cancer. J. Urol. *99,* 740 (1968)
4. Edsmyr, F., Boman, J.: Instillation of thiotepa in vesical papillomatosis. Acta Radiol. *9,* 395 (1971)
5. E.O.R.T.C. Cooperative Group for Leukemias and Haematosarcomas. Clinical screening of epipodophyllotoxin VM 26 in malignant lymphomas and solid tumors. Br. Med. J. *1972/II,* 744
6. Esquivel, E. C., Mackenzie, H. R., Whitmore, W. F.: Treatment of bladder tumors by instillation of thiotepa and 5-fluorouracil. Invest. Urol. *2,* 381 (1965)

7. Greene, L. F., Hanash, K. A., Farrow, G. M.: Benign papilloma or papillary carcinoma of the bladder? J. Urol. *110,* 205 (1973)
8. Jones, H. C., Swinney, J.: thiotepa in the treatment of tumors of the bladder. Lancet *1961/II,* 615
9. Maltry, E.: Benign and malignant tumors of the urinary bladder. New York: Med. Examin. Publ. 1971
10. Marshall, V. F.: Current clinical problems regarding bladder tumors. In: Bladder Tumors: A symposium, p. 2. Philadelphia: J. B. Lippincott 1956
11. Mitchell, R.: Intravesical thiotepa in the treatment of transitional cell carcinoma. Br. J. Urol. *43,* 181 (1971)
12. O'Flynn, J. D., Smith, J. M., Hanson, J. S.: Transurethral resection for the assessment and treatment of vesical neoplasms. A review of 840 consecutive cases. Eur. Urol. *1,* 38 (1975)
13. Pavone-Macaluso, M., Caramia, G., Rizzo, F. P.: Chimiothérapie locale dans les néoplasies vésicales. J. Radiol. Electrol. *55,* 844 (1974)
14. Pavone-Macaluso, M., Caramia, G., Rizzo, F. P., Messana, V.: Preliminary evaluation of VM 26, a new epipodophyllotoxin derivative in the treatment of urogenital tumors. Eur. Urol. *1,* 53 (1975)
15. Peto, R.: Design and analysis of randomized clinical trials requiring prolonged observation of each patient, II. Analysis and examples. BR. J. Cancer *35,* 1 (1977)
16. Potthoff, R. F., Whittinghill, M.: Testing for homogeneity II. The poisson distribution. Biometrika *53,* 183 (1966)
17. Schulman, C. C. et al.: EORTC randomized trial for the adjuvant therapy of T1 bladder carcinoma. Eur. Urol. *2,* 271 (1976)
18. Staquet, M.: The randomized clinical trial: a prerequisite for rational therapy. Eur. Urol. *2,* 265 (1976)
19. UICC (International Union Against Cancer). TNM Classification of Malignant Tumors. 2nd ed. p. 79. Geneva: G. de Buren 1974
20. Veenema, R. J.: Bladder carcinoma treated by direct instillation of thio-TEPA. J. Urol. *88,* 60 (1962)
21. Veenema, R. J., Dean, A. L., Uson, A. C., Roberts, M., Longo, F.: Thiotepa bladder instillation: therapy and prophylaxis for superficial bladder tumors. J. Urol. *101,* 711 (1969)
22. Westcott, J. W.: The prophylactic use of thiotepa in transitional cell carcinoma of the bladder. J. Urol. *96,* 913 (1966)

I. Melanoma

Adjuvant Chemotherapy or Chemoimmunotherapy in the Management of Primary Malignant Melanoma of Level III, IV, or V

C. Jacquillat, P. Banzet, J. Civatte, A. Puissant, F. Cottenot, L. Israel, S. Belaich, Cl. Chastang, and J. Maral

Introduction

The majority of patients with malignant melanoma die within 10 years from dissemination of disease. Significant improvement in overall survival may be expected from treatment that can control subclinical metastasis present at the time of primary treatment. The level of invasion and stage of malignant melanoma are the most important prognostic factors. McGovern reported 5-year survival rates ranging from 85% for level II (Clark's classification) to 23% for level V [16].

Adjuvant Chemotherapy in the Management of Primary Malignant Melanoma: Protocol 2 NK 73

Many chemotherapeutic agents have been evaluated in the treatment of malignant melanoma. We selected currently available drugs of demonstrated activity against this type of malignancy. We undertook a randomized study of the efficacy of a combination of Velban, thiotepa, rufocromomycin, methotrexate, and procarbazine used as an adjuvant after surgery for Clark's level III, IV, and V malignant melanoma. When possible, intra-arterial infusion of DTIC was performed [22]. This paper reports the latest computer analysis of March 1978, which suggests that this form of chemotherapy may be of some use in prolonging disease-free survival.

Material and Methods

Between April 1973 and June 1976, 117 patients undergoing treatment at Saint-Louis Hospital were entered in the present study, following histologic diagnosis of level III, IV, or V malignant melanoma of either Superficial Spreading Melanoma (SSM) or nodular type. All patients were free of metastases. Work-up included history, physical examination, chest X-ray, blood chemistry, test for melanuria, and skin tests. Patients were stratified into two categories, according to the site of the primary melanoma (Table 1).

Table 1. Distribution of patients (Protocol 2 NK 73)

	Limbs			Trunk and head	
	Chemotherapy				
	Control	Systemic	Local + systemic	Control	Chemotherapy
Men	11 (6)	3 (0)	2 (1)	18 (7)	14 (3)
Women	16 (5)	20 (5)	13 (3)	10 (4)	10 (3)
Total	27 (11)	23 (5)	15 (4)	28 (11)	24 (6)

Numbers of recurrences are given in parentheses.

Patients with malignant melanoma of the extremities were assigned to surgical treatment only, to surgical resection plus systemic chemotherapy, or to the above plus preoperative intra-arterial chemotherapy. Patients with the primary located on the trunk or head and neck were assigned to surgical treatment either alone or followed by adjuvant systemic chemotherapy.

Surgical Treatment

To achieve adequate local control of malignant melanoma, wide surgical excision was performed. The area of the excision extended to 4 cm in all directions from the lesion and to the deep fascia, which was not included in the excision specimen. Closure of the excised wound was by split-thickness skin grafting [14]. The International Group for Clinical Study of Melanoma reported identical 3-year survival rates of patients with primary melanoma whether lymph node dissection was performed or not, and we preferred to abstain from any prophylactic lymph node dissection [2, 3].

Chemotherapy Protocols

Systemic chemotherapy was started 1 month after surgery and consisted of 7-day courses of daily oral procarbazine (30 mg/m^2/day), with an IV injection of vinblastine (6 mg/m^2), thiotepa (6 mg/m^2), rufocromomycin (60 μg/m^2), and methotrexate (15 mg/m^2) on day 1; this regimen was started 4 weeks after surgery; the courses were repeated every other week for the first 3 months, and then every 4 weeks up to 18 months.
Intra-arterial chemotherapy consisted of IA administration of DTIC and vincristine, vincristine 1 mg/m^2 was infused intra-arterially on days 1 and 8, DTIC 80 mg/m^2/day was given daily as a 3-h infusion on days 3–7 and 10–14; the vial containing the drug was protected from light. Surgery was performed 4 weeks after completion of this regimen.
Drug doses were modified according to the presence and degree of toxicity (according to white cell and platelet count) recorded before the onset of each course of chemotherapy. If no toxicity occurred, the patient received 100% of the calculated dose. If there was a decrease in white cell count to between 60,000 and 100,000, 50% of the calculated dose was given. When the white cell count was <2000 and the platelet count $< 60{,}000$, therapy was discontinued and only resumed upon evidence of increase of these counts. Fifteen of the patients took less than their prescribed amount as a result of their own failure to comply.

Intra-arterial chemotherapy was very well tolerated. Systemic chemotherapy did not induce severe hematologic toxicity: mean values were: white cells count of $3800/mm^3 \pm 1200$ (SD) with 1500 ± 500 polymorphonuclear leukocytes/mm^3, 10 ± 3 g hemoglobin/100 ml, $140{,}000 \pm 80{,}000$ platelets/mm^3. There was some degree of gastrointestinal toxicity: nausea (80% of patients), vomiting (12% of patients) essentially during the first 3 months and the last 6 months of treatment. We did not observe alopecia or weight losses. No patients interrupted work or daily activities due to chemotherapy.

Follow-up

Frequent clinical examinations were performed and CBC and chemistry were entered every other month on the flow sheets. Treatment failure was defined by local recurrence and/or regional or distant metastatic disease, confirmed by biopsy whenever possible by routine clinical radioisotopic investigations or by postmortem examination. Time to recurrence was taken as the time from surgical resection to the first clinical evidence of recurrence. Median follow-up time of patients was 30 months, ranging 10—48 months. Statistical analyses were performed by the life table and the t-test for comparison of proportions [4].

Results

Of 117 patients entered in the study, 37 developed local recurrence and/or metastatic disease following surgery. Table 2 shows the time and site distribution of these recurrences. A total of 62 patients were treated by operation and adjuvant chemotherapy. Of this group 47 patients remained disease-free throughout the study. Only 33 of the 55 patients in the non-chemotherapy group remained free of disease. Statistical analysis by the actuarial life table method revealed a significant difference between the two disease-free survival rate curves at every point between 8 and 36 months ($p < 0.05$) (Fig. 1).

Table 3 shows the age distribution of the 117 patients, emphasizing a peak of incidence in the 30—60 year old groups. Survival curves failed to show significant differences between the age groups during the follow-up period. Distribution by histologic type (56 SSM, 45 nodular, 16

Table 2. Distribution of first recurrence of malignant melanoma (29/117 patients) (Protocol 2 NK 73)

	Men		Women		All patients	
	Control	Chemo θ	Control	Chemo θ	Control	Chemo θ
Local recurrence	2	–	1	1	3	1
Metastasis : regional lymph node	9	3	8	9	17	12
Distant lymph node	1	–	–	–	1	–
Visceral	1[a]	1[b]	–	1[b]	1	2
No recurrence	16	15	15	32	31	47

[a] Pulmonary.
[b] Brain.

Table 3. Distribution of patients according to age (Protocol 2 NK 73)

	Control[a]	Chemo θ[b]
<30 years	2	10
30–40 years	13 (3)	11 (6)
40–50 years	7 (6)	16 (5)
50–60 years	9 (4)	14 (2)
60–70 years	17 (7)	4
>70 years	6 (2)	4 (1)

[a] Mean: 51 years old.
[b] Mean: 48 years old.
Numbers of recurrences are given in parentheses.

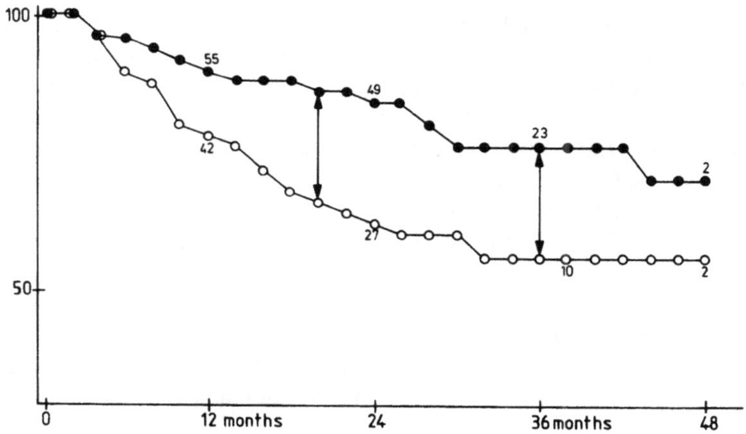

Fig. 1. Protocol 2 NK 73. Disease-free survival rate according to treatment. ○: surgery alone (55 patients, 22 recurrences); ●: chemotherapy (62 patients, 15 recurrences). $P < 0.05$

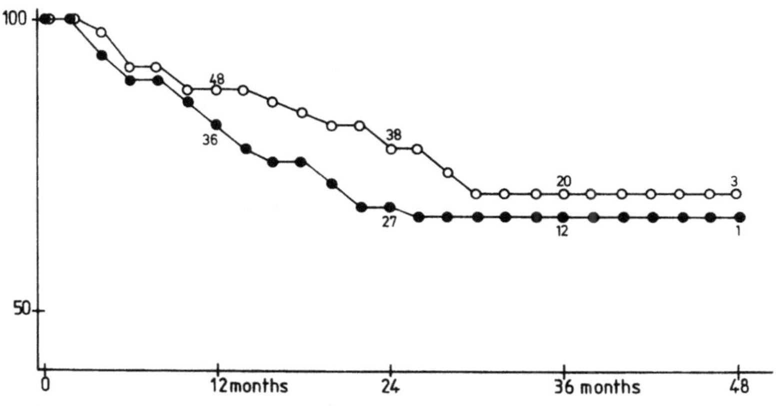

Fig. 2. Protocol 2 NK 73. Disease-free survival rate according to histologic type. ○: superficially spreading melanoma (56 patients, 15 recurrences); ●: nodular melanoma (45 patients, 15 recurrences)

Table 4. Distribution of patients according to site of primary at time of presentation (Protocol 2 NK 73)

	Men		Women	
	Control	Chemo θ	Control	Chemo θ
Head and neck	4	1	1	6
Trunk	15	12	9	4
Upper limb	1	2	3	6
Lower limb (except leg)	8	3	7	10
Leg	1	1	6	17

unclassified) also failed to show a significantly different disease-free survival rate (69% at 36 months in the SSM group vs. 67% at 24 months in the nodular group (Fig. 2).
The rate of response to chemotherapy was the same in SSM and nodular melanoma types. Table 4 shows the distribution of the 117 patients according to level of invasion of malignant melanoma. Only 45% of patients with level V malignant melanoma were free of disease at 36 months, vs. 66% and 68% of patients with levels III and IV, respectively, the difference not being statistically significant owing to the small number of patients with level V malignant melanoma (Fig. 3). The distribution of 117 patients according to the site of the primary at the time of presentation appears in Table 4.
The commonest site of malignant melanoma in males was the trunk and in females the extremities, especially the lower, as in other series [7, 8, 17, 18]. When we drew curves of disease-free survival rates of patients with upper limb malignant melanoma, lower limb malignant melanoma, trunk malignant melanoma, and head and neck malignant melanoma,

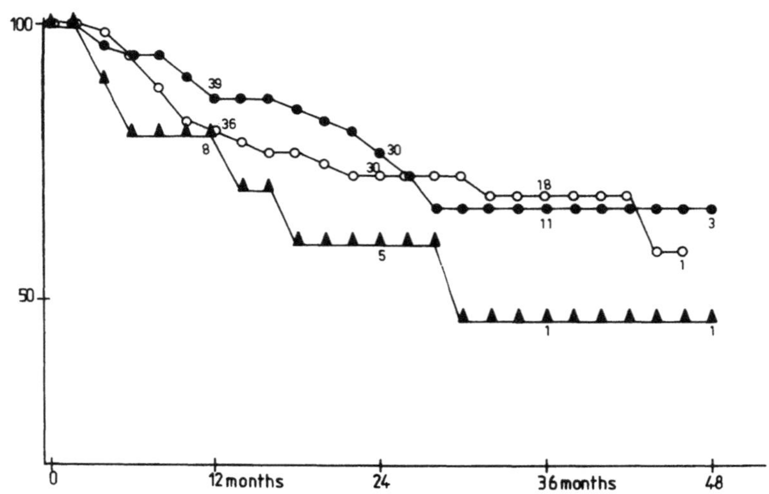

Fig. 3. Protocol 2 NK 73. Disease-free survival rate according to histologic level. ○: level III (46 patients, 15 recurrences); ●: level IV (46 patients, 14 recurrences); ▲: level V (10 patients, 5 recurrences)

there was no significant difference. When we drew disease-free survival rate curves for patients with malignant melanoma of the extremities according to treatment, there was no additional benefit from intra-arterial preoperative chemotherapy compared with postoperative adjuvant systemic chemotherapy alone (Fig. 4).

The sex ratio was of 0.71 (48 men and 69 women). We found that women fared better than men; the disease-free survival rate at 24 months was 76% for women versus 70% for men (Fig. 5). This better prognosis of female patients has been reported in other studies [3, 7, 17, 18]. As a consequence, results of chemotherapy were very different according to sex. In male patients disease-free survival rate curves showed a highly significant difference: at 36 months 83% of the patients who had chemotherapy remained disease-free, compared with only 53%

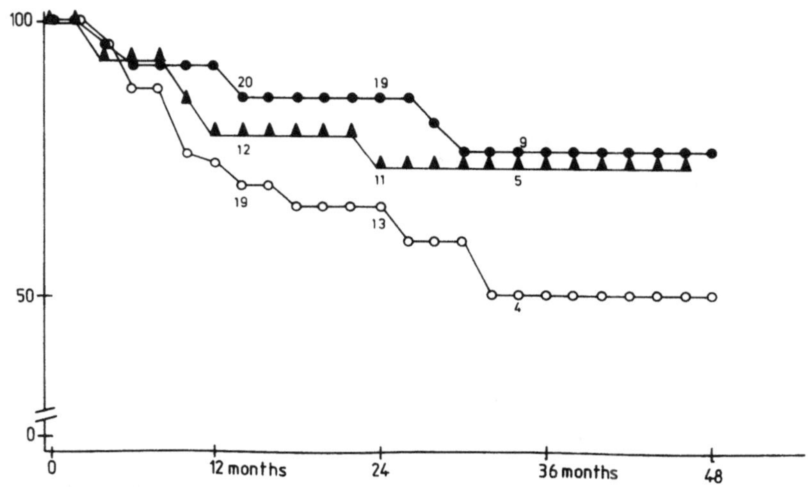

Fig. 4. Protocol 2 NK 73. Patients with melanoma on limbs. ○: surgery alone (27 patients, 11 recurrences); ●: general chemotherapy (23 patients, 3 recurrences); ▲: intra-arterial plus general chemotherapy (15 patients, 4 recurrences)

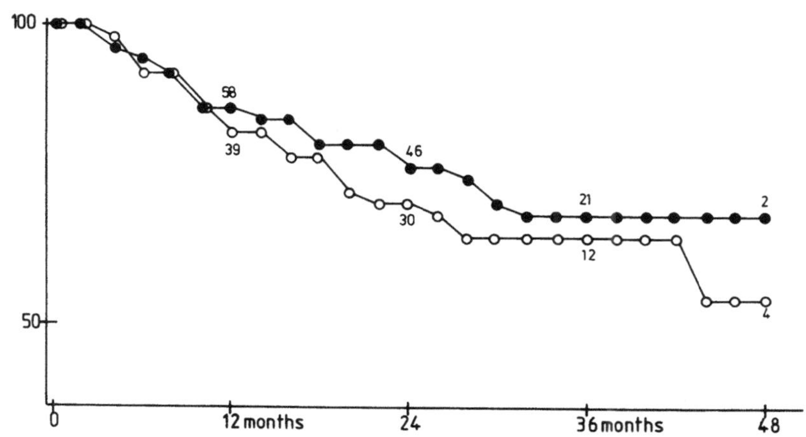

Fig. 5. Protocol 2 NK 73. Disease-free survival rate according to sex. ○: men (69 patients, 20 recurrences); ●: women (48 patients, 17 recurrences)

of patients treated by resection alone ($P < 0.05$). In women, no difference was found; the two curves were quite similar (Figs. 6 and 7). We found that sex distribution in the different groups of the protocol was not homogeneous, especially for patients with melanoma of the extremities.

To test whether a difference between treatment by surgery alone and by chemotherapy might be due merely to random allocation of more of the good-prognosis patients to chemotherapy, we performed a log rank test on patients stratified according to sex and level of invasion, which is not biased by chance correlation [20]. The relative recurrence rate of patients treated by surgery plus adjuvant chemotherapy was 0.69, as against 1.59 for patients treated by surgery alone. The difference between observed recurrences and extent of exposure to risk is significant $-X^2 = 4.82$, $P < 0.03$, suggesting that chemotherapy is indeed effective in preventing recurrence of malignant melanoma. However, for women patients alone, the log rank test is not significant.

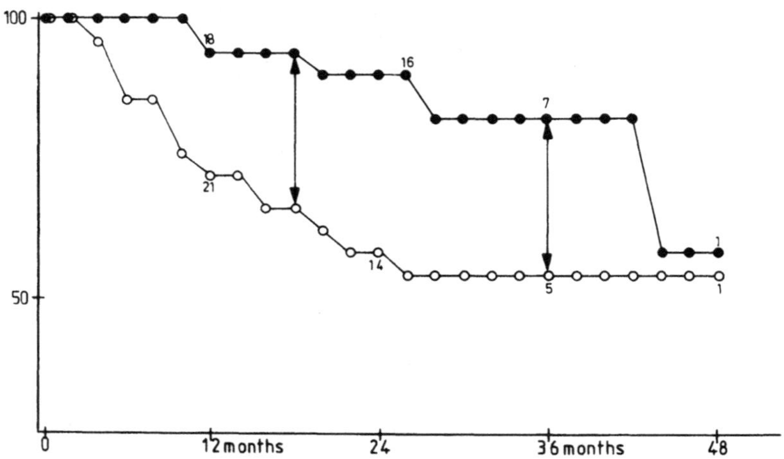

Fig. 6. Protocol 2 NK 73. Disease-free survival rate of men according to treatment. O: surgery alone (29 patients, 13 recurrences); ●: chemotherapy (19 patients, 4 recurrences). $P < 0.04$

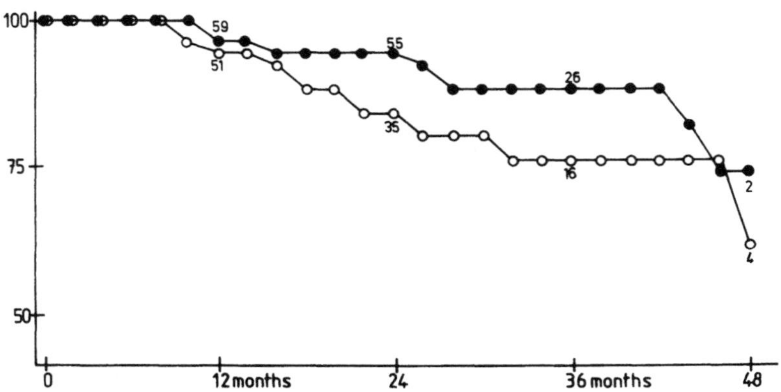

Fig. 7. Protocol 2 NK 73. Disease-free survival rate of women according to treatment. O: surgery alone (26 patients, 9 recurrences); ●: chemotherapy (43 patients, 11 recurrences)

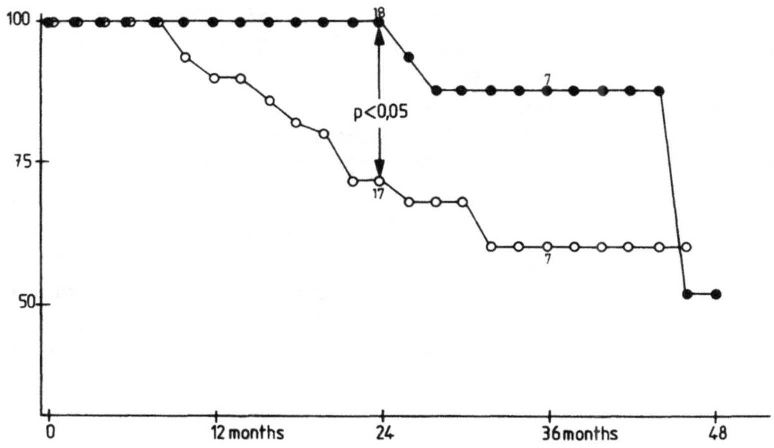

Fig. 8. Protocol 2 NK 73. Survival rate according to treatment. ○: surgery alone (55 patients, 12 deaths); ●: chemotherapy (62 patients, 9 deaths)

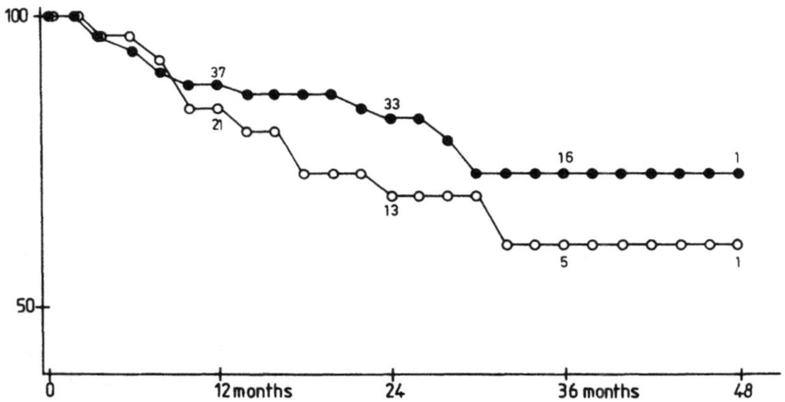

Fig. 9. Protocol 2 NK 73. Survival rate of men according to treatment. ○: surgery alone (29 patients, 11 deaths); ●: chemotherapy (19 patients, 3 deaths)

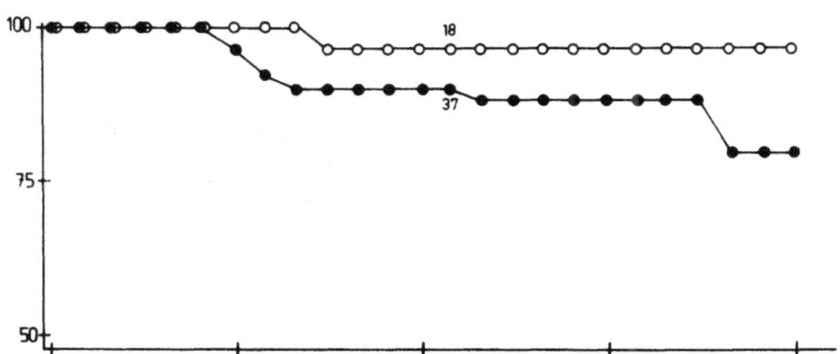

Fig. 10. Protocol 2 NK 73. Survival rate of women according to treatment. ○: surgery alone (26 patients, 1 death); ●: chemotherapy (43 patients, 6 deaths)

During the study, 21 patients died, 20 from dissemination of the disease and one from a nonrelated disorder (myocardial necrosis). In the chemotherapy group, 9 of 62 patients died versus 12 in the group of 55 patients treated by surgery without chemotherapy. Survival rate curves showed a nonsignificant difference in favor of chemotherapy (3-year survival rate of 76% and 88% in the control and chemotherapy group, respectively) (Fig. 8). For men patients the difference was highly significant (Fig. 9) but not for women (Fig. 10).
In this randomized study, patients with level III, IV, or V melanoma were found to benefit significantly from postoperative adjuvant chemotherapy in lengthening the disease-free interval, at least for male patients. However, the influence of sex on the response to treatment has led us to undertake a new randomized prospective trial with stratification for sex, histologic type, and level of invasion to confirm the results of our prior study and to study the effects of immunotherapy, which have been considered to be effective in melanoma [8, 9, 10].

Adjuvant Chemotherapy in the Management of Primary Malignant Melanoma: Protocol 4 NK 76

This new trial, now currently in progress, was started in June 1976. Its objectives are to confirm and eventually improve the results of our preceding study, while keeping to a comparable schedule.

Materials and Methods

Between June 1976 and March 1978, when our latest computer analysis was made, 149 patients were entered in this study. Protocol entry criteria were the same as for 2 NK 73.
Two main groups were chosen for randomization: women patients were assigned to surgical treatment only or to surgical resection plus chemotherapy and immunotherapy; men patients were assigned to surgical resection plus chemotherapy or to surgical resection plus chemotherapy and immunotherapy. Patients were stratified according to histologic type and level of invasion (Table 5). Surgical treatment was identical with that of 2 NK 73.

Chemotherapy Protocol

Systemic chemotherapy was identical with that of 2 NK 73 except for additional DTIC 300 mg/m^2 IV on day 1 of each course.

Immunotherapy Protocol

Immunotherapy consisted in BCG intradermally 0.1 ml in both groins and both axillary areas every 4 weeks and Corynebacterium parvum SC 2 ml every week.

Table 5. Distribution of patients (Protocol 4 NK 76)

Men	Chemo θ	34 (6)
	Chemo θ + immuno.	33 (2)
Women	Control	43 (7)
	Chemo θ + immuno.	39 (1)

Numbers of recurrences are given in parentheses.

Results

Of 149 patients entered in the study, 16 developed local recurrence and/or metastatic disease following surgery. For women patients, 7 of the 43 in the control group had a relapse, as against 1 of the 39 patients treated by chemotherapy and immunotherapy. Disease-free survival rate curves showed a significant difference ($P < 0.05$) throughout the follow-up (Fig. 11).

For men patients, disease-free survival rate curves of patients treated with chemotherapy and patients treated with chemotherapy and immunotherapy showed a difference in favor of immunotherapy but this was not significant (1-year disease-free survival rate of 75% and 87%, respectively) (Fig. 12).

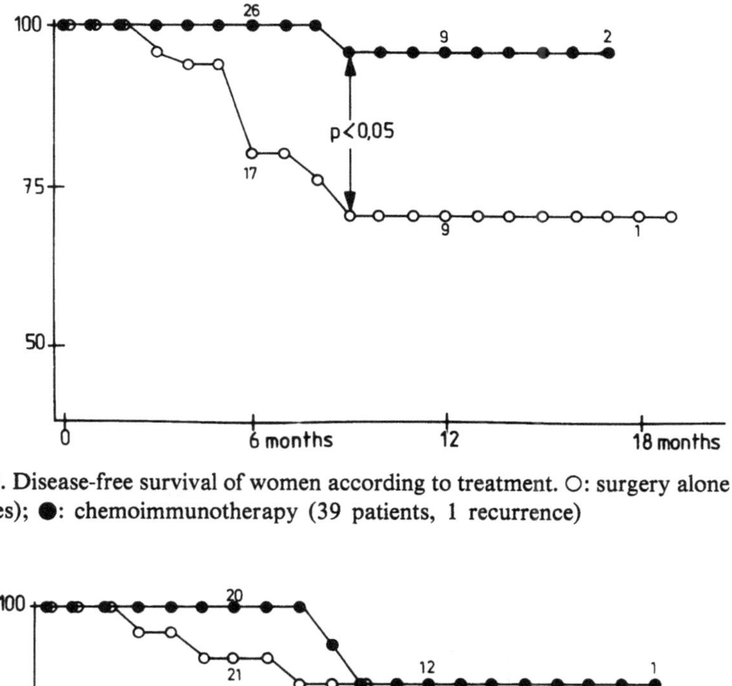

Fig. 11. Protocol 4 NK 76. Disease-free survival of women according to treatment. ○: surgery alone (43 patients, 7 recurrences); ●: chemoimmunotherapy (39 patients, 1 recurrence)

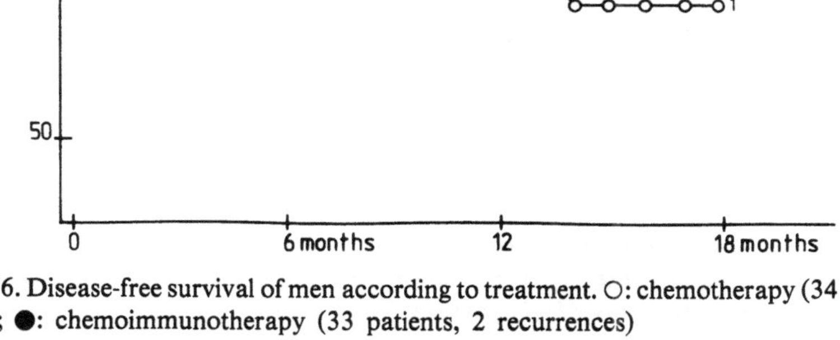

Fig. 12. Protocol 4 NK 76. Disease-free survival of men according to treatment. ○: chemotherapy (34 patients, 6 recurrences); ●: chemoimmunotherapy (33 patients, 2 recurrences)

Table 6. Distribution of patients according to site of primary at time of presentation (Protocol 4 NK 76)

	Men		Women	
	Chemo θ	Chemo-immuno θ	Control	Chemo-immuno θ
Head and neck	6 (1)	3 (0)	3 (0)	–
Upper limb	6 (2)	6 (0)	6 (0)	3 (0)
Lower limb without leg	8 (0)	5 (0)	2 (0)	16 (2)
Leg	1 (0)	2 (0)	15 (0)	12 (0)
Trunk	11 (3)	16 (2)	7 (2)	14 (0)

Numbers of recurrences are given in parentheses.

Table 7. Distribution of patients according to histology (Protocol 4 NK 76)

	Level of invasion			Type	
	III	IV	V	SSM	Nodular
Men					
Chemo θ	16 (1)	15 (3)	3 (2)	24 (3)	10 (3)
Chemoimmuno θ	16 (1)	11 (1)	6 (0)	24 (0)	8 (1)
Women					
Control	21 (0)	20 (6)	2 (1)	26 (6)	27 (1)
Chemoimmuno θ	18 (0)	19 (1)	2 (0)	26 (0)	13 (1)

Numbers of recurrences are given in parentheses.

The distribution of patients according to site of the primary is comparable to that of 2 NK 73 (Table 6). In this study patients with leg melanoma fare worse (4 recurrences in 27 patients). Distribution of histologic type and level of invasion is shown in Table 7. This distribution is homogeneous in the different groups of the study. We did not find any significant difference in disease-free survival rates according to histologic type. Only 38% of the patients with level V melanoma were free of disease at 12 months, as against 72% and 95% for level IV and V melanoma, respectively, confirming the very poor prognosis of level V melanoma (Fig. 13).

Conclusion

In spite of the short follow-up period, the results of 4 NK 76 confirm our prior study: adjuvant therapy as performed seems to improve the disease-free interval of patients with primary malignant melanoma of level of invasion III, IV, or V, even in women patients. The effect of

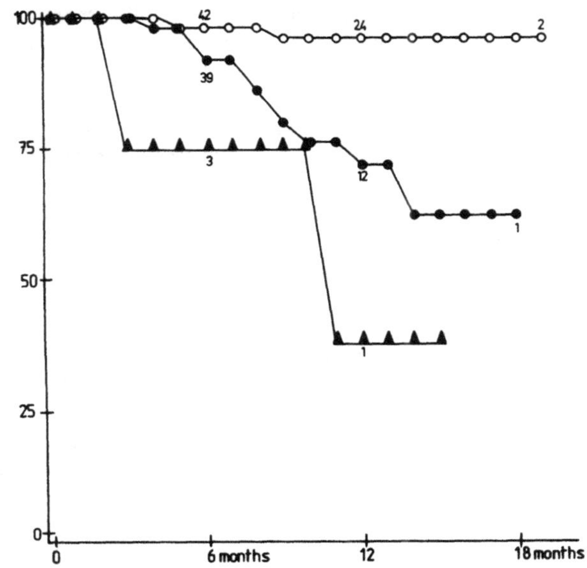

Fig. 13. Protocol 4 NK 76. Disease-free interval according to histologic level. ○: level III MM (71 patients, 2 recurrences); ●: level IV MM (65 patients, 11 recurrences); ▲: level V MM (13 patients, 3 recurrences)

our form of immunotherapy on the disease-free interval and survival cannot yet be evaluated. A prognosis-related staging of malignant melanoma based on histologic findings (type, level of invasion, thickness of lesion), sex, and localization of the primary might give useful guidelines for therapy: i.e., type of drug, doses, and time schedule, and improve the benefit that can be obtained from adjuvant therapy in the management of primary malignant melanoma.

References

1. Banzet, P., Jacquillat, C., Civatte, J., Puissant, A., Maral, J., Chastang, C., Israel, L., Belaich, S., Jourdain, J. C., Weil, M., Auclerc, G.: Adjuvant chemotherapy in the management of primary malignant melanoma. Cancer *41,* 1240–1248 (1978)
2. Banzet, P., Ricbourg, B., Jacquillat, C., Dufourmentel, M.: Traitement des mélanomes malins. Essai d'utilisation du DTIC en infusion intra-arterielle. Nouv. Presse Méd. *4,* 1477–1480 (1975)
3. Beardmore, G. L., Quinn, R. L., Little, J. H.: Malignant melanoma in Queensland: pathology of 105 fatal cutaneous melanoma. Pathology *2,* 277–286 (1970)
4. Berkson, J., Gage, R. P.: Calculation of survival rates for cancer. Mayo Clin. Proc. *25,* 270–286 (1950)
5. Clark, W. H., Ainsworth, A. M., Bernardino, E. A., Yang, C. H., Mihm, M. C., Reed, R. J.: The developmental biology of primary human malignant melanomas. Semin. Oncol. *2,* 83–103 (1975)
6. Clark, W. H., From, L., Bernardino, E. A., Mihm, M. C.: The histogenesis and biologic behavior of primary human malignant melanomas of the skin. Cancer Res. *29,* 705–726 (1969)
7. Elwood, J. M., Lee, J. A. H.: Recent data on the epidemiology of malignant melanoma. Semin. Oncol. *2,* 1949–1954 (1975)
8. Franklin, J. D., Reynolds, V. H., Page, D. L.: Cutaneous melanoma: a twenty years retrospective study with clinico-pathologic correlation. Plast. Reconstr. Surg. *56,* 277–285 (1975)

9. Gutterman, J. U., Mavligit, G., Reed, R., Richmann, S., McBride, C. E., Hersh, E. M.: Immunology and immunotherapy of human-malignant melanoma: historic review and perspectives for the future. Semin. Oncol. *2,* 155–174 (1975)
10. Gutterman, J. U., Mavligit, G., Gottlieb, J. A., Burgess, M. A., McBride, C. E., Einhorn, L., Freireich, E. J., Hersh, E. M.: Chemoimmunotherapy of disseminated malignant melanoma with dimethyl triazeno imidazole carboxamide and bacillus Calmette Guérin. N. Engl. J. Med. *291,* 592–597 (1974)
11. Israel, L.: Effect of intra-nodular BCG in 22 melanoma patients. Panminerva Med. *17,* 187–188 (1975)
12. Jacquillat, C., Auclerc, G., Weil, M., Israel, L., Banzet, P.: Chimiothérapie des mélanomes malins. Rev. Prat. *25,* 4057–4059 (1975)
13. Johnson, F. D., Jacobs, E. M.: Chemotherapy of metastatic malignant melanoma. Experience with 73 patients. Cancer *27,* 1306–1312 (1971)
14. Knutson, C. O., Mori, J. M., Spratt, J. S.: Melanoma. Curr. Probl. Surg. *12,* 3–55 (1971)
15. Luce, J. K.: Chemotherapy of malignant melanoma. Cancer *30,* 1604–1615 (1972)
16. McGovern, V. J.: The classification of melanoma and its relationship to prognosis. Pathology *2,* 89–98 (1970)
17. McLeod, G. R., Beardmore, G. L., Little, J. H., Quinn, R. L., Davis, N.: Results of treatment of 361 patients with malignant melanoma in Queensland. Med. J. Austr. *1,* 1211–1216 (1971)
18. McLeod, R., Davis, N. C., Heron, J. J., Caldnell, R. A., Little, J. H., Quinn, R. L.: A retrospective survey of 498 patients with malignant melanoma. Surg. Gynecol. Obstet. *126,* 99–108 (1968)
19. Nathanson, L., Wolter, J., Horton, J., Colshig, J., Schnider, B., Schilling, A.: Characteristics of prognosis and response to an imidazole carboxamide in malignant melanoma. Clin. Pharmacol. Ther. *12,* 955–962 (1971)
20. Olsen, G.: The malignant melanoma of the skin. New theories based on a study of 500 cases. Acta Chir. Scand. *365* [Suppl.], 128–136 (1966)
21. Stehlin, J. S., Clark, R. L., Vickers, W. E., Monges, A.: Perfusion for malignant melanoma of the extremities. Am. J. Surg. *105,* 607–614 (1963)
22. Veronesi, U. et al.: Clinical trial for treatment of malignant melanoma. International Group for Clinical Study of Melanoma, 1975

Immunotherapy for Recurrent Malignant Melanoma: Efficacy of BCG in Prolonging the Postoperative Disease-Free Interval and Survival

J. U. Gutterman, S. P. Richman, C. M. McBride, M. A. Burgess, S. L. Bartold, A. Kennedy, E. A. Gehan, G. Mavligit, and E. M. Hersh

In this report, we summarize updated results with adjuvant immunotherapy with bacillus Calmette-Guérin (BCG) for patients with recurrent malignant melanoma. This program was initiated in 1971. Preliminary reports have been published elsewhere [5, 6].

Materials and Methods

Between November 1971 and March 1976, 107 patients with regional lymph node metastases were entered in the study. All patients had recurrent melanoma in regional lymph nodes and were eligible for the study after surgical removal of all clinical evidence of tumor. Forty-two patients were entered into the first trial that was conducted between November 1971 and October 1974. Twenty patients received high dose Tice strain BCG and 22 patients received low dose Tice BCG, as described earlier. In the second trial that was conducted between October 1974 and March 1976, 40 patients received fresh frozen Pasteur strain BCG. Twenty-five patients were included in another trial conducted between October 1974 and March 1976. These patients received chemotherapy with DTIC, 250 mg/m^2 daily for 5 days, as well as fresh frozen Pasteur strain BCG, 6×10^8 viable units on days 7, 12, and 17. Cycles were repeated every 21 days.

The surgical control group consisted of 260 patients with stage IIIB melanoma who had been treated with surgery alone at M. D. Anderson Hospital between January 1965 and October 1971. Variables of these patients were examined in a comparable fashion to that of the patients in our study. The natural histories of these surgical control patients will be examined in detail in another report. The statistical methods used included the generalized Wilcoxon test and a one-tailed analysis for testing differences between disease-free or survival curves, (4) and the methods of Kaplan and Meier for calculating and plotting disease-free and survival curves [7].

Results

The postoperative disease-free interval for the surgically treated control and the BCG-treated groups of stage IIIB patients with less than five involved nodes is shown in Figure 1. There has been a statistically significant prolongation of the postoperative disease-free interval for patients treated with either high dose Tice or fresh frozen Pasteur strain BCG compared with the control group. No benefit was derived for those patients treated with low dose Tice BCG. The survival for the group of patients with less than five involved nodes is shown in Figure 2. Patients treated with the high doses of BCG (Tice or fresh frozen Pasteur BCG) have had a highly significant prolongation of survival. Only four of ten patients treated with high dose Tice and 7 of 40 treated with fresh frozen Pasteur BCG have died.

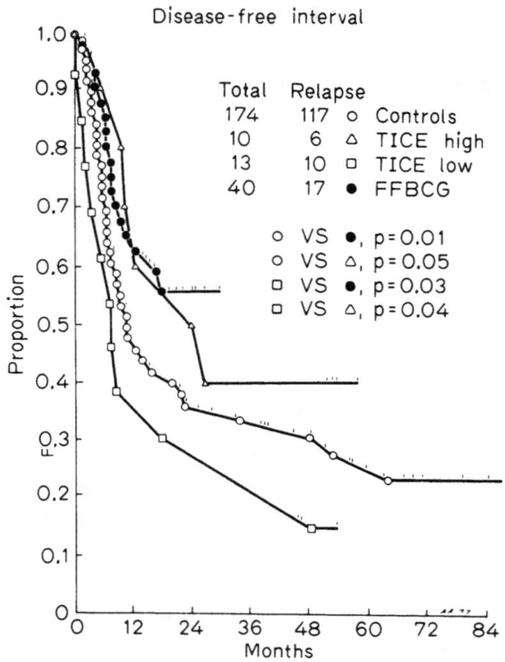

Fig. 1. Postoperative disease-free interval for surgically treated control and BCG-treated groups of stage IIIB patients with less than five involved nodes

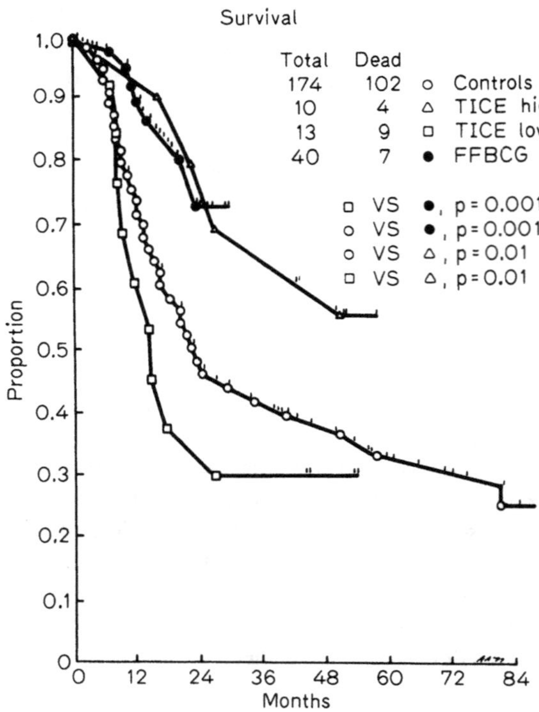

Fig. 2. Postoperative survival for patients with less than five involved nodes

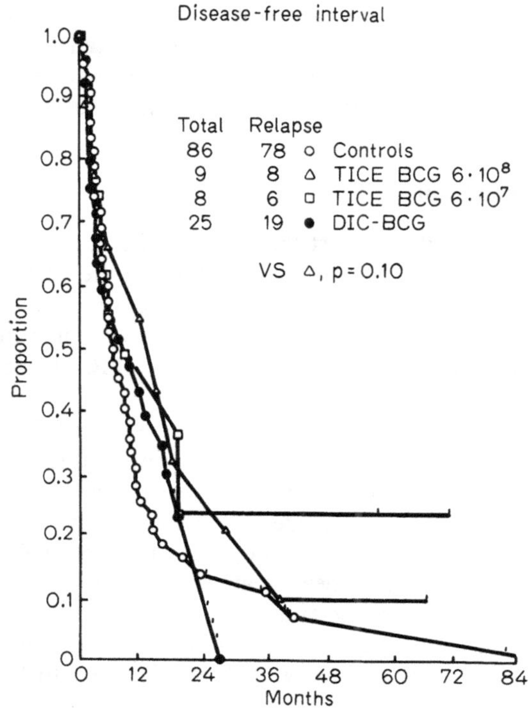

Fig. 3. Postoperative disease-free interval for patients treated with BCG alone or DTIC plus BCG

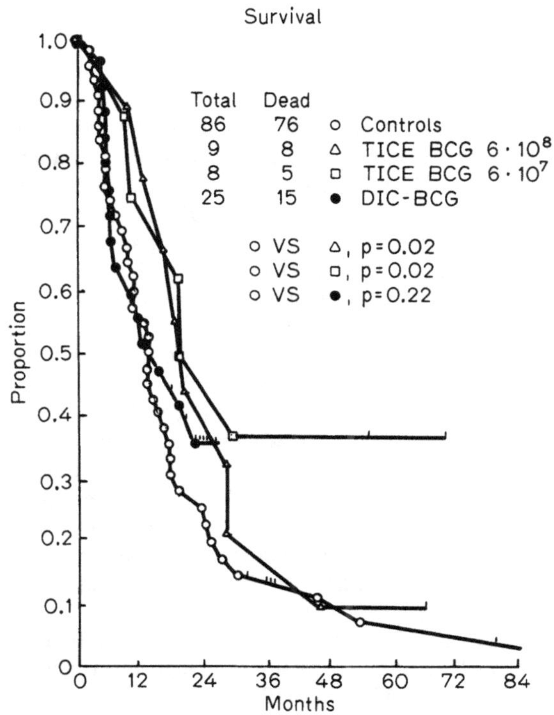

Fig. 4. Postoperative survival for patients treated with BCG alone or DTIC plus BCG

In contrast to these encouraging results, little benefit has been derived for patients with five or more involved nodes. There has been no statistical improvement in the postoperative disease-free interval for patients treated with BCG alone or DTIC plus BCG (Fig. 3). There has been little improvement in the postoperative survival time (Fig. 4).

Discussion

These results suggest that viable BCG given in doses of approximately 6×10^8 colony-forming units is capable of prolonging the postoperative disease-free interval and survival among patients with small amounts of residual tumor. Patients with five or more nodes, in which the natural history is considerably worse, appeared to have benefited only slightly or not at all, even with the addition of DTIC chemotherapy to the adjuvant immunotherapy regimen.

Several groups have now reported successful prolongation of postoperative disease-free interval and survival, particularly among patients with small numbers of positive lymph nodes [1–3, 8]. The original work of MORTON and EILBER and ourselves have been confirmed as noted in this conference by several groups.

Despite the promising results, it is clear that BCG immunotherapy for patients with positive nodes is still not ideal treatment since the majority of patients continue to relapse and eventually die of their tumor. Earlier application of BCG therefore seems indicated. Preliminary results of adjuvant BCG in patients with primary melanoma of the trunk in our own experience is promising. This would seem to be the ideal clinical situation in which to investigate adjuvant immunotherapy. Clearly, adjuvant immunotherapy is safe and it appears that benefit has been achieved. Further trials will need to be carried out with other immunotherapeutic modalities to maximize the clinical benefit.

References

1. Beretta, A.: Controlled study for prolonged chemotherapy, immunotherapy, and chemotherapy plus immunotherapy as adjuvant to surgery. In: Immunotherapy of cancer. Present status of trials in man. Terry, W. D., Windhorst, D. (eds.). New York: Raven Press 1978
2. Bluming, A. Z., Vogel, C. L., Ziegler, J. L.: Immunological effects of BCG in malignant melanoma: Two modes of administration compared. Ann. Intern. Med. *76,* 405–411 (1972)
3. Eilber, F. R., Morton, D. L., Holmes, E. C., Sparks, F. C., Ramming, K. P.: Adjuvant immunotherapy with BCG in treatment of regional lymph node metastases from malignant melanoma. N. Engl. J. Med. *294,* 237–240 (1976)
4. Gehan, E. A.: A generalized Wilcoxon test for comparing arbitrarily singlycensored samples. Biometrika *52,* 203–223 (1965)
5. Gutterman, J. U., Mavligit, G. M., McBride, C. M., Frei, E., Freireich, E. J., Hersh, E. M.: Active immunotherapy with BCG for recurrent malignant melanoma. Lancet *1973 I,* 1208–1212
6. Gutterman, J. U., Mavligit, G. M., Burgess, M. A., Cardinos, J. D., Blumenschein, G. R., Gottlieb, J. A., McBride, C. M., McCredie, K. B., Bodey, G. P., Rodriquez, V., Freireich, E. J., Hersh, E. M.: Immunotherapy of human solid tumors and acute leukemia with BCG: Prolongation of disease free interval and survival. Cancer Immunol. Immunother. *1,* 99–107 (1976)
7. Kaplan, E. L., Meier, P.: Nonparametric estimation from incomplete observations. J. Am. Stat. Assoc. *53,* 457–481 (1958)
8. Morton, D. L., Eilber, F. R., Holmes, E. C., Hunt, J. S., Ketcham, A. S., Silverstein, M. J., Sparks, F. C.: BCG immunotherapy of malignant melanoma: Summary of a seven year experience. Ann. Surg. *180,* 635–643 (1974)

Results of a Nonrandomized Trial in Malignant Melanoma Patients (Clark's Stages III–V) Treated by Post-Surgical Chemoimmunotherapy

B. Serrou, H. Pujol, J. Domas, and L. Gauci

Introduction

Malignant melanoma is a poor prognosis disease when centered in the trunk region and whenever node infiltration has occurred [7, 14]. For this reason, we initiated in 1972 a nonrandomized study of complementary chemoimmunotherapy treatment following radical surgery. Chemoimmunotherapy was modulated according to postchemotherapeutic observations concerning immunologic restoration and overshoot phenomena [8, 12]. This therapeutic practice has subsequently been confirmed experimentally.

Patients, Materials, and Methods

Choice of Patients

From 1972 to 1975, we selected untreated patients who had had exeresis biopsy within the preceding 2 months. Previously treated cases (local excision) with secondary regional lymph node metastases, whether or not associated with a local recurrence were also included in this trial. In all cases, patients were at Clark's grade III–V and had malignant melanomas of the trunk region (with or without node involvement), and/or other localizations where node infiltration had been histologically confirmed. The patients in this group were compared with a historical group treated from 1962 to 1972 by the same surgical team and matched with the test group receiving chemoimmunotherapy. The following were the exclusion criteria: patients less than 15 years of age or older than 70 years of age at the time of presentation; patients with a previous history of cancer or a symptomatic disease; patients having received previous chemo- and/or immunotherapy; patients showing evidence of visceral and/or distant metastases.

Treatment

All patients, including those of the historical group, were treated by radical surgery extending at least 5 cm beyond the primary lesion with verification of the peripheral resected region. This excision was followed by a skin graft. In all cases, node excision was effected at the same time, except for trunk malignant melanoma, where lymph node dissection was performed only for clinically infiltrated nodes. The complementary treatment consisted of chemotherapy with vincristine (1 mg/m^2 IV) on days 1 and 2, DTIC (200 mg/m^2 IV) on days 3 and 4, and CCNU (50 mg/m^2 PO) on days 5 and 6. Chemotherapy was followed by BCG immunotherapy (fresh or immuno BCG-F; Institut Pasteur) on days 7, 14, 21 and 28, which was administered at 150 mg per heaf-gun application. This cycle was repeated every 42 days. The total length of treatment was 2 years.

Evaluation Criteria

Disease-free survival time was employed as the criterion of therapeutic efficacy.

Results (Fig. 1)

We were unable to demonstrate any significant statistical difference due to age or sex between the historical group and the chemoimmunotherapy group, nor was there any difference due to Clark's grade, localization of the disease, or lymph node involvement in the trunk disease patients. The historical group includes 89 patients while the treated group contains 35 patients: 10 grade III, 17 grade IV and, 8 grade V. There were 7 with localization in the trunk, 9 with involvement of the head and neck, 8 with superior limb and 11 with inferior limb localizations. Of the seven patients with trunk involvement, five did not demonstrate clinical lymph infiltration and were therefore not considered for lymph node dissection.

Evolution in the treated group was as follows: nine locoregional recurrences, four brain metastases, four pleuropulmonary metastases, and two liver metastases. Two patients died of intercurrent causes, one of a cerebrovascular accident and the other of myocardial infarct. These patients were included in the analysis. Disease-free survival studies show a significant difference after 2 years in favor of the chemoimmunotherapy group, with a plateau at 45% between the 42nd and 54th month. This is significantly ($P < 0.001$) different from the historical group (12%). A discontinuity of the treated group curve is noted at 2 years, i.e., at cessation of chemotherapy.

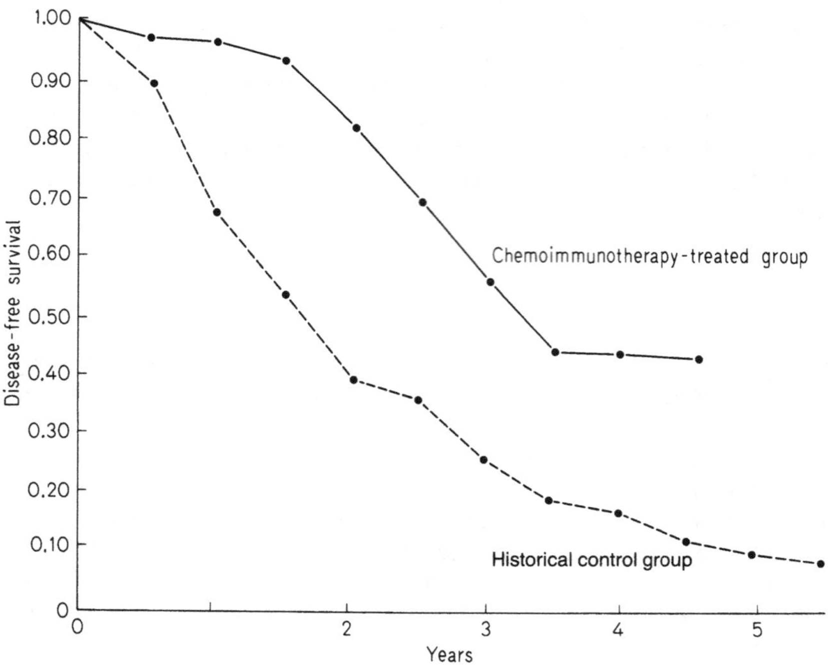

Fig. 1. Comparative results for malignant melanoma patients (Clark's stages III–V)

Discussion

Clark's grades III–V of malignant melanoma localized in the trunk or with lymph node involvement have a very poor 5-year prognosis (approximately 15%), which is noted in the literature [7, 14] and agrees well with the values noted in our historical control group. The use of combined chemoimmunotherapy significantly prolongs the disease-free survival by 4.5 years, with a plateau at 45%. It is pointed out that this treatment is well tolerated and, as we have shown [6, 13], does not elicit any major toxicity.

An interesting point in our opinion is the discontinuity observed around the 2nd year at the cessation of chemoimmunotherapy. Two groups seemed to emerge: patients who relapse in the following year and those who do not relapse, which explains the plateau after the 42nd month. Moreover, we have already reported on the immunologic modifications within these two groups [6, 13], relapse patients being characterized by a reduced number of circulating monocytes, a reduced serum lysozyme concentration, and a decreased number of B-lymphocytes, with increased B-lymphocyte response to PWM, increased levels of IgM, of antigen-antibody complexes, and of β-2-microglobulin. We also observed a decreased number of autorosetting cells [2, 3], whereas E rosettes and skin tests [6, 13] do not correlate with the prognosis.

Our results, therefore, confirm the efficacy of chemotherapy, immunotherapy [1, 4, 5, 9–11], or chemoimmunotherapy [1 and GUTTERMANN] in high-risk malignant melanoma patients. In the light of these results, it seems that in all probability certain patients require a more intensive complementary therapy while others are most probably overtreated. Such matters as prolongation of this treatment, intensification of chemotherapy over a short period of time, and possibly associated with immunorestorative therapy (Levamisole, thymosin) require further study. The immunologic modifications observed argue in favor of modulation of the immune response in cases of high-risk malignant melanoma.

References

1. Beretta, G.: Controlled study for prolonged chemotherapy, immunotherapy and chemotherapy plus immunotherapy as an adjuvant to surgery in stage I–II malignant melanoma: preliminary report. In: Immunotherapy of cancer: present status of trials in man. Terry, W. D., Windhorst, D. (eds.), p. 19. New York: Raven Press 1978
2. Caraux, J., Serrou, B.: The binding of autologous erythrocytes by human lymphocytes. Biomedicine (in press) (1978)
3. Caraux, J., Thierry, C., Serrou, B.: Human autologous rosettes. II. Prognostic significance of variations in autologous rosette forming cells in the peripheral blood of cancer patients. J.N.C.I. (in press) (1978)
4. Cunningham, T. J., Schoenfeld, D., Nathanson, L., Wolter, J., Patterson, W. B., Cohen, M. H.: A controlled study of adjuvant therapy in patients with stage I and II malignant melanoma. In: Immunotherapy of cancer: present status of trials in man. Terry, W. D., Windhorst, D. (eds.), p. 19. New York: Raven Press 1978
5. Eilber, F. R., Morton, D. L., Holmes, E. C., Sparks, F. C., Ramming, K. P.: Adjuvant immunotherapy with B.C.G. in treatment of regional lymph-node metastases from malignant melanoma. N. Engl. J. Med. *294*, 237–240 (1976)
6. Gauci, L., Caraux, J., Thierry, C., Pujol, H., Serrou, B.: Modifications of the immune status induced in malignant melanoma patients by chemo-immunotherapy and immunotherapy. In: Human lymphocyte differentiation. Its application to cancer. Serrou, B., Rosenfeld, C. (eds.). New York: North-Holland 1978 (in press)

7. Gupta, T. K. D.: Results of treatment of 269 patients with primary cutaneous melanoma: a five-year prospective study. Ann. Surg. *186,* 201–209 (1977)
8. Hersh, E. M., Whitecar, J. P., Mc Credie, K. B., Bodey, G. P., Freireich, E. J.: Immunocompetence, immunosuppression and prognosis in acute leukemia. N. Engl. J. Med. *1211,* 285–291 (1971)
9. Jewell, W. R., Thomas, J. H., Sterchi, J. M., Morse, P. A., Humphrey, L. J.: Critical analysis of treatment of stage II and stage III melanoma patients with immunotherapy. Ann. Surg. *183,* 543–548 (1976)
10. Morton, D. L., Holmes, E. C., Eilber, F. R., Sparks, F., Ramming, K. P.: Adjuvant immunotherapy of malignant melanoma: preliminary results of a randomized trial in patients with lymph node metastases. In: Immunotherapy of cancer: present status of trials in man. Terry, W. D., Windhorst, D. (eds.), p. 57. New York: Raven Press 1978
11. Pinsky, C. M., Hirshaut, Y., Wanebo, H. J., Hilal, E. Y., Fortner, J. G., Mike, V., Schottenfeld, D., Oettgen, H. F.: Surgical adjuvant immunotherapy with B.C.G. in patients with malignant melanoma: results of a prospective randomized trial. In: Immunotherapy of cancer: present status of trials in man. Terry, W. D., Windhorst, D. (eds.), p. 27. New York: Raven Press 1978
12. Serrou, B., Dubois, J. B.: Immunological overshoot phenomenon following cancer chemotherapy: significance in prognosis evaluation of solid tumors. Biomedicine *23,* 41–45 (1975)
13. Serrou, B., Caraux, J., Domas, J., Grenier, J., Thierry, C., Pujol, H.: Value of some immunological parameters to evaluate the prognosis of melanoma patients treated by chemo-immunotherapy Proc. ASCO *19,* 349 (Abs. C-170) (1978)
14. Veronesi, U., Cascinelli, N., Preda, F.: Prognosis of malignant melanoma according to regional metastases. Am. J. Roentgenol. *111,* 301–309 (1971)

Value of Adjuvant Therapy With Bacille Calmette Guerin (BCG) or Dimethl Triazeno Imidazole Carboximide (DTIC) in the Control of Minimal Residual Disease in Stage II Melanoma

H. H. Peter, K. E. M. Deutschmann, J. Deinhardt, and H. Deicher

Introduction

Besides several encouraging initial reports on the value of BCG adjuvant immunotherapy (BCG-AIT) in recurrent malignant melanoma [1, 8, 10, 12, 13, 15, 17, 21, 25, 26], recently ineffective therapeutic attempts with this regimen have also been reported [7, 23]. A main criticism was directed against conclusions drawn from nonrandomized studies with historical control groups, since a better understanding of the biology of the tumor [2, 4, 9] and its prognostic factors [2, 11, 19] has led to an improved surgical treatment resulting in longer remission durations for melanoma patients treated by surgery only [24]. Moreover, the successful introduction of dimethyl triazeno imidazole carboximide (DTIC) to the treatment of disseminated melanoma [5, 18, 20] has raised the question whether this drug either alone, in multiple drug combinations [5], or associated with immunotherapy [14, 16] might not be a more promising adjuvant regimen for treating residual minimal disease in stage II melanoma than BCG alone. The WHO Melanoma Cooperative Group in Milano is currently examining this question in a prospective chemo- and/or immunotherapy trial (protocol No. 6) [6] and is regularly preparing progress reports. So far from our hospital, 36 stage II melanoma patients have been entered into this trial. A considerable number of patients were, however, not eligible for the prospective study. It is the purpose of this presentation to report on the fate of these patients. Following radical surgery they received either standard BCG-AIT or DTIC, when the drug became commercially available in Germany. For the BCG-AIT group the remission duration was related to preexisting tuberculin hypersensitivity. The disease-free intervals of both the BCG-AIT and the DTIC group have been compared to a nonrandomized control group of 38 patients.

Material and Methods

During the clinical staging of our patients according to protocol 6 of the WHO Melanoma Group, we realized that stage II melanoma is a less well-defined condition than it might appear at first glance. Problems arise particularly when it comes to classifying local recurrences, in transit metastases, satellite disease, regional recurrences, and lymph node metastases of unknown primaries. It was reasonable to exclude these patients from the prospective chemoimmunotherapy trial 6 together with stage II melanoma patients who had previously received prophylactic local radiotherapy after the excision of the primary tumor [6]. However, it appears from our experience that the excluded patients have an overall similarly poor prognosis than typical stage II patients with regional lymph node involvement. We adopted, therefore, a new definition of clinical stage II melanoma, which allows classification of all "high risk" patients (Table 1), including the previous stage 1A [9, 24] and the trunk melanomas of Clark's grade IV and V.

Table 1. Clinical staging of cutaneous malignant melanoma

Stage	Involvement	TNM
I	Primary melanoma of extremities, head and neck level 1–5, of the trunk level 1–3	T1–5(3)N0M0
IIA	Primary melanoma of the trunk level 4,5; satellite tumors local recurrences; in transit metastases regional micrometastases	TxN0–micrM0
IIB	Clinically apparent regional lymph node metastases, microscopical involvement of less than 4 nodes	TxN1–4M0
IIC	Massive regional lymph node involvement with more than 4 positive nodes, extracapsular growth; recurrent regional tumor	TxN>4M0
III	Distant metastases; disseminated disease	TxNxM1–x

In the present study, 28 high risk melanoma patients (28–78 years of age, 14 females, 14 males), with regional lymph node involvement (No. = 20), in transit metastases, (No. = 1) locoregional recurrences (No. = 5), or invasive trunk melanoma of Clark's grade IV and V (No. = 2) received BCG-AIT for 3–35 months, starting 2–24 weeks after radical surgery. A nonrandomized group of 17 stage II melanoma patients (24–69 years of age, 8 females, 9 males) were postoperatively treated by 3–17 cycles of DTIC starting within 6 weeks after surgery. On 5 consecutive days, 200 mg/m^2 of DTIC were injected intravenously as a bolus, and the subsequent treatment courses were started on days 29, 57, 85, etc. Leukocytes and platelets were counted every 2 weeks; when the values dropped below 3000/mm^3 and 100,000/mm^3, respectively, the treatment-free interval was prolonged until the patient had recovered from toxicity. In no case was prolongation of more than 1 week necessary. Throughout the follow-up period, a thorough physical check-up was performed every month. Complete blood counts, liver and renal function studies, urinanalysis, and appropriate radiologic and scintigraphic studies [22] were done every 3–5 months. Ten patients in the BCG group and one patient in the DTIC group had previously received prophylactic local radiotherapy after excision of the primary melanoma. No further radiotherapy was given to any one of the patients after surgical excision of the secondaries and during the subsequent BCG-AIT or DTIC treatment. Before the first BCG treatment, each patient was tested intradermally with 10 IU (0.2 μg) of tuberculin (PPD, Behring Werke AG, Marburg, Germany). BCG was then applied as follows: 37.5 mg of lyophilized Pasteur BCG (approximately 10^8 viable bacilli) were dissolved in 0.3 ml of saline, and four drops of the suspension were placed on a thoroughly cleaned 5 × 12 cm skin area on the right upper arm. One Heaf gun shot (20 needles, 2 mm deep; Impfstempel, Fa. Ulrich, Ulm, Germany) was fired through each of the four drops of vaccine. The vaccination sites were allowed to dry for 15–20 min and washing was avoided at the sites for 48 h. Subsequent vaccinations were performed in a clockwise schedule continuing on the left upper arm, the left hip, the right hip, and again on the right upper arm. Skin reactions were first read after 1 week and graded into: negative, 1+ (faint redness, no swelling), 2+ (redness, slight swelling), 3+ (strong redness, swelling, and confluence of adjacent puncture sites), 4+ (strong redness, swelling, complete confluence, pustules, strong perifocal reaction, or generalized skin rash). BCG was given weekly until 2+ and 3+ skin reactions were observed; thereafter, vaccinations were performed monthly. In patients with 4+ reactions, subsequent BCG applications were delayed for 1–3 months, depending on the persistence of the vaccination sites. As a rule, it was attempted to maintain permanently at least four 2+ to 3+ reaction sites. The treatment end point was reached after 2 years or when the tumor recurred. Patients who relapsed under BCG-AIT were subsequently put on DTIC, usually after additional surgery, whereas patients relapsing under DTIC received either CCNU (150 mg/m^2 every 5–6 weeks) or radiotherapy plus radiosensitizer (ICRF). The remission duration curves of the BCG-AIT group and the DTIC group were compared to a nonrandomized control group of 38 stage II melanoma patients (23–80 years of age; 21 females, 17 males) including both historical controls treated during 1969–1973 in our radiotherapy department (28 cases) and patients who did not receive any adjuvant treatment for various reasons (10 cases).

Results

The analysis of the three groups of patients according to sex and localization of the primary tumor is presented in Table 2. With the exception of a slight prevalence of trunk melanomas in the BCG group, the three groups of patients are well balanced. Remission durations of stage II melanoma patients are illustrated in Figure 1. The mean tumor-free intervals of patients treated postoperatively with either BCG or DTIC are identical; compared to the control group, however, both are significantly prolonged ($P < 0.01$ after the 10th month). Within the BCG-AIT group there was a close relationship between the PPD skin test and the first BCG reaction (Table 3). As a rule, patients exhibiting strong tuberculine sensitivity started with 3+ and 4+ initial BCG reactions, indicating a previous sensitization to mycobacterial antigens. PPD-negative patients, on the other hand, started usually with negative or weakly positive initial BCG reactions (Table 3) and had to be immunized for several weeks until 2+ and 3+ reactions appeared. The previously reported trend that patients with weak initial BCG reactions, showing gradual positivity after several vaccinations, have longer remissions than patients with strongly positive initial BCG reactions [8] was again confirmed

Table 2. Distribution of stage II melanoma patients according to sex and localization of the primary tumor

Type of adjuvant treatment	Males (No.)	Females (No.)	Head, neck, extremities	Trunk
BCG	14	14	11	17
DTIC	9	8	9	8
None	17	21	20	18

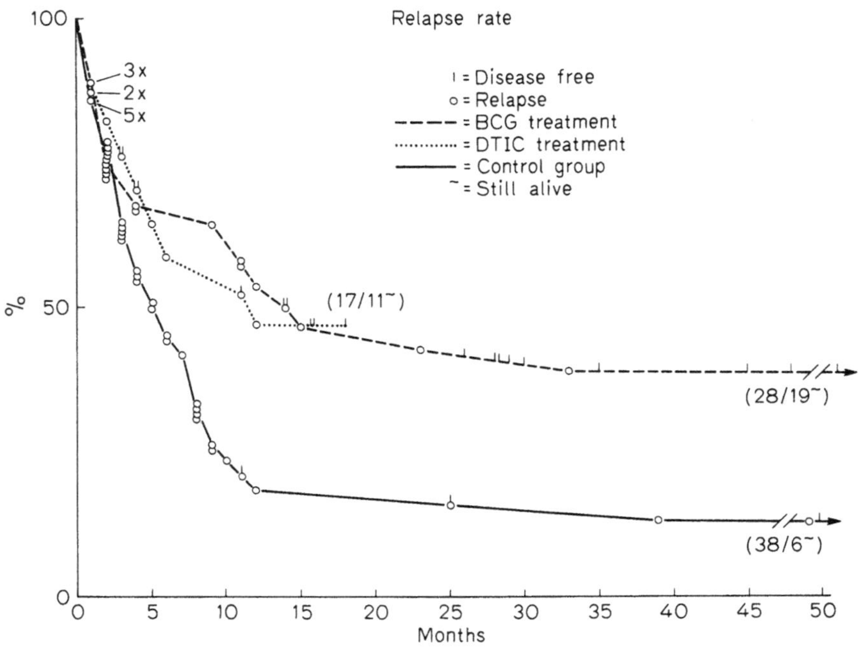

Fig. 1. Remission duration of stage II melanoma patients treated after radical surgery either with epicutaneous BCG adjuvant immunotherapy or with DTIC adjuvant chemotherapy. In comparison to a nonrandomized control group of 38 patients treated either by surgery alone or by surgery plus irradiation, there is a significant difference ($P < 0.01$) after the 10th month

in this study. The mean remission periods for both groups were calculated to be 23.6 and 11.2 months, respectively (Table 3), the difference being significant at the $P < 0.05$ level. It may be stated that the group of patients with weak initial BCG reactions did by no means represent lower risk patients, as judged by the number of regional lymph nodes involved and the size of the primary tumor (thickness, Clark's grading, presence of satellites).

Table 3. Relationship between initial BCG reactivity and remission duration in stage II melanoma treated with systemic BCG adjuvant immunotherapy

Intensity of 1st BCG reaction	No.	PPD skin test[a]		Relapsed (%)	Mean remission duration in months ± 1 SE
		Positive	Negative		
0/+/++	15[b]	7[b]	8[b]	54	23.6 ± 4.5[c]
+++/++++	13	11	2	68	11.2 ± 3.0

[a] Intradermal skin test with 0.2 μg of Behring PPD prior to first BCG vaccination. Positive reaction, induration ⩾ 16 mm ∅ at 72 h.

[b] Number of patients.

[c] Student's t test; difference is statistically significant at $P < 0.05$.

Table 4. Treatment and survival of melanoma patients after relapse under BCG adjuvant immunotherapy in stage II

Patient sex, age	Metastases	Treatment	Objective response to chemotherapy	Survival (months)
OD, F, 70	Locoreg.	S[a], DTIC	Yes	11
CS, F, 62	Bone, skin	S, DTIC, irradiation	Yes	13 →[b]
HG, M, 43	Pleura, lung	DTIC, CCNU[c]	Yes	5 →
GW, M, 45	Skin, lung	S, DTIC	Yes	14 →
WR, M, 29	Lung, viscera	S, DTIC	Yes	7 →
IM, F, 48	Skin	S, DTIC	No	5 →
MR, F, 62	Skin, liver	S, DTIC	No	16
SH, M, 49	Brain	DTIC, methotrexate	No	7
MS, F, 55	Locoreg.	S, DTIC	Uncertain	16 →
CS, F, 28	Locoreg.	S, DTIC-BCG	Uncertain	31 →
HW, M, 48	Skin, brain	S, VCPM[d], irradiation	No	10
HM, M, 41	Locoreg., brain	S, VCPM, irradiation	No	15
WO, M, 47	Pleura	VCPM	No	1
WL, M, 36	Liver, skin	S, VCPM, irradiation	No	14
JT, M, 60	Liver, skin	VCPM, irradiation	No	3
DN, M, 36	Locoreg.	S, CCNU	Too early	1

[a] S, more surgery.
[b] Patient still alive.
[c] CCNU, 250 mg every 6 weeks.
[d] VCPM, vincristine, 1 mg day 2 and 5, cyclophosphamide 300 mg IV day 1 and 5, procarbacin 150 mg day 1–5, methotrexate 50 mg day 1 and 4.

Table 4 summarizes the follow-up treatment of 15 stage II melanoma patients who relapsed under BCG-AIT. After additional surgery, these patients were usually put on DTIC, at least as soon as the drug became available in Germany. As can be seen, five of ten patients treated with DTIC showed an objective tumor regression whereas among the patients relapsing under DTIC (not shown in Table 4) in only one case could a partial remission be induced by subsequent CCNU treatment. It thus appears that unresponsiveness of a melanoma developing under chemotherapy confronts the physician with greater therapeutic problems than the recurrence of a tumor under immunotherapy, leaving still the potential weapon of chemotherapy.

Discussion

The presented preliminary study on adjuvant therapy in stage II melanoma surveys 4 years of experience with BCG and 2 years with DTIC. During July 1973 and May 1978, patients seen in our hospital were divided into two groups according to their eligibility for a prospective trial [6]. It was the purpose of this presentation to report on the noneligible patients who received, after radical surgery, either BCG-AIT or DTIC in monthly intervals. Their remission durations have been compared to a nonrandomized, historical control group of 38 patients, most of whom had been irradiated after surgery. So far the tumor-free intervals of the BCG- and the DTIC-treated patients did not significantly differ but both exhibited significantly prolonged remission periods compared to the control group of patients. It will be of interest to see whether these data will be confirmed by the prospective trial 6 of the WHO Melanoma Cooperative Group [6] from which the dosage schedules for BCG and DTIC have been adopted. Only a comparison with this trial may allow definite conclusions as to the value of BCG-AIT and DTIC in stage II melanoma; moreover, the value of a nonrandomized clinical study performed in one center may then be compared to a prospective multicenter trial.

Despite an eventual discordance with the upcoming data of the controlled trial, several interesting conclusions may be drawn from our local study. Thus, the introduction of BCG and DTIC has improved the remission durations of stage II melanoma patients in our hospital, may it just be by earlier diagnosis, better understanding of the tumor biology, refined surgical techniques, and regular postoperative follow-ups. The role of radiotherapy prior to active BCG-AIT needs further evaluation. So far the group of BCG-treated patients having received local irradiation after excision of the primary tumor is too small (No. = 10) to draw meaningful conclusions. Within the BCG-AIT group the previously reported trend for longer remissions in patients with weak initial BCG reactions [8] has become significant by now. Provided this observation will be confirmed on a greater number of patients, it would indicate that preexisting hypersensitivity to BCG or to cross-reacting mycobacterial antigens can predict noneffectiveness of BCG-AIT in stage II melanoma patients. Other adjuvants or vaccination schedules may then be used. In a recent report on BCG-sensitized melanoma patients, Buckley et al. [3] noted a relationship between the HLA-B7 phenotype and a specific delayed cutaneous hyporesponsiveness to tuberculin before and after attenuated tuberculosis infection. Whether this genetic linkage of the tuberculin responsiveness also affects the prognosis of BCG-treated melanoma patients is not yet known but needs to be tested.

An important observation in view of a strategical approach to adjuvant therapy in high risk melanoma patients is the fact that five of ten patients who relapsed under BCG-AIT showed objective responses under subsequent DTIC treatment (Table 4). Taking into consideration the identical remission durations of BCG and DTIC-treated stage II patients (Fig. 1), different susceptibilities of individual melanomas to both regimens have to be assumed. This would suggest that in stage II melanoma adjuvant therapy to surgery should start with BCG, particularly in tuberculin-negative patients and in stages IIA and IIB. Once the tumor has relapsed, DTIC is then still at disposition. In melanoma of stage IIC and in strongly tuberculin-positive patients, adjuvant therapy may be started with DTIC. Alternatively, DTIC and BCG may be combined from the beginning as has been reported for the treatment of stage III melanoma [14, 16]. In view of the considerable toxicity (nausea) of DTIC, the combined immunochemotherapy regimen is, however, only justified if a prolonged survival can be demonstrated for stage II melanoma patients treated by DTIC-BCG as compared to patients treated first by BCG and then by DTIC once the tumor has recurred.

Summary

Preliminary results of a nonrandomized study on adjuvant therapy in stage II melanoma are reported, surveying 4 years of experience with BCG adjuvant immunotherapy (BCG-AIT) and 2 years of experience with DTIC adjuvant chemotherapy. Stage II melanoma was newly defined as that group of melanoma patients with a high risk of recurrent disease. Compared to a predominantly historical control group of 38 cases, 28 high risk melanoma patients treated by BCG-AIT and 17 patients receiving DTIC showed a significantly improved remission duration. In the BCG group, patients with weak initial BCG reactions becoming gradually positive after several vaccinations seem to get more benefit from the adjuvant immunotherapy than do patients with strongly positive initial BCG reactions. Five of ten patients who relapsed under BCG-AIT showed objective tumor regressions under a subsequent DTIC chemotherapy, whereas unresponsiveness developing under DTIC appeared to be more resistant to subsequent treatments.

References

1. Bluming, A. Z., Vogel, C. L., Ziegler, J. L., Mody, N., Kamja, G.: Immunological effect of BCG in malignant melanoma: two modes of administration compared. Ann. Int. Med. *76*, 405–411 (1972)
2. Breslow, A.: Thickness, cross-sectional areas, and depth of invasion in the prognosis of cutaneous melanoma. Ann. Surg. *172*, 902 (1970)
3. Buckley III, C. E., White, D. H., Seigler, H. F.: HLA-B7 associated tuberculin hyporesponsiveness in BCG treated melanoma patients. Mongr. Allergy *11*, 97–105 (1977)
4. Clark, W. H., From, L., Bernadnino, E. A., Mihm, M. C.: The histogenesis and biologic behaviour of primary human malignant melanoma of the skin. Cancer Res. *29*, 705–726 (1969)
5. Comis, R. L.: DTIC (NSC-45388) in malignant melanoma: A perspective. Cancer Treat. Rep. *60*, 165–176 (1976)
6. Controlled study for prolonged chemotherapy immunotherapy and chemotherapy plus immunotherapy as an adjuvant to surgery. International Group for the Clinical study of Melanoma; Chairmen: U. Veronesi, G. Bonadonna, Milan.
7. Currie, G. A., McElwain, T. J.: Active immunotherapy as an adjunct to chemotherapy in the treatment of disseminated malignant melanoma: a pilot study. Br. J. Cancer *31*, 143–156 (1975)
8. Deutschmann, K. E. M., Peter, H. H., Schultheis, W., Deicher, H.: Experience with BCG adjuvant immunotherapy in stage II malignant melanoma. Tumori *63*, 303–307 (1977)
9. Devita, V. T., Fisher, R. I.: Natural history of malignant melanoma as related to therapy. Cancer Treat. Rep. *60*, 153–157 (1976)
10. Eilber, F. R., Morton, D. L., Holmes, E. C., Sparks, F. C., Rammig, K. P.: Adjuvant immunotherapy with BCG in treatment of regional-lymph node metastases from malignant melanoma. N. Engl. J. Med. *294*, 237–240 (1976)
11. Everall, J. D., Dowd, P. M.: Diagnosis, prognosis and treatment of melanoma. Lancet *1977/II*, 286–289
12. Grant, R. M., Mackie, R., Cochrane, A. J., Murray, E. L., Hoyle, D., Ross, C.: Results of administering BCG to patients with melanoma. Lancet *1974/II*, 1096–1100
13. Gutterman, J. U., Mavligit, S. M., McBride, C. M. et al.: Active immunotherapy with BCG for recurrent malignant melanoma. Lancet *1973/I*, 1208–1212
14. Gutterman, J. U., Mavligit, G. M., Gottlieb, J. A.: Chemoimmunotherapy of disseminated malignant melanoma with dimethyl triazeno imidazol carboxymide and Bacillus Calmette-Guérin. N. Engl. J. Med. *291*, 592–597 (1974)
15. Gutterman, J. U., Mavligit, G. M., Reed, R. C., Burgess, M. A., McBride, C. M., Hersh, E. M.: Adjuvant immunotherapy with BCG for recurrent malignant melanoma. Behring Inst. Mitt. *56*, 199–206 (1975)

16. Gutterman, J. U., Mavligit, G. M., Reed, R., Burgess, M. A., Gottlieb, J., Hersh, E. M.: Bacillus Calmette-Guérin Immunotherapy in combination with DTIC (NSC 45388) for the treatment of malignant melanoma. Cancer Treat. Rep. *60,* 177–182 (1976)
17. Ikonopisov, R. L.: The use of BCG in the combined treatment of malignant melanoma. Behring Inst. Mitt. *56,* 206–214 (1975)
18. Luce, I. K.: Chemotherapy of malignant melanoma. Cancer *30,* 1604–1615 (1972)
19. McGovern, V. I.: The classification of melanoma and its relationship with prognosis. Pathology *2,* 85–98 (1970)
20. Nathanson, L., Wolter, I., Horton, I.: Characteristics of prognosis and response to an Imidazol Carboxamide in malignant melanoma. Clin. Pharmacol. Ther. *12,* 955–962 (1971)
21. Nathanson, L.: Experience with BCG in malignant melanoma. Proc. Ann. Ass. Cancer Res. *12,* 99 (1971)
22. Peter, H. H., Brase, A., Meyer, P. B., Gisbertz, A., Dragojevic, D.: Die ^{67}Gallium Scintigraphie in der präoperativen Diagnostik des malignen Melanoms. Langenbecks Arch. Chir. *338,* 181–200 (1975)
23. Pinsky, C. M.Hirshaut, Y., Oettgen, H. F.: Treatment of malignant melanoma by intratumoral infection of BCG. Natl. Cancer Inst. Monogr. *39,* 225–228 (1973)
24. Rosenberg, S. A.: Surgical treatment of malignant melanoma. Cancer Treat. Rep. *60,* 159–163 (1976)
25. Spitler, L. E., Levin, A. S., Wybran, J.: Combined immunotherapy in malignant melanoma. Cell. Immunol. *21,* 1–19 (1976)
26. Thomas, J. W., Plenderleith, J. H., Clements, D. V., Landi, S.: Observations in immunotherapy of lymphoma and melanoma patients. Clin. Exp. Immunol. *21,* 82–96 (1975)

Controlled Study for Prolonged Chemotherapy, Immunotherapy, and Chemotherapy Plus Immunotherapy as an Adjuvant to Surgery in Malignant Melanoma (Trial 6): Preliminary Report[1]

U. Veronesi and G. Beretta[2, 3]

The International Group for the Clinical Study of Melanoma started in 1974 a controlled study to evaluate the effects of long-term adjuvant therapies on the disease-free period and survival in patients radically operated for primary or recurrent high-risk cutaneous melanoma. Preliminary data were presented in 1977 in Washington [1].

After radical surgery of primary melanoma of regional lymph nodes, all patients with primary melanoma of the skin located in the head and neck, in the extremities, and in the trunk with histologically positive regional adenopathies (N^+) were eligible for the trial. In addition, patients with melanoma of the trunk, Clark's levels III, IV, V, with histologically negative regional lymph nodes were included.

Only patients geographically accessible and providing an informed consent were accepted into the trial. Patients presenting any one of the following conditions were also excluded: previous chemotherapy or immunotherapy, fixation of lymph nodes, in transit metastases, younger than 15 or older than 75 years, concomitant neoplasia, major allergic disease, or symptomatic systemic diseases such as cardiovascular, renal, pulmonary, or hepatic diseases (i.e., patients at high risk for surgical procedure and prolonged follow-up).

All slides of primary melanoma and of regional dissected nodes were routinely reviewed by the panel of pathologists of the group. The Clark's grade of primary melanoma [2] and the number of examined and metastatic lymph nodes had to be specified and were recorded. Location of metastatic growth (intra- or extracapsular) also had to be specified.

After surgery, patients were stratified according to sex, primary site, nodal involvement (head and neck N^+, limbs N^+, trunk N^+, trunk N^-), and previous surgical treatment (indicated patient, including cases with an excisional biopsy within 6 weeks; previously treated cases, submitted to excision of the primary melanoma without concomitant regional lymph node

---

1 Supported by Contract NO1-CM-43726 NIH NCI-Bethesda.

2 Statistical analysis was performed by Dr. A. Morabito, Statistician WHO Collaborating Centers on Melanoma, Istituto Nazionale Tumori, Milan (Italy).

3 *Participants:* Dr. J. Adamus, Oncological Institute, Gliwice (Poland), Dr. C. Aubert, Institut Paoli Calmettes, Marseille (France), Dr. E. Bajetta, Istituto Nazionale Tumori, Milan (Italy), Dr. G. Beretta, Istituto Nazionale Tumori, Milan (Italy), Dr. G. Bonadonna, Istituto Nazionale Tumori, Milan (Italy), Dr. N. Cascinelli, Istituto Nazionale Tumori, Milan (Italy), Dr. A. Cochran, University of Glasgow, Western Infirmary Glasgow (United Kingdom), Dr. J. De Marsillac, Institut Nacional de Cancer, Rio de Janeiro (Brazil), Dr. J. Durand, Fondation Curie, Paris (France), Dr. R. L. Ikonopisov, Oncological Research Institute, Sofia (Bulgaria), Dr. B. Kiss, State Institute of Oncology, Budapest (Hungary), Dr. A. Kulakowski, Oncological Institute, Cracow (Poland), Dr. F. Lejeune, Institut Jules Bordet, Brussels (Belgium), Dr. Z. Mechl, Oncological Institute, Brno (Czechoslovakia), Dr. G. W. Milton, University of Sydney, Dept. of Surgery, Sydney (Australia), Dr. H. H. Peter, Abteilung für Klinische Immunologie, Medizinische Hochschule, Hannover (Federal Republic of Germany), Dr. J. Priario, Hospital de Clinicas "M. Quintela", Montevideo (Uruguay), Dr. P. Rumke, Het Nederlands Kankerinstituut, Amsterdam (The Netherlands), Dr. R. Tomin, Institute of Oncology, Beograd (Yugoslavia), Dr. U. Veronesi, Istituto Nazionale Tumori, Milan (Italy).

Table 1. Outline of adjuvant study in malignant melanoma

Stratification		Randomization
Site and nodal status	*Sex*	
N +	Male	No further therapy
Limbs	Female	DTIC
Head and neck		
Trunk	Previous treatment	
Trunk (N-) (Clark's III–IV–V)	Untreated	BCG
	Previous surgery	DTIC + BCG

Table 2. Treatments[a]

DTIC	200 mg/m²/day × 5 consecutive days, IV; every 4 weeks
BCG	3.2 ± 1.6 × 10^8 living units (2 vials of 37.5 mg of lyophilized vaccine. Pasteur Institute) in 0.5 ml saline, percutaneously by heaf-gun technique: 4 shoots at 2 mm deep; weekly on one site of proximal region of limbs, in rotation clockwise, excluding the limb in which lymphadenectomy was performed
DTIC + BCG	Same doses and frequency; BCG was started on day 5 of the cycle

[a] To be started 10–30 days after surgery and to be administered until the end of the 2nd year after surgery.

dissection, in which regional node metastases were the first relapse of disease with or without local cutaneous recurrence at the time of entering the trial (Table 1).

After stratification, patients were randomized to no further therapy (control group) or one of three adjuvant treatments (Table 2) to be performed during 2 years or until relapse was documented. The dose modifications according to myelosuppression or to different intensity of BCG reaction are reported in Table 3.

A physical examination and blood count were repeated for all in-trial patients every 4 weeks (routine laboratory tests and chest radiogram were performed every 2–3 months), and liver and brain scans, bone X-rays, or other special examinations were repeated whenever indicated by the patient's symptoms or after the end of the treatment.

The end point of study was considered the first evidence of treatment failure, such as the appearance of tumor in local, regional, or distant sites, confirmed by biopsy or needle aspiration cytology whenever possible, or by unequivocal clinical, radiologic, or radioisotopic methods. After relapse, an accurate record of treatments and of clinical events was made to assess any factor influencing survival.

Table 3. Dose modification of adjuvant treatments

DTIC-induced myelosuppression (blood counts performed on day 1 of every course)

WBC[a]	PLT[a]	Further DTIC dose
>4	>100	100 %
3.9–2.5	99–75	50 %
<2.5	<75	Wait 1–2 weeks

BCG skin reaction (read 1 week after each administration)

Skin reaction	Evaluation	Further BCG dose	Heaf-gun	Timing
No reaction or erythema (–, +)	Negative	100% 2 vials	4 shots	weekly
Infiltration (++, +++)	Positive	100% 2 vials	4 shots	every 4 weeks
Ulceration or necrosis (++++)	Strongly positive	50% 1 vial	2 shots	every 4 weeks

[a] Number $\cdot 10^3/mm^3$.

Table 4. Characteristics of 466 evaluable patients, according to stratification parameters

	Controls	DTIC	BCG	DTIC + BCG
No. of evaluable	107	124	114	121
Males	60	70	69	72
Females	47	54	45	49
Limbs, head and neck	55	69	58	63
Trunk N^+	32	34	36	44
Trunk N^-	20	21	20	14
Untreated	49	56	60	63
Previous surgery	58	68	54	58
Median age (years)	47	48	46	52

From 15 June 1974 to 31 December 1977, 540 patients were entered into the trial from 16 participating institutions. At present, 466 patients are evaluable according to the protocol criteria.

The main characteristics of evaluable patients are reported in Table 4. Patient distribution among the four treatment groups is well balanced according the stratification parameters.

Table 5. Percent disease-free at 18 months according to treatments (actuarial analysis)

	Controls	DTIC	BCG	DTIC + BCG
N^+				
Limbs, head and neck	27	54	50	40
Trunk	29	58	44	58
Males	23	47	37	45
Females	37	63	53	53
Untreated	32	54	39	52
Previous surgery	24	56	48	45
Total (N^+)	27	55	44	48
Trunk (N^-)	53	72	61	77

Table 6. Percent survival at 18 months according to treatments (actuarial analysis)

	Controls	DTIC	BCG	DTIC + BCG
N^+				
Males	64	58	62	61
Females	59	63	72	65
Limbs, head and neck	57	58	78	51
Trunk (N^+)	70	66	54	75
Untreated	62	64	78	66
Previous surgery	61	57	64	60
Total (N^+)	62	60	69	62
Trunk (N^-)	69	90	93	79

However, more detailed analysis taking into consideration the number of involved nodes in relation to treatment groups shows that DTIC-treated cases have a higher incidence (37.7%) of patients with three or more involved nodes, as compared with other groups considered (22.6%–27.5%).

The analysis of data presently available according to different treatment groups is detailed in Tables 5 and 6. Table 5 reports the percentage of patients disease-free at 18 months (actuarial analysis), and the estimated survival at 18 months is reported in Table 6.

As to toxicity, no life-threatening side-effects were recorded. Treatments were usually acceptably tolerated. The incidence of myelosuppression remained less than 20% and did not significantly modify the planned treatments. The association of both DTIC and BCG did not show different toxicity from single-agent treatments.

References

1. Beretta, G.: Controlled study for prolonged chemotherapy, immunotherapy and chemotherapy plus immunotherapy as an adjuvant to surgery in stage I–II malignant melanoma: preliminary report. In: Immunotherapy of cancer: present status of trials in man, Terry, W. D., Windhorst, D. (eds.), pp. 65–72. New York: Raven Press 1978
2. Clark, W. H. Jr.: A classification of malignant melanoma in man correlated with histogenesis and biological behaviour. In: Advances in biology of the skin Vol. VIII: The pigmentary system, Montagna, W., Hu, F. (eds.), pp. 621–647. Elmsford, N.Y.: Pergamon Press 1967

Adjuvant Therapy in Malignant Melanoma: A Trial of Immunotherapy, Chemotherapy, and Combined Treatment

S. D. Kaufman, A. B. Cosimi, W. C. Wood, and R. W. Carey

Introduction

Two hundred thirteen patients with malignant melanoma who underwent resection with curative intent were studied retrospectively at the Massachusetts General Hospital, and a group at high risk of recurrence was identified. The patients were classified by pathologic criteria utilizing CLARK's levels. All of the patients in this group had lesions of levels III, IV, or V with vertical thickness exceeding 1.5 mm [2, 3] and/or metastases to regional lymph nodes. This corresponds to stage II of the 1977 American Joint Commission For Cancer Staging and End Results Reporting. The observed recurrence rate in this group of patients was 25% at 1 year and 50% at 5 years. Many of these patients had distant metastases without evidence of local failure. This finding strongly suggests, though it does not prove, the presence of subclinical metastatic disease at the time of initial surgical treatment. The concept of clinically undetectable micrometastases with an important role for adjuvant treatment with chemotherapy is exemplified in the treatment of other solid tumors, notably carcinoma of the breast.

Dimethyl triazeno imidazole carboxamide (DTIC) has been found to be an effective chemotherapeutic agent in the treatment of advanced malignant melanoma. Recent trials of combination chemotherapy, however, have not shown significantly greater benefit than programs utilizing DTIC alone [15, 16]. The Central Oncology Group has recently reported experience in a randomized study using DTIC as an adjunct to surgery for primary melanoma [11].

A decade ago, MORTON and his colleagues [17] pioneered the use of bacillus Calmette-Guerin (BCG) in the treatment of malignant melanoma. Subsequent clinical studies have confirmed the susceptibility of malignant melanoma to immune attack [18, 19, 21]. In the treatment of unresectable cutaneous and subcutaneous nodules in purified protein derivative (PPD)-sensitive patients, tumor regression has been observed in 90% of the lesions injected with BCG and 17% of the uninjected cutaneous lesions [6]. Numerous studies of adjuvant immunotherapy using BCG following surgical resection have been undertaken. Some of these studies have reported apparent benefit [8, 9], but several others have failed to demonstrate any beneficial effect of the immunotherapeutic agent [14, 20].

It is well-known that patints with visceral metastases rarely exhibit significant regression following treatment with BCG immunotherapy [13]. GUTTERMAN et al. [10] reported results utilizing the combination of immune stimulation with BCG with chemotherapy in the form of DTIC. This combination resulted in a tumor remission rate of greater than 50% in patients with disseminated but nonvisceral melanoma and of over 20% of patients with visceral metastases. Our experience at the Massachusetts General Hospital with the combination of BCG and DTIC in patients with advanced malignant melanoma has been quite similar. This combination of chemotherapy and immunotherapy, our most effective program for advanced disease, seemed an appropriate avenue for the investigation of its possible role in adjuvant treatment. The major question posed by this study was as follows: In patients with high risk malignant melanoma, which type of adjuvant treatment is most effective – chemotherapy, immunotherapy, or a combination of both?

Method

To be eligible for inclusion in this study, patients must have undergone resection of all clinically detectable tumor including regional lymph node dissection provided that a single nodal drainage area could be identified clinically. A full battery of screening blood tests, X-rays, and radioactive scans were obtained as part of the staging procedure. Informed consent was obtained and patients were then randomly assigned to one of three treatment arms: (1) chemotherapy with DTIC, (2) immunotherapy with BCG, or (3) the combination of chemotherapy and immunotherapy with both DTIC and BCG. Patients whose treatment began more than 2 months after surgery were put in the category of delayed adjuvant treatment. In the 1st year of the study, all patients were skin tested with common recall antigens and dinitrochlorobenzene. This testing was discontinued after it became evident that no patient with primary melanoma was anergic. Stratification by age, sex, site, level, and nodal status was monitored in an effort to detect any imbalance that might be brought on by the randomization procedure.

All adjuvant treatment was administered in an ambulatory setting. Nearly all patients were able to continue their usual occupations during the 2-year period of treatment. DTIC was given intravenously (200 $mg/m^2/day$) for 3 consecutive days each month for 6 months then every 2 months for 6 months, then every 3 months for the 2nd year. Hematocrit, platelet, and white cell counts were examined just prior to each course of therapy. There were very few instances of bone marrow depression on this regimen but in those cases, dosage was reduced until counts returned to normal levels. The main toxicity observed was nausea and vomiting following the first of each series of injections. For the most part, the gastrointestinal symptoms began 1–2 h after the intravenous course of treatment and lasted for the next several hours with abrupt onset and equally abrupt disappearance of the symptoms. Four patients, two in each of the arms receiving chemotherapy, suffered gastrointestinal toxicity severe enough to require that the drug be discontinued. These patients were treated with an alternative program of phenylalanine mustard (0.15 mg/kg orally daily for 5 days a month for 6 months then every 2 months for a total of 24 months). These patients are not included in the analysis of results.

Immunotherapy was performed by the tine multiple-puncture technique. The skin of the mid-back was chosen to allow stimulation of axillary and inguinal lymph node groups. Acetone was used to degrease the skin. One ampule of lyophilized BCG vaccine (Tice strain, Chicago Research Foundation) was suspended in 1 ml of diluent and placed as rows of small droplets over a rectangle of skin about 4 × 8 cm. A sterile tine plate, held by a magnet (Chicago Research Foundation) was then impressed quickly into the skin 16 times to cover the area of the vaccination. The area was then dried with a cold air hairdryer. No dressing was applied and the skin was not washed for 24 h. BCG was administered every 2 weeks for 12 weeks, then every 4 weeks for a total of 2 years. Those who developed a maximal reaction, with blistering or weeping, received one-half or one-quarter ampule to maintain a strong reaction.

The toxicity of BCG included malaise, diffuse lymphadenopathy, and low grade fever. These symptoms usually were limited to early treatment courses. Alkaline phosphatase, bilirubin, and serum glutamic oxaloacetic transaminase (SGOT) were monitored bimonthly, as granulomatous hepatitis has been reported with intralesional injection of BCG [22]. Only one patient developed rising transaminase. Her SGOT was elevated mildly before the initiation of therapy. She received a brief course of steroids for poison ivy and had a slowly rising SGOT and malaise. BCG therapy was discontinued and she was begun on isonizad with resolution of symptoms and return of her transaminase toward normal.

Chemoimmunotherapy combined both of the individual programs. Immunotherapy was administered the 1st week, DTIC followed the 2nd week, immunotherapy the 3rd week, and no treatment the 4th week.

The follow-up examinations were done with particular care for detecting early disease recurrence. Physical examination and a series of routine blood studies including tests of kidney and liver function were carried out on a bimonthly basis. A chest X-ray was obtained at intervals of 4 months and brain, liver, or bone scans were obtained for any clinical indication. Patients whose disease recurred on either chemotherapy alone or immunotherapy alone were switched to combination chemotherapy. Patients who developed intracranial disease were given no further chemotherapy or immunotherapy. They were treated with oral corticosteroids and, when clinically indicated, brain irradiation.

Statistical evaluation was performed by Robert Lew. The life tables for survival and recurrence were computed according to the actuarial method of Cutler and Ederer [5]. These were compared using the test described by Mantel [12].

Results

Analysis of stratification was performed by comparing the three treatment arms for evidence of skew in randomization for each of the following characteristics: sex, age, delay in initiation of therapy, nodal status, level of invasion, and site of the primary (Table 1). The three arms were found to be balanced without significant difference for any characteristic, except sex, in the DTIC arm. Recurrence has been equal, with 16% of men and 16% of women showing recurrence.

The data was analyzed in terms of nodal status of patients. In the DTIC only group, there were eight patients with positive nodes, eight with negative nodes, and four who did not undergo node dissection at the time of surgery. In the BCG-treated group, 11 patients had positive nodes, 17 had negative nodes, and 4 did not undergo node dissection. In the combined treatment group, there were 8 patients with positive nodes, 13 with negative nodes, and 2 who did not have a resection. It is of great importance that only 1 of the 38 patients with negative nodes has had a recurrence. This was a patient in the BCG-treated group who had the appearance of metastatic brain disease 23 months following the initiation of treatment. All of the other recurrences were in those patients with positive draining lymph nodes. This may have great importance in the rationale of treatment in later studies, but the number of patients in this study is still too small and the follow-up too short to make a definite determination as to whether patients with negative nodes should continue to be treated.

Table 2 lists the results of the group with positive nodes. In the DTIC group, of the eight patients with positive nodes, six have recurred and two who did not have node dissections have recurred. In the BCG group, 7 of the 11 patients with positive nodes have recurred as have one who did not have node dissection carried out and one patient with negative nodes. In the combined group, of the eight patients with positive nodes, there were recurrences in two patients.

Table 1. Patient distribution

	DTIC		BCG		Both	
	No.	(%)	No.	(%)	No.	(%)
Sex						
Male	14	(70)	15	(47)	12	(52)
Female	6	(30)	17	(53)	11	(48)
Age						
20–39 yr	6	(30)	9	(28)	8	(35)
40–59 yr	9	(45)	16	(50)	11	(48)
60+ yr	5	(25)	7	(22)	4	(17)
Delay						
<2 mo	16	(80)	27	(84)	15	(65)
>2 mo	4	(20)	5	(16)	8	(35)
Nodes						
Positive	8	(40)	11	(34)	8	(35)
Negative	8	(40)	17	(53)	13	(56)
No dissection	4	(20)	4	(13)	2	(9)
Level						
III	2	(10)	5	(16)	2	(9)
IV	16	(80)	22	(68)	17	(74)
V	2	(10)	5	(16)	3	(13)
Not classifiable	0		0		1	(4)
Site						
Extremity	12	(60)	18	(56)	15	(65)
Trunk	4	(20)	11	(34)	7	(31)
Head and neck	4	(20)	3	(10)	1	(4)

Table 2. Recurrence rate in patients with positive node dissections

Treatment	No. with positive nodes	Recurrences
DTIC	8	6
BCG	11	7
Combined	8	2

The benefit of each arm was first evaluated for prevention of recurrence (Table 3). Eight of 20 patients in the DTIC arm have recurrent disease. Nine of 32 patients have recurrence in the BCG arm. There have been two recurrences in the 23 patients receiving combined chemoimmunotherapy. Figure 1 illustrates the disease-free interval from the time of primary surgery for each group of patients. Statistical evaluation shows the difference between the combined

Table 3. Evaluation of prevention of recurrence

Treatment	Total	Recurrences	Death	Alive without recurrence (%)
DTIC	20	8 (40%)	6	60%
BCG	32	9 (28%)	3	72%
Both	23	2 (8%)	0	91%
Total patients	75	19	9	

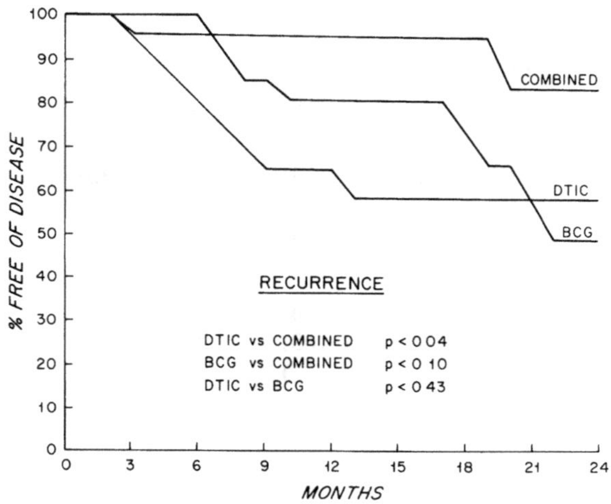

Fig. 1. Disease-free interval from the time of primary surgery for each group

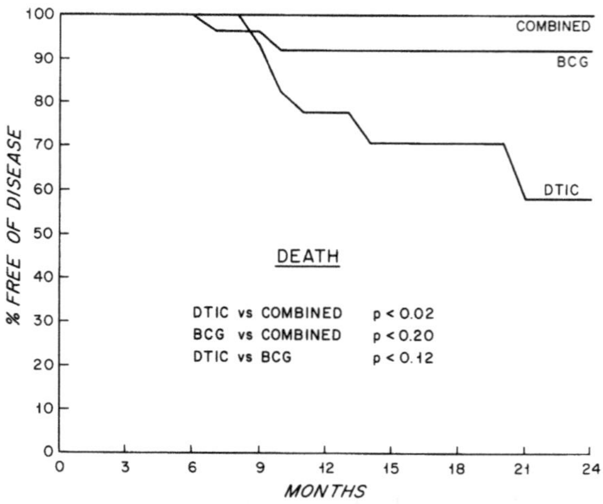

Fig. 2. Survival curves and comparison of chemoimmunotherapy and adjuvant chemotherapy alone

treatment arm and the chemotherapy arm to be highly significant. The combined treatment arm also was significantly superior to immunotherapy alone in prevention of early recurrent disease. As indicated, all recurrences have been in patients with lymph node metastases at the time of primary treatment with the exception indicated above. Recalculation of the data to consider only patients with positive lymph nodes diminished the number of patients evaluable considerably but the benefit of chemoimmunotherapy compared with chemotherapy alone was still significant ($P < 0.05$). Parallel analysis by the method of Cox [4] indicates the same pattern of significant results.

The data were evaluated with survival as the end point. In the DTIC arm, 6 of 20 patients have died and in the combined treatment group, there have been no deaths. Figure 2 demonstrates the survival curves and illustrates the benefit of chemoimmunotherapy as compared with adjuvant chemotherapy alone. Combined therapy is less clearly superior to immunotherapy alone at this point in the study.

Discussion

The data presented on these 75 patients are the results of early follow-up ranging 4—35 months and averaging 18 months. There is demonstrated benefit with adjuvant chemotherapy and immunotherapy in preventing early recurrence and early death. It is still too soon to say whether the time to recurrence and time to death are merely prolonged or if the rate of cure is being influenced by treatment. The therapy cutoff point of 2 years is arbitrary. If micrometastases are being suppressed by treatment rather than eliminated, longer periods of treatment may be necessary.

This study did not directly address the question of adjunctive therapy versus no adjuvant treatment. The concern might arise that, rather than suggesting benefit from immunotherapy or combined chemoimmunotherapy, these data demonstrate detriment from chemotherapy alone. Three facts may alleviate this concern. First, recurrence and survival in the DTIC arm are equivalent to those in the retrospective analysis of cases at the Massachusetts General Hospital. Second, the Central Oncology Group performed a prospective, randomized study comparing DTIC adjuvant therapy with nontreatment and found no significant difference in the two arms. Third, the National Cancer Institute of Italy recently reported their experience with a randomized study similar to ours but including a fourth arm: no treatment control. Patients receiving DTIC alone appear to be benefited as compared with the nontreatment control group, although these results are not yet significant.

It is interesting to note that, although adjuvant immunotherapy failed to demonstrate significant prevention of early recurrence compared with adjuvant chemotherapy, it may prolong survival. This can only be answered by a longer period of follow-up observation.

As many patients remain in the period at high risk of recurrence, close follow-up must continue. Patient accrual to the immunotherapy and combined treatment arms continues but the DTIC alone arm has been discontinued.

References

1. Beretta, G.: Controlled study for prolonged chemotherapy, immunotherapy, and chemotherapy plus immunotherapy as an adjuvant to surgery in Stage I—II malignant melanoma: Preliminary report. In: Immunotherapy of cancer. Present status of trials in man. Terry, W. D., Windhorst, D. (eds.). New York: Raven Press 1978

2. Breslow, R.: Tumor thickness, level of invasion and node dissection in Stage I cutaneous melanoma. Ann. Surg. *182,* 572 (1975)
3. Clark, W. M. (Jr.), From, L., Bernadino, E. A., Mihm, M. C.: The histogenesis and biologic behavior of primary human malignant melanomas of the skin. Cancer Res. *29,* 705 (1969)
4. Cox, D. R.: Regression models and life tables (with discussion). J. R. Statist. Soc. B *34,* 187 (1972)
5. Cutler, S. F., Ederer, F.: Maximum utilization of the life table method in analyzing survival. J. Chronic. Dis. *8,* 699 (1958)
6. Eilber, F. R., Holmes, E. C., Morton, D. L.: Immunotherapy as an adjunct to surgery in the treatment of cancer. World J. Surg. *1,* 547 (1977)
7. Eilber, F. R., Holmes, E. C., Ramming, K. P., Sparks, F. C., Morton, D. L.: Adjuvant immunotherapy of Stage II malignant melanoma. N.E.J.M. *294,* 237 (1976)
8. Eilber, F. R., Morton, D. L., Holmes, E. C., Sparks, F. C. et al.: Adjuvant immunotherapy with BCG in treatment of regional-lymph-node metastases from malignant melanoma. N.E.J.M. *294,* 237 (1976)
9. Gutterman, J. U., Mavligit, G., Gotlieb, J. A., Burgess, M. A. et al.: Chemoimmunotherapy of disseminated malignant melanoma with dimethyl triazeno imidazole carboxamide and bacillus Calmette-Guerin. N.E.J.M. *291,* 592 (1974)
10. Gutterman, J. U., Mavligit, G. M., McBride, C., Frei, E. et al.: Active immunotherapy with BCG for recurrent malignant melanoma. Lancet *1973/I,* 208
11. Hill, G. J., Grage, J. B., Minton, J. P., Krementz, E. T. et al.: DTIC-melanoma randomized surgical adjuvant study. A.S.C.O. Abs. 1007 (1975)
12. Mantel, N.: Evaluation of survival data and two rank order statistics arising in its consideration. Cancer Chemother. Rep. *50,* 163 (1966)
13. Mastrangelo, M. J., Bellet, R. E., Berkelhammer, J., Clark, W. H. (Jr.): Regression of pulmonary metastatic disease associated with intralesional BCG therapy of intracutaneous melanoma metastases. Cancer *36,* 1305 (1975)
14. McIllmurray, M. B., Embleton, M. J., Reeves, W. C., Langman, M. J. S. et al.: Controlled trial of active immunotherapy in management of Stage II-B malignant melanoma. Br. Med. J. *1977/I,* 540
15. McKelvey, E. M., Luce, J. K., Talley, R. W., Hersh, E. M. et al.: Combination chemotherapy with Bis chloroethyl nitrosurea (BCNU), vincristine and dimethyl triazeno imidazole carboxamide (DTIC) in disseminated malignant melanoma. Cancer *39,* 1 (1977)
16. McKelvey, E. M., Luce, J. K., Vaitkevicius, V. K., Talley, R. W. et al.: Bis chloroethyl nitrosurea, vincristine, dimethyl triazeno imidazole carboxamide and chlorpromazine combination chemotherapy in disseminated malignant melanoma. Cancer *39,* 5 (1977)
17. Morton, D. L., Eilber, F. R., Malmgren, R. A., and Wood, W. C.: Immunological factors which influence response to immunotherapy in malignant melanoma. Surgery *68,* 158 (1970)
18. Nathanson, L.: Regression of intradermal malignant melanoma after intralesional injection of mycobacterium bollis strain BCG. Cancer Chemother. Rep. *56,* 659 (1972)
19. Pinsky, C., Hirshaut, Y., Oestgen, H.: Treatment of malignant melanoma by intralesional injection of BCG. Proc. Am. Assoc. Cancer Res. *13,* 21 (1972)
20. Pinsky, C. M., Hirshaut, Y., Wanebo, W. J., Fortner, J., et al.: Surgical adjuvant immunotherapy in patients with malignant melanoma: A prospective, randomized trial. In: Immunotherapy of cancer Present status of trials in man. Terry, W. D., Windhorst, D. (eds.). New York: Raven Press 1978
21. Seigler, H. F., Shingleton, W. W., Metzgar, R. S., Buckley, C. E. et al.: Nonspecific and specific immunotherapy in patients with melanoma. Surgery *72,* 162 (1972)
22. Sparks, F. C., Silverstein, M. J., Hunt, J. S., Morton, D. L.: Complications of BCG immunotherapy in patients with cancer. N.E.J.M. *289,* 827 (1973)

Malignant Melanoma (Stage 1): A Clinical Trial of Adjuvant BCG Immunotherapy

A. H. G. Paterson, D. Willans, L. M. Jerry, and T. A. McPherson

Introduction

The possible role of immunotherapy in the treatment of human cancer is currently being evaluated in centres all over the world. In this paper we present the preliminary results of a randomized prospectively controlled trial of BCG immunotherapy in early operable malignant melanoma. It is clear from a variety of animal experiments that immunotherapy is generally most successful in the situation of "minimum residual disease", where the immune mechanism of the host is intact and the number of malignant cells is small [13]. One human cancer in which an immunotherapeutic phenomenon is frequently observed is the regression of malignant melanoma with the injection of intralesional and occasionally intradermal BCG [4, 12]. It was our hypothesis that if the above phenomenon was to be maximally exploited, then patients with minimal residual malignant melanoma would be the most likely group to benefit in terms of disease-free survival.

Stage 1B (M. D. Anderson staging system) malignant melanoma, that is, patients with disease localised to the skin with no apparent in-transit or lymph node metastases, and treated by wide surgical excision with or without grafting, are a group with a reasonably well-defined expected risk of recurrence. Several investigators have shown that risk of recurrence in malignant melanoma is related to the depth of invasion of the primary [9]. These studies were developed by Clark who has defined five levels of invasion [3]. Levels 3, 4 and 5 are associated with a significantly higher risk of recurrence than levels 1 or 2, and the 5-year survival has been correlated by McGovern to be in the region of 30% for level 5 lesions, 50% for level 4 lesions and 65% for level 3 lesions [11]. Other factors influencing the risk of recurrence are depth of invasion, the presence of ulceration and anatomical location of the primary.

The value of BCG in more advanced malignant melanoma involving the regional lymph nodes was demonstrated by Eilber et al. in 1975, but the trial used concurrent, non-randomized patients as a control group [6]. In a retrospectively controlled trial, Gutterman demonstrated improved disease-free survival in patients with malignant melanoma compared to a group of historical control patients [8]. We found this evidence exciting, but in view of the difficulties of interpretation of these trials, we thought it desirable to launch a prospectively controlled randomized clinical trial using a combination of intradermal and oral BCG as a post-surgical adjuvant in stage 1 malignant melanoma (Clark's level 3—5).

Methods

Patients with stage 1B (Clark's level 3—5) malignant melanoma aged less than 75 years old were eligible for entry. The histology of the lesion was reviewed by the trial pathologist (D.W.) and a level of invasion indicated. Superficial spreading, nodular and lentigo maligna melanoma types were eligible. Other factors such as depth of invasion, lymphoid infiltration, mitotic activity, presence of vascular or lymphatic invasion or ulceration of the lesions were also

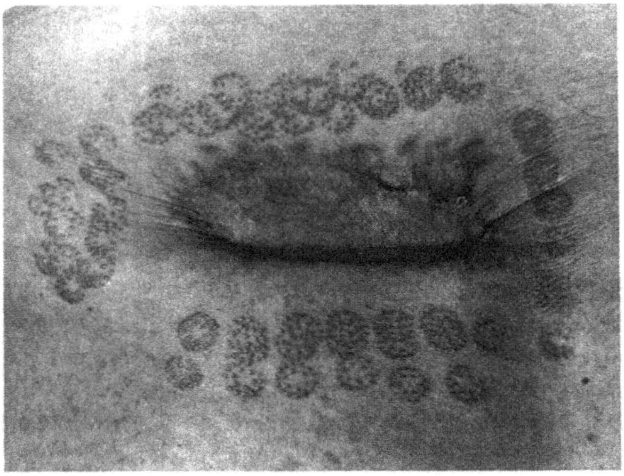

Fig. 1. Immunotherapy technique: BCG is injected by Heaf gun around the site of wide excison of the primary. Treatment with oral BCG follows 1 month later

examined and the radial/vertical growth parameters were indicated. However, for the purpose of this trial eligibility depended on the Clark's level of invasion 3–5. The patient then signs a consent form, which outlines the statistical risk of recurrence, the experimental nature of the treatment of BCG, and that the patient may be randomized to either a control or a treatment group. Randomization was carried out by sealed envelopes. BCG (Connaught) 40 mg in 1 ml of diluent was applied around the site of wide excision and multiple punctures using a 20-needle Heaf gun were made (Fig. 1).

Oral BCG, 40 mg daily for 5 days each month was then started 1 month after the first intradermal injection and was continued for 2 years. A further intradermal injection of 40 mg BCG around the site of wide excision was made after year's treatment with oral BCG. Most of the patients start immunotherapy within 4 months of surgery although some of the earlier patients admitted to the trial had a longer interval between surgery and start of immunotherapy.

The patients are followed up at 3-month intervals and underwent clinical examination with complete blood count and SMA 12 panel. A chest X-ray is performed at 5-month intervals and a liver scan is performed annually; skin testing is repeated every 3 months. Recurrence is defined as local if within the site of excision or up to 5 cm around the site of excision, regional if in-transit intradermal or regional lymph node metastases are present, and distant if distant metastases are present. Statistical analysis was performed by the Department of Research and Development (Mr. John Hansen), Cross Cancer Institute. The significance of the disease-free survivals was compared by the modified Wilcoxon test [7].

Results

The trial was activated in May 1975 and to date 107 patients have been entered into the study. Fifty-eight patients have been randomized to the control group and 49 patients to the treatment group. The Clark's levels of invasion of the entered patients are shown in Table 1. It can been seen that a few more patients have been randomized to the control group with level 4

Clark's level	Treatment group	Control group
Level 3	32	34
Level 4	15	19
Level 5	2	5
Total	49	58

Table 1. Clark's level of invasion of the patients randomised to treatment and control groups. There is a slight bias in favour of the immunotherapy group with more level 4 lesions in the control arm

Table 2. Randomization by site of disease. There is a slight bias in favour of the control group with relatively more patients with extremity lesions in the control group

	Total patients	Site of disease			
		Arm	Leg	Trunk	Head and neck
Immunotherapy group	49	9	18	18	5
Control group	58	11	26	17	4

Table 3. Recurrences of disease; 5 of 49 patients in the immunotherapy group have relapsed compared to 10 of 58 patients in the control group

	Treatment group (49 patients)	Control group (58 patients)
Level 3	2	5
Level 4	2	5
Level 5	1	0
Total recurrences	5 of 49 pts.	10 of 58 pts.
Total deaths	1	2

and 5 lesions, thereby introducing a slight bias in favour of the immunotherapy group at this point in time. However, it will be seen that none of the level 5 patients in the control group have yet had progressive disease.

All entered patients have been analysed for disease-free survival. A second analysis has been made of all 102 fully assessable patients. Reasons for non-assessability were: in the control group, one patient refused further attendance; in the immunotherapy group, one patient refused further attendance, two patients refused further BCG after initial vaccination, one patient had a severe myocardial infarction and G.P. stopped treatment. Sites of disease of the 107 entered patients are shown in Table 2. There are more patients in the control group with the more favourable limb melanomas.

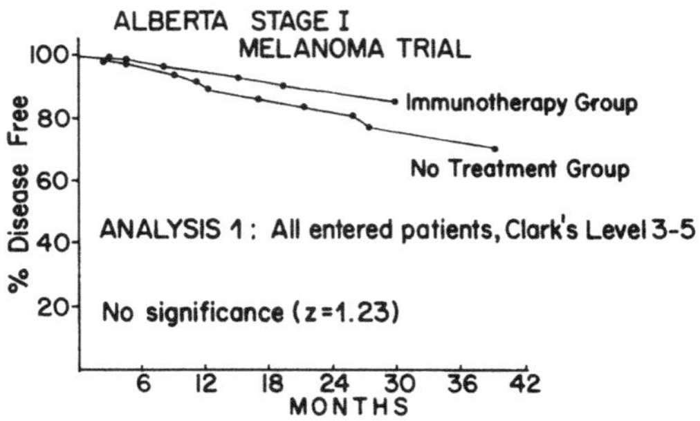

Fig. 2. Analysis 1: all entered patients. The observed trend in favour of the BCG group is not yet statistically significant ($P = 0.17$) at median follow-up of 20 months

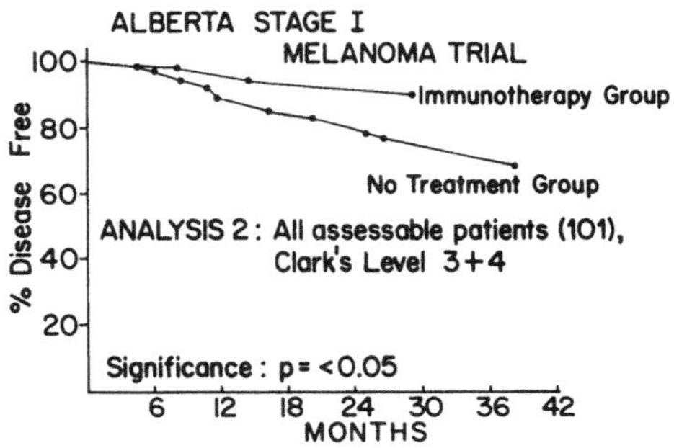

Fig. 3. Analysis 2: all evaluable patients with lesions of Clark's level 3 and 4. The observed trend in favour of the BCG group is statistically significant ($P = 0.05$) at median follow-up of 20 months

Table 3 outlines the recurrences of disease. Five of 49 patients in the immunotherapy group have had progression of disease compared to ten of 58 patients in the control group. This includes one woman with a level 4 lesion randomised to the immunotherapy group who refused further BCG after the first vaccination and relapsed 18 months later. One death has occurred in the treatment group compared to two deaths in the control group. Analysis 1 (Fig. 2) of all entered patients shows a trend in favour of the immunotherapy group that is, however, not significant at the 5% level)$P = 0.17$). A second analysis (Fig. 3) was performed comparing all fully assessable patients with Clark's level 3 and 4 lesions. Here there appears to be a definite trend in favour of the immunotherapy group ($P < 0.05$) at a median duration of follow-up of 20 months.

Discussion

There is little doubt that the phenomenon of regression of certain clinical patterns of malignant melanoma with the intralesional and occasionally intradermal injection of BCG exists [4, 12]. Whether this effect is specific or non-specific is uncertain since it has been difficult to correlate any immune function tests with clinical results [10]. It has been difficult, however, to satisfactorily prove that BCG is of definite clinical benefit. Earlier trials of BCG in malignant melanoma have suffered from criticism of inadequate control data. Thus, GUTTERMAN et al. demonstrated improved disease-free survival in stage 3 patients compared to historical control patients [8] and EILBER et al. showed improved disease-free survival in stage 3 patients using BCG compared to current but non-randomly selected control patients [6].

It was our postulate that, to utilise the phenomenon of BCG-induced regression of melanoma, close proximity of the organisms to any microscopic foci of malignant cells was required. Therefore, perilesional injection of BCG after surgery was used to deliver organisms to areas of possible microscopic in-transit and nodal disease. For systemic therapy, oral BCG was selected. This was the original route of administration used by CALMETTE and GUÉRIN [2]. Using this route, sensitisation to the organisms occurs and it can be demonstrated, using radionuclide labelling techniques, that organisms are present in the liver and lungs as well as other sites [1]. This mode of administration is also very convenient to manage.

This trial is a prospective randomized controlled trial and in this first report, 3 years after its activation, we have demonstrated a trend that is not yet significant at the 5% level, in favour of the immunotherapy group. If, however, fully assessable patients with only level 3 and 4 lesions are analysed, there is a significant trend in favour of the BCG group ($P < 0.05$). There are three reasons why we believe this separate analysis is justifiable. Firstly, level 5 lesions are often associated with significant volumes of sub-clinical disease, which may be beyond the means of immune mechanisms to cope with. Indeed, many oncologists feel it justifiable to treat these patients with adjuvant chemotherapy. Secondly, the number of patients in the level 5 group is small and may introduce a statistical bias that is difficult to control. Thirdly, in the treatment group of analysis 1, there are included two patients who withdrew from the trial after only one injection of intradermal BCG and therefore do not allow us to assess the value of 2 years of immunotherapy on the course of the disease. In fact, one of these patients did relapse with pulmonary metastases 18 months after the BCG injection.

The ECOG have recently published a preliminary communication on their randomized study using BCG in melanoma [5]. Several points must be made about this study, which has shown no detectable difference in favour of the immunotherapy group at a median duration of follow-up of a little over 1 year. Firstly, patients with stage 1, 2 and 3 disease are eligible for entry. This has resulted in a bias of patients with proven positive nodes randomized to the treatment group (20 cases in BCG group and 14 cases in control group). No analysis has been made of the sub-group of stage 1 patients. Secondly, the follow-up period is short. If there is a threshold of tumour load beyond which immunotherapy is not effective, then patients with a high tumour load will relapse at the same rate as control patients and this is most likely to occur in the first 2 years of follow-up.

This report of the Alberta Stage 1 Malignant Melanoma Immunotherapy Trial is necessarily prelimary but demonstrates a very encouraging trend in disease-free survival in the BCG-treated group, suggesting that in post-surgical "minimal residual disease" the known phenomenon of BCG-induced regressions of disease may be utilised as post-surgical adjuvant therapy to the patient's benefit.

Summary

A prospectively controlled randomized clinical trial of adjuvant BCG immunotherapy in patients with stage 1B malignant melanoma (Clark's level 3–5) is described. The combination of intradermal and oral BCG allows approximation of the bacilli to any microscopic foci of residual disease. The trial was activated in May 1975 and to date 107 patients have been admitted to the trial, 49 patients being randomized to the treatment group and 58 patients to the control group. To date, of all entered patients, there have been five relapses of 49 patients in the treatment group and ten relapses of 58 patients in the control group. This encouraging trend is not yet statistically significant at the 5% level ($P = 0.17$). If evaluable patients with

Clark's level 3 and 4 lesions are assessed separately, there is a significant trend in favour of the immunotherapy group ($P < 0.05$) with three relapses in the treatment group and ten relapses in the control group.

References

1. Blasi, A., Curci, G.: Indigini Sperimentale sulla vaccinazione autibuberuleare con BCG per via orale secundo le metodiche di A de Assis. Arch. di Tisiologia *10,* 96 (1955)
2. Calmette, A., Boquet, A., Negre, L.: Essais de vaccination contro l'infection tuberculeus par voie buccale chez les petis animaux du laboratoine. Ann. Inst. Pasteur *38,* 399 (1924)
3. Clark, W. H. (Jr.), Ainsworth, A. M., Bernardino, E. A., Yong, C. H., Milm, M. C. (Jr.), Reed, R. J.: The developmental Biology of primary human malignant melanomas. Semin. Oncol. *2,* 83–104 (1975)
4. Coates, A. S., Peters, M.: Complete remission of metastatic malignant melanoma following immunotherapy with BCG. Report of a case. Aust. N. Z. J. Surg. *47,* 362–365 (1977)
5. Cunningham, T. J., Schoenfeld, D., Nathanson, L., Wolter, J., Patterson, W. B., Cohen, M. H.: A controlled study of adjuvant therapy in patients with stage 1 and 2 malignant melanoma. In: Immunotherapy of cancer: Present status of trials in man. Terry, W. D., Windhorst, D. (eds.), New York: Raven Press 1978
6. Eilber, F. R., Morton, D. L., Holmes, E. C., Sparks, F. C., Ramming, K. P.: Adjuvant immunotherapy with BCG in treatment of regional lymph node metastases from malignant melanoma. N. Engl. J. Med. *294,* 237–240
7. Geeham, E. H.: Statistics. Biometrika (London) *52,* 203–223
8. Gutterman, J. U., Mavligit, G. M., McBride, C. M., Frei, E., Freireich, E. J., Hersh, E. M.: Active immunotherapy with BCG for recurrent malignant melanoma. Lancet *1973/I,* 1208–1212
9. Lane, N., Lattes, R., Malm, J.: Clinico-pathological correlation in a series of 117 malignant melanomas of the skin of adults. Cancer *11,* 1025–1043 (1958)
10. Mavligit, G. M., Gutterman, J. U., Hersh, E. M.: Effect of BCG (Tice strain) on primary sensitisation to 2–4 dinitrochlorobenzene and on established delayed hypersensitivity in human malignant melanoma. J. Natl. Cancer Inst. *57,* 749–751
11. McGovern, V. J.: The classification of melanoma and its relationship with prognosis. Pathology *2,* 85–98 (1970)
12. Morton, D. L.: Immunotherapy of human melanoma and sarcomas. Natl. Cancer Inst. Monogram *35,* 375 (1972)
13. Oettge, H. F.: Immunotherapy of Cancer. N. Engl. J. Med. *297,* 484–491

J. Neurological Tumors

Adjuvant Chemotherapy With Nitrosourea Compounds Following Surgery Plus Radiotherapy in Glioblastoma Multiforme[1]

S. Monfardini, C. Brambilla, C. L. Solero, A. Vaghi, P. Valagussa, G. Morello, and G. Bonadonna

Natural History of Glioblastoma Multiforme

The outlook for patients with glioblastoma multiforme is almost uniformly fatal. Patients with this highly malignant tumor usually survive 2–4 months from the time of diagnosis with no intervention. Glioblastoma multiforme does not metastasize to distant sites but leads to death by uncontrolled growth in a confined space. Surgery reduces the bulk of the tumor and relieves the compressive symptoms, thus prolonging survival without necessarily influencing the malignancy. As a consequence, the effectiveness of therapy must be judged in terms of survival rather than of objective response. Usually, the duration of initial neurologic symptoms is very short since the majority of patients have symptoms of 1–3 months' duration.

Conventional treatment of glioblastoma multiforme consists primarily in surgical intervention. The median survival from operation ranges from 4.5 to 6 months, [4, 19] while approximately 20% of patients are alive at 12 months and less than 10% at 24 months [20]. Survival is related to the extent of surgery. Extensive resection is superior to partial resection, while external decompression provides very poor results [4]. Radiation therapy (RT) following surgery does not consistently affect survival in patients with glioblastoma multiforme, since it can only increase survival for 3–4 months. Furthermore, it appears that the extra survival attributable to RT only occurs in the 1st year following surgery [5]. It has, in fact, been reported that the difference in survival between patients treated with surgery alone and cases receiving surgery plus RT tends to disappear at 15–18 months [5].

In conclusion, the local treatment modality, i.e., surgery with or without radiotherapy, does not appear to influence the ultimate course of glioblastomas. This leaves to chemotherapy the theoretical possibility of further improving survival after initial local treatment.

Effective Drugs in Brain Tumors

Measurement of tumor response to chemotherapy is a major problem in brain tumors. Objective assessment of tumor regression, as determined by angiogram, brain scan, and

1 Supported in part by contract No. N01-CM-337414 with DCT, NCI, NIH.

computerized axial tomography do not lend themselves to exact definitions that can then be used to denote drug efficacy. This, then, would leave the objective evaluation of response mainly to neurologic examination. For these reasons, studies on the efficacy of chemotherapy in brain tumors must rely mainly upon survival. Extensive reviews of the chemotherapy of glioblastoma multiforme have been recently made by BRODER and RALL [1], GOLDSMITH and CARTER [5] and LEVIN and WILSON [13].

To our current knowledge, nitrogen mustards do little to affect the eventual course of the disease [1]. Among the antimetabolites, methotrexate has been employed as an intra-arterial or intraventricular infusion, showing some activity in medulloblastoma. However, the data available in the adult population are not sufficient for any adequate evaluation of methotrexate clinical activity on glioblastoma multiforme [1]. The vinca alkaloids seem to produce responses without prolonging survival. In the treatment of brain tumors, it would appear that vincristine is more active than vinblastine [1, 5].

Among the antitumor antibiotics, mithramycin was originally reported to be an active drug. However, after the failure to induce prolongation of survival in a controlled trial by a Brain Study Group [11], this compound has not been further studied. Preliminary data suggesting that bleomycin could have some activity in gliomas have not yet been confirmed [1]. The data obtained with procarbazine seem promising but need further confirmation [13]. Recently, epipodophyllotoxin VM-26 has been tested in a pilot study [14]. Preliminary results indicate that it may be a useful agent in glioma multiforme.

In the miscellaneous class of anticancer agents, the most interesting drugs are the lipid-soluble agents that are capable of crossing the blood-brain barrier, such as procarbazine, epipodophyllotoxin (VM-26, VP-16), and dibromodulcitol and nitrosoureas. Among the lipid-soluble agents, the nitrosourea compounds are the class of anticancer agents most extensively studied in brain tumors. In fact, in several studies 1, 3-bis-(2-chloroethyl)-1-nitrosourea (BCNU) and 1-(2-chloroethyl)-3-cyclohexyl-1-nitrosourea (CCNU) have shown definite activity against experimental as well as human malignant gliomas [4, 7, 8, 12, 18, 19]. BCNU was reported to produce a 46%–51% response rate in patients with advanced glioblastoma multiforme [5, 13]. Fewer patients have so far been studied following treatment with CCNU and methyl CCNU (MeCCNU), but the responses are roughly similar [5].

In glioblastoma multiforme there have been few studies with drug combinations, probably because the number of drugs with known activity is still very limited. All combinations have included a nitrosourea as a drug component. Procarbazine was combined with CCNU and vincristine [6], methotrexate was combined with CCNU and vincristine [9], while adriamycin, VM-26, and CCNU were combined in a pilot study [15]. However, it appears unlikely that all the above-mentioned multiple drug regimens are significantly superior to BCNU or CCNU alone.

Results of Current Studies with Adjuvant Nitrosourea Compounds

As recalled in the introduction, neither surgery nor RT influences the ultimate course of glioblastoma multiforme. The uniformly fatal outlook of this brain tumor has prompted several investigators to utilize chemotherapy after definitive surgical resection in conjunction with irradiation. It has been properly stated by WALKER [20] that the major problem with adjuvant chemotherapy in the treatment of brain tumors lies in defining its efficacy in a comparative way so that anyone will be convinced that such adjuvant chemotherapy is efficacious. Only the use of controlled, prospective, randomized clinical trials can provide statistically meaningful data to serve as a basis for further progress. Due to the difficulty in the evaluation of objective tumor response to therapy in brain tumors, there is general agreement at the moment that survival after operation is currently the only clear way to demonstrate an improvement in the treatment of malignant brain tumors.

The first two randomized trials with adjuvant chemotherapy in glioblastomas were conducted with agents such as 5-fluorouracil [2] and mithramycin [11]. In both studies no difference in survival could be detected between patients treated with chemotherapy and those who were treated only by surgery and RT. This is not surprising, since no definite evidence of clinical activity of either 5-fluorouracil and mithramycin had ever been clearly proved in inoperable or recurrent glioblastomas.

Since nitrosourea compounds are essentially the only drugs with significant activity against inoperable or recurrent glioblastoma multiforme, their use appears most appropriate in patients who have received both surgery and irradiation to reduce the tumor burden to destroy residual neoplastic cells. The first important randomized study on adjuvant chemotherapy with nitrosourea compounds for glioblastoma multiforme was that conducted in the United States by the Brain Tumor Study Group [18]. Two hundred twenty-three patients received conventional neurosurgical care including tumor resection with adequate decompression. They were randomized within 3 weeks from operation into four groups: controls, irradiation (6000 rad to the whole head in 6–8 weeks); BCNU (80 mg/m^2/day for 3 days and cycles repeated every 6–8 weeks); and BCNU plus RT. The survival analysis was calculated in weeks. Patients who received conventional care without RT or BCNU had a median survival of 17 weeks, while median survival was 25 weeks after BCNU alone, 37 weeks after RT alone, and 40 weeks after RT plus BCNU. This study was the first investigation to report prolongation of survival as a result of adjuvant treatment.

Following this trial, several prospective randomized adjuvant studies have been carried out in the attempt to evaluate the relative efficacy of other nitrosourea compounds. Table 1

Table 1. Value of adjuvant chemotherapy in glioblastoma multiforme: median survival according to the modality of treatment in the principal controlled studies

Treatment	Evaluable cases	Median survival (months)	Author
Surgery		3.7	Walker et al. [20]
BCNU		5.8	
RT	223	8.6	
RT + BCNU		9.3	
RT	22	11.5	Reagan et al. [16]
CCNU	22	6.6	
RT + CCNU	19	12.0	
RT	32	10.5	Solero et al. [17]
RT + BCNU	34	12.0	
RT + CCNU	36	17.0	
RT		8.2	Walker et al. [21]
MeCCNU	332	7.1	
RT + MeCCNU		7.1	
RT + BCNU		11.7	

summarizes the effect upon survival of the principal combined modality studies. For the sake of uniformity, survival has been expressed in months.

REAGAN et al. [16] reported a controlled study on 63 patients who were randomly assigned to one of three treatment regimens within 2 weeks of surgery. One group received radiation therapy alone, the second group received CCNU 130 mg/m^2 at intervals of 8 weeks, and the third group received combined RT and CCNU. In patients who received RT with or without CCNU, survival was significantly longer than in those who received the drug alone. There was no difference in survival between the two treatment groups who received RT and RT plus CCNU. The authors concluded that CCNU did not seem to be effective when used as adjuvant agent in the therapy of glioblastomas.

A series of 102 consecutive patients operated on at the Istituto Neurologico "C. Besta" and treated in cooperation with the Istituto Nazionale Tumori of Milan [17] have been randomized to receive either irradiation alone or irradiation plus BCNU 80 mg/m^2 day IV. for 3 days every 6–8 weeks or irradiation plus CCNU 130 mg/m^2 PO every 6–8 weeks. In the group treated with RT alone, the median survival was 10.5 months while in the groups also treated with BCNU and CCNU, the median survival was 12 and 17 months, respectively. In patients treated with RT plus CCNU, the prolongation of the survival was statistically significant ($P = 0.02$) over that of patients who received radiotherapy alone. However, no significant difference in survival was noted between patients receiving RT plus BCNU and RT plus CCNU (Fig. 1).

In a preliminary report presented by WALKER et al. [21] on 332 patients randomized to receive, after surgery, irradiation alone, MeCCNU (220 mg/m^2 every 6–8 weeks), RT plus MeCCNU, RT plus BCNU (80 mg/m^2/day for 3 days every 6–8 weeks), no advantage was shown to result from adding MeCCNU to irradiation, while RT plus BCNU was found to achieve a better survival than irradiation alone.

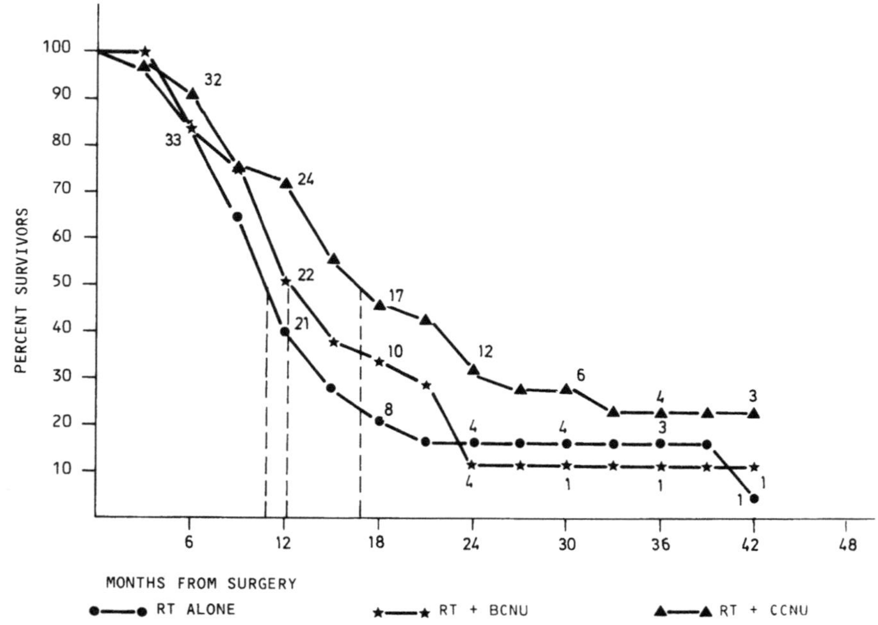

Fig. 1. Resectable glioblastoma multiforme. Comparative overall survival in 102 patients treated with different combined modalities. From SOLERO et al. [17]

Table 2. Nitrosoureas in glioblastoma multiforme: adjuvant treatment versus treatment after recurrence

Treatment	Evaluable cases	Median survival (months)	Author
RT + early BCNU	18	9.3	Kessinger et al. [10]
RT + late BCNU	8	16.5	
RT + early CCNU	36	11.6	EORTC brain tumor group [3]
RT + late CCNU	45	17.9	

[a] Nonrandomized study. [b] Randomized study.

The proven efficacy of nitrosourea compounds in recurrent glioblastoma, which is apparently in contrast to the somewhat contradictory evidence of the activity of these agents when used as adjuvant chemotherapy after a local treatment modality, has prompted some authors to compare adjuvant chemotherapy against chemotherapy after primary treatment failure (Table 2). The EORTC Brain Tumor Group has reported the results of a trial on 81 patients randomized to receive CCNU 130 mg/m^2 every 6 weeks beginning 3 weeks after the neurosurgical procedure or, alternatively, CCNU at the same dosage only after relapse [3]. All patients received RT after surgery. In patients receiving "late" CCNU, the median survival was 17.9 months, while in cases treated with "early" CCNU survival was only 11.6 months. The authors concluded that CCNU should be administered only after relapse, at least in patients with a disease-free interval. A similar nonrandomized study performed by Kessinger et al. [10] on a limited number of patients treated with BCNU showed similar results in favor of patients receiving late BCNU.

Comments

Although malignant gliomas have traditionally been the most frequent indication for neurosurgery, the only surgical progress in the past 20 years has been the reduction of operative morbidity and mortality. RT following surgery affects survival favorably for only a few months. Neither surgery nor RT appears to influence the course of glioblastomas, and this leaves to chemotherapy an open field for the evaluation of possible clinical activity.
At present, nitrosourea compounds appear moderately effective as a palliative treatment of recurrent disease but cannot successfully replace postoperative RT. The results available would indicate that CCNU and BCNU have slightly improved the overall survival. The apparent discrepancy on survival among available series treated with a combined modality approach is most probably due to patient selection and extent of surgery. Although single-agent treatment with modest improvement may be understandable, experience in other tumor areas indicates more strongly the need for combination chemotherapy as adjuvant treatment in the future, even if multiple-agent chemotherapy has not proved superior to nitrosoureas used as single agents in advanced glioblastomas.

References

1. Broder, L. E., Rall, D. P.: Chemotherapy of brain tumors. In: Recent advances in brain tumor research. Bingham, W. G. (Jr.) (ed.), p. 373. Basel, Munich, Paris, London, New York, Sydney: S. Karger 1972

2. Edland, R. W., Javid, M., Ansfield, F. J.: Glioblastoma multiforme. An analysis of the results of postoperative radiotherapy alone versus radiotherapy and concomitant 5-fluorouracil. Am. J. Roentgenol. *3,* 337–342 (1971)
3. EORTC Brain Tumor Group: Effect of CCNU on survival, rate of objective remission and duration of free interval in patients with malignant brain glioma. First evaluation. Eur. J. Cancer *12,* 41–45 (1976)
4. Frankel, S. A., German, W. J.: Glioblastoma multiforme (Review of 219 cases with regard to natural history, pathology, diagnostic methods, and treatment). J. Neurosurg. *15,* 489–503 (1958)
5. Goldsmith, M. A., Carter, S. K.: Glioblastoma multiforme. A review of therapy. Cancer Treat. Rev. *1,* 153–165 (1974)
6. Gutin, P. H., Wilson, C. B., Kumar, A. R. W., Boldrey, E. B., Levin, V., Powell, M., Enot, K. J.: Phase II study of procarbazine, CCNU and vincristine combination chemotherapy in the treatment of malignant brain tumors. Cancer *35,* 1398–1404 (1975)
7. Hansen, H. H., Selawry, O. S., Muggia, F. M., Walker, M. D.: Clinical studies with 1-(2 chloroethyl)-3-cyclohexyl-1-nitrosourea. Cancer Res. *31,* 223–227 (1971)
8. Hansen, H. H., Muggia, F. M., Walker, M. D., Rosenblum, M. C.: The treatment of malignant brain tumors with nitrosoureas. Cancer Chemother. Rep. *55,* 99–100 (1977)
9. Hildebrand, J., Brihaye, J., Wageknecht, L., Michel, J., Kenis, Y.: Combination chemotherapy with CCNU, vincristine and methotrexate in primary and metastatic brain tumors. Eur. J. Cancer *11,* 585–587 (1975)
10. Kessinger, A., Lemon, M. L., Foley, J. F.: Sequential and adjuvant chemotherapy of malignant astrocytoma of the brain. Proc. Am. Soc. Clin. Oncol. *19,* (Abst. C-140) (1978)
11. Leventhal, C. M., Walker, M. D.: Chemotherapy of malignant glioma: a collaborative study. Amsterdam: Excerpta Medica Foundation. Congress Series *193,* 33 (1969)
12. Levin, V. A., Shapiro, W. R., Clancy, T. P., Oliverio, V. T.: The uptake, distribution and antitumor activity of 1-(2-chloroethyl)-3-cyclohexyl-1-nitrosourea in the murine glioma. Cancer Res. *30,* 2451–2455 (1970)
13. Levin, V. A., Wilson, C. B.: Chemotherapy: The agents in current use. Brain tumors. Semin. Oncol. *2,* 63–67 (1975)
14. Muggia, F. M., Selawry, O. S., Hansen, H. H.: Clinical studies with a new podophyllotoxin derivative, epipodophyllotoxin 4′-demethyl-9-(4,6-0-2-thenylidene β-D-Glupyranoside) (NSC-122819). Cancer Chemother. Rep. *55,* 575–581 (1971)
15. Pouillart, T. P., Mathé, G., Pisson, M.: Essai de traitement des glioblastomes de l'adulte et des métastases cerebrales par l'association d'adriamycine de VM26 et de CCNU. Nouv. Presse Méd. *5,* 1571–1576 (1976)
16. Reagan, T. J., Bisel, H. F., Childs, D. S., Layton, D. D., Rhoton, A. L., Taylor, W. F.: Controlled study of CCNU and radiation therapy in malignant astrocytoma. J. Neurosurg. *44,* 186–190 (1976)
17. Solero, C. L., Monfardini, S., Brambilla, C., Vaghi, A., Valagussa, P., Bonadonna, G., Morello, G.: Controlled study with BCNU versus CCNU as adjuvant chemotherapy following surgery plus radiotherapy in glioblastoma multiforme (in press) (1978)
18. Walker, M. D.: Nitrosoureas in central nervous system tumors. Cancer Chemother. Rep. *4,* 21–26 (1973)
19. Walker, M.: Brain and peripheral nervous system tumors. In: Cancer medicine. Holland, J. F., Frei, E. III (eds.), pp. 1385–1407. Philadelphia: Lea and Febiger 1973.
20. Walker, M.: Chemotherapy: Adjuvant to surgery and radiation therapy. Brain tumors. Semin. Oncol. *2,* 69–71 (1975)
21. Walker, M. D., Strike, T. A.: An evaluation of methil-CCNU, BCNU and radiotherapy in the treatment of malignant glioma. Proceedings of the American Association for Cancer Research. Toronto, 4–8 May 1976 (Abst. 652)

Treatment of Adult Malignant Gliomas

P. Pouillart, T. Palangie, M. Poisson, A. Buge, P. Huguenin, P. Morin, and H. Gautier

Introduction

The review of accumulated experience with adult brain tumors indicates a potential efficiency of chemotherapy when associated with surgery and radiotherapy [2]. Some drugs show their abilities to improve the clinical course of resected or partially resectable or nonresectable malignant gliomas in adult patients [4, 6]. Successively vincristine [1], BCNU, CCNU, and more recently VM-26 and procarbazine have been introduced into therapeutic trials [1–5, 12, 14, 15, 16]. Even the potent nitrosources remain merely a palliative form of therapy. Some recent results obtained in animal tumor model systems indicate that some combinations of drugs appear more effective than drugs used alone. This same approach may increase the mean life span of patients with gliomas [7, 9]. We may anticipate that the failure of brain tumor therapy requires research directed at the discovery of additional active drugs and, for the present, attempts to potentiate the activity of nitrosoureas with a rational combination of drugs [8, 13]. The aim of this study was to compare the best sequence of chemotherapy and to determine the best point for the administration of radiotherapy associated with chemotherapy.

Patients and Methods

Two trials were begun simultaneously.

Trial I

We entered 71 patients with partially resectable supratentorial malignant gliomas into a randomized chemotherapy trial between 1 June 1975 and 1 April 1976. Initially, the patients were randomized to four groups of treatment. Because of failures of the fourth therapy

Table 1. Distribution of patients into the four groups of treatment according to age

	Group I	Group II	Group III	Group IV
Number of patients	21	21	23	6
Median age	47	53	53	56
Range	20–68	20–72	26–68	26–67

program, we suspended further entry of new patients into this group. The numbers of patients in each group were thus as follows: 21 patients in group I, 21 patients in group II, 23 patients in group III, and 6 patients in group IV. The median age of the patients was comparable in each group (Table 1). Eight patients were considered nonevaluable because of early death, inadequate treatment, or failure in administration of treatment.

Treatment

Group I: adriamycin at a dose of 45 mg/m^2 on day 1; VM-26 at a daily dose of 60 mg/m^2 on days 2 and 3; CCNU at a daily dose of 60 mg/m^2 on days 4 and 5
Group II: VM-26 at a daily dose of 60 mg/m^2 on days 1 and 19; CCNU at a daily dose of 60 mg/m^2 on days 2 and 20; procarbazine at a daily dose of 100 mg/m^2 on days 2–20
Group III: VM-26 at a daily dose of 60 mg/m^2 on days 1 and 2; CCNU at a daily dose of 60 mg/m^2 on days 3 and 4
Group IV: VM-26 at a daily dose of 60 mg/m^2 on day 1; CCNU at a daily dose of 60 mg/m^2 on day 2
Each sequence of VM-26 and CCNU is given after a free interval of 35 days for hemopoietic recovery. In group IV treatment was given every 20 days. Distribution of patients according to initial treatment in shown in Table 2.

Evaluation of Results

Each patient included in this trial underwent a general, neurologic, and biologic checkup. The patients were classified into four clinical stages:
Stage IV: the patient is in a vegetative state
Stage III: the patient is conscious and his neurologic condition requires constant aid
Stage II: the patient is conscious and can look after his basic needs
Stage I: the patient can assume all activities.
Clinical improvement is defined as a regression of neurologic signs enabling the patient to progress by at least one of the above-described stages within a minimum of 2 months. In 46 patients, radionuclide monitoring was practiced every 3 months. The final overall assessment of the therapeutic effects was based on the evolution of the survival curve for the entire group of patients included in the trial.

Table 2. Distribution of treatment according to initial local treatment

	Patients operated on	Patients with		Patients not operated on	No. of evaluable patients
		relapse after surgery	Surgery + radiotherapy		
Group I	10	4	3	4	19
Group II	10	4	2	5	18
Group III	11	4	0	8	20
Group IV	2	2	2	0	6
	33	14	7	17	63

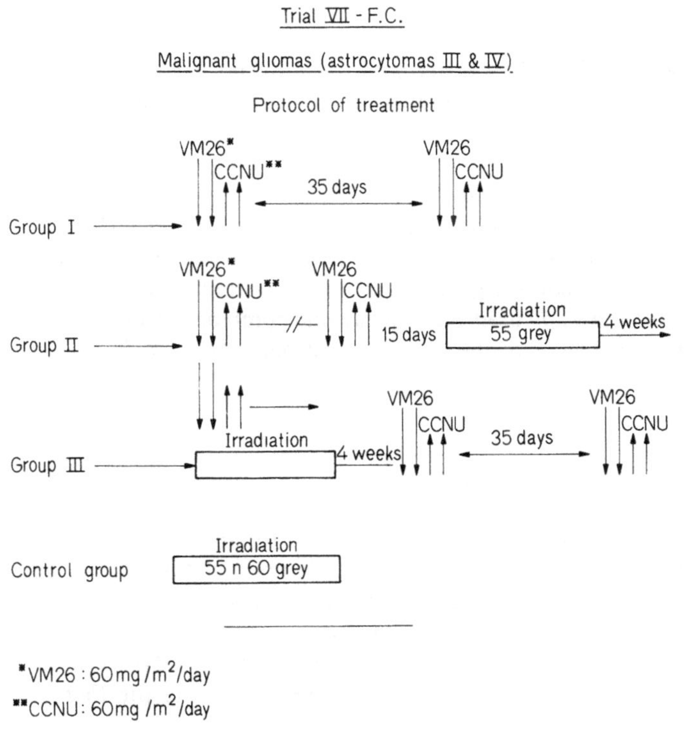

Fig. 1. Protocol of treatment; three treatment groups are proposed

Table 3. Malignant gliomas (astrocytomas III and IV)

	No. of patients	Astrocytomas	
		III	IV
Group I[a]			
chemotherapy	22	7	15
Group II[a]			
chemoradiotherapy chemotherapy	22	9	13
Group III[a]			
radiotherapy chemotherapy	11	2	9
Total	55	18	37
Historical group Radiotherapy alone	36		

[a] All the patients entered this trial 2–6 weeks after surgical resection of the brain tumor.

Trial II

We entered 55 patients with partially resected supratentorial malignant gliomas into a randomized chemotherapeutic trial between 1 January 1976 and 1 March 1977. Three treatment groups were proposed (Fig. 1).

The patients in group I were treated with chemotherapy alone beginning 2–6 weeks after surgical removal of the tumor. *The patients in group II* received three cycles of chemotherapy and then were submitted to radiotherapy. *The patients in group III* were treated with radiotherapy and 4 weeks later with chemotherapy. All the patients were compared with a historical control group of 36 patients treated with radiotherapy alone. The protocol of chemotherapy used was a sequential combination of VM-26 and CCNU. The distribution of the patients to the treatment groups by histologic type of tumor is presented in Table 3.

Adjuvant Therapy

Before undergoing the first cycle of treatment, all patients in both cycles, whatever their neurologic status, were given a daily optimal dose of dexamethasone associated with a daily 100-ml infusion of isotonic mannitol. This adjuvant treatment was progressively reduced to the minimum effective dose and was replaced during the free interval by 0.5 mg three times a week of tetracosactide retard. The reduction and discontinuation of the doses of corticosteroids were taken into account when assessing the therapeutic effect.

Tolerance

Trial I

Administration of CCNU induced in 60% of the patients with gastrointestinal symptoms such as nausea and vomiting beginning 3–4 h after treatment. These difficulties were more intensive and persistent in patients treated with procarbazine. The hematologic tolerance was comparable in groups I and III, and after the second cycle of treatment, significantly altered for patients in group II (Table 4).

Table 4. Average intervals for hematologic recovery between cycles of chemotherapy for malignant gliomas

Cycles of chemotherapy	Chemotherapy combination		
	VM-26–CCNU	ADM–VM-26–CCNU	VM-26–CCNU–PCR
1st cycle	31.8 days	33.45 days	33 days
2nd cycle	31 days	34.4 days	33.6 days
3rd cycle	35.2 days	34.5 days	45.5 days
4th cycle	34.8 days	34.7 days	
5th cycle	40.7 days	40.1 days	
6th cycle	39.5 days	39.8 days	

Trial II

The hematologic tolerance to cycles of chemotherapy was not disturbed by irradiation.

Therapeutic Results

Trial I

The clinical responses we observed are presented in Table 5: 57.8% (11/19) of the patients in group I are objective responders; 58% (10/18) of the patients in group II are objective responders; 60% (12/20) of the patients in group III are objective responders.
As far as neurologic improvement is concerned, the therapeutic effect of each protocol is identical. A parallel improvement of the radionuclide scan used for tumor measurement was noticed in 60% of the patients. The survival curves for each treatment group are presented in Fig. 2. The median survival time for patients in group II is 8.3 months, and 19% of the patients are alive at the 16th month.
The median survival time was comparable in groups I and III: 12 and 12.3 months, respectively. In group I 35% and in group III 25% of the patients are alive at the 16th month (the difference is nonsignificant). The survival curve obtained in patients introduced into the first three groups is represented in Fig. 3. The median survival time is 10 months and 30% of the patients are alive at the 16th month.

Trial II

In this trial, only 43 patients who were alive 6 months after they entered into the trial were evaluated. At the 16th month, the difference in survival between the group treated with

Table 5. Clinical responses in patients treated with chemotherapy

	TR	PR > 50%	PR < 50%	TF
Group I N: 21 evaluable: 19	5	6	6	2
Group II N: 21 evaluable: 18	8	2	4	4
Group III N: 23 evaluable: 20	4	8	6	2
Group IV N: 6 evaluable: 6	0	0	0	6

TR total remission; *PR* partial remission; *TF* total failure.

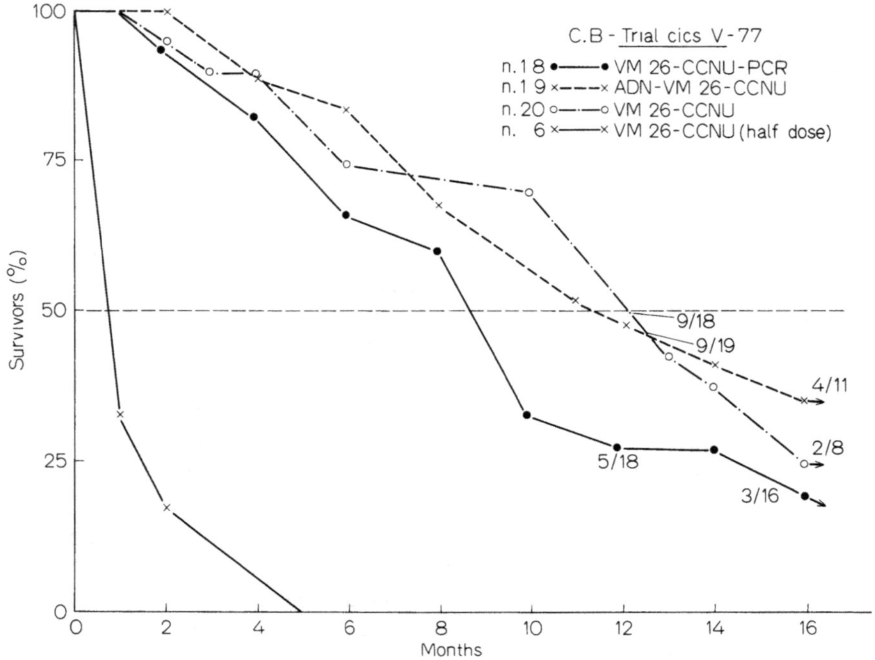

Fig. 2. Survival curves for each treatment group

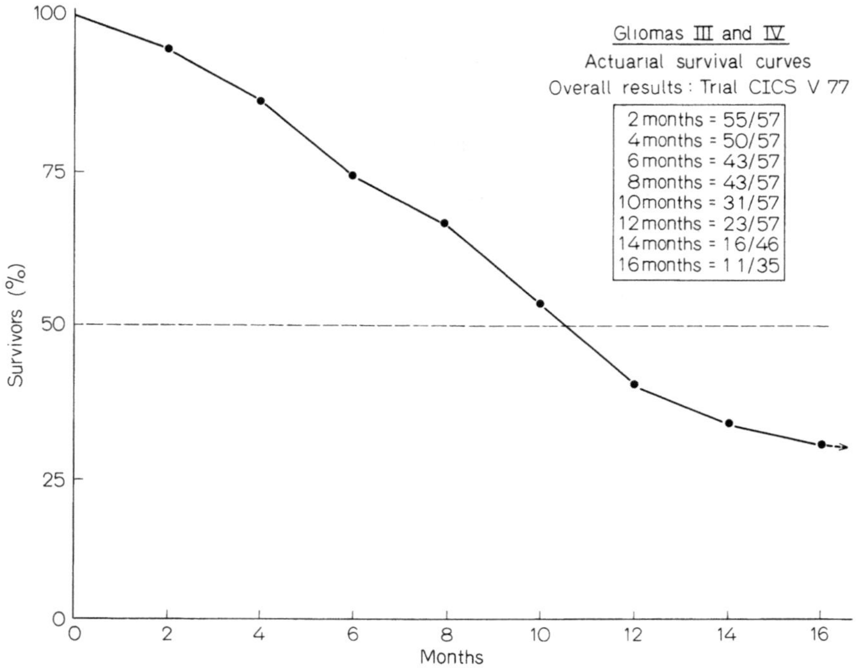

Fig. 3. Actuarial survival curves; overall results for trial I

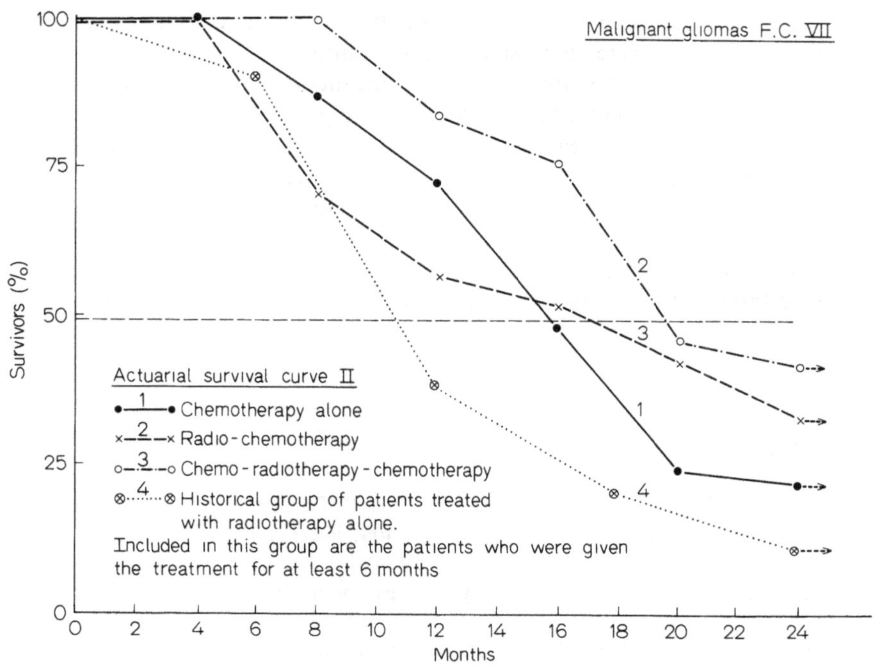

Fig. 4. Actuarial survival curves for trial II

chemoradiochemotherapy (group II) and the group treated with radiochemotherapy (group III) is significant. The median survival time of patients in group II is 20 months and for patients in groups I and III 16 months. At the 24th month, a better effect is observed with the radiochemotherapy program compared to the chemotherapy protocol. The median survival time of patients in the historical control group is 10 months (Fig. 4).

Discussion

We entered 71 patients with partially resectable or relapsed malignant gliomas into a randomized study to compare four different treatment programs including chemotherapy. Some results previously reported demonstrated the therapeutic efficiency of two drug combinations [10, 11]. The results of this trial raise three points for discussion:

1) The *comparison* of the results we obtained in the first and third groupsof patients demonstrated that adriamycin has no effect in the treatment of malignant gliomas. This drug seems unable to exert any different cytolytic effect or to potentiate the activity of an active combination.

2) This trial demonstrates the *efficiency* of the combination of VM-26 and CCNU at full dose. However, the reduction in the dose of CCNU to 60 mg/m^2 per cycle does not appear to improve the course of tumor progression.

3) The second protocol combining the nonefficient sequence of VM-26 and CCNU (half dose) with daily intake of procarbazine for 20 days exhibited an immediately good therapeutic

effect. It appears that such a combination will be effective as a "maintenance" therapy given to patients with complete regression of their tumors.

The preliminary results of this trial let us study the therapeutic role of radiotherapy in patients treated with the better combination of chemotherapy. The first conclusion of the second trial was that radiotherapy increased the survival of patients and that radiotherapy is more effective when applied after three cycles of chemotherapy. Two hypothesis may be proposed to explain this supplementary beneficial effect: either chemotherapy acts as a so-called nonspecific radiosensitizer and then increases the cytolytic effect of radiotherapy at the cellular level or chemotherapy and radiotherapy do not work in the same manner and we observe in this trial the results of their successively cumulative effects. It is too early to choose between these hypotheses.

References

1. Armentrout, S. A., Foltz, E., Vermund, H., Otis, P. T.: Comparison of postoperative irradiation alone and in combinations with BCNU (NSC 409, 962) in the management of malignant gliomas. Cancer Chemother. Rep. *58,* 841–844 (1974)
2. Bloom, H. J. G.: Combined modality therapy for intracranial tumors. Cancer *35,* 111–120 (1975)
3. Fewer, D., Wilson, C. B., Boldrey, E. B., Enot, K. J.: Phase II study of 1 (2-chloroethyl) 3 cyclohexyl-1-Nitrosourea (CCNU-NSC 79037) in treatment of brain tumors. Cancer Chemother. Rep. *56,* 421–427 (1972)
4. Goldsmith, M. A., Carter, St K.: Glioblastoma multiforme. A review of therapy. Cancer Treat. Rev. *1,* 153–156 (1974)
5. Lassman, L., Pearce, G. W., Gang, J.: Sensitivity of intracranial glioblastoma to vincristine sulfate. Lancet *1965 I,* 296–297
6. Levin, V. A., Wilson, Ch. B.: Chemotherapy. The agents in current use. Semin. Oncol. *2,* 63–67 (1975)
7. Levin, V. A., Wilson, Ch. B.: Correlations between experimental chemotherapy in the murine glioma and effectiveness of clinical therapy regimens. Cancer Chemother. Pharmacol. *1,* 41–48 (1978)
8. Levin, V. A., Wilson, Ch. B.: Nitrosourea for primary malignant gliomas. Cancer Treat. Rep. *60,* 719–724 (1976)
9. Pouillart, P., Palangie, T., Poisson, M., Huguenin, P., Morin, P.: Chimiothérapie cytolytique appliquée au traitement des gliomes malins hémisphériques de l'adulte: bases théoriques. Vie Médicale (in press) (1978)
10. Pouillart, P., Mathe, G., Poisson, M., Buge, A., Huguenin, P., Gautier, H., Morin, P., Hoang Thy Huong, T., Lheritier, J., Parrot, R.: Essai de traitement des glioblastomes de l'adulte et des métastases cérébrales par l'association d'Adriamycine, de VM 26 et de C.C.N.U. Résultats d'un essai de type II. Nouv. Presse Méd. *25,* 1571–1576 (1976)
11. Pouillart, P., Mathe, G., Hoang Thy Huong, T., Lheritier, J., Poisson, M., Huguenin, P., Gautier, H., Morin, P., Parrot, R.: Treatment of malignant gliomas and brain métastases in adults with a combination of Adriamycin, VM 26 and C.C.N.U. Results of a phase II trial. Cancer *38,* 1909–1916 (1976)
12. Rosenblum, M. L., Reynolds, A. F., Smith, K. A., Rumack, B. H., Walcker, D.: Chloroethyl-cyclohexyl-nitrosourea (CCNU) in the treatment of malignant brain tumors. J. Neurol. Surg. *39,* 306–324 (1973)
13. Shapiro, W. R.: Malignant brain tumor chemotherapy. Part II. Clin. Bull. *3,* 58–62 (1973)

14. Sklansky, B. D., Mann-Kaplan, R. S., Reynolds, A. F., Rosenblum, M. L., Walker, M. D.: 4′dimethyl-epipodophylotoxin-D-thenylidene glucoside (PT 6) in the treatment of malignant intracranial neoplasms. Cancer *33*, 460–467 (1974)
15. Vasantha-Kumar, A. R., Renaudin, J., Wilson, Ch. B., Boldrey, Ed. B., Jean-Enot, K., Levin, V. A.: Procarbazine hydrochloride in the treatment of brain tumors. Phase II study. J. Neurol. Surg. *40*, 365–371 (1974)
16. Walker, M. D., Hurwitz, B. S.: BCNU (1,3 bis-(2-chloroethyl)-1 nitrosourea-NSC 409962) in the treatment of malignant brain tumors. Cancer Chemother. Rep. *4*, 263–273 (1970)

Adjuvant Chemotherapy in Malignant Brain Gliomas[1]

J. Hildebrand

Since neurosurgery followed by high dose radiation therapy invariably fails to completely remove malignant brain gliomas, these tumors appear to be excellent candidates for adjuvant chemotherapy of the residual disease. At least three parameters can be measured in brain tumor chemotherapeutic trials: (1) prolongation of survival, (2) rate and duration of objective remissions, and (3) prolongation of the disease-free interval (Table 1). As in other neoplasms, these parameters do not necessarily measure the same phenomenon and may give apparently contradictory results, especially when the drugs used are moderately active. Therefore, their results should be considered separately. The therapeutic effects on the residual tumor cells are tested in trials that measure the disease-*free interval* and/or *total survival.*

Randomized trials that investigate the ability of the drugs to prolong the survival time of patients with operated malignant brain gliomas are few. They are listed in Table 2, and their results can be summarized as follows:

a) 5-Fluorouracil and mithramycin are inactive.
b) The activity of CCNU is questionable.
c) BCNU is active when used in combination with radiotherapy.

From the begining the EORTC Brain Tumor Group has tried to measure the effects of chemotherapy on disease-free survival. The group has demonstrated in two consecutive trials that this parameter can be reproducibly measured, with a degree of acceptable accuracy, in selected patients who do not require the administration of steroids and have a normal or minimally abnormal neurologic examination.

Table 1. Types of trials evaluating chemotherapy in malignant brain tumors

Measured parameter	Advantages	Difficulties	Type of patients
Survival time	Short constant median: 24 weeks, easy to measure	Requires prolonged hospitalization	All patients
Objective remission	Hospitalization not required	More difficult to measure than survival time	Recurring primary tumors
Disease-free interval	Measures the quality of survival	Difficult to measure	Selected patients

1 This work is supported by the NCI contract NO1-CM-53840.

Table 2. Effects of single-agent chemotherapy on survival time in malignant gliomas

References	Treatment	No. of patients		Survival (median)		
Edland et al., 1971 [4]	5-Fluorouracil+RT	17		11.5 months		NS
	vs RT alone	15		11.7 months		
Walker et al., 1976 [8]	Mithramycin	52		21 weeks		NS
	vs no chemotherapy	44		26 weeks		
Walker and Gehan, 1972 [9]	RT + BCNU	Total 180		41 weeks		($P<0.01$)
	RT alone			28 weeks		($P<0.01$)
	BCNU alone			20 weeks		NS
	controls			17 weeks		
Armentrout et al., 1974 [1]	RT + BCNU	16		10 months		($P<0.01$)
	vs RT alone	11		3 months		
EORTC Group 1976 [5]	RT + CCNU	11		45 weeks		($P<0.025$)
	vs RT alone	9		17 weeks		
Brisman et al., 1976 [3]	RT+BCNU or CCNU or methyl CCNU *vs* RT alone	Group A 29		12 months	all patients	($P<0.005$)
		Group A 39	(no chemotherapy)	4.2 months		
		Group B 19		12 months	full RT	NS
		Group B 21	(no chemotherapy)	9 months		
		Group C 17		6.1 months	randomized for chemot.	NS
		Group C 16	(no chemotherapy)	6.3 months		
Regan et al., 1976 [7]	RT + CCNU	19		12 months		
	RT alone	22		11.6 months		($P<0.005$)
	CCNU alone	22		6.6 months		
Walker and Strike 1976 [10]	RT + BCNU	332		51 weeks	statistically superior	"statistically superior"
	RT+methyl CCNU			31 weeks		
	RT alone			36 weeks		
	methyl CCNU alone			31 weeks		

In a first trial CCNU given alone at the scheduled dose of 130 mg/m² every 6 weeks (the actual dose received was over 100 mg/m² every 6 weeks) did not affect the duration of the disease-free interval (Fig. 1). To the best of our knowledge, the disease-free interval has been measured in only one other study [2]. The results of this study differed from those obtained in our trial in that the disease-free interval was longer in patients receiving 4500 rad plus CCNU (291 d) than in patients treated by radiotherapy alone (152 d). The total number of patients included in this study was, however, much lower than in the EORTC trial.

In a second trial by the EORTC Group, it was not possible to demonstrate any beneficial effect of the combination VM–26 (given on day 1, 100 mg/m² every 6 weeks) plus CCNU (given on day 2, 130 mg/m² every 6 weeks) on the duration of the disease-free interval after a first evaluation of the study (Fig. 2).

To conclude: although we do have agents, like the nitrosoureas, that are able to produce objective remissions in patients with recurring symptoms due to malignant brain gliomas, their activity when given as adjuvant chemotherapy, as judged by the duration of the disease-free interval and/or total survival, is modest or none.

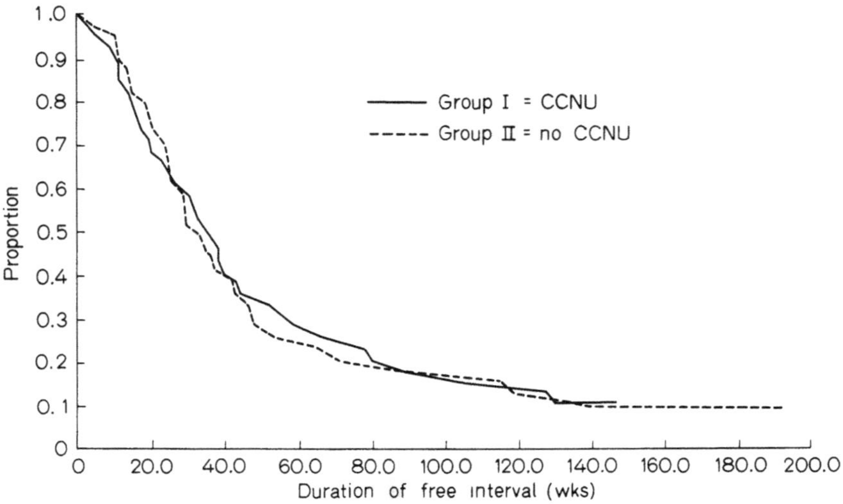

Fig. 1. Study 26741. Disease-free interval length curves in 42 patients receiving CCNU (130 mg/m^2 every 6 weeks, ——) and 39 controls (– – –)

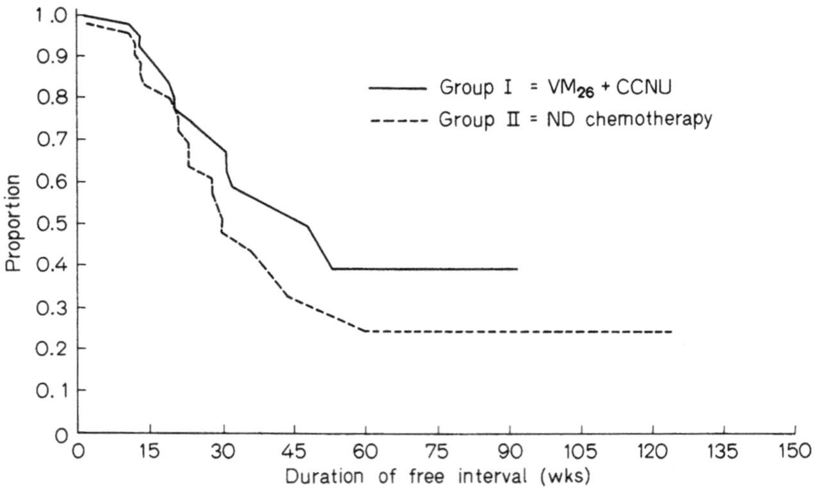

Fig. 2. Study 26751. Disease-free interval length curves in 48 patients receiving VM-26 (100 mg/m^2 every 6 weeks or day 1) plus CCNU (130 mg/m^2 every 6 weeks or day 2, ——) and in 45 controls (– – –)

References

1. Armentrout, S. A., Foltz, E., Vermund, H., Otis, P. T.: Comparison of postoperative irradiation alone and in combination with BCNU (NSC-409962) in management of malignant gliomas. Cancer Chemother. Rep. *58*, 841–844 (1976)
2. Band, P. R., Weir, Urtasun, R. C., Blain, G., McLean, D., Wilson, F., Mielke, B., Grace, M.: Radiotherapy and CCNU in Grade III and IV astrocytoma. ASCO Abs. p. 161 (1974)

3. Brisman, R., Housepian, E. M., Chang, C., Duffy, P., Balis, E.: Adjuvant nitrosourea therapy for glioblastomas. Arch. Neurol. *33*, 745–750 (1976)
4. Edland, R. W., Javid, M., Ansfield, J. F.: Glioblastoma multiforme. An analysis of the results of post-operative radiotherapy alone versus radiotherapy and concomitant 5-Fluorouracil. Am. J. Roentgenol. *3*, 337–342 (1971)
5. EORTC Brain Tumor Group. Effects of CCNU on the survival, rate of objective remission and duration of free interval in patients with malignant brain glioma. First evaluation. Eur. J. Cancer *12*, 41–45 (1976)
6. EORTC Brain Tumor Group. Effects of CCNU on the survival, rate of objective remission and duration of free interval in patients with malignant brain glioma. Final evaluation. Eur. J. Cancer (in press) (1978)
7. Reagan, T. J., Bisel, H. F., Childs, D. S., Layton, D. D., Rhoton, A. L. (Jr.), Taylor, W. F.: Controlled study of CCNU radiation therapy in malignant astrocytomas. J. Neurol. *44*, 186–190 (1976)
8. Walker, M. D., Alexander, E. (Jr.), Hunt, W. E., Leventhal, C. M., Mahaley, M., Mealey, J. S. (Jr.), Norrell, H. A., Owens, G., Ransohoff, J., Wilson, C. B., Gehan, E. A.: Evaluation of mithramycin in the treatment of anaplastic gliomas. J. Neurol. *44*, 655–667 (1976)
9. Walker, M. D., Gehan, E. A.: An evaluation of 1-3-Bis (2-chloroethyl)-1-nitrosourea (BCNU) and irradiation alone and in combination for the treatment of malignant glioma. AACR Abs. p. 67 (1972)
10. Walker, M. D., Strike, T. A.: An evaluation of methyl-CCNU, BCNU and radiotherapy in treatment of malignant glioma. AACR Abs. p. 163 (1976)

Adjuvant Therapy for Residual Disease in Children With Medulloblastoma

H. J. G. Bloom

Introduction

It has been widely recognised for many years that postoperative radiotherapy is essential for the eradication of medulloblastoma. Residual tumor leading to recurrence and to early death is inevitable following surgery alone. To achieve the maximum number of cures, radiotherapy must be meticulously planned and carried out, ensuring coverage of the entire cerebro-spinal contents with the maximum dose in the posterior fossa where tumor recurrence is most frequently seen [9]. It has also become clear that the only real chance of cure depends upon the first treatment: experience has shown that once recurrence occurs, any further treatment is essentially palliative and that a fatal outcome is practically certain. In spite of these observations, the established principles of postoperative radiotherapy for medulloblastoma are not universally applied and very poor results are still being seen in some centres.

In general, current neurosurgical practice is to remove as much of the tumor as possible, without undue risk to life and function, to lower intracranial pressure, preserve vision, restore CSF circulation, obtain tissue for histology and reduce tumor bulk. Following tumor reduction by surgery and the attack on residual disease by radiotherapy, the average 3-, 5- and 10-year survival rates reported from major centres have been approximately 40%, 35% and 25%, respectively [5]. More recently, survival rates of up to 60% at 3 years, 40% at 5 years and 30% at 10 years have been achieved (Table 1). Occasionally, in small series, even higher survival rates have been reported [21]. It is important to point out that results coming from radiotherapy centres are often based on selected material in that deaths, prior to or as a result of operation, have been excluded.

Even with improved radiation techniques and higher maximum tumor doses in the range of 5000–6000 rad, there is a persistent 5-year tumor mortality rate of at least 50%–60%, with the great majority of initial recurrences occurring in the posterior fossa [9, 18] (Fig. 1, Table 2). Since the surgeons can excise no more tumor and since the radiotherapists have virtually reached the limits to which the dose of irradiation can be increased without incuring serious risk of injury, especially in young children, we must turn to other modalities to seek further improvement in treatment results.

Table 1. Medulloblastoma (children) 10-year survival

Author	Cases	10-year survival
Mealey & Hall (1977)	32	22%
Bloom (1977)	68	29%
Harisiadis & Chang (1977)	58	31%[a]

[a] Life table.

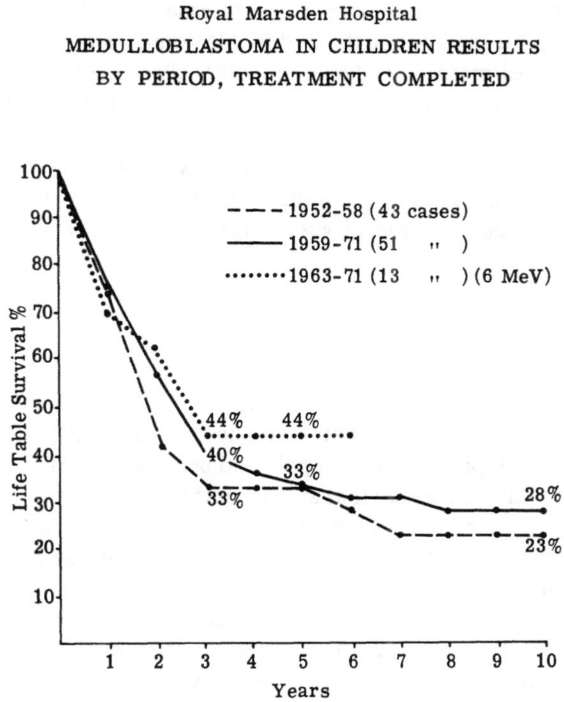

Fig. 1. There was little difference in results following postoperative radiotherapy for the two periods 1952–1958 and 1959–1971. With the introduction of megavoltage X-rays (6 MeV) in 1963, and prior to the use of chemotherapy, survival rates for children with medulloblastoma may be increasing

Table 2. Even with maximum tumor doses in the range of 5000–6000 rad there is still a 5-year mortality rate of at least 50–60%. Medulloblastoma failure by radiation dose

Dose (rads)	Cases	5-year mortality
4000–4500	22	59%
4500–5000	12	66%
5000–6000	18	66%

Bloom et al. (1969).

Dose (rads) to post. fossa	Cases	Recurrence rate	5-year mortality
4000–4700	17	76%	65%
4700–5200	25	52%	55%
5200–6000	13	46%	52%

Harisiadis and Chang (1977).

Problems relating to residual disease in medulloblastoma patients are threefold. First and foremost, although the medulloblastoma is a highly radiosensitive lesion and responds rapidly to treatment, a residue of resistant cells in the primary tumor appears to be the most frequent cause of treatment failure. Second, although seeding along the CSF pathways especially down the spinal cord is commonly associated with posterior fossa recurrence, this type of spread may occur alone [18]. Finally, in about 10% of cases blood-borne metastases develop and this complication may be facilitated by the establishment of ventriculo-atrial and ventriculo-peritoneal shunts [20]. We may try and reduce these problems through the following approaches.

Radiosensitizing Agents

There is evidence that hypoxia is present in tumors largely as a result of the neoplasm outstripping its blood supply and because of the limitation of diffusion of oxygen in tissues. It is widely accepted that at least part of the radioresistance and radioincurability of tumors in general may be explained by the presence of a hypoxic but viable tumor cell population. Such cells may occur in quite small tumor nodules and are certain to be present in larger masses, especially when necrosis is evident, which is a common feature in medulloblastomas. Compared with well-oxygenated tissue, hypoxic cells are more resistant to conventional irradiation by a dose factor of between 2.5 and 3.0.

Efforts have been made to increase tissue oxygen to try and overcome radioresistance by breathing oxygen under raised pressure during treatment or by lowering oxygen consumption by inducing hypothermia. Since normal tissue is considered to be well-oxygenated, its response to irradiation is not affected by such manoevres.

Breathing Oxygen

Hyperbaric oxygen during irradiation with the patient enclosed in a special pressure chamber was used for glioblastoma cases in a controlled study by Chang [14]. The initial survival rates for patients treated in hyperbaric oxygen were not significantly greater than for controls treated in air.

Hypothermia

By lowering body temperature, it is hoped to reduce tissue oxygen consumption through a fall in the general metabolic rate. During hypothermia there is also an increase of dissolved oxygen in plasma and these two factors may result in a significant increase in the oxygen environment of hypoxic tumor tissue. An increased sensitivity to whole body irradiation in mice under mild hypothermia was demonstrated by Bloom and Dawson [8]. A pilot clinical study was initiated in which patients with glioblastoma, maintained at a body temperature of between 33° and 30° C, were treated by whole brain irradiation. Although an apparent increased clinical response of brain tissue to irradiation was observed in these circumstances, the treatment resulted in no benefit for the patients, was difficult to carry out and was associated with considerable risks relating to the periods of hypothermia [4].

Although greater local tumor control following radiotherapy under hyperbaric oxygen has been reported for head and neck cancer [19], the use of physical procedures to increase tissue oxygen do not appear to overcome the oxygen effect sufficiently, and their role in radiotherapy now appears to have been completely superceded by chemical methods involving the administration of electron-affinic radiosensitizing agents.

Chemical Sensitizers

It is the hope of all radiotherapists to find a compound capable of selectively increasing the radiosensitivity of tumor cells relative to normal tissue. The pioneer attempts to treat brain gliomas with this principle using halogenated pyrimidines (BUdR and IUdR) failed to produce results significantly better than those following surgery and radiotherapy alone [22]. In recent years attention has been focussed on a number of electron-affinic agents, principally derivatives of nitroimidazole (e.g. metronidazole) [1, 3] that, like oxygen, sensitize hypoxic cells to irradiation in all phases of the cell cycle. Such agents, not being rapidly metabolised like oxygen, are expected to penetrate deeply into the tumor beyond the capillaries and reach central hypoxic areas. Encouraging observations have been made in both in vitro and in vivo laboratory experiments [2, 17]. URTASUN et al. [28] have reported a brief increase in survival in patients with glioblastoma treated with radiotherapy and metronidazole, compared with radiotherapy alone.

There is evidence that the nitroimidazole drugs, apart from their radiosensitizing action, also possess a *direct* cytotoxic effect on hypoxic tumor cells with little effect on well-oxygenated tissue [15, 16, 27]. This property may be useful in reducing the hypoxic tumor cell population *prior to* radiotherapy. Thus, a remarkable group of agents has become available to the radiotherapist that may go some way towards meeting his need for effective selective adjuvants. These compounds are not only selective radiosensitizers but also selective cytotoxics, aimed specifically at hypoxic cell elements. They have promising pharmacological and, although restrictive, acceptable toxicological properties. They are water-soluble, become widely distributed throughout the body, diffuse into non-vascularised hypoxic areas of the tumor and are not rapidly metabolised. Enhancement ratios of 1.3–2.4 have been obtained in laboratory experiments, depending largely upon the dose of drug and whether single or multiple dose radiation regimes are employed.

The most effective chemical radiosensitising agent to date appears to be misonidazole (Roche 07-0582), another nitroimidazole derivative (Fig. 2). It is well absorbed when given by mouth. The peak plasma level is reached in 4 h and has a half-life of 12 h. The chief side-effects limiting dosage are gastro-intestinal disturbance and especially neurotoxicity: at present it is recommended that the total dose should not exceed 12 g/m^2 (maximum 24 g) over at least 18 days. Clinical trials to assess the value of misonidazole in radiotherapy of brain gliomas are in

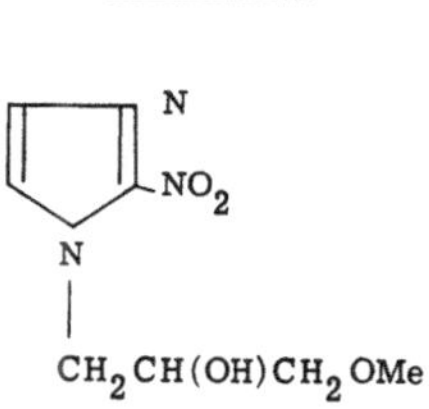

Fig. 2. Misonidazole

progress or being planned at Edmonton (URTASUN), at Cambridge (BLEEHAN), at Vienna (KARCHER), within the EORTC organisation (HILDEBRAND), and at Rochester, New York (SALAZAR). At the Royal Marsden we are developing a three-armed prospective study involving treatment with megavoltage X-rays alone, megavoltage X-rays and misonidazole, and neutrons alone (in conjunction with CATTERALL at the MRC Cyclotron Unit). Preliminary human studies with misonidazole by ASH at the Royal Marsden Hospital have shown that there is good entry of the drug into the CSF and that a concentration in glioblastoma cyst fluid of between 22% and 70% of the blood level is reached at 5 h after administration.

Heavy Particle Beam Irradiation

High LET irradiation, using fast neutrons, is more densely ionising than X-rays or γ-rays and is less dependent on the presence of oxygen and on the phase of the cell cycle for its biological effects. Based on in vitro and in vivo studies, neutron therapy is expected to be 20%–30% more effective than X-rays.

In collaboration with St. George's Hospital Neurosurgical Unit (Atkinson Morley's Hospital) and with CATTERALL of the Medical Research Council Cyclotron Unit in London, we have conducted a randomized pilot study to compare the results of 7.5 MeV neutron irradiation with 6 MeV X-ray therapy in adults with high grade supratentorial cerebral astrocytomas treated initially by substantial tumor excision. The tumor doses used were 1300 or 1560 rad from neutrons given in 12 fractions over 4 weeks, and 5000 or 5500 rad from X-rays in 25–30 fractions over 5–6 weeks. Sixty-three cases entered the study. Far greater tumor destruction appeared to have been produced by neutron irradiation compared with X-rays. Pathological evidence of moderate to gross tumor recurrence was found in six of seven patients (86%) coming to autopsy or second craniotomy after treatment with X-rays, compared with only 5 of 16 patients (31%) treated with neutrons. In 4 of the 16 neutron cases, the tumor appeared to have been totally destroyed by treatment, an event that is extremely rare after megavoltage X-ray therapy. The neutron treatment, however, did not produce an improved survival and was associated with increased degenerative changes in the cerebral white matter, in some cases leading to a clinical picture of progressive dementia [13]. A similar experience has been reported from Seattle by PARKER et al. [25] where treatment with 8 MeV neutrons was compared with an historical series treated with megavoltage X-rays or 60 Co γ-rays (Table 3).

Table 3. Workers in both Seattle and London have obtained similar results with neutron therapy for high grade supratentorial astrocytomas. In both centres the survival rates were no greater than following treatment with megavoltage X-rays or Co 60 γ-rays

Interval (months)	Seattle (Parker et al., 1976)		London (Present series)	
	Survival		Survival	
	Neutrons (21)	Photons (45)[a]	Neutrons (30)	Photons (33)[b]
6	62%	67%	77%	72%
12	23%	33%	30%	36%

[a] Historical. [b] Randomized.

Efforts are now being directed to modify this treatment so that the greater anti-tumor effect of neutrons is retained without excessive damage being inflicted on normal brain tissue. Eventually, a chemical radiosensitizer combined with neutron irradiation may provide the most effective means of overcoming the profound resistance of cerebral glioblastoma to irradiation. Neutron irradiation must first be explored in patients with glioblastomas who have an extremely poor prognosis following conventional treatment, not more than 5% of such patients surviving 5 years, before attempting to introduce this modality in children with medulloblastoma for whom the survival rate with conventional treatment is now about 50%.

Chemotherapy

RALL and ZUBROD [26] enumerated the features required for a compound to cross the blood-brain barrier by diffusion – high lipid solubility, low plasma-protein binding and low ionisation at physiological pH. The nitrosourea drugs have these properties and are the most effective agents discovered to date against cerebral gliomas in both experimental animals and in man. The average response rate among 168 collected cases with various gliomas was 40% [6]; surprisingly, the same figure was found for glioblastomas.

Experience with the nitrosoureas as the sole treatment for recurrent gliomas at the Royal Marsden Hospital has been less encouraging. The overall response rate among 41 cases was 19%. In 23 patients who survived for long enough to receive three or more courses of chemotherapy, the response rate reached 35%. In 6 of these 23 patients, the benefit lasted for 12–46+ months [6].

Controlled studies involving a nitrosourea drug in the postoperative *primary* treatment of high grade astrocytomas have shown such agents to be less effective than irradiation alone and of uncertain value when combined with irradiation. We may conclude that the nitrosoureas undoubtedly cause tumor regression and promote clinical improvement in some recurrent glioma cases, but that their value as adjuvants in the primary treatment of this group of tumors has yet to be established.

The following single drugs have been reported as producing tumor regression in children with recurrent medulloblastoma: CCNU, vincristine, intrathecal methotrexate, procarbazine and VM-26. From scattered reports in the literature, intrathecal methotrexate appears to have a substantial effect on certain recurrent gliomas including medulloblastoma. However, a study at Gustave Roussy Institute, involving the use of intrathecal and intramuscular methotrexate combined with intravenous vincristine as adjuvant therapy in the primary treatment of children with medulloblastoma, produced a 3-year survival rate (46%) that was virtually identical to that of an historical control group without chemotherapy (42%) [23].

Royal Marsden Hospital Clinical Trial

In 1970 we set up a pilot study to explore the feasibility and value of adjuvant multiple agent chemotherapy in children with medulloblastoma following surgery and whole cranio-spinal irradiation. We used oral CCNU, intravenous, vincristine and, in some cases, intrathecal methotrexate. Survival in 25 cases appears better than that for an historical series treated at the same centre without chemotherapy (Fig. 3).

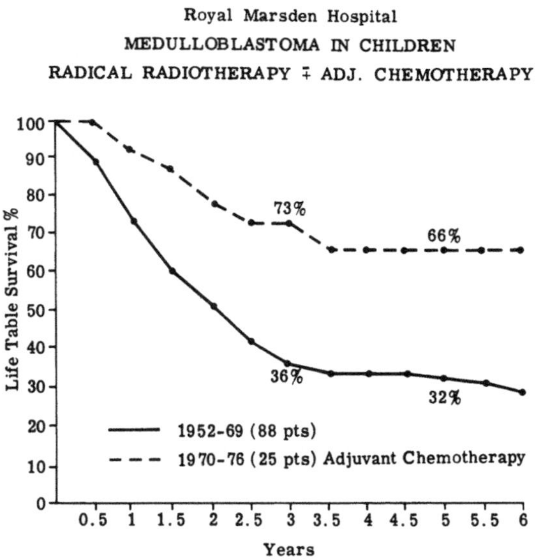

Fig. 3. Survival among a small group of children receiving adjuvant chemotherapy was considerably greater than in an historical series from the same centre treated by surgery and radiation alone

SIOP Trial

These results encouraged a multicentre prospective controlled trial to be sut up in 1975 through the International Society of Paediatric Oncology. So far, some 30 centres, principally in Europe, have contributed over 200 cases that have been randomized between adjuvant chemotherapy (Fig. 4) and no chemotherapy. The results up to 24 months are shown in Table

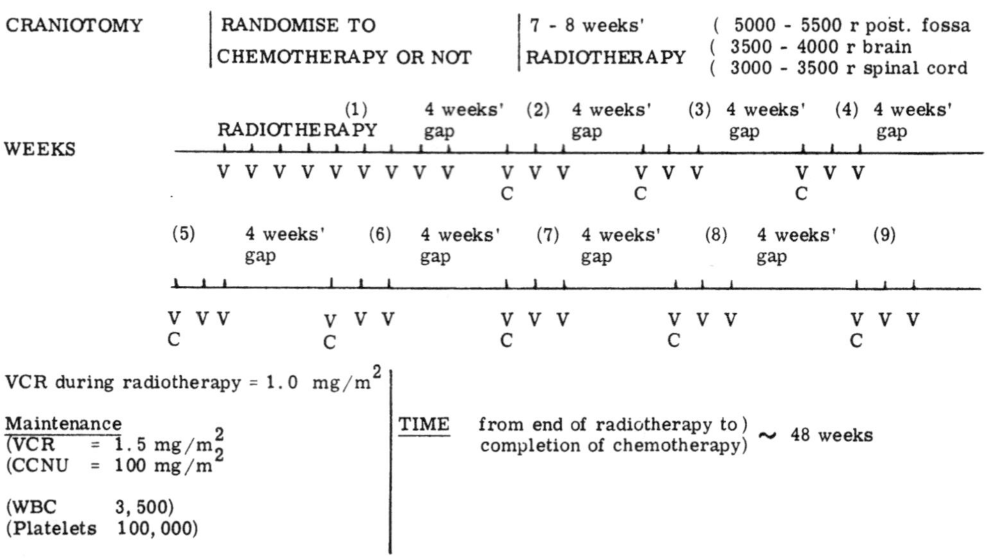

Fig. 4. International society of paediatric oncology (SIOP). Trial of adjuvant chemotherapy in children with medulloblastoma and high grade intracranial ependymoma

Table 4. Early results of a randomized prospective multicentre trial organized by the International Society of Paediatric Oncology. So far, there is no appreciable benefit for children receiving adjuvant chemotherapy according to the protocol shown in Fig. 4. Note the high 2-year survival rate of the *control* group, compared with the generally reported figure of 40–50%. Medulloblastoma, March 1978, survival rates

Interval from op. (mths)	Controls			Chemotherapy		
	Cases	Alive		Cases	Alive	
6	81	64	79%	80	68	85%
12	60	45	75%	60	48	80%
18	43	34	79%	41	33	80%
24	25	18	72%	24	20	83%

4. At present there is no real advantage for the adjuvant chemotherapy group, but with further follow-up a divergence in the survival curves may occur. It is of special interest that the survival rate for the control group following the protocol radiotherapy is remarkably high compared with modern historical series.

Chemotherapy trials for patients with medulloblastoma should be randomized and include a control group without chemotherapy because of the potential additional risks of severe myelosuppression and greater neurological damage following cranio-spinal irradiation, especially in young children. The SIOP Trial shows no increase in the early deaths in the chemotherapy group compared with the controls indicating that, with the usual precautions, chemotherapy following radical cranio-spinal irradiation is feasible and reasonably safe. Apart from the general crude statistical analysis (Table 4), a sequential procedure is also being

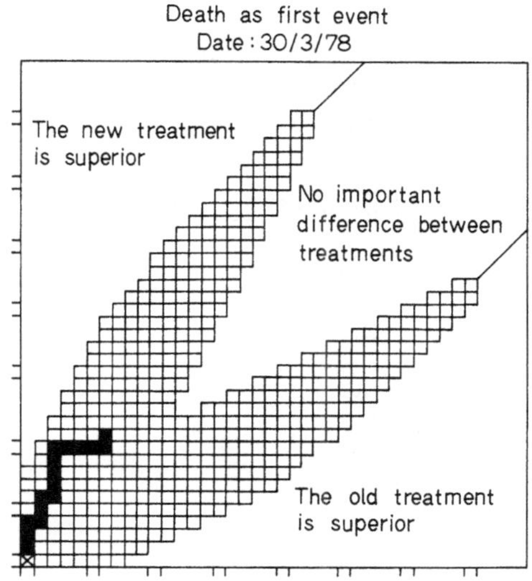

Fig. 5. Sequential analysis shows that the new treatment (adjuvant chemotherapy) in the SIOP Trial is now unlikely to produce results inferior to those of surgery and radiotherapy alone. The graph, however, may soon pass into the area of no significant difference between treatments

used in which the cases are paired by various strata factors and the determinate results, based on death in one of the pairs, are plotted according to the method of BROSS [12] (Fig. 5).

Two other controlled studies of adjuvant multiple agent chemotherapy for children with medulloblastoma are being conducted in the United States. The Children's Cancer Study Group in collaboration with the Radiation Therapy Oncology Group have a trial in which CCNU, vincristine and prednisone are being used (with procarbazine being tested in recurrent cases) and the Southwest Oncology Group is using vincristine together with intrathecal methotrexate and intrathecal hydrocortisone.

Immunotherapy

Our efforts to improve survival in adult patients with high grade gliomas by active immunotherapy using autochthonous tumor tissue in a randomized trial proved unsuccessful [10]. There would seem little to gain by pursuing such an approach further in glioma cases until more effective post-surgical adjuvant measures have been established for reducing tumor cell mass to a minimum.

Conclusion

From this brief review it is evident that a number of potentially useful therapeutic combinations could be proposed for patients with medulloblastoma in an endeavour to eradicate residual disease after surgery. Thus, a nitroimidazole radiosensitizing agent could be used prior to radiotherapy to reduce hypoxic cells. Radiation would then be given using megavoltage equipment to the whole cranio-spinal axis, combined with the administration of a radiosensitizer, followed by a neutron 'boost' to the posterior fossa. Finally, maintenance chemotherapy may be envisaged using CCNU alone or in combination with such agents as vincristine or procarbazine (Fig. 6).

In planning new treatment approaches for children with medulloblastoma caution is necessary. Although laboratory experiments have been promising and some clinical observations are encouraging, the value of the various new post-surgical adjuvants has yet to be established. Cytotoxic drugs and also radiosensitizing chemicals are still under trial, and neutron therapy, in spite of its striking effect on glioblastoma, must be modified to reduce the risk to

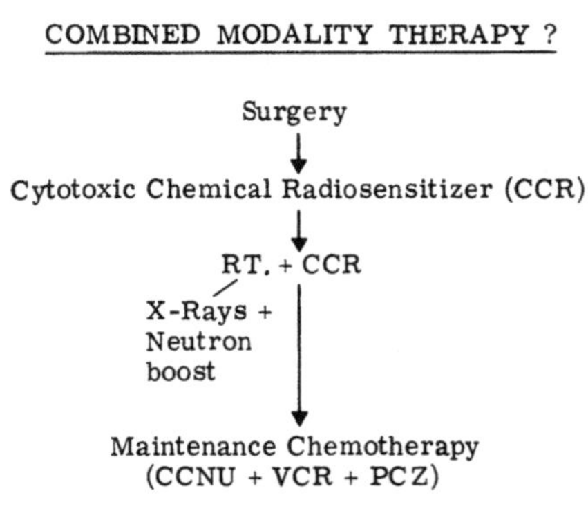

Fig. 6

normal brain tissue. The therapeutic gains achieved in recent years for medulloblastoma cases must not be jeopardised by the premature introduction of untried and potentially dangerous methods of treatment.

From the many options available, it is difficult to select the individual components with which to try and construct the most effective multiagent and multimodality treatment against gliomas including medulloblastoma. We have established a xenograft model in which human gliomas, including medulloblastomas, growing in immune-deprived or nude mice will be used to test newer cytotoxic agents and chemical radiosensitizers. It is hoped to evaluate the timing and the sequence of multimodal treatments and, eventually, to select a suitable programme for clinical trial [11].

References

1. Adams, G. E.: Chemical radiosensitization of hypoxic cells. Br. Med. Bull. *29,* 48–53 (1973)
2. Adams, G. E.: Hypoxic cell sensitizers for radiotherapy. In: Cancer: A comprehensive treatise. Becker, F. F. (ed.), pp. 181–223. New York, London: Plenum Press *6,* 1977
3. Adams, G. E., Flockhart, I. R., Smithen, C. E., Stratford, I. J., Wardman, P., Watts, M. E.: Electron-affinic sensitization. VII. A correlation between structures, one-electron reduction potentials and efficiencies of some nitromidazoles as hypoxic cell radiosensitizers. Radiat. Res. *67,* 9–20 (1976)
4. Bloch, M., Bloom, H. J. G., Penman, J., Walsh, L.: Observations on patients with cerebral astrocytoma (glioblastoma multiforme) treated by irradiation under whole body hypothermia. Br. J. Cancer *20,* 722–728 (1966)
5. Bloom, H. J. G.: Concepts in the natural history and treatment of medulloblastoma in children: increasing survival rates and possible risks with current therapy techniques. C. R. C. Crit. Rev. Radiol. Sci. *2,* 89–143 (1971)
6. Bloom, H. J. G.: New therapeutic perspectives in brain tumours. In: I Tumori Infantili. Bucalossi, P., Veronesi, U., Emanuelli, H., Bellani, F. (eds.), pp. 101–113. Milan: Casa Editrice Ambrosiana 1976
7. Bloom, H. J. G.: Medulloblastoma and Ependymoma: treatment principles and prognosis. Paper presented at 9th Annu. Meet. Int. Soc. Paediatric Oncology (SIOP). Philadelphia, Sept. 1977
8. Bloom, H. J. G., Dawson, K. B.: Enhanced effect of total body X-irradiation in mice under mild hypothermia. Nature *192,* 232–233 (1961)
9. Bloom, H. J. G., Wallace, E. N. K., Henk, J. M.: The treatment and prognosis of medulloblastoma in children – a study of 82 verified cases. Am. J. Roentgenol. *105,* 43–62 (1969)
10. Bloom, H. J. G., Peckham, M. J., Richardson, A. E., Alexander, P. A., Payne, P. M.: Glioblastoma multiforme – a controlled trial to assess the value of specific active immunotherapy in patients treated by radical surgery and radiotherapy. Br. J. Cancer *27,* 253–267 (1973)
11. Bradley, N. J., Bloom, H. J. G., Davies, A. J. S., Swift, S. M.: The growth of human gliomas in immune-deficient mice: a possible model for pre-clinical therapy studies. Br. J. Cancer (in press) (1978)
12. Bross, I.: Sequential medical plans. Biometrics *8,* 188–205 (1952)
13. Catterall, M., Bloom, H. J. G., Uttley, D., Ash, D. S., Lewis, P., Gowing, N. F. C., Chaucer, B.: The treatment of supratentorial high grade astrocytomas with fast neutrons and with megavoltage X-rays – a controlled pilot study (to be published) (1978)
14. Chang, C. H.: Hyperbaric Oxygen and Radiation Therapy in the Management of Glioblastoma. Natl. Cancer Inst. Monogr. *46,* 163–169 (1977)

15. Foster, J. L.: Differential cytotoxic effects of metronidazole and other nitro-heterocyclic drugs against hypoxic tumour cells. Int. J. Radiat. Oncol. Biol. Phys. *4,* 153–156 (1978)
16. Foster, J. L., Conroy, P. J., Searle, A. J., Willson, R. L.: Metronidazole (Flagyl): characterisation as a cytotoxic drug specific for hypoxic tumour cells. Br. J. Cancer *33,* 485–490 (1976)
17. Fowler, J. F., Adams, G. E., Denekamp, J.: Radiosensitizers of hypoxic cells in solid tumours. Cancer Treat. Rev. *3,* 227–256 (1976)
18. Harisiadis, L., Chang, C. H.: Medulloblastoma in children: a correlation between staging and results of treatment. Int. J. Radiat. Oncol. Biol. Phys. *2,* 833–841 (1977)
19. Henk, J. M., Kunkler, P. B., Smith, C. W.: Radiotherapy and Hyperbaric Oxygen in Head and Neck Cancer. Lancet *1977/I* 101–103
20. Hoffman, H. J., Hendrick, E. B., Humphreys, R. P.: Metastasis via ventriculoperitoneal shunt in patients with medulloblastoma. J. Neurosurg. *44,* 562–566 (1976)
21. Hope-Stone, H.: Results of treatment of medulloblastomas. J. Neurosurg. *32,* 83–88 (1970)
22. Hoshino, T., Sano, K.: Radiosensitization of malignant brain tumours with bromouridine. Acta Radiol. *8,* 15–26 (1969)
23. Jundt, M. S.: Essai d'une chimiothérapie systématique dans les médulloblastomes de la fosse posterieure chez l'enfant. Neurochirurgie *20,* 170–171 (1974)
24. Mealey, J., Hall, P. V.: Medulloblastoma in children: survival and treatment. J. Neurosurg. *46,* 56–64 (1977)
25. Parker, R. G., Berry, H. C., Gerdes, A. J., Soronen, M. D., Shaw, C. M.: Fast neutron beam radiotherapy of glioblastoma multiforme. Am. J. Roentgenol. *127,* 331–335
26. Rall, D. P., Zubrod, C. S.: Mechanisms of drug absorption and excretion; passage of drugs in and out of the central nervous system. Annu. Rev. Pharmacol. *2,* 109–128 (1962)
27. Sutherland, R. M.: Selective chemotherapy of non-cycling cells in an in vitro tumour model. Cancer Res. *34,* 3501–3504 (1974)
28. Urtasun, R. C., Miller, J. D. R., Frunchak, V., Koziol, D.: Radiotherapy pilot trials with sensitizers of hypoxic cells: metronidazole in supratentorial glioblastoma. Br. J. Radiol. *50,* 602–603 (1977)

Radiochemotherapy of Postoperative Minimal Residual Disease in Neuroblastoma

J. M. Zucker and E. Margulis

"One might ask whether we have any evidence that survival rate is affected by treatment of any kind" [13].

Introduction

Two-year survival of neuroblastoma patients has not been substantially improved in the last 20 years, either in localized and regional disease or in metastatic tumors (Tab. 1) [1, 16, 19, 23]. As in other tumors of childhood the anatomic extent of the disease is the main prognostic factor (Fig. 1), but host-tumor interrelations seem to be much more decisive in neuroblastoma [7] than the ability of chemotherapeutic agents to eradicate microscopic foci of metastatic deposits as they do in Wilm's tumor and soft-tissue sarcoma. Thus, guidelines for treatment of postoperative minimal residual disease have been found in supervision of the urinary level of the biochemical markers of neuroblastoma by serial assays [14] and in the reappraisal of the various factors influencing survival [1, 4, 6, 9, 12, 23]. Age at diagnosis is the most prominent of these factors (Fig. 2), and infants under 1 year of age have a surprisingly good prognosis compared to children of 1 year or more, whether disease is localized or widespread.
No general agreement on staging childhood tumors has yet been found. For patients with neuroblastoma, the Children's Cancer Study Group A (CCSGA) has proposed an anatomic staging [4] (Table 2) that has been tentatively adopted by several authors, allowing them to compare different series. Stage I tumors are, as a rule, completely resected, and residual disease if any is only microscopic. In stage II tumors, removal is also usually complete but sometimes small macroscopic foci cannot be extirpated. Stage I and II neuroblastomas,

Table 1. Two-year survival of neuroblastoma patients

Author	1st period	2 year survival (No. patients)	2nd period	2 year survival (No. patients)
Localized and regional neuroblastoma				
Sutow 1970 [19]	1956	41% (41)	1962	54% (46)
Breslow 1971 [1]	1947–1967	66% (50)	1966–1968	51% (33)
Zucker 1977 [23]	1950–1960	68% (19)	1961–1970	73% (103)
Metastatic neuroblastoma				
Sutow 1970 [19]	1956	13% (43)	1962	22% (95)
Breslow 1971 [1]	1947–1967	13% (84)	1966–1968	22% (79)
Zucker 1977 [23]	1950–1960	10% (30)	1961–1970	18% (188)

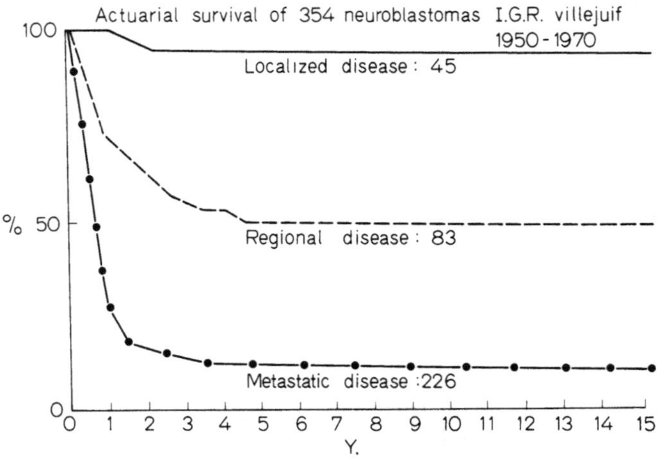

Fig. 1. Anatomic extent of neuroblastomas

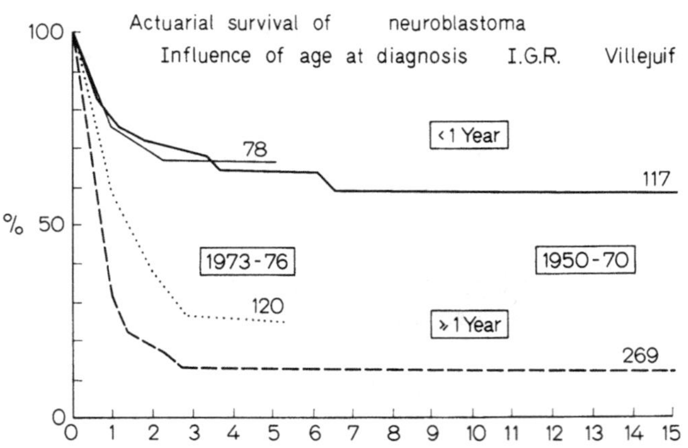

Fig. 2. Influence of age on neuroblastoma prognosis

Table 2. Staging for children with neuroblastoma (according to CCSGA)

Stage I	Tumor confined to the organ or structure of origin
Stage II	Tumors extending in continuity beyond the organ or structure of origin but not crossing the midline; regional lymph nodes on the homolateral side may be involved
Stage III	Tumors extending in continuity beyond the midline; regional lymph nodes may be involved bilaterally
Stage IV	Remote disease involving skeleton, organs, soft tissues, or distant lymph node group
Stage IV-S	Patients who would otherwise be stage I or II, but who have remote disease confined only to one or more of the following sites: liver, skin, or bone marrow (without radiographic evidence of bone metastases on complete skeletal survey)

though frequently pseudoencapsulated, may thus be considered to leave so-called postoperative minimal residual disease, whether in the tumor bed or at clinically undetectable, distant sites.

Retrospective Studies

After the first period of conjectural case-by-case treatment, retrospective studies [12, 21], carried out in Philadelphia and Villejuif on a large number of patients (Fig. 3) permitted an analysis of the prognostic factors and an attempt at assessing the value of radiation and chemotherapy. The 5-year survival in our group was 95% in stage I and 68% in stage II. All stage I patients except one were cured (Table 3) whatever postoperative complementary treatment was given. The survival rate in stage II (Table 4) is high, and again there is no benefit from radio- or chemotherapy. Moreover, five of seven partially resected tumors did not relapse. The same experience was recorded in Philadelphia, with good results (Table 5) whether the tumor was completely resected or not, whether or not subsequent radiotherapy was given. It must nevertheless still be kept in mind that an a posteriori staging of heteroge-

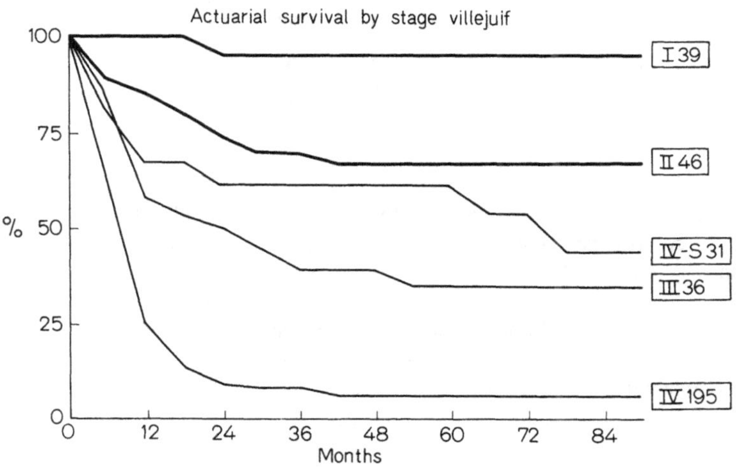

Fig. 3. Neuroblastoma prognosis according to stage

Table 3. Treatment of 35 completely resected stage I neuroblastomas (I.G.R. 1950–1970)

Radiotherapy		Chemotherapy		2 year and 5 year survival
+	17	+	9	9
		–	8	8
–	18	+	11	10
		–	7	7

neous patients and lack of prospective rationale in the treatment are factors limiting an accurate assessment of the efficacy of therapy.

Thus, local postoperative radiotherapy is still under discussion in this group of patients with localized disease since:

Failures are due much more often to metastatic relapses than to local recurrence, which does not exceed 10% (as against 33% in gross residual disease)

Effectiveness of local control is difficult to evaluate when age and host-tumor interaction play such an important role [7]

Radiosensitivity of neuroblastoma is beyond question [2] but varies from one tumor to another and the changes induced are composite: destruction of malignant cells and/or differentiation into ganglioneuroma cells

Table 4. Effect of treatment on the 2-year survival of 40 children with neuroblastoma stage II (I.G.R. Villejuif 1950–1970)

Radiotherapy		Chemotherapy		2-year survival		
+	34	+	26	19	RT+	CT+
		–	8	7	76%	76%
–	6	+	3	3	RT–	CT–
		–	3	2	83%	82%

Table 5. Effect of treatment on the 2-year survival of 20 children with neuroblastoma stage II (adapted from Koop and Johnson [12])

Surgery	Radiotherapy	2-year survival
Complete 4	No	3/4
Partial 6	No	5/6
10	Yes	6/10

Table 6. Radiation therapy in neuroblastoma (adapted from D'Angio [2], Stella [18], Tefft [20])

Age (months)	Tumor dose (grey)	Duration (week)
0–18	15–25	2–3
19–30	25–30	3–4
> 30	30–40	3–5

If radiotherapy is given (Table 6) recommended doses [2, 18, 20] are moderate in young children. The portal that includes the tumoral residue, as demonstrated by the silver clips left by the surgeon, is usually limited but has to encompass the regional nodes if macroscopic or microscopic lymph node involvement has been proved; in abdominal neuroblastoma the question of prophylactic irradiation of mediastinal and/or supraclavicular area is also raised. Opposing anterior and posterior fields must extend across the midline to include the entire width of the epiphyseal plates [2] and avoid critical organs. A milk- and gluten-free diet is effective to prevent intestinal damage, even if a limited part of the small bowel is irradiated [3].

As far as response to chemotherapy is concerned, therapeutic results in metastatic neuroblastoma [11, 16, 22] have been proved helpful for recognizing two groups of patients currently known as "responders" and "nonresponders." Drug response is independant of extent of the disease or age [22] and the most effective agents are vincristine, cyclophosphamide, adriamycin [22], and DTIC [16]. Taking into account the kinetics of neuroblastoma cells may add to the efficacy of chemotherapy [10]. Prophylactic one- or multiple-drug therapy has been used for a long time in localized neuroblastoma that has been completely or nearly completely removed, but there are still no results to confirm its usefulness [13].

Prospective Studies

A randomized study was designed in the CCSGA [5], with an untreated control group, to determine the effect 10 mg/kg/day of cyclophosphamide given orally for 7–10 days every 28 days for 1 year. Postoperative radiotherapy was left to the discretion of investigators in the cooperative group. There were 113 patients with localized and regional neuroblastoma who were at risk for more than 12 months and evaluable. The recurrence rate in stage I was 0/8 in the treated group and 0/19 in the control group; in stage II it was 2/23 and 6/29, respectively. Thus, there is no significant difference between the two groups with this chemotherapy schedule. The 2-year survival of 100% in stage I and 85% in stage II is better than the results of previous studies [4] because prospective staging probably eliminates some metastatic patients.

Since 1973 patients at the Institut Gustave Roussy in Villejuif (Service de Pédiatrie, O. Schweisguth) have also been prospectively staged, and treatment of minimal residual disease (Table 7) has been based on the previous results of our retrospective study. Drug regimens used were according to the age of the children, with low dosages of cyclophosphamide given to infants under 1 year and intensive multichemotherapy including adriamycin to

Table 7. Treatment of minimal residual disease in neuroblastoma (I.G.R. Villejuif 1973–1976)

Stage I	No complementary treatment
Stage II	
Complete removal	No XRT 6 months chemo
Partial removal	XRT 12 months chemo

Table 8. Chemotherapeutic regimens used in postoperative residual neuroblastoma (Institute G. Roussy 1973–1976)

< 1 year	9 · 14 days	
Vincristine	1.5 mg/m²	J_1
Cyclophosphamide	10 mg/kg	J_1 J_2 J_3
> 1 year		
Vincristine	1.5 mg/m²	J_1 J_{21} J_{28}
Adriamycin	60 mg/m²	J_1
Cyclophosphamide	15 mg/kg	J_{21}–J_{27}
followed by a 4-week rest		

Table 9. Effect of treatment in 47 children with minimal residual neuroblastoma (I.G.R. Villejuif 1973–1976)

	No. patients (<1 year) living	Follow-up (months) range median
Stage I	15/15 (12) 100%	18–59 44
Stage II_A	17/19 (12) 89%	20–61 37
Stage II_B	11/13 (6) 84%	21–62 43

children older than 1 year of age (Table 8). Current results in 47 children, with a median follow-up of 37–44 months, show a recurrence rate of 0% in stage I, 11% in stage II after complete removal of the tumor, and 16% in stage II after partial removal of the tumor (Table 9). These numbers are in the same high range as those of the CCSGA. It should be noted that 30 of the 47 patients are under 1 year of age and that in 12 of the 17 other patients the primary was extra-abdominal [8]. Thus, four of five children older than 1 year with stage II abdominal neuroblastoma died, and all the children in the first year of life were cured.

In 11 of 19 patients with stage IIA, regional lymph node status was precisely known. Eight of 11 patients, had a macroscopic or microscopic involvement despite which the six who were under 1 year of age recovered.

Conclusions

Radiochemotherapeutic treatment of minimal residual disease in neuroblastoma must be selective for which two conditions are distinct (Table 10): In *low risk* patients, early or late hazards of therapy are probably higher than the benefit. Therefore, even radiotherapy after a partial removal and chemotherapy in stage II are questionable. In that group, the number of

Table 10. Postoperative complementary treatment of minimal residual disease in neuroblastoma

	XRT	Chemo
Low risk patients		
Complete removal stage I	O	O
Complete removal stage II	O	O/+
< 1 year: all sites		
> 1 year: extra-abdominal		
Partial removal stage II	+/O	+/O
< 1 year		
High risk patients		
Complete removal stage II	+	+
> 1 year: abdominal		
Partial removal stage II	+	+
> 1 year		

patient is small and therapeutic progress could come from new randomized cooperative trials with an untreated group.

In *high risk* patients, the course of disease is so bad that it would not be wise to abandon an intensive complementary treatment.

In the future, chemotherapy of neuroblastoma could be refined to improve results even in apparently limited disease: induction of a cytodifferenciation is already an effect of radio- and chemotherapy in some cases [11]; the specific cytotoxicity for neuroblastoma cells that has been established in vitro with oxidation products of L-dopa [14] will perhaps some day undergo clinical applications.

References

1. Breslow, N., McCann, B.: Statistical estimation of prognosis for children with neuroblastoma. Cancer Res. *31*, 2098–2103 (1971)
2. D'Angio, G. J.: Radiotherapy of children with neuroblastoma. J. Pediatr. Surg. *3*, 110–113 (1968)
3. Donaldson, S., Jundt, S., Ricour, C., Sarrazin, D., Lemerle, J., Schweisguth, O.: Radiation enteritis in children. A retrospective review, clinicopathologic correlation, and dietary management. Cancer. *35*, 1167–1178 (1975)
4. Evans, A. E., D'Angio, G. J., Randolph, J.: A proposed staging for children with neuroblastoma. Cancer *27*, 374–378 (1971)
5. Evans, A. E., Albo, V., D'Angio, G. J., Finklestein, J. Z., Leiken, S., Santulli, T., Weiner, J.: Cyclophosphamide treatment of patients with localized and regional neuroblastoma. A randomized study. Cancer *38*, 655–660 (1976)
6. Evans, A. E., Albo, V., D'Angio, G. J., Finklestein, J. Z., Leiken, S., Santulli, T., Weiner, J.: Factors influencing survival of children with non metastatic neuroblastoma. Cancer *38*, 661–666 (1976)

7. Evans, A. E., Gerson, J. G., Schnaufer, L.: Spontaneous regression of neuroblastoma. J. Natl. Cancer Inst. *44*, 49–54 (1976)
8. Filler, R. M., Traggis, D. G., Jaffe, N., Vawter, G. F.: Favorable outlook for children with mediastinal neuroblastoma. J. Pediatr. Surg. *7*, 136 (1972)
9. Hassenbusch, S., Kaiser, H., White, J. J.: Prognostic factors in neuroblastic tumors. J. Pediatr. Surg. *11*, 287–297 (1976)
10. Hayes, F. A., Mauer, A. M.: Cell kinetics and chemotherapy in neuroblastoma. J. Natl. Cancer Inst. *57*, 697–699 (1976)
11. Helson, L., Helson, C., Peterson, R. F., Dass, K.: A rationale for the treatment of metastatic neuroblastoma. J. Natl. Cancer Inst. *57*, 727–729 (1976)
12. Koop, C. E., Johnson, D. G.: Neuroblastoma. An assessment of therapy in reference to staging. J. Pediatr. Surg. *6*, 595–600 (1971)
13. Koop, C. E., Schnaufer, L.: The management of abdominal neuroblastoma. Cancer *35*, 905–909 (1975)
14. Labrosse, E. H., Comoy, E., Bohuon, C., Zucker, J. M., Schweisguth, O.: Catecholamine metabolism in neuroblastoma. J. Natl. Cancer Inst. *57*, 633–638 (1976)
15. Labrosse, E. H., Belehradek, K., Barski, G.: Cytotoxicity of oxydation products from L-dopa. Specificity for neuroblastoma cells in culture. Proceedings of the Society for Experimental Biology and Medicine (to be published). (1978)
16. Leikin, S., Evans, A., Heyn, R., Newton, W.: The impact of chemotherapy on advanced neuroblastoma. Survival of patients diagnosed in 1956, 1961, and 1966–68 in children's cancer study group A. J. Pediatr. *84*, 131–134 (1974)
17. Leikin, S., Bernstein, I., Evans, A. E., Finklestein, J., Hittle, R., Klemperer, M.: Use of combination Adriamycin and DTIC in children with advanced stage in neuroblastoma. Cancer Chemother. Rep. *59*, 1015–1018 (1975)
18. Stella, J. G., Schweisguth, O., Schlienger, M.: Neuroblastoma. A study of 144 cases treated in the Institut Gustave Roussy over a period of 7 years. Am. J. Roentgenol. *108*, 324–332 (1970)
19. Sutow, W., Gehan, E., Heyn, R., Kung, F. H., Miller, R. W., Murphy, M. L., Traggis, D. G.: Comparison of survival curves, 1956 versus 1962, in children with Wilm's tumor and neuroblastoma. Pediatrics *45*, 800–811 (1970)
20. Tefft, M., Wittenborg, M. H.: Radiotherapeutic management of neuroblastoma in childhood. JAMA *205*, 159–166 (1968)
21. Zucker, J. M.: Retrospective study of 462 neuroblastomas treated between 1950 and 1970. Maandschr. Kindergeneesk. *42*, 369–385 (1974)
22. Zucker, J. M., Mercier, J. C.: Chimiothérapie lourde dans le neuroblastome. Premiers résultats chez 40 enfants porteurs d'une forme métastatique. Arch. Fr. Pediatr. *33*, 555–567 (1976)
23. Zucker, J. M., Hesse, C.: Prognostic factors in neuroblastoma. Proceedings of the International Symposium on Neuroblastoma: Biological Bases and Therapeutic Perspectives. Genova, 8–9 July 1977 (to be published) (1978)

K. Tumors Not Yet Submitted to Adjuvant Chemotherapy and Immunotherapy Trials

Adjuvant Systemic Therapy of Cancer: Rationale for Future Trials

F. M. Muggia and M. Rozencweig

Introduction

The initial reporting of successful adjuvant chemotherapy in osteosarcoma was hailed as a landmark and stimulated many trials in other malignant conditions [10]. With the renewed interest in management of patients with apparently localized disease, there has been an increasing integration of combined modality treatments for curative purposes.

Adjuvant trials bring together all of our knowledge of cancer treatment. Data presently available clearly indicate that surgical adjuvant therapy can prolong survival without evidence of disease over that obtained solely by surgical resection. This observation alone validates the concept of a combined modality approach to primary tumors at a time when dissemination is most likely to be present but cannot be detected by current diagnostic methods. However, whether this control of clinically undetected metastases will improve cure rates in many conditions still remains a matter of conjecture. The problem, therefore, is no longer whether adjuvant therapy has a role but rather how do we correctly design therapeutic trials in early disease to answer the most relevant questions.

Positive results are not easily demonstrated; very careful design and execution are required if these results are to be convincing. The design of adjuvant trials must be based on a correct understanding of the natural evolution of the disease following initial therapy. These trials should be rigorously controlled and involve sufficient numbers of patients. Patient selection and stratification criteria are critical in making comparisons between therapeutic approaches, and a lack of knowledge concerning pertinent risk factors may noticeably obscure the relevance of results. All these difficulties indicate that only centers with extensive experience in cancer treatment should be encouraged to attempt adjuvant trials, and that this effort is most likely to necessitate a polycentric collaboration.

New questions have emerged from the reportedly positive trials. This brief overview will point to new considerations based on our current experience and will outline some of the treatments and concepts presently tested in adjuvant studies sponsored by the National Cancer Institute. It will also be shown that the stage is set for adjuvant trials in an increasing number of tumor types.

Immediate Versus Delayed Chemotherapy

Adjuvant therapy poses difficult dilemmas especially when local measures may be curative and when aggressive systemic treatments are considered for this setting. The actual effectiveness of adjuvant systemic therapy cannot be accurately assessed in individual patients without evidence of disease. The benefits of decreasing the overall rate of recurrence and thereby increasing the chance of cure must be balanced against inherent problems in current systemic therapy such as known acute and potentially life-threatening toxic effects and the less clearly defined potential for inducing second malignancies.

That the effectiveness of systemic chemotherapy may actually be a deterrent rather than a stimulus to early combined approaches is exemplified by experience in *testicular cancer*. With an unprecedented therapeutic effectiveness, treatment regimens employing cis-diamminodichloroplatinum (DDP), vinblastine, and bleomycin appear to salvage all patients carefully followed after relapsing from initial surgical treatment of stage I and II disease [8]. Overall, waiting until relapse may have an advantage since delayed treatment including modalities in addition to chemotherapy may be carried out more aggressively when the progression of the disease is well-established. The feasibility of trials of immediate versus delayed chemotherapy is also partly determined by cell kinetic considerations. In this respect, characteristics of testicular tumors [14] would appear to be most favorable since almost all initial recurrences occur within the first 2 years after resection, a time interval still consistent with a very close follow-up.

In *osteogenic sarcoma*, it has been suggested that the effect of adjuvant chemotherapy is primarily to delay and modify the appearance of clinically obvious metastases [6, 16]. This altered pattern of dissemination would in turn facilitate the treatment of the initial recurrence. To what extent the observed prolongation in survival can be ascribed to such a phenomenon or to an agressive approach to metastases needs to be evaluated. A prospective trial initiated at the Mayo Clinic should provide some insight into this problem. The trial is comparing adjuvant chemotherapy at the outset versus chemotherapy following cytoreductive surgery for metastases (Fig. 1).

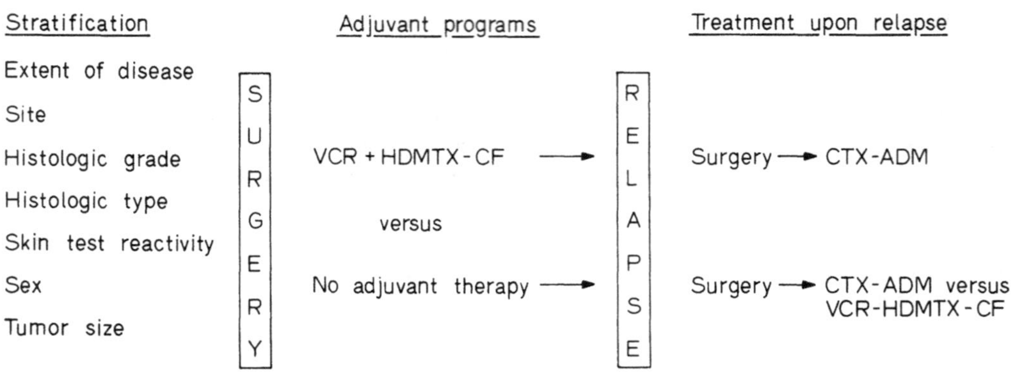

ADM = adriamycin, CTX = cytoxan, HDMTX-CF = methotrexate given at high dose followed by citrovorum factor rescue, VCR = vincristine.

Fig. 1. Mayo Clinic trial of postsurgical adjuvant therapy for osteogenic sarcoma

Chemotherapy and Measures for Local Control

The development of active systemic treatments could provide new bases for selecting local measures. Chemotherapy prior to surgery and postoperative irradiation is now being compared prospectively to local therapy alone in *head and neck cancer*. The trial is about to begin in a number of institutions and includes stratification according to disease site and local therapy will be standardized according to site. Chemotherapy will consist of a DDP and bleomycin combination, a regimen that has given reproducible response rates in these carcinomas [5]. An important question to be answered is whether this chemotherapy will be effective, not only in obtaining better local control, which is already quite effectively achieved by local therapies alone, but also in improving overall survival and preventing deaths from metastatic disease.

Another area to be investigated with similar questions in mind is *soft tissue sarcoma*. Experience recently reported by the Surgery Branch of the National Cancer Institute indicates a favorable outcome with conservative surgery and postoperative irradiation, as well as with radical surgery when both treatments are followed by adjuvant chemotherapy with adriamycin and cyclophosphamide [12]. These treatment options (Fig. 2) yielded highly significant disease-free and overall survival advantage compared with a comparable series of historical controls treated by radical surgery. The many pitfalls in the use of historical controls preclude a correct evaluation of the role of adjuvant chemotherapy in these results. Prospective randomized studies should be undertaken to test the value of conservative surgical approaches plus irradiation and to ascertain the role of adjuvant chemotherapy in this context.

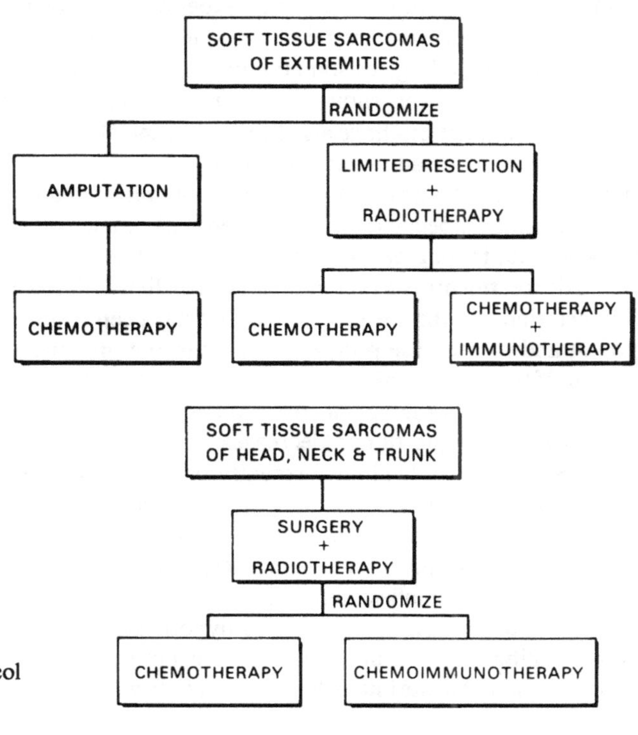

Fig. 2. Outline of the NCI protocol for soft tissue sarcomas

In *breast cancer* with involvement of axillary lymph nodes, modification of surgical approaches and introduction of radiotherapy in modest doses to achieve adequate local control should be explored in combination with currently applied chemotherapies. More conservative, function-sparing, local procedures could conceivably be soon evaluated in additional tumor types such as *bladder cancer*. In the advanced stage of this disease, chemotherapy is beginning to yield reproducibly favorable responses with regimens including adriamycin and cyclophosphamide [19], and particularly DDP [18]. However, chemotherapy programs remain to be investigated in an adjuvant setting.

A novel approach developed at the National Cancer Institute may have potential for adjuvant treatment of stage III *ovarian cancer* where irradiation and chemotherapy have not been easily combined. Pharmacologic and toxicologic studies of intraperitoneal administration of drugs reveal that use of drugs in large volumes of peritoneal dialysate may be beneficial in terms of exposing microscopic intraperitoneal tumors to optimal drug concentration while minimizing systemic concentrations [3]. Administration of methotrexate by this technique is currently being tested at the Medicine Branch of the National Cancer Institute in patients with advanced ovarian cancer in complete remission after chemotherapy. This technique may offer the possibility of eliminating minimal residual disease in patients achieving complete remission through a newly devised local intensification of the treatment.

New Systemic Approaches

Dose schedule and duration of treatment are likely to be critical in adjuvant surgical chemotherapy programs. Intensive regimens and prolonged administrations are widely advocated. New approaches based on experimental data have been proposed. A major cause of relapse in cancers that are initially responsive to chemotherapy seems related to a selection and overgrowth of drug-resistant tumor cells [15]. Sequential administration of effective drug combinations has been shown to circumvent this phenomenon in murine leukemia [15]. Alternate combinations have also been used clinically in advanced solid tumors and should be further explored in adjuvant programs.

Intensive chemotherapy can generally be administered only during the initial phase of the treatment, mainly because of the emergence of cumulative toxicities. This tapering of dose has not been a matter of great concern in the past since it is commonly believed that sensitivity to cytotoxic treatments is a function of the growth fraction of the tumors. In tumors following a Gompertzian growth, the growth fraction has been assumed to be maximum at the onset of growth and to decrease progressively up to the time when the size of the tumor reaches a plateau. If tumoral shrinkage also follows a Gompertzian pattern, this would imply that the sensitivity to chemotherapy is lowest at the start of the treatment and increases progressively when the size of the tumor decreases.

Norton and Simon [11] have recently proposed that the sensitivity to chemotherapy is a function of the growth rate and not of the growth fraction. In a Gompertzian growth, it may be calculated that the growth rate is maximum when the tumor is about 37% of its maximum size, and it is at this point that chemotherapy would produce the greatest cell kill. In contrast, the growth rate is smallest, and resistance to chemotherapy the greatest, for very large and very small tumors. According to this hypothesis, the optimal treatment requires a therapy level that initially is just sufficient to induce tumor regression. This procedure would allow the administration of a late intensification at a time when the cell kill induced by chemotherapy is noticeably diminished. Late intensification programs are being clinically explored and additional investigations based on this rationale should be encouraged.

Long-term risks of adjuvant therapy also warrant considerable attention. The selection of an adjuvant chemotherapy regimen should take these risks into consideration. The possible development of second malignancies induced by chemotherapy also requires efforts directed to prevent carcinogenic effect of anticancer agents.

The adjuvant value of hormonotherapy in *breast cancer* remains controversial [13] and should be further assessed according to relevant hormone receptor data. In the near future, additional hormone responsive tumors should be targets for combined modality approaches at the onset of treatment. In *endometrial carcinoma,* unfavorable prognostic factors may be carefully delineated [4]. These patients should be prime candidates for consideration of additive hormonal therapy with progestins in trials complemented by information on hormone receptors [20]. Furthermore, chemotherapy should also be tested in the most unfavorable, undifferentiated histologic group in view of the effectiveness reported with certain combinations [9].

The role of immunotherapy in the treatment of cancer is being increasingly investigated [7]. Immunotherapy is essentially used with other modalities since experimental models have shown its effectiveness to be dependent upon reduction of tumor cell burden. The potential of immunotherapy would thus appear to be most apparent in a surgical adjuvant situation. Surprisingly, despite increasing knowledge of the mechanism of action of immunotherapeutic agents and the greater scientific basis for their use, most of the current trials remain largely empiric. More thorough information on immunotherapeutic agents is needed to logically build clinical experience that, in turn, should provide some clues to important interactions between a particular immunotherapy, the status of the host immune system, tumor burden, and other therapeutic modalities.

Inclusion of *small cell carcinoma of the lung* in a review of adjuvant trials is justified because chemotherapy now represents the basis for the initial treatment approach in every instance, whether complemented by surgery or irradiation. The lack of durable remissions has been the major disappointment of such aggressive chemotherapeutic approaches [1]. Recently, attempts to prolong these remissions by the addition of thymosin have given rise to startling results that need further confirmation. A trial was designed at the NCI-VA Medical Oncology Branch to add no immunotherapy or thymosin (20 or 60 mg/m^2 twice weekly) to an induction regimen consisting of cyclophosphamide, CCNU, and methotrexate. Following an induction period of 42 days, patients received further chemotherapy with alternating cycles of vincristine-adriamycin-procarbazine, VP-16-ifosphamide, and the induction combination. All patients were restaged to assess the completeness of their tumor regression and both limited and extensive disease categories were included.

The addition of thymosin (60 mg/m^2) appeared to exert a striking effect on the duration of complete remissions [2]. Such an effect was translated into a survival advantage but no enhanced rate of complete remission was observed relative to patients receiving chemotherapy alone. This trial holds great interest but confirmatory studies with immunoreconstituting agents, such as thymosin, in combination with chemotherapy are still needed in small cell carcinoma of the lung as well as in other chemoresponsive tumors.

Conclusion

The impact of systemic therapy on the current concepts of treatment of a malignant disease is discernible in a wide variety of ways and areas. A logical flow is apparent upon close inspection, which depends on the effectiveness of chemotherapy and the characteristics of relapse, whether it is rapid or slow and whether it involves local or hematogeneous spread (Table 1). Where systemic treatment is strikingly effective and has curative potential, the question being posed is one of immediate versus delayed intervention. This is also a valid question with less effective treatment when relapse is expected shortly after the initial local intervention and an agressive approach on clinically obvious metastases may be more rewarding. When systemic chemotherapy is effective, but nevertheless destined to be associated with a considerable relapse rate, the duration and intensity of chemotherapy or the addition of immune stimulation to chemotherapy seem particularly pertinent areas of study. Finally, in the instances where chemotherapy does not have established curative potential, but manifests reproducible activity, its addition to aggressive local therapies is now being evaluated in a wide variety of circumstances. Eventually, modification of local therapies leading to preservation of function and lesser morbidity may be feasible.

Table 1. Examples of questions being asked in trials dealing with minimal residual disease

Cancer	Chemotherapy effectiveness	Predominant characteristics of relapse	Trial question[a]
Testicular	+++	Hematogeneous; rapid	Immediate *vs* delayed CT
Osteosarcoma	+	Hematogeneous; rapid	Immediate *vs* delayed CT after cytoreductive surgery
Breast	++	Local, hematogeneous; slow	Intensified CT *vs* CI-HT
Small cell lung	++	Local, hematogeneous; intermediate	Intensified CT *vs* CI
Ovarian	++	Local, slow	CT *vs* added LT
Head and neck	+	Local, hematogeneous; intermediate	LT and CT *vs* LT only
Soft tissue sarcoma	+	Local, hematogeneous; rapid	LT and CT *vs* LT only
Squamous, adeno, and large cell lung	0 to +	Local, hematogeneous; intermediate	LT and IT *vs* LT only

[a] *CT* chemotherapy; *CI* chemoimmunotherapy; *HT* hormonotherapy; *LT* local therapy; *IT* immunotherapy.

When systemic therapy is of uncertain value, immune stimulation alone has held some appeal and has been tested in some trials. With current immunoadjuvants, this approach is likely to be beneficial only in situations with the most minimal residual disease. Such trials should be confined to situations where the more pertinent therapeutic questions described above are not applicable.

References

1. Bunn, P. A. (Jr.), Cohen, M. H., Ihde, D. C., Fossieck, B. E. (Jr.), Matthews, M. J., Minna, J. D.: Advances in small cell bronchogenic carcinoma. Cancer Treat. Rep. *61,* 333–342 (1977)
2. Cohen, M. H., Chretien, P. B., Ihde, D. C., Fossieck, B. E. (Jr.), Bunn, P. A., Kenady, D. E., Lipson, S. D., Minna, J. D.: Thymosin fraction V prolongs the survival of small cell lung cancer (SCLC) patients treated with intensive combination chemotherapy. Proc. Am. Assoc. Cancer Res. *19,* 117 (1978)
3. Dedrick, R. L., Myers, C. E., Bungay, P. M., DeVita, V. T. (Jr.),: Pharmacokinetic rationale for peritoneal drug administration in the treatment of ovarian cancer. Cancer Treat. Rep. *62,* 1–11 (1978)
4. Gusberg, S. B.: New directions in the control of cancer. Presidential Address. Society of Pelvic Surgeons. Gynecol. Oncol. *5,* 1 (1977)
5. Hong, W. K., Bhutani, R., Shapshay, S., Craft, M. L., Ucmakli, A., Snow, M., Vaughan, C., Strong, S.: Induction chemotherapy of advanced unresectable head and neck cancer with cis-diammine dichloro platinum (II) (DDP) and bleomycin. Proc. Am. Soc. Clin. Oncol. *19,* 321 (1978)
6. Jaffe, N., Frei, E. III, Watts, H., Traggis, D.: High-dose methotrexate in osteogenic sarcoma: A 5-year experience. Cancer Treat. Rep. *62,* 259–264 (1978)
7. Muggia, F. M.: Immunotherapy of cancer. A short review and commentary on current trials. Cancer Immunol. Immunother. *3,* 5–9 (1977)
8. Muggia, F. M.: Adjuvant chemotherapy of testicular carcinoma: The evaluation of curative strategies. Plenary Meeting of the EORTC. Paris, 22–24 June 1978
9. Muggia, F. M., Chia, G., Reed, L. J., Romney, S.: Doxorubicin-cyclophosphamide: Effective chemotherapy for advanced endometrial adenocarcinoma. Am. J. Obstet. Gynecol. *128,* 314–319 (1977)
10. Muggia, F. M., Louie, A. C.: Five years of adjuvant treatment of osteosarcoma: More questions than answers. Cancer Treat. Rep. *62,* 301–305 (1978)
11. Norton, L., Simon, R.: Tumor size, sensitivity to therapy, and design of treatment schedules. Cancer Treat. Rep. *61,* 1307–1317 (1977)
12. Rosenberg, S. A., Kent, H., Costas, J., Webber, B., Young, R., Chabner, B., Baker, A. R., Brennan, M. F., Chretien, P. B., Cohen, M. H., deMoss, E. V., Sears, H. F., Seipp, C., Simon, R.: Prospective randomized evaluation of the role of limb-sparing surgery, radiation therapy, and adjuvant chemoimmunotherapy in the treatment of adult soft tissue sarcomas. Surgery (to be published) (1978)
13. Rozencweig, M., Heuson, J. C., Von Hoff, D. D., Matheiem W. H., Davis, H. L., Muggia, F. M.: Breast cancer. In: Randomized trials in cancer. A critical review by sites. Staquet, M. J. (ed.), pp. 231–272. New York: Raven Press 1978
14. Shackney, S. E., Mc Cormack, G. W., Cuchural, G. J. (Jr.): Growth rate patterns of solid tumors and their relationship to responsiveness to therapy. An analytical review. Ann. Intern. Med. (to be published) (1978)
15. Skipper, H. E.: Adjuvant chemotherapy. Cancer *41,* 936–940 (1978)
16. Sutow, W. W., Gehan, E. A., Dyment, P. G., Vietti, T., Miale, T.: Multidrug adjuvant chemotherapy for osteosarcoma: Interim report of the Southwest Oncology Group studies. Cancer Treat. Rep. *62,* 265–269 (1978)

17. Wittes, R. E., Cvitkovic, E., Shah, J., Gerold, F. P., Strong, E. W.: Cis-dichlorodiammineplatinum (II) in the treatment of epidermoid carcinoma of the head and neck. Cancer Treat. Rep. *61,* 359–366 (1977)
18. Yagoda, A., Watson, R. C., Gonzalez-Vitale, J. C., Grabstald, H., Whitmore, W. F.: Cis-dichlorodiammineplatinum (II) in advanced bladder cancer. Cancer Treat. Rep. *60,* 917–923 (1976)
19. Yagoda, A., Watson, R. C., Grabstald, H., Barzell, W., Whitmore, W. F.: Adriamycin and cyclophosphamide in advanced bladder cancer. Cancer Treat. Rep. *61,* 97–99 (1977)
20. Young, P. C. M., Ehrlich, C. E., Cleary, R. E.: Progesterone binding in human endometrial carcinomas. Am. J. Obstet. Gynecol. *125,* 353–360 (1976)

Some New Chemotherapeutic Agents and Combinations Possibly Available for New Adjuvant Therapies of Minimal Disease

G. Mathé, M. Hayat, J. L. Misset, M. Bayssas, J. Gouveia, F. De Vassal, M. Delgado, M. A. Gil, P. Ribaud, D. Machover, V. Slioussartchouk, and D. Dantchev

There are several new chemotherapeutic agents that, as their combinations, are particularly active in advanced disease and should be considered in trials of adjuvant therapies of minimal residual disease (MRD).

Single Drugs

Antagonists

Methotrexate (MTX) is a compound that deserves reevaluation. In 1969, we obtained a remarkable incidence of complete regressions of advanced diseases (Table 1) with doses then considered high (75 mg/m^2) and followed by folinic acid rescue [21]. We have recently used MTX at the dose of 10–30 mg/kg in combinations, and we could observe a remarkable

Table 1. Are huge doses of methotrexate (MTX) superior to middle-high doses with folinic acid rescue?

	Protocol	Results		Toxicity
MTX folinic acid	Schwarzenberg, Mathé et al. (1969) 75 mg/m^2 IV or IM q 8 h × 6 (48 h)/8 days 25 mg/m^2 IV or IM q 6 h × 16 (96 h) starting 8 h after last dose of MTX	Remission in advanced leukemia: 44% Remission in solid tumors: 62%	No phase III study has compared the oncostatic effects on the three protocols	Nil
MTX folinic acid	Djerassi (1975) 70–1000 mg/m^2 IV infusion in 36–42 h/15 days 40 mg/m^2 q 6 h IV during infusion then 25 mg/m^2 q 6 h per os × 4 (24 h)	Remission in lung carcinoma: 40%		Possibly lethal
MTX folinic acid	Our present protocol (in combination chemotherapy) 10–30 mg/kg IV 10 mg/m^2 IV q 6 h (48 h)	Not yet available		Nil to moderate

oncostatic effect without any lethal toxicity. The serum concentration measured 48 h after the administration of 30 mg/kg is between 10^{-8} and 10^{-7} *M*. There is a need for a randomized trial to compare Djerassi's huge doses of MTX (100–300 mg/kg) [3] and these moderately high dosages as far as their respective efficacies are concerned.

Agents Acting on Tubulin

Within the framework of the poisons of tubulin, *vindesine* (VDN) seems to be active not only in leukemia and lymphosarcomas [14, 15, 18] but also in solid tumors such as breast and bronchus carcinomas [7, 19] and melanoma [20]. The most interesting finding is that the acute lymphoid leukemia patients do not develop cross resistance between VDN and vincristine (VCR) [14, 15, 18].

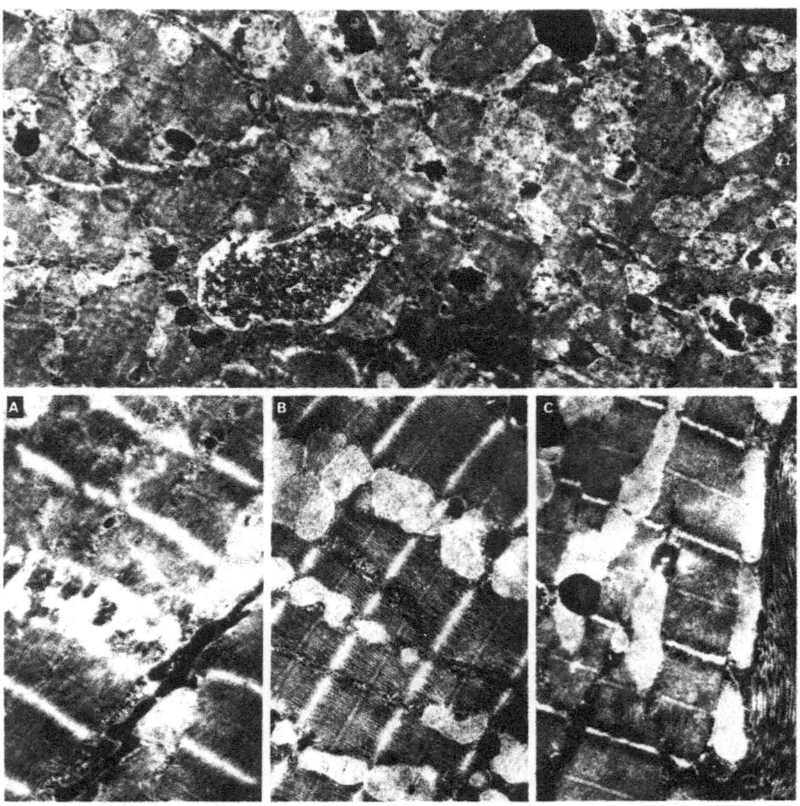

Fig. 1. Myocardium of golden hamster that received, for murine L1210 leukemia, 1/3 of the optimal dose of adriamycin (ADM) (3 mg/kg, 3 times a week IP) (*above*) *and of aclacinomycin* (*ACM*) (*6 mg/kg, 3 times a week IP*) (*below*). View under electron microscope at the end of the 1st week. Note the lesions of mitochondrias of the fibrils after adriamycin (*above*) and the absence of lesions after aclacinomycin (*below*)

Intercalating Agents

We have used some of the anthracyclines in our clinical trials, and we have particularly been comparing the survival of two groups of metastatic breast cancer patients, one treated with VCF [VCR, cyclophosphamide (CPM), and 5-fluorouracil (5-FU)], and the other one with the same combination and *adriamycin* (ADM). The survival is significantly superior when ADM is included (AVCF) [16]. At present, we are conducting with the FIF Group an adjuvant therapy trial with this latter combination applied after surgery. The alopecia and the possible cardiac toxicity are of concern to us. The preliminary study of *aclacinomycine*, a new anthracycline, provides us with the hope of avoiding this problem: it does not cause alopecia and appears less cardiotoxic, as already observed in patients [17] and demonstrated with electron microscopy in cardiopathic golden hamsters (Fig. 1) [2].

Table 2. Phase II trial of peptichemio (single drug) results (clinical screening group of the EORTC)

Diagnosis	No. of cases	No. of evaluable patients	Response			Failure	Response rate
			Complete regression	Regression < 50%	Regression > 50%		
Head and neck	46	43	–	2	2	39	9%
Digestive tract	12	12	–	–	–	12	–
Lung	10	10	–	1	1	8	20%
Bone	5	4	–	–	–	4	–
Soft tissue	7	7	–	1	–	6	14%
Melanoma and skin	7	7	–	–	–	7	–
Breast	11	7	–	1	–	6	14%
Cervix uteri	10	10	1	1	1	7	30%
Ovary	8	7	–	1	1	5	29%
Penis	1	–	–	–	1	–	–
Bladder	3	2	–	–	–	2	–
Kidney	7	7	–	–	–	7	–
Neuroblastoma	7	7	3	1	2	1	86%
Total	134	124	4	8	8	105	16%
AML	1	1	–	–	1	–	–
CML blastic crisis	7	7	1	4	1	1	86%
Reticulosarcoma	1	1	–	–	–	1	–
Hodgkin's disease	2	2	–	–	–	2	–
Total	11	11	1	4	2	3	63%
Total (ST + LHS)	145	135	5	12	10	108	20%

Alkylating Agents

Among the alkylating agents, our attention is turned to *peptichemio*, which proved to be of great value in advanced neuroblastoma (Table 2) [4]. In this series of alkylating cytostatics, we have compared the effects of three new *nitrosoureas:* the French *RFCNU* and *RPCNU* [10] chosen among 20 sugar derivatives synthetized by IMBACH [22] and the American *chlorozotocin* [1]. The alkylating activity is strongest for RPCNU and lowest for RFCNU (Table 3), but RFCNU is experimentally the most frequently active on murine solid tumors [8] and the least toxic for platelets (Table 4) [11]. RPCNU is the only experimentally immunosuppressive compound [6]. In man, RFCNU has given a reasonable proportion of regressions in advanced gastrointestinal tract tumors [12], while chlorozotocin is more active in leukemia and lymphomas [13]. RFCNU seems to be a little less but still toxic enough for platelets (Table 5).
Cis-platinum used by the French-American Cooperative Group in testis and cervix carcinomas (Table 6) [9] induced a reasonable number of regressions without causing severe toxicity. No less interesting is *cytembena,* a drug of unknown mechanism of action. The EORTC Clinical Screening Group has observed its value in carcinoma of the cervix and of the ovary (Table 6) [5].

Table 3. Alkylating activities of RFCNU, RPCNU, and chlorozotocin compared to that of CCNU

$$\text{R–NH–CO–}\overset{\text{NO}}{\overset{|}{\text{N}}}\text{–CH}_2\text{CH}_2\text{Cl}$$

Structure R	Name	Synthesis	Carbamoylating activity % carbamyolated C14-lysine	Alkylating activity (% CNU)	LD_{10} (mol/kg)	$T_{0.5}$ (min)
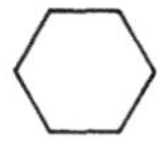	CCNU	Montgomery	90	10	171	117
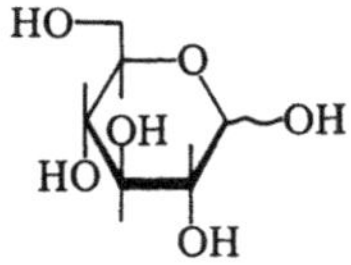	RFCNU	Montero-Imbach, 1974	38	40	210	25
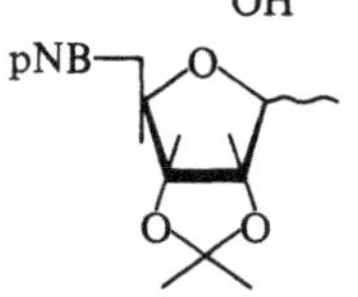	RPCNU	Montero-Imbach, 1974	45	111	–	12,5
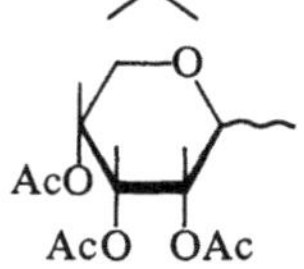	Chlorozotocin	Montgomery 1975	4	64	64	48

Table 4. Experimental (murine) oncopharmacology, hematopharmacology, and immunopharmacology of RFCNU, RPCNU, and chlorozotocin

	RFCNU	RPCNU	Chlorozotocin
L1210 leukemia	+++	+++	+++
E♂ G2	++	–	++
C1498 myeloid leukemia	+	+	–
TM2 mammary	–	+	–
Lewis lung tumor	++	+	–
B16 melanoma	++	++	–
CFUa after 1 injection	↓	↓	→
Platelets in peripheral blood after 11 injections	N	↓	↓
T-cell–dependent antibody production after 1 injection	N	↓	N
Allogeneic skin graft after 1 injection	N	↓	N
Inhibition of activated macrophage cytotoxicity	–	–	–
Activation of macrophages	+	+	+

Table 5. Preliminary evaluation of clinical toxicities of RFCNU, RPCNU, and chlorozotocin

	RFCNU		RPCNU		CZT	
Hematologic	12/38	(31.5%)	13/21	(61%)	11/24[b]	(45%)
Anemia	4/38	(10.5%)	4/21	(19%)	2/24	(8%)
Platelets	10/38	(26.0%)[a]	11/21	(52%)	11/24	(45%)
Leuconeutropenia	2/38	(5.0%)[a]	3/21	(14%)	3/24	(12,5%)
Digestive	2/38	(5.0%)	5/21	(23%)	2/24	(8%)

[a] Only one had nitrosourea before RPCNU 1 cycle, 1 month before RFCNU; lethal: 1/38 (2.5%).
[b] Three patients had aplasia before treatment and were unevaluable.

Combinations

We have established several *combinations* comprising these two drugs. In ovarian tumors combining them with adriamycin, vincristine, 5-fluorouracil, and cyclophosphamide, we have obtained 71% remissions. In a trial concernig all epidermoid carcinomas (combining them with adriamycin, vincristine, and bleomycin), we have achieved more than 50%

Table 6. Oncostatic effects in a phase II trial of cis-platinum. [9]. 100 mg/m²/month IV

Diagnosis	No. of ev. patients	Localization of responses	Complete regression	Regression > 50%	Regression < 50%	Failure	Response rate
Head and neck	11	Lung, nodes		1		10	1/11 (9%)
Esophagus	4	Lung, nodes		1		3	1/4
Bones	4					4	
Soft tissues	4					4	
Melanomas and skin	7	Lung, nodes	1			5	2/7 (28,5%)
		Skin			1		
Lung	1					1	
Breast	7	Lung		1		6	
Uterine cervix	11	Lung	1	1		6	45%
		Nodes		2			
		Local relapse			1		
Uterine endometrium	4	Lung			1	3	
Ovary	6	Pelvic T, nodes		1		5	1/6
Testis no prior chem.	7	Lung	2	1	1		5/7 (55% with 6/13)
Testis with prior chem.		Lung, liver, nod.		1		2	
	13	Lung, abd.		3	3	7	6/13
Kidney	1					1	
Total	80		4	12	7		29%

Table 7. Phase II trial of cytembena results (EORTC clinical screening group)

Diagnosis	No. of cases	No. of evaluable patients	Response			Failure	Response rate
			Complete regression	Regression > 50%	Regression < 50%		
Head and neck	20	13				13	
Digestive tract	6	0					
Lung	3	3				3	
Bone and soft tissues	6	3				3	
Melanoma	2	1				1	
Breast	6	3				3	
Uterine cervix	49	35		2	5	28	20%
Uterine endometrium	2	2				2	
Ovary	8	8			2	6	< 20% (1/8)[a]
Vagina	4	4				4	
Kidney	4	2				2	
Brain	1	1				1	
Hodgkin's disease	1	1				1	
Total	113	76			8		11%

[a] Since this evaluation, we have obtained two more regressions < 50%.

remissions in carcinoma of the cervix, in squamous cell carcinoma of the bronchus, and in head and neck tumors (Table 8). In the latter case, we are already using this combination for an adjuvant therapy comparative trial.

In conclusion, chemotherapy has been enriched in recent years with new active drugs and combinations that seem promising for adjuvant chemotherapy of cancer not yet submitted to postsurgical chemotherapy trials.

Table 8. Squamous cell carcinomas: Effect in term of regression induction of a combination comparising adriamycin, vincristine, bleomycin, cytembena, and cis-platinum

Origin	Stratification	No. of cases	Localization of responders	Complete regression	Partial regression		No change	Progressive disease	Response rate
					> 50%	< 50%			
Lung	Inoperable	8	–	2	2	–	2	2	50%
	Metastatic	10	Hepatic 2 Nodes 2 Control lateral 1	–	2	3	2	3	50%
Cervix	Local relapse	1	–	–	1	–	–	–	1/1
	Metastatic	6	Hepatic Lung; nodes	1	1	1	2	1	50%
Head and neck	Local relapse	13	–	1	2	7	2	1	77%
	Inoperable	6	–	1	3	1	1	–	83%
	Metastatic	4	Lung; thyroid	1	1	1	1	–	75%
Esophagus	Local relapse	1	–	–	–	–	–	1	
Esophagus skin		1	–	–	–	–	–	1	
	Metastatic	1	Nodes	–	2				
Anal		1	Hepatic	–					
Total		52		6 (12%)	14 (27%)	13 (25%)	10 (19%)	9 (17%)	63%

References

1. Anderson, T., McMenamin, M. G., Schein, P. S.: Chlorozotocin, [2-(3-2-)3-(2-chloroethyl)-3-nitrosoureido γ-D-glycopyranose], an antitumor agent with modified bone marrow toxicity. Cancer Res. *35,* 761–765 (1975)
2. Dantchev, D., Paintrand, M., Hayat, M., Umezawa, H., Muggia, G., Mathé, G.: Electron microscopy on Golden hamster of compared cardiotoxicity of several anthracyclines. (In preparation) (1978)
3. Djerassi, I.: High-dose methotrexate (NSC-740) and citrovorum factor (NSC-3590) rescue: background and rationale, Part 3. Cancer Chemother. Rep. *6* 3–6 (1975)
4. EORTC Clinical Screening Group: A phase II clinical trial of peptichemio. Biomedicine *27,* 290–294 (1977)
5. EORTC Clinical Screening Group: A phase II clinical trial of cytembena. Biomedicine *26,* 392–395 (1977)
6. Florentin, I., Mathé, G.: Comparative experimental immunopharmacology of three nitrosoureas: RFCNU, RPCNU and chlorozotocin. (In preparation) (1978)
7. Gralla, R. J., Young, C. W.: A phase II trial on vindesine in nonsmall cell carcinoma of the lung. International Workshop on Vindesine. Frankfurt, 7. July 1978
8. Hayat, M., Mathé, G.: Comparative experimental oncostatic pharmacoly of three nitrosoureas: RFCNU, RPCNU and chlorozotocin. (In preparation) (1978)
9. Hayat, M., Brule, G., Clavel, B., Chauvergne, J., Cappelaere, P., Cattan, A., Guerrin, J., Pommatau, E., Bayssas, M., Gouveia, J., Mathé, G.: Essai thérapeutique clinique phase II du cisplatinum. Nouv. Presse Méd. (1978) (in press)
10. Imbach, J. L., Montero, J. L., Moruzzi, A., Serrou, B., Chenu, E., Hayat, M., Mathé, G.: The oncostatic and immunosuppressive action of new nitrosourea derivatives containing sugar radicals. Biomedicine *23,* 410–413 (1975)
11. Jasmin, C., Mathé, G.: Comparative experimental hematopharmacology of three nitrosoureas: RFCNU, RPCNU and chlorozotocin. (In preparation) (1978)
12. Mathé, G., Serrou, B., Hayat, M., De Vassal, F., Misset, J. L., Schwarzenberg, L., Machover, D., Ribaud, P., Belpomme, D., Jasmin, C., Musset, M., Montero, J. L., Imbach, J. L.: Preliminary results of phase I and II clinical trials of RFCNU, a new nitrosourea sugar derivative in digestive tract tumours. Biomedicine *27,* 294–297 (1977)
13. Mathé, G., Bayssas, M., De Vassal, F., Gouveia, J.: Phase II trials of three oncostatic nitrosoureas: RFCNU, RPCNU and chlorozotocin. (In preparation) (1978)
14. Mathé, G., Misset, J. L., De Vassal, F., Hayat, M., Gouveia, J., Machover, D., Belpomme, D., Schwarzenberg, L., Ribaud, P., Pico, J. L., Musset, M., Jasmin, C., De Luca, L.: Traitement de leucémies et hématosarcomes par la vindésine. Résultats d'un essai phase II en termes d'induction de rémission. Nouv. Presse Méd. *7,* 525–528 (1978)
15. Mathé, G., Misset, J. L., De Vassal, F., Gouveia, J., Hayat, M., Machover, D., Belpomme, D., Pico, J. L., Schwarzenberg, L., Ribaud, P., Musset, M., Jasmin, C., De Luca, L.: Phase II clinical trial with vindesine for remission induction in acute leukemia, blastic crisis of chronic myeloid leukemia, lymphosarcoma and Hodgkin's disease: absence of cross-resistance with vincristine. Cancer Treat. Rep. *62,* 805–809 (1978)
16. Mathé, G., Misset, J. L., Bayssas, M., Gouveia, J., De Vassal, F., Hayat, M., Delgado, M., Gil, M. A., Machover, D.: Does adriamycin increases survival in metastatic breast patients? Preliminary evaluation. Cancer Chemother. Pharmacol. (1978) (in press)
17. Mathé, G., Bayssas, M., Gouveia, J., De Vassal, F., Dantchev, D.: A propos de la Revue Générale de Jacquillat et al.: l'aclacynomyciine, une nouvelle anthracycline non alopéciante et moins cardiotoxique que l'adriamycine. Nouv. Presse Méd. (1978) (in press)
18. Misset, J. L., De Vassal, F., Hayat, M., Machover, D., Belpomme, D., Schwarzenberg, L., Ribaud, P., Musset, M., Jasmin, C., Mathé, G.: Phase II clinical trial with vindesine for remission induction in acute leukaemia, blastic crisis of chronic myeloid leukaemia, lymphosarcoma and Hodgkin's disease. Absence of cross resistance with vincristine. Med. Oncol. *3,* S21 (1977)

19. Powles, T., Smith, I. E.: Vindesine in the treatment of breast cancer. International Workshop on Vindesine. Frankfurt, 7. July 1978
20. Retsas, S., Newton, K. A., Westbury, G.: Vindesine in treatment of advanced malignant melanoma. International Workshop on Vindesine. Frankfurt, 7. July 1978
21. Schwarzenberg, L., Mathé, G., Hayat, M., De Vassal, F., Amiel, J. L., Cattan, A., Schneider, M., Schlumberger, J. R., Jasmin, C., Ngo Minh Man: Une nouvelle combinaison de méthotrexate-acide folinique pour le traitement des cancers (leucémies et tumeurs solides). Presse Méd. *77*, 385 (1969)
22. Serrou, B., Imbach, J. L., Hayat, M., Mathé, G., Macieira-Coelho, A. M.: Experimental screening and pharmacology of new sugar derivatives of nitrosourea. Proc. Am. Assoc. Cancer Res. *18*, 223 (Abs. 892) (1977)

Third Generation of Systemic Adjuvants of Immunity: Experimental Basis for Adjuvant Combinations

G. Mathé, I. Florentin, J. I. Schulz, M. Bruley-Rosset, and N. Kiger

We already discussed in another paper in this Volume the rational experimental and clinical basis of specific and nonspecific immunotherapy [15]. We have compared the respective value of BCG and that of agents making up the second generation of systemic adjuvants of immunity including *Corynebacterium parvum*, levamisole, synthetic polynucleotides, and polysaccharides such as krestin, etc. All these adjuvants have been the object of intensive studies on their mode of action, [6, 12] and they have been used in clinical trials of cancer immunotherapy [3, 12]. We underlined that, despite their unquestionable antitumoral activity, these agents in some cases may exert deleterious actions. Side-effects due to toxicity are often not negligible. Overall, many adjuvants may induce suppressor cells thought to play a role in tumor enhancement.

Table 1. Effects of a chronic administration of thymosin to 6-month-old mice until the 15th month[a]

Immune response tested		
Spleen cell response to		
PHA	0.28[b]	
Con A	0.40	
DS	1.23	
LPS	0.71	
T cell (nylon nonadherent cell) response to		
PHA	0.72	
Con A	0.73	
Test for suppressor cell detection, mitogen response of normal spleen cells cocultivated with thymosin-treated cells		
PHA	*1.08*	*(–)*
Con A	*0.97*	*(–)*
Antibody response to SRBC	*3.21*	
Macrophage cytostatic activity in vitro, inhibition of tumor cell proliferation (%)	*85%*	

[a] Mice were given weekly IP injections of 100 μg thymosin.

[b] $\frac{\text{Response of thymosin-treated mice}}{\text{Response of untreated mice}}$.

We shall deal here with new agents that can be considered as the third generation of systemic immunity adjuvants. We postulated that it will include agents that share the following characteristics: (1) they will be, preferentially, well-defined chemical compounds or at least well-quantifiable agents; (2) their action will be limited to stimulation of one or a few populations of cells; (3) they will not induce suppressor cells; and (4) their side-effects will be minimal. We think that after taking into account their respective mode of action, these adjuvants may be combined judiciously in such a way that a maximal antitumoral effect could be obtained without stimulation of suppressor cells.

Table 2. Effects of a chronic administration of bestatin to 14-month-old mice until the 20th month

Immune response tested	Dose of bestatin per injection	
	10 μg	100 μg
Spleen cell response to		
PHA	1.16 →[b]	1.33 ↗
DS	1.52 ↗	1.72 ↗
T cell (nylon nonadherent cell) response to		
PHA	1.37 ↗	1.48 ↗
Test for suppressor cell detection, mitogen response of spleen cells from 2-month-old mice cocultivated with		
Unfractionated Bestatin-treated cells		
PHA	0.80 → (–)	0.78 → (–)
DS	1.81 ↗ (–)	1.48 ↗ (–)
Nylon nonadherent Bestatin-treated cells		
PHA	1.46 ↗ (–)	0.91 → (–)
DS	1.09 → (–)	1.11 → (–)
Plastic-adherent Bestatin-treated cells		
PHA	1.45 ↗ (–)	1.35 ↗ (–)
DS	1.09 → (–)	1.29 ↗ (–)
Macrophage cytostatic activity, inhibition tumor cell proliferation (%)	4% →	83% ↗
Antibody response to SRBC	2.40 ↗	1.34 →
Delayed-type hypersensitivity reaction to oxazolone	0.40 ↘	2.17 ↗
Antibody-dependent cell-mediated cytotoxicity, specific lysis (%) (effector cell to target cell ratio 1:100: antibody dilution 1:2000)	70% aged controls 86% young controls 65%	65%

[a] Mice were given weekly injections of 10 or 100 μg of bestatin.

[b] $\frac{\text{Response of bestatin-treated mice}}{\text{Response of untreated mice}}$.

We shall discuss here some agents that, on the basis of experimental results, fulfill at least some of the critera described above. Thymosin, as shown in Table 1, when chronically administered to age-immunodepressed mice, restored their antibody response to a thymus-dependent antigen (sheep red blood cells, SRBC) and induced macrophage activation presumably by the intermediary of T-lymphocyte stimulation. Examination of spleen cell mitogen responsiveness allowed us to demonstrate that no suppressor cells were induced by thymosin administration [4]. CHRETIEN [7] recently reported that thymosin in combination with chemotherapy increased survival of patients with oat cell lung carcinoma, but only if they were immunodepressed.

Bestatin, an antibotic that was isolated by UMEZAWA et al. [22] from actinomycetes and exhibited immunostimulating properties [23], was also examined for its ability to restore the immune capacity of aged mice. Results summarized in Table 2 demonstrated that T cell functions were potentiated by the repeated administration of this compound. Small doses (10 μg per injection) were more effective in restoring humoral response to SRBC rather than delayed-type hypersensitivity reaction, whereas larger doses (100 μg per injection) acted in

Table 3. Effect of 2-[2-cyanaziridinyl-(1)]-[2-carbamoylaziridinyl-(1)]-propane (or BM 12 531) on immune responses of 2-month-old mice

	Day of BM 12 531 administration[a]			
	0	– 3	– 7	– 10
Spleen cell response to				
PHA	NT	1.00[b]	0.47	0.47
Con A	NT	1.03	0.74	0.40
LPS	NT	0.53	0.85	0.55
T cell (nylon nonadherent cell) response to				
PHA	NT	1.29	1.20	*1.33*
Con A	NT	1.05	1.09	1.03
Test for suppressor cell detection, mitogen responses of normal spleen cell cocultivated with BM-treated cells				
PHA	NT	*1.19 (–)*	*1.09 (–)*	*1.98 (–)*
Con A	NT	*0.88 (–)*	*1.49 (–)*	*1.45 (–)*
LPS	NT	1.40 (–)	0.98 (–)	1.52 (–)
Delayed-type hypersensitivity reaction to oxazolone	*1.6*	*1.3*	1.0	1.1
Antibody response to				
TNP-KLH	*1.2*	*1.4*	1.1	0.9
TNP-POL	1.0	0.9	1.0	0.8
Macrophage cytostatic activity, inhibition of tumor cell proliferation (%)	NT	0%	*50%*	*65%*

[a] BM 12 531 was given IV at the dose of 25 mg/kg

[b] $\frac{\text{Response of BM 12 531-treated mice}}{\text{Response of untreated mice}}$.

the opposite way. Macrophage activation was observed only after treatment with the large doses, suggesting that it resulted from a T-cell-mediated immune response. No suppressor cells were induced. Antibody-dependent cell cytotoxic activity of spleen cells against antibody-coated chick erythrocytes, which was markedly increased in aged mice when compared to yound adult mice, returned to this normal value after bestatin treatment.

A new aziridine derivative, 2-[2-cyanaziridinyl-(1)-]-propane (Boehringer Mannheim: BM 12 531) [1], was tested for its immunostimulating properties in young adult mice. As shown in Table 3, it selectively potentiated immune responses involving T-lymphocytes: delayed

Table 4. Effect of heat-killed Pseudomonas aeruginosa on immune responses of 2-month-old mice

Immune response tested	Day of Pseudomonas administration[a]	
	3	7
Spleen cell response to		
PHA	0.92[b]	0.59
DS	5.74	2.48
T cell (nylon nonadherent cell) response to		
PHA	1.07	1.03
Test for suppressor cell detection, mitogen response of normal spleen cell cocultivated with		
Unfractionated		
Pseudomonas-treated cells		
PHA	1.50 (–)	1.04 (–)
DS	1.64 (–)	1.37 (–)
Nylon nonadherent		
Pseudomonas-treated cells		
PHA	0.97 (–)	0.92 (–)
DR	0.86 (–)	0.86 (–)
Macrophage cytostatic activity, inhibition tumor cell proliferation (%)	35%	36%
Antibody responses to		
TNP-KLH	1.17	0.99
TNP-POL	1.53	1.98
Delayed-type hypersensitivity reaction to oxazolone	0.85	0.78
Antibody-dependent cell-mediated cytotoxicity, specific lysis (%) (effector cell to target cell ratio 1:100; antibody dilution 1:40,000)	27.5% control : 40.2%	33.5% control : 31.2%

[a] Mice were given 10^8 heat-killed organisms IV 3 or 7 days before testing.

[b] $\frac{\text{Response of Pseudomonas-treated mice}}{\text{Response of control mice}}$.

hypersensitivity to oxazolone [19] and antibody response to a thymus-dependent antigen (trinitrophenylhemocyanin: TNP-KLH). Macrophage cytostatic activity for tumor cells was detected only after preceding evidence of a stimulati†n0of T-lymphocyte0functions suggesting that these latter cells played a role in macrophage activation. Antibody response to a thymus-independent antigen (trinitrophenyl-polymerized flagellin: TNP-POL) was not potentiated, and suppressor cells were not detected in the spleen of the animals whatever the time of BM 12 531 administration. Recently, Bicker demonstrated that BM 12 531 induced leukocytosis in normal rats and restored cyclophosphamide-induced leukopenia [2]. Thus, an action of BM 12 531 on hematopoietic stem cells may be expected.

With a preparation of Pseudomonas aeruginosa (mixture of ten serotypes of bacteria, Pasteur Institute, Paris), we think that we have at our disposal an adjuvant that acts mainly on B-lymphocytes (Table 4) [9]. Indeed, potentiation of antibody response to TNP-POL in vivo and stimulation of lymphocyte response to a B cell mitogen (dextran sulfate: DS) in vitro were observed after injection of 10^8 heat-killed bacteria. In contrast, antibody formation against TNP-KLH and contact hypersensitivity reaction to oxazolone were not influenced by this adjuvant. Macrophage cytostatic activity for tumor cells was only slightly increased. Antibody-dependent cell-mediated cytotoxicity against antibody-coated chick erythrocytes was depressed 3 days after Pseudomonas injection. This adjuvant was capable of delaying the development of L1210 lymphoid leukemia in an immunoprophylaxis trial, but the antitumoral effect was strongly dependent upon the number of bacteria injected and the time of administration [13]. In clinical trials, Pseudomonas aeruginosa restored delayed-type hypersensitivity reactions in 50% of anergic cancer patients [14]. It was reported by Oettgen [16]

Table 5. Effect of various systemic adjuvants on macrophage activation in mice

Adjuvant	Day	Dose	Maximal cytostatic activity[a] maximal inhibition of tumor cell proliferation (%)
BCG	14	0.2 mg	33
		0.1 mg	93
		0.5 mg	99
Levamisole	3		
	7	75 µg	0
	14		
Pseudomonas aeruginosa	3	10^8 organisms	36
	7		
Bestatin	7	100 µg	44
BM 12 531	7	500 µg	65
	14		
Glucan	7	500 µg	93
Tuftsine	7	400 µg	97

[a] Percent inhibition =

$$\left[100 - \frac{^3\text{H-TdR uptake by tumor cells incubated on treated macrophages}}{^3\text{H-TdR uptake by tumor cells incubated on normal macrophages}}\right] \times 100 .$$

that lipopolysaccharide (LPS) from Pseudomonas aeruginosa, when administered before remission induction in patients with acute myeloid leukemia, prolonged the duration of the remission.

Since activated macrophages seem to play a major role in defense against neoplasia, we compared some of the new agents to BCG and levamisole for their capacity to render macrophages cytostatic for tumor cells. In addition to Pseudomonas and BM 12 531, we have tested bestatin, glucan (β-1-3 polyglucose extracted from yeast wall) [8], and tuftsine, a basic tetrapeptide synthetized by MARTINEZ et al. [11]. As shown in Table 5, glucan and tuftsine were as effective as BCG in inducing macrophage activation, whereas levamisole did not render macrophage cytostatic whatever the time of its administration. Pseudomonas, BM 12 531, and bestatin gave an intermediary level of macrophage activation.

Thus, at the present time, we have in our hands various adjuvants that act rather selectively on one type of cells involved in immune responses (Table 6). We can attempt to combine them with the aim to obtain additive, if not synergistic immunostimulating effects because they are more cell population-specific in their stimulatory activities than BCG and hence they might not result in suppressor cell induction. Should suppressor cells be still stimulated, we will search for such modalities of combinations that hopefully will be able to dissociate the respective kinetics of the different cell populations and then attempt to apply chemotherapy capable of neutralizing the suppressor cells [17]. There are several other ways in which one could, at least theoretically, deal with this problem: (a) thymectomy to eliminate short-lived T suppressor cells, (b) application of antibodies directed against cell surface antigens of suppressor cells as demonstrated in the sera of patients with active juvenile rheumatoid arthritis [20], and (c) potential use of thymic hormones for differentiation of immature T cells shown to exert a suppressive activity that can be converted in this way into mature antitumoral effector T cells [21]. This latter hypothesis has been partially supported by PATT's observation [18] of inhibition by thymosin of suppressor cell induction in cancer patients; however, in our own experiments, thymosin was not able to neutralize suppressor cells induced by BCG.

Combinations of adjuvants may also be envisaged with the objective to stimulate a particular mechanism of antitumoral activity. CARSWELL et al. [5] described the presence in the serum of mice given sequentially BCG, or other macrophage-activating agents, then LPS, at a factor that induced necrosis of some experimental tumors (tumor necrosis factor, TNF). Since LPS is strongly toxic, we have tried to induce TNF by injection of entire bacilli that are better tolerated in man [14] than its LPS [10]. We have observed necrosis of P 815 mastocytoma in mice given serum from animals injected with BCG followed by Pseudomonas aeruginosa

Table 6. New immunity adjuvants and their combinations

Immunologic state of the host	T-lymphocytes	B-lymphocytes	Macrophages
Immunocompetent	Aziridine derivative (BM 12 531)	Pseudomonas aeruginosa	Glucan Krestin Tuftsine
Immunodepressed	Thymosin Levamisole Bestatin		

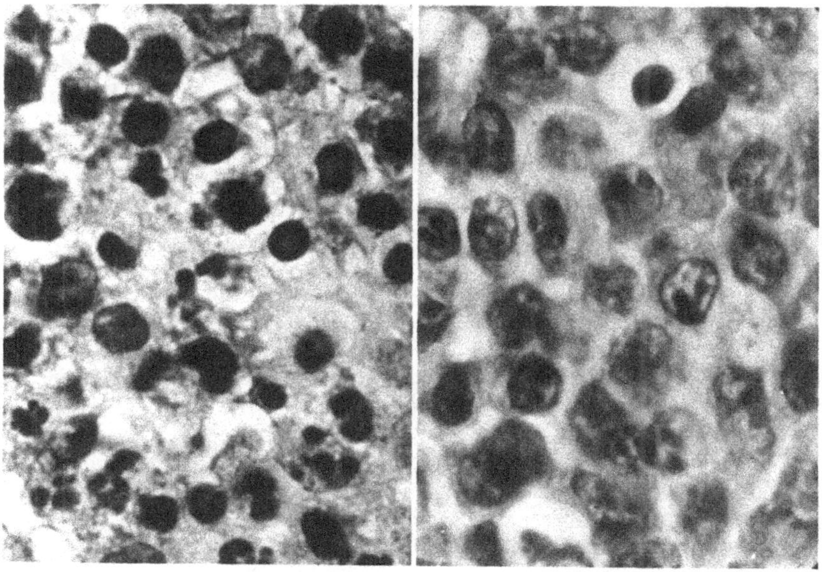

Fig. 1. Effects of tumor necrosis factor (TNF) on P 815 mastocytoma. On the *left*, marked necrosis of the tumor in the animal treated with TNF serum (0.5 ml IV) obtained from mice given BCG (1 mg IV) followed 14 days later by Pseudomonas aeruginosa (5.10^8 bacilli). On the *right*, same tumor treated

Table 7. Effect of a treatment by BCG and Pseudomonas aeruginosa on the growth of a methylcholanthrene-induced fibrosarcoma (Mc C3–2) transplantated SC in C57BL/6 mice

Treatment	Mean tumor diameter ± S.D. (mm) at day 22[a]	P value[b]	Mean tumor diameter ± S.D. (mm) at day 28	P value
Group 1 (control): 10 mice, 4.10^5 tumor cells sc day 0	11.32 ± 2.76		15.11 ± 3.01	
Group 2: 8 mice, idem control + BCG 1 mg IV day 1	10.74 ± 3.41	N.S.	15.93 ± 4.05	N.S.
Group 3: 8 mice, idem control + Pseudomonas 0.01 ml IV day 14	12.08 ± 2.81	N.S.	17.83 ± 3.49	0.05 P 0.1 N.S.
Group 4: 10 mice, idem control + BCG day 1 and Pseudomonas day 14	9.14 ± 1.27	$0.02 < P < 0.05$	11.81 ± 1.62	$0.001 < P < 0.01$

[a] The mean tumor diameter is calculated from measurements of two tumor dimensions at right angles to each other.

[b] The significance of the differences between each group and the control group was assessed by the Student's *t* test.

(Fig. 1). In another experiment, mice grafted with a chemically induced fibrosarcoma were directly treated with BCG and Pseudomonas. As shown in Table 7, a significant reduction of the tumor size was observed in animals receiving both BCG and Pseudomonas. BCG alone was ineffective and Pseudomonas alone enhanced tumor growth in this particular experiment. This interesting adjuvant combination could serve as an example of potentially advantageous use of multiple adjuvants in the therapy of cancer.

References

1. Bicker, O., Ziegler, B. E., Hebold, G.: 2-[2-cyanaziridinyl-(1)-]-2-[-2-carbamocyl aziridinyl-(1)]-propane BM 12 531. A new substance with immune stimulating action. I.R.C.S. Med. Sci. *5,* 299 (1977)
2. Bicker, U., Hebold, G., Ziegler, A. E., Maus, W.: Animal experiments on the compensation of the immunosuppressive action of cyclophosphamide by 2-[-2-cyanaziridinyl-(1)-]-2-[-2-carbamocyl aziridinyl-(1)-]-propane BM 12 531. (in press) (1978)
3. Bonadonna, G., Mathé, G., Salmon, S. E. (eds.): Adjuvant therapies and markers of post-surgical minimal residual disease I. Berlin, Heidelberg, New York: Springer 1979
4. Bruley-Rosset, M., Florentin, I., Kiger, N., Goldstein, A., Mathé, G.: Prevention of aged-induced immunodepression in mice by chronic treatment with thymosin and systemic adjuvants of immunity. Cancer Immunol. Immunother. (in press) (1978)
5. Carswell, E. A., Old, L. J., Kassel, R. L., Green, S., Fiore, N., Williamson, B.: An endotoxin-induced serum factor that causes necrosis of tumors. Proc. Natl. Acad. Sci. USA *72,* 3666 (1975)
6. Chirigos, M. A. (ed.): Immune modulation and control of neoplasia by adjuvant therapy. Cancer Treat. Rep. (in press) (1978)
7. Chretien, P.: The effects of thymosin in vitro on lymphocytes from cancer patients responding to thymosin immunotherapy. In: Human lymphocyte differentiation, its application to human cancer. Serrou, B., Rosenfeld, C. (eds.), Vol. 1. Amsterdam: Elsevier North-Holland (1978) (in press)
8. Diluzio, N.: An overview of glucan activity. In: Immune modulation and control of neoplasia by adjuvant therapy. Chirigos, M. A. (ed.). Cancer Treat. Rep. (in press) (1978)
9. Florentin, I., Kiger, N., Bruley-Rosset, M., Schulz, I. J., Mathé, G.: Effect of seven immunomodulators on different types of immune responses in mice. In: Human lymphocyte differentiation, its application to human cancer. Serrou, B., Rosenfeld, C. (eds.), Vol. 1. Amsterdam: Elsevier North-Holland (in press) (1978)
10. Hortobagyi, G. N., Gutterman, J. U., Richman, S. P., Hersh, E. M.: Pseudomonas aeruginosa vaccine: a phase I evaluation for cancer immunotherapy. Cancer Immunol. Immunother. (in press) (1978)
11. Martinez, J., Winternitz, F., Vindel, J.: Nouvelles synthèses et propriétés de la tuftsine. Eur. J. Med. Chem. (in press) (1978)
12. Mathé, G.: Cancer active immunotherapy, immunoprophylaxis and immunorestoration. Vol. 1. Heidelberg, New York: Springer 1976
13. Mathé, G., Florentin, I., Bruley-Rosset, M., Hayat, M., Bourut, C.: Heat-killed pseudomonas aeruginosa as a systemic adjuvant in cancer immunotherapy. Biomedicine *27,* 368 (1977)
14. Mathé, G., de Vassal, F., Gouveia, J., Simmler, M. C., Misset, J. L.: Comparison of the restoration effect of pseudomonas aeruginosa, BCG and poly I: poly C on cancer patients non responsive to recall antigen delayed hypersensitivity. Biomedicine *27,* 328 (1977)
15. Mathé, G., Olsson, L., Florentin, I., Kiger, N.: Post-surgical systematic active immunotherapy: rational, experimental and clinical basis on non solid tumors. In: Adjuvant therapies and markers of post-surgical minimal residual disease I. Bonadonna, G., Mathé, G., Salmon, S. E. (eds.). RRCR Vol. 67, pp. 132–150. Berlin, Heidelberg, New York: Springer 1979

16. Oettgen, H. F.: Effects of endotoxin and endotoxin-induced mediators on cancer and on the immune system. In: The role of nonspecific immunity in the prevention and treatment of cancer. Study Week of the Pontifical Academy of Sciences. Vatica City, (in press) (1978)
17. Orbach-Arbouys, S., Castes, M., Berardet, M.: Enhancement of immunological responses by methotrexate pretreatment as a result of an eventual elimination of suppressor cells. In: Experimental hematology today. Berlin, Heidelberg, New York: Springer (in press) (1978)
18. Patt, Y. Z., Hersh, E. M., Goldman, R., Washington, M.: Suppressor cells in cancer patients and possible effects of thymic hormone. In: Immune modulation and control of neoplasie by adjuvant therapy. Chirigos, M. A. (ed.). Cancer Treat. Rep. (in press) (1978)
19. Schulz, J. I., Florentin, I., Bourut, C., Bicker, O., Mathé, G.: Delayed-type hypersensitivity response and humoral antibody formation in mice treated. A new immunostimulant 2-2-cyanaziridinyl-(1)-2-2-carbamoyl aziridinyl-(1)-propane BM 12 531. I.R.S.C. Med. Sci. *6,* 215 (1978)
20. Strelkauskas, A. J., Schauf, V., Wilson, B. S., Chess, L., Schlossman, J. F.: Isolation and characterization of naturally occuring subclasses of human peripheral blood T cells with regulatory functions. J. Immunol. *120,* 1278 (1978)
21. Trainin, N., Small, M., Gabizon, A.: Thymic humoral factor (THF) as modulator of T cell differentiation involved in antitumor reactivity. In: Human lymphocyte differentiation, its application to human cancer. Serrou, B., Rosenfeld, C. (eds.), Vol. 1. Amsterdam: Elsevier North-Holland (in press) (1978)
22. Umezawa, H., Aoyagi, T., Suda, H., Hamada, M., Takeuchi, T.: Bestatin, a new amino-peptidase B inhibitor produced by actinomycetes. J. Antibiotics *29,* 97 (1976)
23. Umezawa, H., Ishisuka, M., Aoyagi, T., Takeuchi, T.: Enhancement of delayed-type hypersensitivity by Bestatin, an inhibitor of aminopeptidase B and leucine aminopeptidase. J. Antibiotics *29,* 857 (1976)

Interrelationship Between Chemotherapy and Immunotherapy in the Treatment of Disseminated Disease

A. Goldin, A. Nicolin, and E. Bonmassar

There are a number of important factors that may contribute to a decrease in effectiveness of therapy against disseminated disease. A primary factor is the absolute increase in body burden of tumor cells [14, 25]. With an increase in the number of tumor cells a greater demand is made on the amount of drug that is necessary to elicit the desired therapeutic response. It was demonstrated with leukemia L 1210, for example, that as the inoculum level was increased, the dose of methotrexate also had to be increased to maintain a given level of therapeutic response (ED_{50}; 50% cures [14]. In another study it was observed that the number of cures that could be obtained on treatment with cyclophosphamide or 1,3-bis-(2-chloroethyl)-1-nitrosourea (BCNU) was diminished as the inoculum size was increased [7]. As the disease becomes more advanced there may be a reduction in the percentage cures that can be obtained over a variety of treatment schedules. Delay in treatment with cytosine arabinoside until the leukemia L 1210 disease was advanced (7 days following leukemic inoculation) resulted in a decrease in percentage cures as compared with treatment initiated early (day 3) on a variety of treatment schedules including treatment four times daily, twice daily, daily, every 2 days, or every 4 days as well as single treatment [8].

In the treatment of Lewis lung carcinoma with cyclophosphamide, delay in therapy until the disease was advanced (8th day following tumor inoculation) was considerably less effective in increasing the life span of the animals and in eliciting cures [9]. The decreased effectiveness on delay in therapy was attributable not only to the increase in size of a local tumor mass at the site of intramuscular inoculation of the tumor but also to the metastatic spread to the lungs from the local tumor.

Another important contributing factor to the reduction in therapeutic effectiveness against advanced disseminated disease is the increased demand for generalized drug distribution to widely disseminated metastatic foci of tumor growth. There is the need for the drug to reach the various metastatic sites at a sufficiently high concentration and for a requisite period of time ($C \times T$). The dosage of drug administered has to be sufficiently high to treat the largest metastases successfully.

A further complication results from dissemination of tumor to sequestered sites not readily available to the action of a drug. For example, manifestation of meningeal leukemia during therapy with methotrexate or cycloposphamide would necessitate the need for some other type of therapy. These drugs have shown reduced effectiveness against intracerebrally inoculated leukemia L 1210 [5, 26]. The lung also represents a somewhat sequestered metastatic site as evidenced in the sudy cited above with Lewis lung carcinoma, where tumor dissemination to the lung resulted in diminished drug effectiveness.

Another important factor that may contribute to reduced effectiveness of drugs against disseminated disease is the possibility for the occurrence of a higher incidence of spontaneous or drug-induced mutants, because of an increased number of tumor cells in a greater variety of metabolic loci. Such resistance could result, for example, from heritable alteration in permeability or transport or increased alteration of active enzymatic or metabolic sites.

As the disseminated disease becomes more extensive, there may be a decrease in the immune capacity of the host and decreased tolerance to the toxicity of therapy. This is complicated further since most of the antitumor agents have demonstrated immunosuppressive properties. Decrease in the immune capacity of the host could result in (a) increased tumor growth and dissemination, (b) reduced tolerance to the drug, (c) increased susceptibility to infection.

The question arises as to the possible ways in which the difficulties in treating advanced disseminated disease may be overcome. Various procedures may be outlined as follows:

Treatment of Advanced Disseminated Tumor

1) Search for drugs with greater specificity of action, including the capability of reaching metastatic sequestered sites
2) Drug action to prevent metastasis
3) Stimulation of nondividing tumor cell pool (Go cells)
4) Combination chemotherapy: drugs with differing mechanisms
A) Reduction of limiting toxicity
B) Permits use of higher effective dosage
C) Delay in origin and treatment of resistant tumor cells
D) Action at differing target sites
E) Second drug to improve distribution, prevent detoxification, maintain tissue levels
F) Priming dose therapy to reduce tumor mass, followed by more prolonged treatment with a second drug
5) Surgery or X-irradiation of tumor mass plus chemotherapy
6) Reduction host toxicity without concomitant loss of antitumor effect
A) Appropriate drug scheduling
B) Metabolite plus antimetabolite
C) Supportive measures for host
7) Increase action of host against tumor
A) Nonspecific immunologic stimulants
B) Adoptive immunologic procedures
C) Active or passive immunization
8) Combination of chemotherapy plus immunotherapy
A) Prevention immunosuppression by chemotherapeutic agent or other means
B) Nonspecific immunostimulants plus chemotherapy
C) Chemotherapy plus adoptive immunotherapy
D) Passive immunization plus chemotherapy
E) Active immunization plus chemotherapy
F) Alteration tumor cell antigenicity and collateral sensitivity

Although there is abundant evidence that the combined modalities of single or multiple drug polychemotherapy plus surgery and/or irradiation may result in improved therapeutic response, it is also clear that appropriate addition of immunotherapy may lead to a further and most important increment of therapeutic effectiveness and result in a higher incidence of total tumor cell eradication. This may be particularly so where the immunotherapy results in an increase in specificity of cytotoxic action against residual disseminated disease.

It has been demonstrated in animal tumor model systems that an increase in the immune reaction of the host against tumor growth, even a mild one, may result in significant augmentation of chemotherapeutic effectiveness. This observation underlies and emphasizes the potential importance of the combined modality of chemotherapy and immunotherapy. An important potential means for increasing the immunogenicity of the host involves the alteration of the antigenicity of tumor cells, and it is worthwhile discussing this approach in relation to the phenomenon of collateral sensitivity. The term collateral sensitivity refers to the situation in which the origin of tumor cell resistance to therapy with one drug results in an improved therapeutic response to a different chemotherapeutic agent. In early studies it was observed, for example, that a subline of leukemia L 1210 that had become resistant to 6-mercaptopurine and to 8-azaguanine had become more sensitive to treatment with methotrexate than the parent line [17, 28]. The phenomenon of collateral sensitvity was initially considered to be attributable to some biochemical or pharmacologic alteration of the tumor cells, occurring during the appearance of resistance and making the tumor cells more vulnerable to attack by a drug with a differing mechanism of action. However, it is now considered that collateral sensitivity may also result from a contribution to therapy stemming from alteration of the antigenicity of the tumor cells. Immunologic-collateral sensitivity may be distinguished from biochemical-pharmacologic-collateral sensitivity since with the former, in general, the improved therapeutic response may be at least partially overcome by immunosuppression of the host. An immunologic contribution to the phenomenon of collateral sensitivity has been demonstrated in several laboratories [2, 3, 18, 20, 21, 23] where it has been indicated that accompanying the origin of tumor cell resistance there may be some antigenic alteration of the tumor cells and that the immunologic response of the host to these cells when coupled with chemotherapy may result in a favorable form of immunochemotherapy. Bonmassar et al. [2] treated leukemia L 1210 with 5-(3,3-dimethyl-1-triazeno)-imidazole-4-carboxamide (DTIC) over a series of generations and observed that this resulted in an alteration of the antigenicity of the tumor cells. The tumor cells were not capable of growing in the CDF-1 host of origin unless the animals were treated with DTIC. Growth and survival of the cells were attributable to the origin of tumor cell resistance to DTIC, accompanied by immunosuppressant action of the drug, which interfered with the ability of the host to eradicate the tumor cells. Immunosuppression of the animals by treatment with cyclophosphamide prior to inoculation of the DTIC-altered tumor resulted in progressive tumor growth, indicating that the failure to grow in nonimmunosuppressed animals was attributable to alteration of the antigenicity of the tumor cells.

It is worthy of note that the origin of tumor cell resistance is not a necessary requirement for the alteration of tumor cell antigenicity. It was demonstrated that a line of leukemia L 1210 naturally resistant to DTIC evidenced high immunogenicity after treatment with the drug [3]. In addition, the drug 3-(or 5-)amino pyrazole-4-carboxamide, an analog of purine precursors, although inactive as a chemotherapeutic agent for the treatment of leukemia L 1210, could alter the immunogenicity of the tumor cells [21]. Studies by Nicolin et al. [20] have suggested that the contribution of altered tumor cell antigenicity to the observation of collateral sensitivity may be a somewhat generalized phenomenon. They examined a number of sublines of leukemia L 1210 that had become resistant to a variety of drugs and made the following observations:

a) In general when the animals received equivalent inoculum levels, untreated controls of the resistant sublines died moderately later than the animals inoculated with the sensitive line.

b) When the animals were pretreated with cyclophosphamide, there was usually a reduction in the survival time of the animals bearing the resistant sublines.

c) With the various resistant sublines, there was increased sensitivity to treatment with BCNU (collateral sensitivity) as reflected in extensive increases in survival time relative to the sensitive line, and many of the animals appeared to be cured of disease.

d) The augmentation of therapeutic response was diminished when the animals were pretreated with cyclophosphamide.

Another approach to alteration of the immunogenicity of tumor cells involves exposure of the cells to neuraminidase [1, 24]. The treatment with neuraminidase may unmask antigenic sites on the tumor cells, thereby exposing them to interaction with the host. It should be pointed out that for the DTIC-treated sublines the antigenic alteration is heritable whereas it is necessary to expose the tumor cells to neuraminidase in each instance that antigenically altered cells are desired.

An interesting approach for investigation of the influence of immunologic differences between tumor and host in chemotherapy involves the utilization of a host that differs genetically from the tumor. It has been observed in such studies that a minor immune reaction of the host against the growth of tumor may make a marked contribution to an increased response to chemotherapy. Examples include the following:

a) Treatment of experimental leukemia L 1210 in first generation hybrids of the parent DBA/2 mouse is in general more effective than treatment in the DBA/2 host [6, 16].

b) Treatment of advanced leukemia L 1210 with the halogenated derivatives of methotrexate, 3′5′-dichloromethotrexate (DCM) or 3′chloro5′bromomethotrexate (BCM) resulted in immunity of the mice to reinoculation of the tumor [10, 11, 13]. By taking advantage of the immune response of the host against the sensitive line, it was possible to effectively treat a subline of leukemia L 1210 resistant to folic acid antagonists [12]. This was accomplished by the treatment of animals harboring advanced sensitive leukemia L 1210 that were also inoculated with the resistant subline at the time therapy was initiated or at a subsequent time.

c) When a subline of leukemia L 1210 resistant to methotrexate was inoculated subcutaneously into BALB/c mice, differing from the parent DBA/2 line by the presence of multiple minor histocompatibility loci (MMHL), the tumor grew initially and then regressed. However, on treatment with methotrexate, which was apparently mildly suppressive for the BALB/c animals, the tumors grew progressively and all of the animals succumbed [16]. When the immunosuppressive effect of methotrexate was blocked by concomitant administration of citrovorum factor, again the tumor grew initially and then regressed, as in the control animals.

d) Riccardi et al. [22] compared the effectiveness of a number of drugs in the treatment of leukemia L 1210 in compatible (BALB/c X DBA/2) F1 (CD2F1) mice with treatment in H-2-compatible BALB/c recipients incompatible for MMHL. Markedly enhanced effects were found in BALB/c mice treated with 1-(2-chloroethyl)-3-cyclohexyl-1-nitrosourea (CCNU), methyl CCNU, nitrogen mustard, adriamycin, and methotrexate. With the two nitrosourea derivatives, long-term survival was observed over a narrow dose range in compatible CD2F1 mice, whereas in BALB/c mice long-term survivors were observed over a broad dose range, including dose levels at which the nitrosoureas were essentially inactive in the treatment of the leukemia in CD2F1 mice. Although nitrogen mustard was only minimally active in the treatment of compatible CD2F1 mice, it yielded a high percentage of long-term survivors over a wide range of doses in the BALB/c mice. Adriamycin was only moderately active in increasing survival time in CD2F1 mice and elicited no long-term survival. In BALB/c mice it produced a high percentage of long-term survivors over a wide dose range. Methotrexate treatment also resulted in only a moderate increase in survival time in CD2F1 mice, and although its behavior was somewhat erratic in the BALB/c mice, it did yield a high percentage of long-term survival at a number of dose levels. Actinomycin-D showed weak and equivalent activity in CD2F1-mice and BALB/c mice. Bleomycin was essentially inactive in the CD2F1 and BALB/c mice.

It is of interest to note that, although the nitrosourea derivatives were highly active in the treatment of leukemia L 1210 in CD2F1 mice, whereas nitrogen mustard was only weakly active, both the nitrosourea derivatives and nitrogen mustard elicited markedly enhanced activity in the BALB/c mice. Also, although nitrogen mustard and actinomycin-D showed approximately comparably low activity in the treatment of CD2F1 mice, with nitrogen mustard in contrast to actinomycin-D, there was extensively increased therapeutic response in the BALB/c mice. Thus, the increased efficacy of antineoplastic agents in the presence of antitumor immune responses in mice does not appear to be totally dependent upon the extent of antineoplastic efficacy of the drug in compatible mice but to some other as yet unidentified properties.

The studies involving the combined effects of chemotherapy and antilymphoma allograft responses with leukemia cells incompatible for MMHL were extended to additional drugs including BCNU, cyclophosphamide, DTIC, and hexamethylmelamine [C. Riccardi, A. Bartocci, F. Spreafico, A. Goldin) unpublished data]. The studies were conducted in CD2F1 and in MMHL-incompatible BALB/c mice with leukemia L 1210 Cr, and in compatible CD2F1 and MMHL-incompatible (C57B1/6 × DBA/2) F1 (BDF1) or B10.D2 mice with leukemia LSTRA. BCNU and cyclophosphamide produced marked increases in survival time of compatible mice. Synergistic effects between chemotherapy and allograft responses were more evident for BCNU than for cyclophosphamide in the allogeneic hosts, which were cured by low doses of BCNU scarcely effective in compatible recipients. DTIC was moderately active0in compatible mice and there was no enhancement of activity in allogeneic hosts. Vincristine was only moderately effective in increasing the survival time of compatible leukemic mice. However, it was highly effective when administered to allogeneic recipients, where optimal doses of the drug were capable of curing most of the MMHL-incompatible leukemic hosts. Hexamethylmalamine was ineffective in prolonging the survival time of either compatible or allogeneic mice. These studies again stress that there would appear to be no obvious relationship between the antileukemic activity of different drugs in the treatment of tumors in compatible hosts and their antineoplastic effectiveness when combined with antitumor immunoresponses.

Thus, it has been demonstrated that it is possible for a moderate immune reaction of the host to the tumor to result in a marked improvement in therapeutic response to at least a number of drugs. The question presents itself as to whether it may be possible to employ antigenically altered tumor cells to improve the therapeutic effectiveness of drugs against the original tumor. In one study by Houchens et al. [15], immunochemotherapy of the LSTRA lymphoma, induced by Moloney leukemia virus, was attempted with a combination of a DTIC-antigenically altered subline of LSTRA and BCNU. Therapeutic synergism was observed when animals bearing the LSTRA lymphoma received a single injection of viable antigenically altered LD-1 tumor cells 1 day after inoculation of LSTRA and this was followed by BCNU treatment on day 3. With this combined modality of therapy there resulted a high percentage of long-term survivors. No synergism occurred when the LD-1 subline was administered after BCNU therapy or when an unrelated allogeneic L5MF-22 lymphoma was administered before or after BCNU treatment. Tolerance studies indicated that there are novel antigens and parental tumor antigens associated with the drug-treated subline [15].

It has been shown in additional studies that mice that had rejected DTIC-treated sublines that originated either in conventional or athymic mice were relatively resistant to a subsequent inoculum of the parental lines [4]. This observation indicated that the DTIC-treated sublines retained at least a portion of the antigenic makeup of parental lymphomas. It led to the suggestion that if the immunogenic character of human tumors could be altered by treatment in athymic mice this might serve as a potential approach to clinical immunotherapy.

Nicolin et al. demonstrated that animals that were sensitized with viable DTIC cells were more resistant to tumor challenge than animals sensitized by X-ray inactivated parental cells [19]. Presensitization of syngeneic hosts with antigenically altered tumor cells resulted in increased survival with subsequent inoculation of L 1210 Cr cells, but inoculation of these cells was ineffective when they were inoculated after tumor challenge with the parental line. However, when preinoculation or postinoculation of DTIC-antigenically altered tumor cells was employed in conjunction with conventional therapy, curative synergism was elicited. An increase in the survival time of the leukemic animals was also obtained on adoptive transfer of immune lymphocytes that had been previously sensitized either in vivo or in vitro to DTIC cells. Combination of the immune lymphocytes with cyclophosphamide or BCNU resulted in further benefit to the host. It was concluded from the study that DTIC cells elicited host immune response to both novel DTIC-induced antigens and to tumor-associated transplantation antigens (TATA), the latter being shared with the original drug-untreated tumor. Also, it would appear that viable DTIC cells are capable of eliciting a stronger host-immune reaction to TATA than do inactivated cells.

Thorpe and Rosenberg [27] have provided evidence that serum from patients bearing osteogenic sarcoma contain antibodies that are active against both fetal and tumor-specific antigens expressed on osteogenic sarcoma cells in tissue culture. It was observed that the reactivity against the osteogenic sarcoma antigens was relatively specific for the autologous tumor, lacking in reactivity with osteogenic sarcoma obtained from most of the other patients. The identification of tumor-specific antigens on human tumor cells, present without specific induction by drugs, encourages the possibility for further alteration of antigenicity of human tumors by means of appropriate drug application. The establishment of antigenically altered sublines of human tumors would be of considerable interest for further investigation and potential therapeutic application. Such immunotherapeutic procedures conceivably could provide the necessary appropriate specificity in conjunction with chemotherapy to result in the total eradication of residual metastatic disease.

References

1. Bekesi, J. G., Holland, J. F., Fleminger, R., Yates, J., Henderson, E. S.: Immunotherapeutic efficacy of neuraminidase treated allogenic myeloblasts in patients with acute myelocytic leukemia. In: Control of neoplasia by modulation of the immune mechanism. Chirigos, M. (ed.), pp. 573–592. New York: Raven Press 1977
2. Bonmassar, E., Bonmassar, A., Vadlamudi, S., Goldin, A.: Immunological alteration of leukemic cells in vivo after treatment with antitumor drug. Proc. Natl. Acad. Sci. USA *66,* 1089–1095 (1970)
3. Bonmassar, E., Bonmassar, A., Vadlamudi, S., Goldin, A.: Antigenic changes of L 1210 leukemia in mice treated with 5-(3,3-dimethyl-1-triazeno) imidazole-4-carboxamide. Cancer Res. *32,* 1446–1450 (1972)
4. Campanile, F., Houchens, D. P., Gaston, M., Goldin, A., Bonmassar, E.: Increased immunogenicity of two lymphoma lines following drug treatment in athymic (nude) mice. J. Natl. Cancer Inst. *55,* 207–209 (1975)
5. Chirigos, M. A., Humphreys, S. R., Goldin, A.: Effectiveness of cytoxan against intracerebrally and subcutaneously inoculated mouse lymphoid leukemia L 1210. Cancer Res. *22,* 187–195 (1962)
6. Glynn, J. P., Humphreys, S. R., Trivers, G., Bianco, A. R., Goldin, A.: Studies on immunity to leukemia L 1210 in mice. Cancer Res. *23,* 1008–1015 (1963)
7. Goldin, A.: Preclinical methodology for the selection of anticancer agents. In: Methods in cancer research. Busch, H. (ed.), pp. 193–254. New York, London: Academic Press 1968

8. Goldin, A.: Factors pertaining to complete drug-induced remission of tumor in animals and man. Cancer Res. *29,* 2285–2291 (1969)
9. Goldin, A.: Effects of drugs on disseminated tumor. In: Chemotherapy of cancer dissemination and metastasis. Garattini, S., Franchi, G. (eds.), pp. 341–354. New York: Raven Press 1973
10. Goldin, A., Humphreys, S. R.: Studies of immunity in mice surviving systemic leukemia L 1210. J. Natl. Cancer Inst. *24,* 283–300 (1960)
11. Goldin, A., Humphreys, S. R., Chapman, G. O., Chirigos, M. A., Venditti, J. M.: Immunity of mice surviving leukemia (L 1210) to antifolic resistant variants of the disease. Nature *185,* 219–221 (1960)
12. Goldin, A., Humphreys, S. R., Chapman, G. O., Venditti, J. M., Chirigos, M. A.: Augmentation of therapeutic efficacy of 3′5′-dichloroamethopterin against an antifolic-resistant variant of leukemia (L 1210-M46R) in mice. Cancer Res. *20,* 1066–1071 (1960)
13. Goldin, A., Humphreys, S. R., Venditti, J. M., Mantel, N.: Prolongation of the lifespan of mice with advanced leukemia (L 1210) by treatment with halogenated derivatives of amethopterin. J. Natl. Cancer Inst. *22,* 811–823 (1959)
14. Goldin, A., Venditti, J. M., Humphreys, S. R., Mantel, N.: Influence of the concentration of leukemic inoculum on the effectiveness of treatment. Science *123,* 840 (1956)
15. Houchens, D. P., Bonmassar, E., Gaston, M. R., Kende, M., Goldin, A.: Drug-mediated immunogenic changes of virusinduced leukemia in vivo. Cancer Res. *36,* 1347–1352 (1976)
16. Humphreys, S. R., Chirigos, M. A., Milstead, K. L., Mantel, N., Goldin, A.: Studies on the suppression of the homograft response with folic acid antagonists. J. Natl. Cancer Inst. *27,* 259–276 (1961)
17. Law, L. W., Taormina, V., Boyle, B. J.: Response of acute lymphocytic leukemias to the purine antagonist 6-mercaptopurine. Ann. N.Y. Acad. Sci. *60,* 224–250 (1954)
18. Mihich, E.: Synergism between chemotherapy and immunity in the treatment of experimental tumors. In: Proc. 5th Int. Congr. Chemotherapy. Spitzy, Haschek (eds.), Vol. III, pp.. 327–331. Wien: Wiener Medizinische Akademie 1967
19. Nicolin, A., Cavalli, M., Marelli, O., Goldin, A.: Tumor resistance induced in a syngeneic host by viable DTIC-Cells. Proc. Am. Assoc. Cancer Res. *19,* 108 (1978)
20. Nicolin, A., Vadlamudi, S., Goldin, A.: Antigenicity of L 1210 leukemic sublines induced by drugs. Cancer Res. *32,* 653–657 (1972)
21. Nicolin, A., Vadlamudi, S., Goldin, A.: Increased immunogenicity of murine lymphatic tumors by pyrazole-4-carboxamide, 3(or 5)-amino (NSC-1402; PCA). Cancer Chemother. Rep. *57,* 3–10 (1973)
22. Riccardi, C., Kline, I., Peruzzi, L., Goldin, A.: Increased efficiency of antineoplastic agents in presence of antitumor immune responses in mice. Proc. 5th Pharmacology-Toxicology Symposium, p. 56 (1977)
23. Schmid, F. A., Hutchison, D. J.: Collateral sensitivity of resistant lines of mouse leukemias L 1210 and L 5178Y. Proc. Am. Assoc. Cancer Res. *12,* 23 (1971)
24. Simmons, R. L., Rios, A.: Immunotherapy of cancer: Immunospecific rejection of tumors in recipients of neuraminidase-treated tumor cells plus BCG. Science *174,* 591–593 (1971)
25. Skipper, H. E., Schabel, F. M. (Jr.), Bell, M., Thomson, J. R., Johnson, S.: On the curability of experimental neoplasms I. Amethopterin and mouse leukemia. Cancer Res. *17,* 717–726 (1957)
26. Thomas, L. B., Chirigos, M. A., Humphreys, S. R., Goldin, A.: Development of meningeal leukemia (L 1210) during treatment of subcutaneously inoculated mice with methotrexate. Cancer *17,* 352–360 (1964)
27. Thorpe, W. P., Rosenberg, S. A.: Identification of tumor specific antigens on human osteogenic sarcoma. Proc. Am. Assoc. Cancer Res. *19,* 107 (1978)
28. Venditti, J. M., Goldin, A.: Drug synergism in antineoplastic chemotherapy. In: Advances in chemotherapy. Goldin, A., Hawking, F. (eds.), Vol. 1, pp. 397–498. New York: Academic Press 1964

Concluding Remarks

L. Lajtha

It is my privilege in the name of the Council of the EORTC to conclude this meeting and I am quite sure that you do not expect me to try to summarize the results of this marathon of papers presented during the last 3 days. I think both the organizers and the audience are to be congratulated for embarking upon such an ambitious, high pressure meeting, but clearly the gamble has paid off. We had a great deal of information and the vigor of discussions amply demonstrated the recognition of the problems we are facing in the therapy of cancer.

Many of you who are working in clinical trials may not appreciate that what is accepted today as the natural and normal way of studying the problem has not been accepted as such always. Equally, it may not be appreciated by all that we are only beginning the study of clinical trials. With increasing sophistication of treatment methods and the increasing number and complexity of the monitoring methods available, I can imagine that future clinical trials will be far more difficult to organize and to run than those that we are running today. All the more reason why we should recognize the problem and criteria of the framework that will be essential for carrying out the new developing trials. I cannot overemphasize enough the degree of sophistication that I can foresee emerging. I am quite sure that there will be very few cancer centers, if any, that will have *all* the techniques available for all kinds of trials and monitoring at any one time, and also enough patient material. Consequently, in the future we will depend more and more on the cooperative clinical trials. This, of course, is the main task of the EORTC: the organization and facilitation of cooperative clinical work. In these trials appropriate documentation, data retrieval, and analysis will, of course, be sine qua non. The progress is satisfactory but I warn you that the work is going to be more arduous requiring greater effort and manpower investment.

Finally, I wish to thank the speakers and discussants for their participation and I am sure you will join with me in expressing our very special thanks to Professor Mathé who organized and made this highly instructive and productive meeting possible.

Recent Results in Cancer Research

Sponsored by the Swiss League against Cancer. Editor in Chief: P. Rentchnick, Genève

For information about Vols. 1–9, please contact your bookseller or Springer-Verlag

10 NELSON, R. S.: Radioactive Phosphorus in the Diagnosis of Gastrointestinal Cancer.
11 FREEMAN, R. G. and J. M. KNOX: Treatment of Skin Cancer.
12 LYNCH, H. T.: Hereditary Factors in Carcinoma.
13 Tumours in Children, 2nd Edition. Edited by H. B. MARSDEN and J. K. STEWARD.
14 ODARTCHENKO, N.: Production Cellulaire Erythropoïétique.
15 SOKOLOFF, B.: Carcinoid and Serotonin.
16 JACOBS, M. L.: Malignant Lymphomas and Their Management.
17 Normal and Malignant Cell Growth. Edited by R. J. M. FRY, M. L. GRIEM, and W. H. KIRSTEN (Symposium).
18 ANGLESIO, E.: The Treatment of Hodgkin's Disease.
19 BANNASCH, P.: The Cytoplasm of Hepatocytes during Carcinogenesis. Electron- and Lightmicroscopical Investigations of the Nitrosomorpholineintoxicated Rat Liver.
20 Rubidomycin. A new Agent against Cancer. Edited by J. BERNARD, R. PAUL, M. BOIRON, C. JACQUILLAT, and R. MARAL.
21 Scientific Basis of Cancer Chemotherapy. Edited by G. MATHÉ (Symposium).
22 KOLDOVSKÝ, P.: Tumor Specific Transplantation Antigen.
23 FUCHS, W. A., J. W. Davidson, and H. W. FISCHER: Lymphography in Cancer. With contributions by G. JANTET and H. RÖSLER.
24 HAYWARD, J.: Hormones und Human Breast Cancer. An Account of 15 Years Study.
25 ROY-BURMAN, P.: Analogues of Nucleic Acid Components. Mechanisms of Action.
26 Tumors of the Liver. Edited by G. T. PACK and A. H. ISLAMI.
27 SZYMENDERA, J.: Bone Mineral Metabolism in Cancer.
28 MEEK, E. S.: Antitumour and Antiviral Substances of Natural Origin.
29 Aseptic Environments and Cancer Treatment. Edited by G. MATHÉ (Symposium).
30 Advances in the Treatment of Acute (Blastic) Leukemias. Edited by G. MATHÉ (Symposium).
31 DENOIX, P.: Treatment of Malignant Breast Tumors. Indications and Results.
32 NELSON, R. S.: Endoscopy in Gastric Cancer.
33 Experimental and Clinical Effects of L-Asparaginase. Edited by E. GRUNDMANN and H. F. OETTGEN (Symposium).
34 Chemistry and Biological Actions of 4-Nitroquinolin 1-Oxide. Edited by H. ENDO, T. ONO, and T. SUGIMURA.
35 PENN, I.: Malignant Tumors in Organ Transplant Recipients.
36 Current Concepts in the Management of Lymphoma and Leukemia. Edited by J. E. ULTMANN, M. L. GRIEM, W. H. KIRSTEN, and R. W. WISSLER (Symposium).
37 CHIAPPA, S., R. MUSUMECI, and C. USLENGHI: Endolymphatic Radiotherapy in Malignant Lymphomas. With contributions by G. BONADONNA, B. DAMASCELLI, G. FAVA, F. PIZZETTI, U. VERONESI.
38 KOLLER, P. C.: The Role of Chromosomes in Cancer Biology.
39 Current Problems in the Epidemiology of Cancer and Lymphomas. Edited by E. GRUNDMANN and H. TULINIUS (Symposium).
40 LANGLEY, F. A. and A. C. CROMPTON: Epithelial Abnormalities of the Cervix Uteri.
41 Tumours in a Tropical Country. A Survey of Uganda (1964–1968). Edited by A. C. TEMPLETON.
42 Breast Cancer: A Challenging Problem. Edited by M. L. GRIEM, E. V. JENSEN, J. E. ULTMANN, and R. W. WISSLER (Symposium).
43 Nomenclature, Methodology and Results of Clinical Trials in Acute Leukemias. Edited by G. MATHÉ, P. POUILLART, L. SCHWARZENBERG (Symposium).
44 Special Topics in Carcinogenesis. Edited by E. GRUNDMANN (Symposium).
45 KOLDOVSKÝ, P.: Carcinoembryonic Antigens.
46 Diagnosis and Therapy of Malignant Lymphoma. Edited by K. MUSSHOFF (Symposium).
47 Investigation and Stimulation of Immunity in Cancer Patients. Edited by G. MATHÉ and R. WEINER (Symposium).
48 Platinum Coordination Complexes in Cancer Chemotherapy. Edited by T. A. CONNORS and J. J. ROBERTS (Symposium).
49 Complications of Cancer Chemotherapy. Edited by G. MATHÉ and R. K. OLDHAM (Symposium).
50 Cancer Registry, Edited by E. GRUNDMANN and E. PEDERSEN (Symposium).

51 Gliomas. Current Concepts in Biology, Diagnosis and Therapy. Edited by J. Hekmatpanah (Symposium).

52 The Ambivalence of Cytostatic Therapy. Edited by E. Grundmann and R. Gross (Symposium).

53 A. Clarysse, Y. Kenis, and G. Mathé: Cancer Chemotherapy.

54 Malignant Bone Tumors. Edited by E. Grundmann.

55 Mathé, G.: Cancer Active Immunotherapy, Immunoprophylaxis, and Immunorestoration.

56 Lymphocytes, Macrophages, and Cancer. Edited by G. Mathé, I. Florentin, and M.-C. Simmler (Symposium).

57 Breast Cancer: A Multidisciplinary Approach. Edited by G. St. Arneault, P. Band, and L. Israël (Symposium).

58 B. S. Schoenberg: Multiple Primary Malignant Neoplasms.

59 Selective Heat Sensitivity of Cancer Cells. Edited by A. Rossi-Fanelli, R. Cavaliere, B. Mondovi, and G. Moricca.

60 Tumors of the Male Genital System. Edited by E. Grundmann and W. Vahlensieck (Symposium).

61 D. Metcalf: Hemopoietic Colonies.

62 Tactics and Strategy in Cancer Treatment. Edited by G. Mathé (Symposium).

63 Antitumor Antibiotics. Edited by S. K. Carter, H. Umezawa, J. Douros, and Y. Sakurai (Symposium).

64 Lymphoid Neoplasias I: Classification, Categorization, Natural History.

65 Lymphoid Neoplasias II: Clinical and Therapeutic Aspects.
Lymphoid Neoplasias I & II. Proceedings of the 1977 CNRS-EORTC International Colloquium. Editors: G. Mathé, M. Seligmann, M. Tubiana. Devided into two volumes.

66 Carcinogenic Hormones. Edited by C. H. Lingeman.

67/68 Adjuvant Therapies and Markers of Post-Surgical Minimal Residual Disease I & II. Proceedings of the 1978 Annual Plenary Meeting of the EORTC. Editors: G. Bonadonna, G. Mathé, S. E. Salmon. Divided into two volumes:

67 Markers and General Problems of Cancer Adjuvant Therapies.

68 Adjuvant Therapies and Markers of the Various Primary Tumors.

GPSR Compliance
The European Union's (EU) General Product Safety Regulation (GPSR) is a set of rules that requires consumer products to be safe and our obligations to ensure this.

If you have any concerns about our products, you can contact us on

ProductSafety@springernature.com

In case Publisher is established outside the EU, the EU authorized representative is:

Springer Nature Customer Service Center GmbH
Europaplatz 3
69115 Heidelberg, Germany

www.ingramcontent.com/pod-product-compliance
Lightning Source LLC
Chambersburg PA
CBHW061152240926
51846CB00006B/990
* 9 7 8 3 6 4 2 8 1 3 3 4 4 *